Case Studies in

UVEITIS

Real Cases & Practical Insights

Under the Aegis of International Uveitis Study Group

Case Studies in UVEITIS Real Cases & Practical Insights

IUSG International Uveitis Study Group 1978

Editors

Alejandra de-la-Torre MD PhD
Professor
Immunology Unit
Neuroscience Research Group (NEUROS)
Neurovitae Center for Neuroscience
Institute of Translational Medicine (IMT)
School of Medicine and Health Sciences
Universidad del Rosario
Bogotá, Colombia

Meghan Berkenstock MD
Rose Parapiglia Endowed Professor of Ophthalmology
Associate Professor and Medical Director
Wilmer Eye Institute
The Johns Hopkins School of Medicine
Baltimore, Maryland, USA

Germán Mejía-Salgado MD MSc
Research Assistant
Immunology Unit
Neuroscience Research Group (NEUROS)
Neurovitae Center for Neuroscience
Institute of Translational Medicine (IMT)
School of Medicine and Health Sciences
Universidad del Rosario
Bogotá, Colombia
Ophthalmology Resident
Health Sciences Faculty
Universidad Autónoma de Bucaramanga (UNAB)
Bucaramanga, Colombia

John H Kempen MD MPH MHS
Senior Scientist and Surgeon
Director of Epidemiology for Ophthalmology
Director of Global Surgery and Health-Ophthalmology
Schepens Eye Research Institute, Massachusetts Eye and Ear
Boston
Professor of Ophthalmology, PT, and Associate
Global Health and Social Medicine
Harvard Medical School
Boston, Massachusetts, USA

Reema Bansal MD PhD FAMS
Professor
Uveitis and Vitreo-Retina Services
Advanced Eye Centre
Postgraduate Institute of Medical Education
and Research
Chandigarh, India

Vishali Gupta MD
Professor
Department of Ophthalmology
Advanced Eye Centre
Postgraduate Institute of Medical Education and Research
Chandigarh, India
President, International Uveitis Study Group

Forewords

James T Rosenbaum, Amod Gupta, Philip Ian Murray,
Manabu Mochizuki, Rubens Belfort Jr

JAYPEE

JAYPEE BROTHERS MEDICAL PUBLISHERS
The Health Sciences Publisher
New Delhi | London

Jaypee Brothers Medical Publishers (P) Ltd

Headquarters
EMCA House, 23/23-B
Ansari Road, Daryaganj
New Delhi 110 002, India
Landline: +91-11-23272143, +91-11-23272703
+91-11-23282021, +91-11-23245672
e-mail: jaypee@jaypeebrothers.com

Corporate Office
4838/24, Ansari Road, Daryaganj
New Delhi 110 002, India
Phone: +91-11-43574357
Fax: +91-11-43574314
e-mail: jaypee@jaypeebrothers.com

Overseas Office
JP Medical Ltd.
83, Victoria Street, London
SW1H 0HW (UK)
Phone: +44-20 3170 8910
e-mail: info@jpmedpub.com

EU GPSR Authorised Representative
Logos Europe, 9 rue Nicolas Poussin
17000, La Rochelle, France
Phone: +33 (0) 6 67 93 73 78
e-mail: contact@logoseurope.eu

Website: www.jaypeebrothers.com
Website: www.jaypeedigital.com

Case Studies in Uveitis: Real Cases & Practical Insights

First Edition: **2026**

ISBN: 978-93-6616-023-8

Printed at: Samrat Offset Pvt. Ltd.

Dedication

All patients whose journeys through uveitis have inspired deeper understanding and better care. The mentors, colleagues, and trainees who, with compassion and curiosity, advance the science of ocular inflammation daily.

Alejandra de-la-Torre dedicates her work on this book to her daughters, Andrea and Gabriela, and her granddaughters, Antonia and Emilia, with her deepest love.

Meghan Berkenstock would like to dedicate her work with much love to all of her children: Isabella, Daniel, Julianna, and Martin Dobkin.

Germán Mejía-Salgado dedicates his work on this book to his parents, Germán Alberto Mejía Estupiñán and Yasmina Salgado Páez, with deep gratitude.

John H Kempen would like to dedicate his work on this book to his late parents, Harold M Kempen and Frances Elliot Kempen, with much love and cherished memories.

Reema Bansal dedicates her work on this book to her late mother, Saroj Goyal, sister Dr Seema Kumar, and children, Naman and Dhwani, with deepest love and affection.

Vishali Gupta dedicates this work to her husband Rajesh and daughter Sarakshi, whose steadfast support has been the foundation of her professional journey.

Contributors

Talluri Ronnie Abhishek MS
Consultant
Uveitis and Medical Retina Services
LV Prasad Eye Institute (LVPEI)
Kode Venkatadri Chowdary Campus
Vijayawada, Andhra Pradesh, India

Massimo Accorinti MD PhD
Consultant
Uveitis Service
IRCCS Fondazione Bietti
Rome, Italy

Manisha Agarwal MD DNB FMRF
Director
Vitreoretina and Uvea Services
Dr. Shroff's Charity Eye Hospital
New Delhi, India

Anita Agarwal MD
Vitreo Retinal and Uveitis Consultant
West Coast Retina Medical Group
San Francisco, California, USA
Adjoint Professor of Ophthalmology
Vanderbilt Eye Institute
Vanderbilt University Medical Center
Nashville, Tennessee, USA

Rupesh Agrawal
MD (Res) (UCL) MMed (Singapore)
FRCS (Glasgow) FAMS DNB DO
Senior Consultant
Ophthalmologist–Clinician Scientist and Head of Research
Department of Ophthalmology
National Healthcare Group Eye Institute
Tan Tock Seng Hospital, Singapore
Co-Lead, Ocular Anti-Infective and Inflammation Research Group
Singapore Eye Research Institute, Singapore
Associate Professor
Lee Kong Chian School of Medicine
Nanyang Technological University
Singapore
Associate Professor
Department of Ophthalmology
National University of Singapore, Singapore
Associate Professor
Eye ACP Program, Duke NUS Medical School, Singapore

Radgonde Amer MD
Clinical Professor and Director of Uveitis and Ocular Immunology Service
Department of Ophthalmology
Hadassah Medical Center
Jerusalem, Israel

Sofia Androudi MD PhD
Professor and Head
Department of Ophthalmology
University of Thessaly
University Hospital of Larissa
Mezourlo, Larissa, Greece

Anshukita MD FMRF (Uvea)
Anterior Segment and Uvea Consultant
Department of Ophthalmology
All India Institute of Medical Sciences
Bhopal, Madhya Pradesh, India

J Fernando Arevalo MD PhD
Professor and Chairman
Department of Ophthalmology
Johns Hopkins Bayview Medical Center
Retina Division
Wilmer Eye Institute, The Johns Hopkins University School of Medicine
Baltimore, Maryland, USA

Atul Arora MBBS MS MCh
Consultant
Department of Ophthalmology
Post Graduate Institute of Medical Education and Research
Chandigarh, India

Figen Bezci Aygun MD
Assistant Professor
Department of Ophthalmology
Hacettepe University School of Medicine
Ankara, Turkey

Shravya Choudhary Bala MBBS MS
Fellow in Uveitis and Medical Retina
Department of Uveitis and Retina
Saroja A Rao Center for Uveitis
LV Prasad Eye Institute (LVPEI)
Kallam Anji Reddy Campus
Hyderabad, Telangana, India

Reema Bansal MD PhD FAMS
Professor
Uveitis and Vitreo-Retina Services
Advanced Eye Centre
Postgraduate Institute of Medical Education and Research
Chandigarh, India

Soumyava Basu MS
Network Head, Uveitis Services
Saroja A Rao Center for Uveitis
LV Prasad Eye Institute (LVPEI)
Kallam Anji Reddy Campus
Hyderabad, Telangana, India

Meghan Berkenstock MD
Rose Parapiglia Endowed Professor of Ophthalmology
Associate Professor and Medical Director
Wilmer Eye Institute
The Johns Hopkins School of Medicine
Baltimore, Maryland, USA

Shruthika Bhimewar MBBS MS
Consultant
Department of Ophthalmology
Vasan Eye Care Hospital
Hubli, Karnataka, India

Jyotirmay Biswas MS FMRF FAMS FIC Path FAICO FNAsc FRCS (Ed) FACS
Senior Consultant
Department of Uveitis and Ocular Pathology
Sankara Nethralaya
Chennai, Tamil Nadu, India
Emeritus Professor
Department of Ophthalmology
National Academy of Medical Sciences
Chennai, Tamil Nadu, India

Bahram Bodaghi MD PhD FEBOph
Professor and Chair
Department of Ophthalmology
IHU FOReSIGHT, AP-HP Sorbonne University
Paris, France

Lawrence Chan MD
Vitreoretinal Surgeon
Department of Retina Surgery
West Coast Retina
San Francisco, California, USA

Jonathan Malcolm Chavan MBBS MS DNB Fellowship in Uvea
Specialist Ophthalmologist
Department of Ophthalmology
KIMSHEALTH Medical Center
Dubai, UAE

Luca Cimino MD
Director and Associate Professor
Ocular Immunology Unit
AUSL-IRCCS Reggio Emilia
University of Modena and Reggio Emilia
Emilia, Emilia-Romagna, Italy

Miguel Cordero-Coma MD PhD FEBOphth
Medical Retina and Uveitis Consultant
Department of Ophthalmology
Hospital Regional Universitario
Málaga, Andalucía, Spain

Andre Luiz Land Curi MD PhD
Senior Researcher in Public Health and Head
LaPClin Ophthalmology Laboratory
Instituto Nacional de Infectologia
Evandro Chagas–INI, Fundação Oswaldo Cruz
Manguinhos, Rio de Janeiro-RJ, Brazil

Janet Davis MD MA
Leach Distinguished Professor
Department of Ophthalmology
Bascom Palmer Eye Institute
University of Miami Miller School of Medicine
Miami, Florida, USA

Alejandra de-la-Torre MD PhD
Professor
Immunology Unit
Neuroscience Research Group (NEUROS)
Neurovitae Center for Neuroscience
Institute of Translational Medicine (IMT)
School of Medicine and Health Sciences
Universidad del Rosario,
Bogotá, Colombia

Marc de Smet MD CM BSc (Hon) PhD FRCSC FRCOphth FARVO FEBO FMH
Invited Researcher
Université libre de Bruxelles, Belgium
Honorary Professor
Department of Ophthalmology
University of Leiden, Netherlands
Adjunct Professor
Department of Ophthalmology
New York Eye and Ear Infirmary of Mt Sinai, Icahn School of Medicine, NYC, USA
Director
MIOS sa/Helvetia Retina Associates
Lausanne, Switzerland

Wenbo Ding BS
Medical Student
Department of Ophthalmology
Drexel University College of Medicine
Philadelphia, Pennsylvania, USA

Russel Dinh MD
Attending Physician
Department of Ophthalmology
Vanderbilt Eye Institute
Nashville, Tennessee, USA
Attending Physician
Department of Ophthalmology
The Retina Group of Washington
Washington, Columbia, USA

James P Dunn MD
Uveitis Unit/Retina Division
Wills Eye Hospital
Professor of Ophthalmology
Sydney Kimmel Medical College
Philadelphia, PA
USA

Armin Taghavi Eraghi MD
Assistant Physician
Department of Ophthalmology
Campus Benjamin Franklin (CBF)
Campus Virchow-Klinikum (CVK)
Eye Clinic
Charité Campus Virchow Clinic
Charité - University Medicine Berlin
Berlin, Germany

Claudia Fabiani MD PhD
Consultant
Uveitis and Inflammatory Ocular Diseases Center
Ophthalmology Unit
University Hospital of Siena
Siena, Tuscany, Italy
Co-Founder, AIDA Network

Shahin Faghihi MD
International Retina Fellow
Department of Ophthalmology
UCLA Jules Stein Eye Institute
Los Angeles, California, USA

Maggie Feng MD
Research and Senior Resident
Department of Ophthalmology
Drexel University College of Medicine
Philadelphia, Pennsylvania, USA

Alessandro Feo MD
Clinical Research Fellowship in Uveitis
Department of Ophthalmology
UCLA Stein Eye Institute
Los Angeles, California, USA

Lisia Barros Ferreira MD PhD
Ophthalmologist
Department of Ophthalmology
Centro de Medicina Humanizado
Curitiba, Brazil

Alejandro Fonollosa MD PhD
Ophthalmology Consultant
Department of Ophthalmology
Biocruces Bizkaia Health Research Institute
Cruces University Hospital
University of the Basque Country
Barakaldo, Basque, Spain
Ophthalmology Consultant
Department of Retina
Instituto Oftalmológico Bilbao
Berástegui, Bilbao, Spain

Sapna Gangaputra MD MPH
Associate Professor
Associate Vice Chair for Clinical Research
Vanderbilt Eye Institute
Nashville, Tennessee, USA

Miranda Gehrke MD
Assistant Physician
Department of Ophthalmology
Eye Clinic and Polyclinic
LMU University Hospital
LMU Munich, City Campus
München, Germany

Pietro Gentile MD PhD
Medical Doctor
Ocular Immunology Unit
AUSL-IRCCS Reggio Emilia
Reggio Emilia, Italy

Daniele de Geronimo MD
Ophthalmologist and Researcher
Uveitis Service
IRCCS Fondazione Bietti
Rome, Italy

Pallavi Goel DNB FVRS
Consultant
Vitreo Retina and Uvea Services
Dr Shroff's Charity Eye Hospital
New Delhi, India

Vishali Gupta MD
Professor
Department of Ophthalmology
Advanced Eye Centre
Postgraduate Institute of Medical Education and Research
Chandigarh, India
President
International Uveitis Study Group

Carsten Heinz MD FEBO
Professor
Department of Ophthalmology
St Franziskus Hospital, Muenster, Germany
Department of Ophthalmology
University Essen
Essen, Germany

Jacob S Heng MD PhD
Assistant Professor
Department of Clinical Ophthalmology
UC San Diego, Shiley Eye Institute and Viterbi Family
San Diego, California, USA

Jennifer Hu MD MS
Clinical Fellow
Ocular Immunology Service
Massachusetts Eye and Ear Infirmary
Harvard Medical School
Boston, Massachusetts, USA

Jia-Horung Hung MD PhD
Instructor in Ophthalmology
Spencer Center for Vision Research
Byers Eye Institute
Stanford University School of Medicine
Palo Alto, California, USA

Sara Abdel Jalil MD
Clinical Fellow
Uveitis and Ocular Immunology Service
Department of Ophthalmology
Hadassah Medical Center
Jerusalem, Israel

Yanny Pérez Jimenez MD
Ophthalmology Consultant
Uveitis Services
Fundonal
Bogotá, Colombia

Ramesh Jois MBBS MD MRCP CCT
Consultant Rheumatologist
RheumaCARE
Bengaluru, Karnataka, India

Rubens Belfort Jr MD PhD MBA
Head Professor
Department of Ophthalmology
Hospital São Paulo
Federal University of São Paulo
President Vision Institute
Brazilian Academy of Medicine
Brazilian Academy of Sciences

Sibel Kadayifcilar MD
Professor and Head
Department of Ophthalmology
Hacettepe University School of Medicine
Ankara, Turkey

John H Kempen MD MPH PhD MHS
Senior Scientist and Surgeon
Director of Epidemiology for Ophthalmology
Director of Global Surgery and Health-Ophthalmology
Schepens Eye Research Institute
Massachusetts Eye and Ear
Boston
Professor of Ophthalmology, PT, and Associate
Global Health and Social Medicine
Harvard Medical School
Boston, Massachusetts, USA

Moncef Khairallah MD
Professor
Department of Ophthalmology
Fattouma Bourguiba University Hospital
Faculty of Medicine
University of Monastir
Monastir, Tunisia

Maria Carolina Kuba MD
Research Lab of Ophthalmology
Instituto Nacional de Infectologia Evandro Chagas - Fiocruz
Brazil

Katerina Lazari MD PhD
Ophthalmologist
Department of Ophthalmology
University of Thessaly
University Hospital of Larissa
Larissa, Thessaly, Greece

Aurélie Le MD
Medical Doctor
Department of Ophthalmology
CHU St-Pierre, Université Libre de Bruxelles
Brussels, Belgium

Panayiotis Maghsoudlou MBBS PhD
Academic Clinical Lecturer
Department of Ophthalmology
Bristol Eye Hospital and University of Bristol
Bristol, England, UK

Padmamalini Mahendradas DO DNB
Head
Uveitis and Ocular Immunology
Narayana Nethralaya
Bengaluru, Karnataka, India

Neofytos Mavris MD
Clinical Fellow
Department of Ophthalmology
Hadassah Medical Center
Jerusalem, Israel

Peter McCluskey MD DSc FRANZCO
Professor
Specialty of Ophthalmology
Faculty of Medicine and Health
The University of Sydney, Sydney
Director
Save Sight Institute
Faculty of Medicine and Health
The University of Sydney
Sydney, New South Wales, Australia

Charlotte van Meerwijk MD
Faculty of Medical Sciences
Department of Ophthalmology
University Medical Center Groningen (UMCG)
Groningen, Netherlands

Germán Mejía-Salgado MD MSc
Research Assistant
Immunology Unit
Neuroscience Research Group (NEUROS)
Neurovitae Center for Neuroscience
Institute of Translational Medicine (IMT)
School of Medicine and Health Sciences
Universidad del Rosario
Bogotá, Colombia
Ophthalmology Resident
Health Sciences Faculty
Universidad Autónoma de Bucaramanga (UNAB)
Bucaramanga, Colombia

Israel Mendez MD MPH
Assistant Professor
Department of Ophthalmology
University of Puerto Rico
San Juan, Puerto Rico, USA

Matteo Menean MD
Research Clinical Fellow
Department of Ocular Oncology and Retina
Bascom Palmer Eye Institute
University of Miami Health System
Miami, Italy

Elisabetta Miserocchi MS
Professor
Department of Ophthalmology
Chief
Ocular Immunology and Uveitis Service
San Raffaele Scientific Institute San Raffaele, University Vita-Salute
Milan, Lombardy, Italy

Kalpana Babu Murthy
DO MRCOphth (Lon)
Head
Department of Uveitis and Ocular Inflammation
Prabha Eye Clinic and Research Centre
Vittala International Institute of Ophthalmology
Bengaluru, Karnataka, India

Wijden Nabi MD
Assistant Professor
Department of Ophthalmology
Fattouma Bourguiba University Hospital
Faculty of Medicine
University of Monastir
Monastir, Tunisia

Piergiorgio Neri MD PhD MBA
Full-Professor
Cleveland Clinic Lerner College of Medicine
Case Western Reserve University
Cleveland, Ohio, USA
Senior Uveitis Consultant
Department of Ophthalmology
Cleveland Clinic Abu Dhabi
Abu Dhabi
United Arab Emirates

Alexander Newman
MD Mmed (OphthSci)
Fellow of the Royal Australia and New Zealand
College of Ophthalmologists (FRANZCO)
Consultant Ophthalmologist and Comprehensive Eye Surgeon
Department of Ophthalmology
Conrad Eye Care, Vision for Life Institute
Royal Brisbane and Women's Hospital (RBWH) and Surgical Treatment, and Rehabilitation Service (STARS)
Griffith University
Auchenflower, Queensland, Australia

Quan Dong Nguyen
MD MSc FAAO FARVO FASRS
Professor of Ophthalmology
Medicine (Immunology and Rheumatology), and Pediatrics
Spencer Center for Vision Research
Byers Eye Institute
Stanford University School of Medicine
Palo Alto, California, USA

Agustina Nieddu MD
Head
Department of Uveitis Section
Santa Lucía Eye Hospital
Caba, State: Buenos Aires, Argentina
Fellows Instructor
Department of Uveitis Section
Hospital Universitario Austral
Pilar, Buenos Aires Province, Argentina

Pinar Ozdal MD
Professor
Department of Ophthalmology
Ulucanlar Eye Research and Training Hospital, Uvea Academy Eye Clinic
Ankara, Turkey

Alessandra Pagliara MD
Medical Doctor
Ophthalmology Unit
Department of Medicine
Surgery and Neurosciences
University of Siena
Siena, Tuscany, Italy

Araniko Pandey MD
Clinical Rotation
Department of Ophthalmology
AdventHealth Central Florida
Orlando, Florida, USA

Athanasios Pappas MD MSc
Chief Resident
Department of Ophthalmology
University Hospital of Larissa
Larissa, Thessaly, Greece

Nimesh Patel MD
Assistant Professor and Director
Pediatric Retina Service
Massachusetts Eye and Ear Infirmary
Harvard Medical School
Boston, Massachusetts, USA

Carlos Pavesio MD FRCOphth
Professor of Ocular Inflammation and Infection, UCL and Consultant Ophthalmologist
Department of Ophthalmology
Moorfieds Eye Hospital
London, England, UK

Francesco Pichi MD
Associate Professor
Department of Ophthalmology and Vision Sciences
University of Toronto
Toronto, Ontario, Canada

Uwe Pleyer MD FEBO
Professor
Department of Ophthalmology
Campus Virchow Klinikum and Berlin Institute of Health, Charité Universitätsmedizin Berlin
Berlin, Germany

Sara Prischak MD
Resident
Department of Ophthalmology
Loyola Stritch School of Medicine
Maywood, Illinois, USA

Athimalaipet V Ramanan
MBBS FRCPCH FRCP
Professor of Paediatric Rheumatology and Consultant Paediatric Rheumatologist
Department of Paediatric Rheumatology
University Hospitals Bristol and Weston NHS Foundation Trust
Bristol, England, UK

Laura Camila Ramírez-Márquez MD
Voluntary Teacher and Surgeon
Department of Ophthalmology
São Geraldo Hospital
Belo Horizonte
Retina, Cataract Surgeon and Teacher
Department of Ophthalmology
Hilton Rocha Eye Hospital
Belo Horizonte, Minas Gerais, Brazil

Eugenia Ramos-Davila MD
Clinical Fellow
Division of Ocular Immunology
Wilmer Eye Institute
The Johns Hopkins School of Medicine
Baltimore, Maryland, USA

SR Rathinam FAMS PhD
Principal, Professor, and Head
Department of Uveitis Service
Aravind Eye Hospital and PG Institute of Ophthalmology
Madurai, Tamil Nadu, India

Jose Manuel Cachero Rodríguez MD
Ophthalmology Consultant
Department of Ophthalmology
Cruces University Hospital
Barakaldo, Spain
Ophthalmology Consultant
Department of Ophthalmology
Instituto Oftalmológico Etxeandia
Galdakao, Spain

James T Rosenbaum MD
Emeritus Senior Scientist and Chief
Department of Ophthalmology
Legacy Devers Eye Clinic
Portland, Oregon, USA

Sudharshan S DNB
Senior Consultant
Department of Uvea
Sankara Nethralaya
Chennai, Tamil Nadu, India

Ahmed Sallam MD PhD FRCOphth
Professor
Department of Retina and Uveitis Services
University of Arkansas for Medical Sciences
Little Rock, Arkansas, USA

David Sarraf MD
Clinical Professor
Department of Ophthalmology
UCLA Stein Eye Institute
Los Angeles, California, USA

Maria Carmela Saturno MD
Ophthalmologist
Department of Ophthalmology
MVM Microsurgery Villa Massimo
Rome, Lazio, Italy

Ariel Schlaen MD PhD
Medical Doctor and Director
Department of Uveitis Section
Hospital Universitario Austral
Pilar
Medical Doctor and Sub-Director
Department of Uveitis Section
Hospital de Clínicas "José de San Martín", Universidad de Buenos Aires
Pilar, Buenos Aires Province, Argentina

Ahana Sen DNB FMRF
Consultant
Department of Uvea and Medical Retina
Aditya Birla Sankara Nethralaya
Kolkata, West Bengal, India

Ahmed Shakarchi MD MPH
Vitreoretinal and Uveitis Fellow
Department of Ophthalmology
University of Arkansas for Medical Sciences
Little Rock, Arkansas, USA

Derrick Smit
MBChB MMed Ophth FC Ophth (SA) PhD
Associate Professor
Division of Ophthalmology
Department of Surgical Sciences
Faculty of Medicine and Health Sciences
Stellenbosch University
Stellenbosch, Western Cape Province, South Africa

Justine R Smith FRANZCO PhD
Matthew Flinders Distinguished Professor
Flinders Health & Medical Research Institute and College of Medicine & Public Health
Flinders University
Adelaide, South Australia, Australia

Lucia Sobrin MD MPH
Professor of Ophthalmology, Associate Director of the Retina Service
Massachusetts Eye and Ear Infirmary
Harvard Medical School
Boston, Massachusetts, USA

Guilherme Macedo Souza MD
Uveitis Assistant
Department of Ophthalmology and Visual Science
Federal University of Sao Paulo
Sao Paulo, Brazil

Radhika Sriram MBBS DNB
Consultant
Department of Uvea and Medical Retina
Dr Agarwals Eye Hospital
Mumbai, Maharashtra, India

Jie Sun MD PhD
Retina and Uveitis Specialist
Department of Retina and Uveitis
Retina Group of Florida
Lakewood Ranch, Florida, USA

Emebet Getahun Tabor MD
Assistant Professor and Director
Department of Ophthalmology
MyungSung Medical College
Addis Ababa, Ethiopia

Merve Inanç Tekin MD FEBO
Associate Professor and Senior Assistant
Department of Ophthalmology
University of Health Sciences
Ulucanlar Eye Hospital
Ankara, Turkey

Jennifer Thorne MD PhD FARVO
The Cross Family Professor of Ophthalmology
Director, Division of Ocular Immunology
Professor of Epidemiology
The Wilmer Eye Institute
The Johns Hopkins School of Medicine
Baltimore, Maryland, USA

Stephan Thurau MD
Senior Physician
Department of Ophthalmology
Eye Clinic and Polyclinic
LMU University Hospital
LMU Munich, City Campus
München, Germany

Ilknur Tugal-Tutkun MD
Professor and Director
Department of the Uveitis Service
Istanbul Faculty of Medicine
Eye Protection Foundation
Bayrampasa Eye Hospital, Uveitis Service
Istanbul, Turkey

Ngoc Trong Tuong Than MD
Medical Consultant
Spencer Center for Vision Research
Byers Eye Institute
Stanford University School of Medicine
Palo Alto, California, USA

Mudit Tyagi MS
Consultant and Head of Services
Smt. Kanuri Santhamma Center for Vitreoretinal Diseases
Anant Bajaj Retina Institute
Hyderabad
Consultant
Saroja A Rao Center for Uveitis
LV Prasad Eye Institute
Hyderabad, Telangana, India

Cristhian Urzúa MD MSc
Director
Laboratory of Ocular and Systemic Autoimmune Diseases
Faculty of Medicine, University of Chile
Santiago, Chile

Daniel Vitor Vasconcelos-Santos MD PhD
Associate Professor and Chairman
Department of Ophthalmology and Otorhinolaryngology
Faculty of Medicine, Federal University of Minas Gerais
Belo Horizonte, Minas Gerais, Brazil

Marcelo Vega-Codd MD
Researchers and Clinicians
Laboratory of Ocular and Systemic Autoimmune Diseases
Faculty of Medicine
University of Chile
Santiago, Chile

Linda Visser MBChB MMed (Ophth)
Associate Professor
Department of Ophthalmology
Stellenbosch University
Stellenbosch, South Africa

Mark Westcott MD FRCOphth
Consultant
Uveitis Service
Moorfields Eye Hospital NHS Trust
London
Consultant
Uveitis Service
Barts Health
London, UK
Visiting Adjunct Professor
Uveitis Service
University of Pittsburgh
Pennsylvania, USA

François Willermain MD PhD
Chef de Service
Department of Ophthalmology
CHU St-Pierre, Université Libre de Bruxelles
Brussels, Belgium

Charlotte Wortmann MD PhD
Medical Doctor and Resident Physicians
Department of Ophthalmology
St. Franziskus Hospital
Muenster, North Rhine-Westphalia, Germany

Foreword

Case Studies in Uveitis: Real Cases & Practical Insights is an invaluable resource for anyone who evaluates and treats patients with intraocular inflammation. The book is based on a series of grand rounds presented by the International Uveitis Study Group (IUSG). Each chapter is multiauthored so that the guidance represents a broad perspective. Although undoubtedly not every uveitis expert was asked to participate in the lectures and writing, the list of authors reads like a who's who in the pantheon of uveitis experts. The format is unique, based on cases, and intended to provide practical information. Practitioners at all levels of experience will find these 400 pages to be of immense value.

My own interest in uveitis began around 1978 from a chance observation in laboratory rodents who "misbehaved" by "refusing" to develop arthritis and instead developing uveitis. My limited knowledge of the IUSG in the 1970s led me falsely to believe that it was an elitist organization that acted like a fraternity with an elected membership and only sporadic impact on understanding eye inflammation. I was wrong, or maybe the passage of time has changed the IUSG, or perhaps, both concepts are true.

The IUSG course to teach an understanding of uveitis to international ophthalmologists with limited access to educational opportunities is a marvelous, visionary success that supports knowledge and equity. Delphi panels, scoping reviews, and meta-analyses sponsored by the IUSG are bringing clarity to important issues relevant to uveitis such as retinal vasculitis. The Webinar series promotes a sharing of scholarship which is extremely welcome.

Five decades ago, I might have described the IUSG as stodgy. I should not have been so judgmental in the 1970s as I really had limited interactions with the IUSG at that time. Today, the IUSG is characterized by leadership, innovation, curiosity, and motivation to educate and share. This book is an excellent example of what can be achieved.

James T Rosenbaum MD
Emeritus Senior Scientist and Chief
Department of Ophthalmology
Legacy Devers Eye Clinic
Portland, Oregon, USA

Foreword

The field of uveitis and ocular inflammation has always demanded a rare combination of scientific rigor, keen insight, clinical skills, and humility. Unlike many other medical disciplines, where the diagnosis of an ailment is often obvious to an experienced clinician and confirmed by laboratory tests and scans, the practice of uveitis very often begins and ends with uncertainty. A patient presents with a limited set of eye symptoms, yet these may represent imminent, sight-threatening inflammation of the sclera, uvea, retina, choroid, retinal vessels, or the optic nerve, or even a life-threatening masquerade. The uveitis expert is often challenged to connect disparate symptoms, ocular signs, and systemic clues that may appear unrelated to the uninitiated, with precision and urgency. Standard textbooks can provide only a framework, but it is the real patients and real discussions in the classroom/bedside setting that impart the most enduring lessons.

It is precisely this philosophy that makes *Case Studies in Uveitis: Real Cases & Practical Insights* such a timely and valuable contribution.

This volume emerges from an exceptional academic initiative by the International Uveitis Study Group (IUSG), a globally respected collaborative platform that has brought together clinicians, surgeon-scientists, educators, and basic scientists and researchers committed to advancing the understanding and management of ocular inflammatory diseases. Through its year-long grand rounds and webinar discussions in 2025, the IUSG created a vibrant forum where challenging cases from around the world were presented, debated, and dissected by experts with remarkable openness and intellectual honesty. This book represents the finest distillation of those discussions.

Across 18 thoughtfully curated chapters, readers will encounter some of the most complex and intriguing cases in ocular inflammation, ranging from common diagnostic dilemmas to rare masquerade syndromes and emerging therapeutic challenges. What makes this work distinctive is its format. Each chapter begins with foundational knowledge, followed by real-world clinical cases, each systematically discussed by a roster of internationally recognized experts who bring both evidence-based reasoning and decades of practical wisdom.

The editorial leadership behind this volume reflects the truly global nature of modern uveitis practice. The editors, Drs Alejandra de-la-Torre, Meghan Berkenstock, Germán Mejía-Salgado, John H Kempen, Reema Bansal, Vishali Gupta, have brought together an extraordinary range of contributors from North and South America, Europe, Asia, Australia, Africa, and the Middle East. Their collective expertise spans infectious uveitis, autoimmune disorders, pediatric inflammation, ocular imaging, immunology, translational research, epidemiology, and therapeutics. This diversity of contributors ensures that readers benefit from both regional perspectives and universal principles of care.

The strength of this book lies not only in the depth of its discussions but also in its practical design. It is richly illustrated with outstanding clinical photographs, color fundus images, fluorescein and indocyanine green angiography, OCT scans, slit-lamp photographs, and tables, algorithms, and flowcharts that simplify complex decision-making. The inclusion of detailed question-and-answer sections mirrors the dynamic learning environment of grand rounds and addresses the very questions trainees and practitioners often hesitate to ask. Each chapter is further strengthened by current references and an updated review of the contemporary literature, ensuring that readers are exposed not merely to established doctrines but also to evolving concepts and emerging therapies.

I strongly recommend this book to anyone involved in the care of patients with ocular inflammation. Fellows in training will find it an invaluable resource, bridging textbook knowledge and clinical reality. Comprehensive ophthalmologists and retinal specialists will benefit from its diagnostic frameworks. Rheumatologists, infectious disease specialists, internists, and physician-scientists will appreciate its multidisciplinary perspective. Even seasoned uveitis specialists will find pearls that refine their practice.

I believe this learning model will serve as a torchbearer for future medical education. I believe it already has. Medicine is increasingly moving toward collaborative, case-based, digitally connected learning ecosystems. This book captures that transition beautifully, transforming live global discussions into a permanent educational resource.

Above all, this volume reminds us that every challenging case is not merely a diagnostic puzzle; it is a patient seeking clarity, vision, and hope. If this book helps clinicians navigate that journey with greater confidence and wisdom, it will have achieved something truly enduring.

Amod Gupta MBBS MS DSc (Hon) FAMS
Emeritus Professor
Advanced Eye Centre
Postgraduate Institute of Medical Education and Research
Chandigarh, India

Foreword

Uveitis remains a field that continues to challenge, even after many years in practice. What appears, at first glance, to be a straightforward inflammation within the eye often proves to be anything but. Similar clinical signs may arise from entirely different underlying processes—infectious, immune-mediated, systemic or, often, idiopathic. The task for the ophthalmologist is not only to recognize patterns, but also to question them, to test assumptions, and to remain alert to what does not fit. It is this need for careful judgment, often in the face of uncertainty, that defines uveitis and makes it such a demanding and rewarding area of ophthalmology.

In my experience, uveitis is learnt by seeing patients. Each case presents a sequence of decisions—what to ask, what to look for, what to investigate, and when and how to treat. These decisions evolve as new information emerges. A well-presented clinical case captures this process far better than any didactic text, and through this approach, ophthalmologists develop confidence and sound clinical judgment.

This book covers the main anatomical types of uveitis: Anterior, intermediate, posterior, and panuveitis and their many disease associations, as well as specific chapters on infections: Toxoplasmosis, tuberculosis, syphilis, herpes, RNA viruses, and HIV. Systemic diseases are well represented, with chapters on juvenile idiopathic arthritis (JIA), Behçet disease, plus white dot syndromes, local and systemic therapy, and drug-induced uveitis. There is also a chapter on scleritis. It is built around real cases that illustrate not only the diversity of uveitis but also how clinical reasoning unfolds in practice. The breadth of contributors, with international authorship and the wisdom of world-renowned uveitis gurus, brings together experience from around the world, which is an important strength. Uveitis is influenced by geography, population, and disease patterns, and exposure to these differing perspectives broadens understanding in ways highly relevant to modern clinical practice.

A particular strength of the book is its clear focus on hands-on application, with practical tips and diagnostic and treatment algorithms that help structure thinking. The figures are well laid out, clear, and highly accessible. There are abundant, well-chosen, high-quality color and black-and-white clinical images that reinforce key diagnostic features. Importantly, management is presented as a dynamic process. Treatment is not portrayed as a fixed pathway but as something that must be adapted to disease activity, response, and the individual patient. This is entirely consistent with the realities of uveitis care. Chapters conclude with "Pearls from the experts on frequently asked questions", which reflect issues that arise repeatedly in everyday clinical practice. A "Final wrap-up" succinctly summarizes each chapter.

The discussion of anterior uveitis offers a clear example of this approach. The reader is guided from initial clinical questions—such as epidemiology and systemic associations—through detailed examination findings and targeted investigations to the principles of treatment escalation. The emphasis throughout is on asking the right questions and interpreting findings in context. This mirrors clinical decision-making and reinforces the importance of a structured yet flexible approach.

What, in my view, most clearly distinguishes this book from others is that it teaches a way of thinking. It encourages the reader to consider not only what is most likely, but also what must not be missed. It prompts reflection on whether the clinical picture truly fits the presumed diagnosis, when infection must be excluded before escalating therapy, and how best to balance the risks and benefits of treatment. These are the questions that underpin safe and effective care, and they are often the most difficult to teach. By embedding them in real cases, the authors have provided a framework that can be readily applied in clinical practice.

Another important aspect emerging from these cases is the need to view the patient as a whole. Uveitis does not exist in isolation. It frequently reflects systemic disease and often requires collaboration with colleagues in other specialties.

Recognizing when to extend the assessment beyond the eye and when to involve others is a key part of good clinical practice. The cases presented here repeatedly and appropriately highlight that principle.

This book will be of value to a wide range of readers. For trainees and fellows, it offers a clear and practical guide to tackling complex clinical problems. For more experienced ophthalmologists, it provides an opportunity to reflect on established practices and refine decision-making. Above all, it serves as a reminder that experience in uveitis is built gradually, through careful observation, thoughtful interpretation, and ongoing learning from patients.

Perhaps most importantly, the book teaches a way of thinking. It encourages the reader to ask the right questions: What is the most likely diagnosis? What else could this be? Which features do not fit? When should infection be excluded before escalating therapy? When is it appropriate to treat aggressively, and when is it safer to observe? These are the judgments that define experienced ophthalmologists, and they are difficult to convey in conventional textbooks. By grounding these questions in real cases, the authors provide a framework that readers can apply directly to their own patients.

Ultimately, the strength of this book lies in its ability to bridge knowledge and practice. In a field where uncertainty is unavoidable, clarity of thought is the ophthalmologist's most important tool. This book supports the development of that clarity and, in doing so, makes a valuable contribution to the teaching and practice of uveitis. It is a resource that will be both read and used and will undoubtedly benefit those involved in the care of patients with intraocular inflammation.

Philip Ian Murray MBBS DO (RCS) PhD FRCP FRCS FRCOphth FRSM
Emeritus Professor of Ophthalmology
University of Birmingham, UK

Foreword

An amazing book appears now in the uveitis world, that is, *Case Studies in Uveitis: Real Cases & Practical Insights* edited by the International Uveitis Study Group (IUSG).

It is my great honor and privilege to introduce this book as a member of IUSG for over 30 years. The book has a number of unique features as follows.

What is unique and new about this book?

The book emphasizes "real-world" clinical insights and practical wisdom rather than theoretical concepts. This means that the book will be greatly helpful in daily clinical situations for managing patients with uveitis, not only for young ophthalmologists but also for uveitis experts. For this purpose, the book comprises 18 chapters, and each chapter features a keynote contribution from an eminent uveitis expert, followed by case presentations of three instructive cases with detailed discussions. In addition, a question-and-answer section, "pearls from experts on frequently asked questions", is a unique feature of the book and provides practical answers to simple but essential questions which you may often ask yourself.

The 18 chapters of this book include 5 chapters on different anatomical types of uveitis and scleritis, 11 chapters on specific entities of uveitis, and 2 chapters on therapies. The 11 chapters on specific uveitis entities include ocular toxoplasmosis, ocular tuberculosis, ocular syphilis, herpetic anterior uveitis, acute retinal necrosis, RNA viruses and uveitis, ocular complications of HIV and AIDS, juvenile idiopathic arthritis-associated uveitis, Behçet's disease, white dot syndrome, and drug-induced uveitis, all of which are common and clinically important diseases all over the world and sight-threating unless managed appropriately.

How shall we use this book?

This book can be used in many ways, depending on each clinician's clinical problems. It is educational as a textbook on uveitis. Needless to say, it can be used as a practical resource book in our daily practice managing uveitis patients. In real-life clinical practice, patients suffering from uveitis present a variety of symptoms and signs without a definitive diagnosis. In such cases, we will review the medical history and perform ocular examinations, followed by an anatomical diagnosis where the major site of inflammation is located in the eye, such as anterior uveitis, intermediate uveitis, posterior uveitis, panuveitis, or scleritis. Thus far, the steps are relatively straightforward; then further assessment is needed to obtain more information from the eye and the systemic organs. At this step, the first five chapters of this book can be used to clarify how to proceed and to reach a final diagnosis and its management. Once the diagnosis is made, further detailed information will be provided in other chapters on specific uveitis entities of this book.

How this book was born?

This book is based on the Grand Rounds Webinar Seminars conducted by IUSG.

The IUSG Webinar Seminar on Basic Uveitis started in 2021 amid the COVID-19 pandemic under the leadership of late Dr Manfred Zierhut, previous President of IUSG. The webinar series has been successful and continues to be held monthly. The "Grand Rounds" Webinar Seminars, which are the basis of this book, were held between 2024 and 2025 under the leadership of Dr Vishali Gupta, President of IUSG; Dr Marc de Smet, Secretary of IUSG; and Dr John H Kempen, Chair of Education Program Committee.

What is IUSG?

IUSG is an international organization formed in 1978 and incorporated in Belgium. It comprises both clinicians and researchers committed to improving the standards of care in uveitis, teaching state-of-the-art diagnostics and therapeutics, and fostering through individual and collaborative efforts in preclinical, translational, and clinical research. The goals of IUSG are prevention of the blinding complications of uveitis and improve outcomes (from IUSG Home Page).

Finally, I have long been hoping for a practical resource book of this kind, emphasizing real-world clinical insights and practical approaches, and it is now available.

Manabu Mochizuki MD PhD
Emeritus Professor
Department of Ophthalmology & Visual Science
Graduate School of Medical and Dental Sciences
Institute of Science Tokyo
Tokyo, Japan

Foreword

Uveitis has always occupied a particularly demanding place within ophthalmology. It is a field that requires scientific rigor, technical precision, clinical intuition, patience, and the wisdom acquired through years of direct experience with complex patients. While textbooks and guidelines provide essential foundations, much of the true art of uveitis is transmitted through the real cases, reflective clinical judgment, and the collective local and international experience.

It is therefore a great pleasure and honor to introduce this remarkable volume prepared by the International Uveitis Study Group (IUSG). This work represents far more than a conventional academic textbook. It reflects the living spirit of a global community committed to improving the understanding and management of ocular inflammatory disease through collaboration, education, and open exchange

Since the 1980s, as a member of the IUSG, I have had the privilege of accompanying its development and witnessing its growth for over a half century. I remember well the aspirations that inspired the strengthening of this truly international society: The dream of creating a global forum where specialists—including regions historically underrepresented—could share their concepts, observations, and clinical experiences in an integrated and respectful manner.

Over the years, the IUSG transformed that vision into reality. The society became not only a center for scientific discussion, but also a bridge connecting generations, nations, and different schools of thought in ophthalmology. It fostered an environment in which experienced leaders and younger colleagues could openly discuss difficult cases, challenge concepts, and collectively refine the understanding of inflammatory eye disease. This spirit of collegiality and intellectual generosity remains one of the defining strengths of the IUSG.

This book beautifully demonstrates the success of that vision. Its structure is particularly valuable and innovative. Each chapter begins with a comprehensive review prepared by internationally recognized experts, offering readers an updated and practical overview of important uveitis entities and management strategies. These discussions are enriched by illustrative clinical cases that highlight diagnostic reasoning, therapeutic decision-making, and subtle complexities that often define successful patient care in real-world practice. The inclusion of frequently asked questions and concise practical discussions further enhances the educational value of the text for specialists, comprehensive ophthalmologists, fellows, residents, and trainees alike.

Equally important is the diversity of perspectives represented throughout this volume. Uveitis varies across populations and geographic regions, influenced by local epidemiology, infectious diseases, genetics, socioeconomic conditions, and healthcare access. By bringing together experts from around the world, this book reflects the richness and complexity of global ophthalmology itself.

I congratulate the editors and contributors for creating a work that will undoubtedly become an important educational resource for our field. More importantly, this volume stands as a testimony to the enduring ideals of the International Uveitis Study Group: International collaboration, scientific openness, friendship, and the shared commitment to preserving vision and improving patients' lives throughout the world.

Rubens Belfort Jr MD PhD MBA
Head Professor
Department of Ophthalmology
Hospital São Paulo
Federal University of São Paulo
President Vision Institute
Brazilian Academy of Medicine
Brazilian Academy of Sciences

Preface

Case Studies in Uveitis: Real Cases & Practical Insights was conceived as a collaborative initiative of the International Uveitis Study Group to address the need for a case-based learning resource in ocular inflammation. Uveitis often presents diagnostic and therapeutic challenges requiring a nuanced and patient-centered approach. Through real-world clinical cases contributed by global experts, this book aims to provide ophthalmologists, fellows, and trainees with practical insights into the complexities of uveitis. Each case highlights the importance of detailed clinical reasoning, differential diagnosis, and tailored management strategies. We hope this work serves as a learning tool and an inspiration to continue advancing care for patients with uveitis worldwide.

Alejandra de-la-Torre, Meghan Berkenstock, Germán Mejía-Salgado,
John H Kempen, Reema Bansal, Vishali Gupta

Message from IUSG Executive Committee

It is a moment of great pleasure and pride for us to present this unique book, *Case Studies in Uveitis: Real Cases & Practical Insights*, authored by members of the IUSG from across the globe.

The International Uveitis Study Group (IUSG) began in 1978 as a small society of clinicians united by a common interest in uveitis. In its early days, the core of IUSG meetings revolved around case discussions. Uveitis cases, by their very nature, are challenging, and there has always been an intrinsic need to discuss them with peers—seeking diverse perspectives and learning collectively. Indeed, no amount of textbook knowledge can truly replace the practical wisdom gained from the experience of world-renowned uveitis experts.

As the society grew, meetings evolved and became more structured, with increasing emphasis on cutting-edge advances in diagnostics and therapeutics. While this progress has been invaluable, the simplicity and richness of interactive case-based learning was something we deeply missed.

Education has remained a central mission of IUSG. In 2021, we initiated a series of online virtual courses comprising monthly webinars that addressed all aspects of uveitis. Building on this, in January 2024, we introduced a novel format—*Uveitis Grand Rounds*. Each session focused on a major theme, beginning with an expert lecture followed by three illustrative cases—simple, moderate, and complex—covering the full spectrum of disease. These cases, presented by fellows and discussed by mentors, highlighted real-world challenges and practical decision-making. The sessions concluded with interactive discussions, where attendees engaged directly with experts.

This series of 18 webinars has been thoughtfully compiled into this book—a process that required immense dedication and effort. We extend our sincere gratitude to all the editors and especially to Alejandra de-la-Torre and Meghan Berkenstock, for their invaluable contributions to bringing this project to fruition.

The result is a timeless resource that showcases cases from around the world, offering rich practical insights, management challenges, and diverse approaches reflective of global practice.

We sincerely hope that readers will not only enjoy this book but also gain pearls of wisdom that cannot be fully captured in textbooks, journals, or even artificial intelligence platforms.

Vishali Gupta, Marc de Smet, Massimo Accorinti,
Ilknur Tugal Tutkun, Sapna Gangaputra
(IUSG Executive Committee)

Acknowledgments

We express our heartfelt gratitude to the members of the International Uveitis Study Group (IUSG) for their continuous commitment to advancing the field of uveitis. Special thanks to all the contributing authors and case presenters, whose clinical insights and dedication to patients' care made this book possible. We are especially thankful to our families and institutions for their unwavering support throughout the development of this project.

We would also like to thank Shri Jitendar P Vij (Group Chairman) and Mr Ankit Vij (Managing Director), along with the entire team of M/s Jaypee Brothers Medical Publishers (P) Ltd, New Delhi, India, for their invaluable support in bringing this project to completion.

Contents

CHAPTER 1

Anterior Uveitis

Alejandra de-la-Torre, Rupesh Agrawal, Miranda Gehrke, Stephan Thurau, Armin Taghavi Eraghi, Uwe Pleyer, Jonathan Malcolm Chavan, SR Rathinam, Germán Mejía-Salgado, Meghan Berkenstock, Reema Bansal, Vishali Gupta, John H Kempen

INTRODUCTION

Anterior uveitis (AU) is the most common form of uveitis.[1-3] However, its diagnostic and therapeutic approach can be a clinical challenge even for a uveitis specialist. Throughout its management, it is important to always keep in mind the following principles:

- Preserving vision
- Controlling inflammation
- Managing the recurrence of episodes
- Preventing new recurrences with prophylactic management
- Avoiding complications

To achieve these principles, the patient's diagnostic and therapeutic regimen must be dynamic. The frequency, route of administration, and dosage of medications should vary according to the evolution of the disease.[4] For example, new therapeutic schemes, such as immunosuppressants or biologic therapies, can be added when activity is not controlled with previous treatment. On the contrary, in a patient with long-term inflammation control, we can gradually reduce medications until achieving the objectives with the least possible number of drugs.[5]

PRACTICAL TIPS IN THE MANAGEMENT OF ANTERIOR UVEITIS

When addressing a patient with AU, we must ask ourselves several questions:

1. What geographical location am I in? Where is my patient from?

Knowing the epidemiology of uveitis is essential, as it allows for directing diagnoses according to geographic region. Uveitis generally has a prevalence ranging from 9 to 730 cases per 100,000 inhabitants, with an incidence ranging from 17.40 to 111.28 per 100,000 persons per year.[6] Geographic variation, as seen in a meta-regression analysis, is a significant factor explaining the high heterogeneity among epidemiological studies of uveitis. Populations have different geographical factors and environmental exposures that result in varying diagnoses between regions.[6,7]

The anterior segment is the most common location of uveitis worldwide, with AU prevalence ranging from 29.6 to 92.2% of all uveitis patients.[1,8] In the Western world, non-infectious AU appears to be the main cause.[7] In recent updates from regions such as South America, where idiopathic or infectious uveitides were the most frequent etiologies of AU, there has been an increase in non-infectious diseases, such as human leukocyte antigen (HLA)-B27+ associated AU.[9] This trend has also been observed in European and Asian countries.[10,11] Some factors that might explain this change include improvements in technology, imaging, and laboratory capabilities, which have enhanced our diagnostic ability and reduced the number of idiopathic uveitis cases.[4,12]

Additionally, migratory processes between regions are important to consider, given that some pathologies related to AU are still underdiagnosed, hence the importance of epidemiological studies.[4,12] An example is leptospiral uveitis, an infectious process that should be considered a probable diagnosis in patients with non-granulomatous AU who have migrated from an endemic region.[13]

2. What is the most likely diagnosis?

As with any disease, the key lies in conducting a thorough review of systems and physical examination, in which one must ask questions that elucidate the most probable diagnosis.[4] For this purpose, questionnaires or registration platforms such as the Ocular Autoimmune Systemic Inflammatory Infectious Study (OASIS) may be useful,[4,14] allowing for systematic questioning of patients and ensuring no detail is overlooked, thus obtaining as much information as possible.

In the slit-lamp examination, it is important to evaluate:

- Corneal sensitivity
- The pattern of keratic precipitates (KPs)
- Pupillary reflexes
- *Cellularity and flare in the anterior chamber:* This should always be done before dilating the patient and with a 1 × 1 mm conical light. It is also important to remember to evaluate all four quadrants and note the worst value
- Evaluate cells in the anterior vitreous

Note: All these evaluations should be performed in a dark environment to see these details.

Figures 1 and 2 show common slit-lamp findings in patients with AU.

Systematically carrying out a history and physical examination allows us to discern the possible etiology of the uveitis. For example, as we will see later in this chapter from the patient cases presented, a recurrent bilateral, non-granulomatous, non-hypertensive AU is different from acute unilateral uveitis with an elevated ocular pressure,

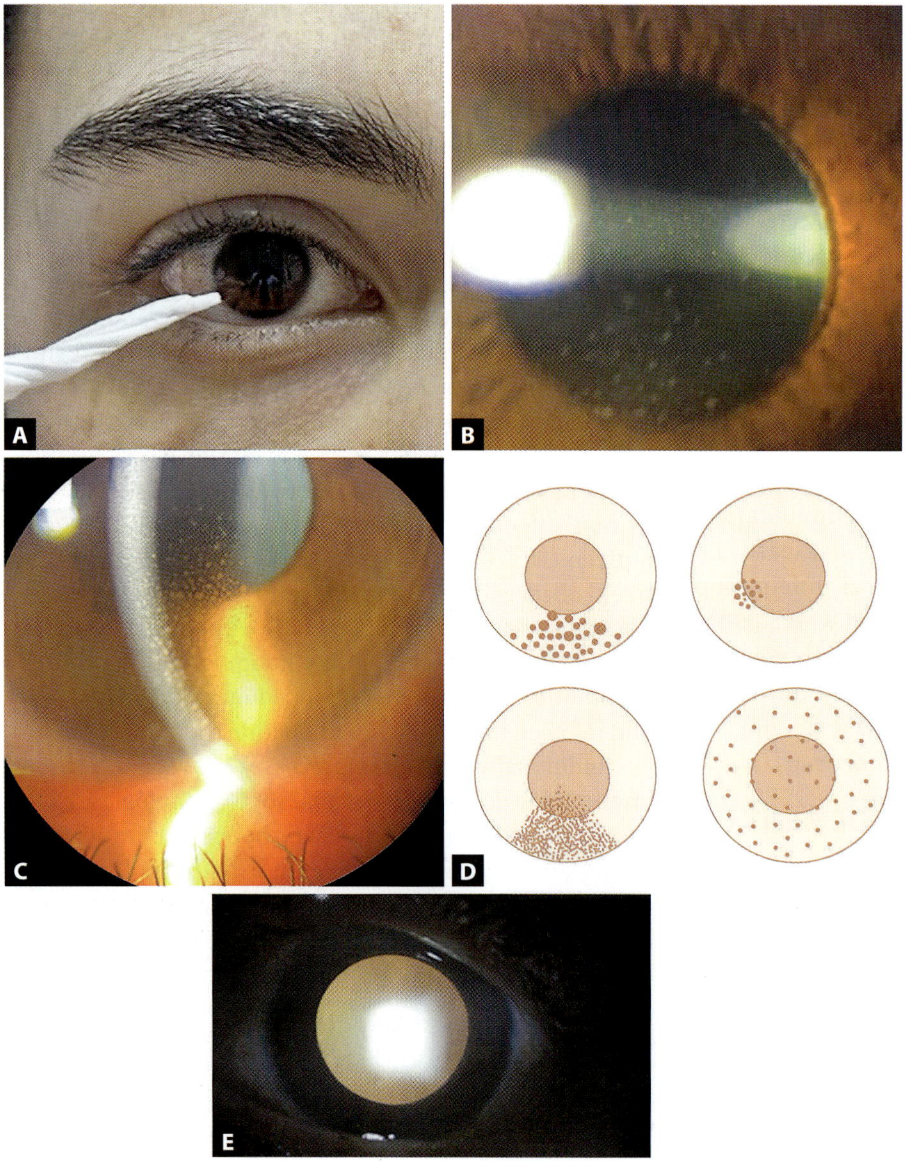

Figs. 1A to E: Physical and slit-lamp examination of patients with anterior uveitis: (A) Corneal sensitivity evaluation; (B) Correct method of assessing cellularity in the anterior chamber with a 1 × 1 mm diameter parallelepiped in a dark room; (C) Granulomatous keratic precipitates (KPs) distributed predominantly in the lower sector (Arlt's triangle); (D) Distribution patterns of KP: Pigmented KP in Arlt's triangle (top-left) suggestive of ocular toxoplasmosis and sarcoidosis, central or paracentral (top-right) suggestive of viral herpetic infection, dusty fine KP in Arlt's triangle (bottom-left) suggestive of HLA-B27-associated anterior uveitis, and small diffuse KP from the limbus to the limbus (bottom-right) suggestive of Fuchs' uveitis syndrome; (E) Pupil retroillumination technique to evaluate iris trans-illumination (not seen here). (HLA: human leukocyte antigen, KP: Keratic precipitates)

Source: Uveitis Webinar - Grand Round 1. International Uveitis Study Group (IUSG). 2025. https://youtu.be/zjP2f03Lqms?si=loNshiovs2Ew2tuJ.

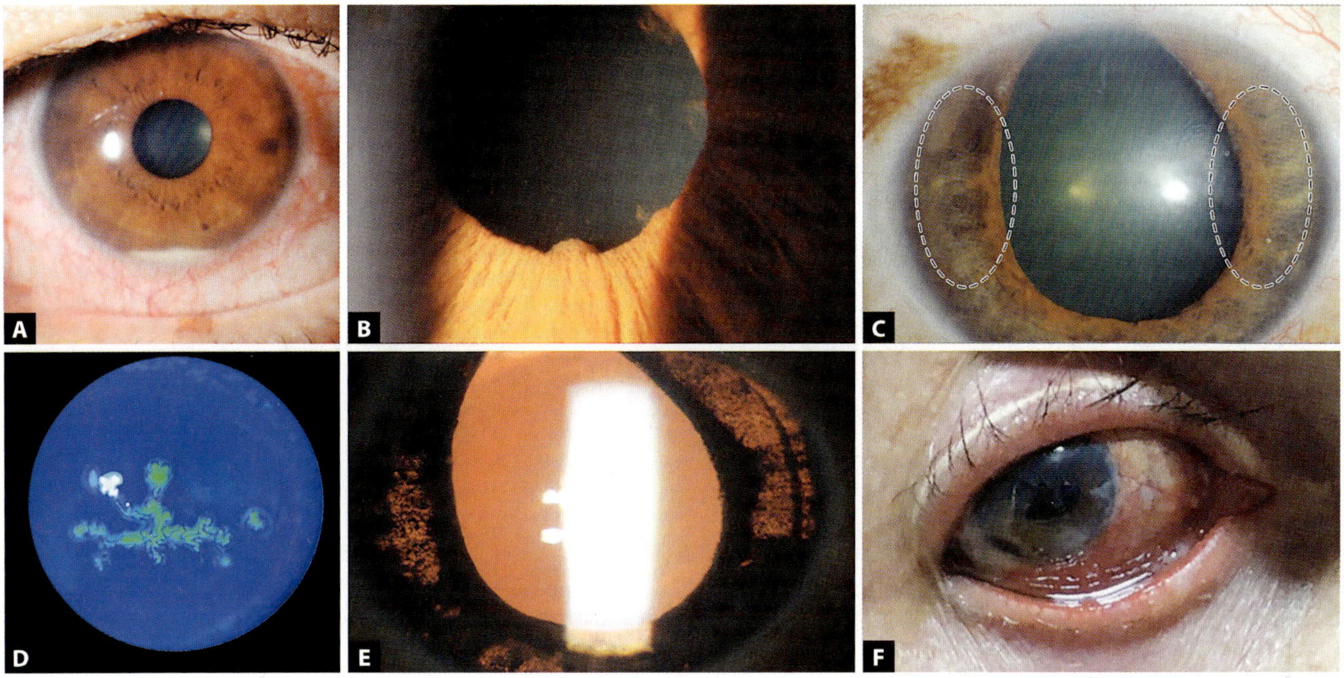

Figs. 2A to F: Biomicroscopy findings in patients with anterior uveitis:[4] (A) Hypopyon grade I (<one-third height of the anterior chamber); (B) Iris nodules; (C) Sectoral or generalized differences in iris color (white ovals); (D) Dendritic epithelial defect typical of herpes simplex virus infection; (E) Transillumination defect (same eye as in C); (F) Scleral involvement.
Source: Uveitis Webinar - Grand Round 1. International Uveitis Study Group (IUSG). 2025. https://youtu.be/zjP2f03Lqms?si=IoNshiovs2Ew2tuJ.

with different etiologies and management.[4] In the future, registration on these platforms will allow for the creation of algorithms with artificial intelligence that provide the most probable diagnosis and the most appropriate treatment according to the patient's clinical characteristics.[15]

Another key aspect is to view the patient as a whole; ophthalmologic assessment is important but not the only consideration. When facing a patient with AU, we must investigate symptoms of any origin (gastrointestinal, neurologic, rheumatologic, and dermatologic, amongst others) and evaluate every part of the body. A uveitis specialist must search for any clues that may guide the diagnosis **(Figs. 3A to C)**.[4]

There are different diagnostic approach algorithms for patients with uveitis.[16-18] These involve conducting basic tests for every uveitis patient at the first instance, including a complete blood count (to identify an increase or decrease in cell counts; for example, leukopenia is commonly seen in sarcoidosis); acute phase reactants (when elevated, they indicate systemic inflammation); HLA-B27 testing in areas with high prevalence (to help detect spondyloarthritis); chest radiographs, and syphilis detection (Treponemal tests because, indirect or non-treponemal assays may become negative years after the initial infection), followed by a series of infectious or non-infectious tests according to the epidemiology and clinical characteristics of the patient. These algorithms have been shown to be more cost-effective compared to when laboratory tests are ordered without any specific approach. They also reduce the use of more specific tests, such as the polymerase chain reaction (PCR), for use in cases of high diagnostic doubt.[16-18]

3. How do I manage a patient with anterior uveitis?

The first step is to define the patient's degree of inflammation and assess whether it is isolated AU or associated with a systemic disease.[4,19,20] Once this is defined, the next step is to rule out infectious pathologies. The third step is to establish clear objectives; we must reduce inflammation, always aiming to achieve "zero inflammation" as soon as possible. According to the Standardization of Uveitis Nomenclature (SUN), improving inflammation is defined as a decrease of two levels on the anterior chamber cellularity scale or a reduction from 0.5+ to 0+.[21] The fourth step is to initiate treatment. For infectious uveitis, specific treatment is given regarding the pathogen. For non-infectious uveitis, it is necessary to perform escalated anti-inflammatory management **(Flowchart 1)**.[4,19,20,22]

The starting point of this escalated anti-inflammatory management begins with the use of corticosteroids to induce control of the uveitis, for which there are different

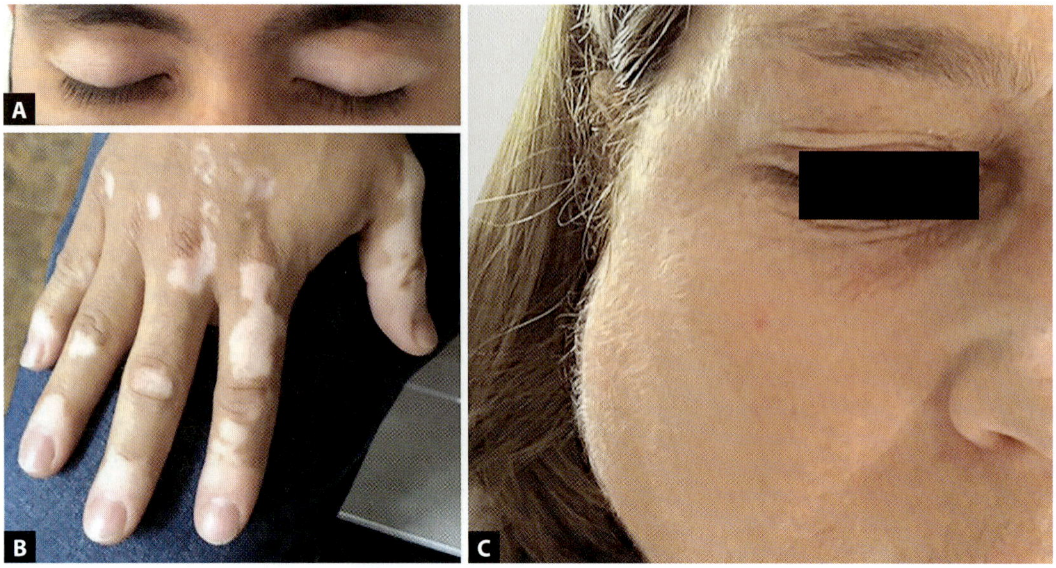

Figs. 3A to C: Systemic findings suggestive of diseases associated with anterior uveitis: (A) Vitiligo in superior eyelids; (B) Vitiligo on the hands (A and B both are suggestive of Vogt–Koyanagi–Harada disease); (C) Diffuse swelling and enlargement of the parotid gland, suggestive of sarcoidosis.
Source: Uveitis Webinar - Grand Round 1. International Uveitis Study Group (IUSG). 2025. https://youtu.be/zjP2f03Lqms?si=loNshiovs2Ew2tuJ.

Flowchart 1: Escalated treatment of anterior uveitis.

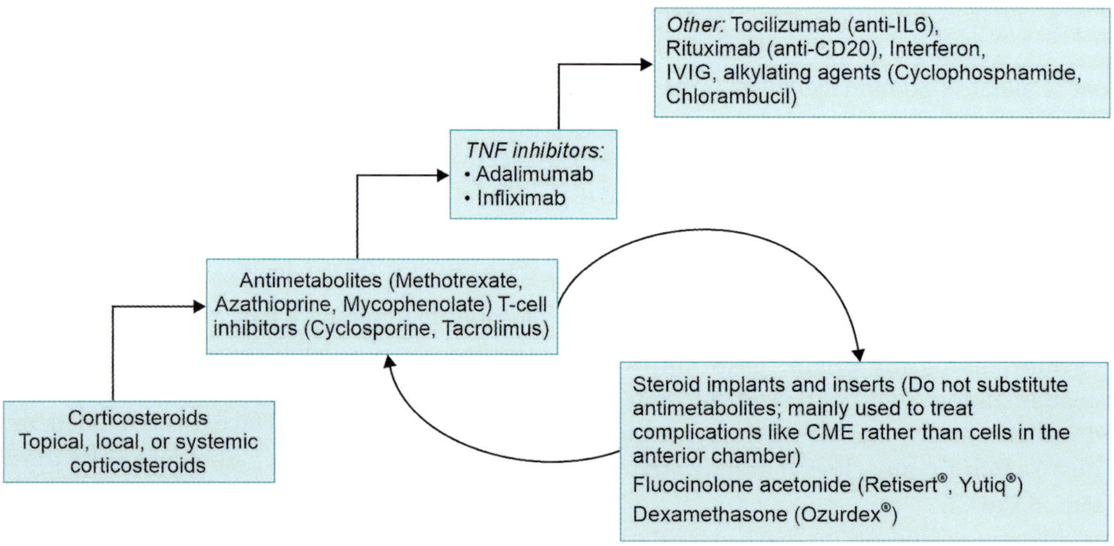

(CME: cystoid macular edema; IL: interleukin; IVIG: intravenous immunoglobulin; TNF: tumor necrosis factor)
Source: Uveitis Webinar - Grand Round 1. International Uveitis Study Group (IUSG). 2025. https://youtu.be/zjP2f03Lqms?si=loNshiovs2Ew2tuJ.

routes of administration, including topical, local, or systemic. Although corticosteroid management is associated with the development of complications, such as ocular hypertension and cataracts, it must be initiated as soon as possible. Corticosteroid dosing frequency and strength must be sufficient to penetrate into the anterior chamber. Complications, although they must be considered, should not be a limitation to administering corticosteroid medications.[4,19,20,22,23] Papaliodis et al. recently demonstrated that high doses of topical corticosteroids did not increase the risk of cataract formation in cases of active uveitis. Presumably, the cataractogenic effect of the corticosteroids was balanced against the same outcome from continued inflammation.[23] Topical corticosteroid frequency is guided by the severity of the inflammation, clinical characteristics, and response to treatment.[4,19,20,22]

It is also important to administer adjuvant medications, such as mydriatics, along with topical corticosteroids. These medications relax the iris sphincter muscle and the ciliary muscle, alleviating symptoms, promoting the breaking of formed synechiae, and preventing the formation of new ones.[4,19,20,22] Other topical adjuvant medications are topical non-steroidal anti-inflammatory drugs (NSAIDs), which can be useful in patients with recurrent AU with macular edema, sometimes helping to reduce central macular thickness.[24,25]

Systemic corticosteroids are rarely used in patients with AU, and if used, should primarily be administered initially in severe cases and for a short period of time. They should be avoided as the primary therapy to reduce long-term inflammation.[4,19,20,22] In addition, they should be administered with a calcium supplement: 1,500 mg/day and vitamin D: 400–800 IU.[26]

4. When to initiate immunomodulatory therapy?[26]

The initiation of systemic immunomodulatory therapy is indicated in the following scenarios:

- Failure of topical and systemic corticosteroid therapy to control inflammation
- Lack of adequate inflammation control in <1 month with high doses of prednisolone
- Maintaining control of the inflammation while preventing complications from corticosteroids (corticosteroid-sparing)
- Cases where high doses of corticosteroids are contraindicated (or rejected by the patient)

In cases of therapeutic failure or in those difficult to treat, always reassess if the working diagnosis is correct. Therefore, considering an alternative diagnosis is also important. Lastly, not all patients with AU require systemic immunosuppression. It is important to consider the aforementioned indications, as the use of immunosuppressive therapy is associated rarely with the development of adverse events, such as cytopenias.[26] Therefore, immunosuppression should only be administered in patients where the benefit outweighs the risk. Likewise, before their use, a pregnancy test should be performed on women of childbearing age. If the ophthalmologist lacks expertise to prescribe and monitor for adverse events associated with use of the immunosuppressive agent, a multidisciplinary approach involving internal medicine and rheumatology should be employed. It is important for other specialties to understand the significance of immunosuppression in cases of persistent intraocular inflammation, even when the disease is systemically controlled.[19,20,22]

The goal of using systemic immunosuppressive therapy is to control inflammation with the lowest possible daily dose of corticosteroids. An acceptable goal is to achieve a prednisone dose of less than or equal to 7.5 mg/day and less than or equal to one drop of prednisolone acetate 1% without the occurrence of any adverse events.[26] Regarding the decision of which systemic immunosuppressant to choose, methotrexate or mycophenolate mofetil are a good first-line options.[20,27] However, the cost of mycophenolate may limit its use in developing countries.[28]

Biologic therapy is the next step after failing to control inflammation in patients with non-infectious uveitis, showing a faster, recurrence-free period in AU than in other anatomic locations.[29] Indications for use include:

- Failure of non-biologic, corticosteroid-sparing therapies to control inflammation
- Worsening of inflammation with the use of high doses and/or two non-biologic, corticosteroid-sparing therapies
- Recurrent disease

It is important to rule out latent infections such as tuberculosis, syphilis, hepatitis B or C, and human immunodeficiency virus (HIV) and treat them (if applicable) before initiating biologic therapy.[4,19,20,22] Likewise, biologic therapy is contraindicated for patients with demyelinating diseases, heart failure, or malignant neoplasms.[4,19,20,22] Tumor necrosis factor (TNF) inhibitors are the most popular biologic agents for the treatment of non-infectious uveitis, although they are only United States Food and Drug Administration (FDA) approved for the treatment of intermediate, posterior, and panuveitis, as well as for uveitis associated with systemic diseases with approved indications, such as juvenile idiopathic arthritis.[30]

Regarding infectious AU, just like non-infectious uveitis, the goal is to obtain the uveitis diagnosis through medical history and risk factor questioning, examination, and testing.[4] It is always important to rule out major imitator diseases, such as syphilis and tuberculosis.[4]

Regarding viral AU, it is essential to note that treatment against infection after an acute attack is important, as well as suppressive, virus specific regimens [(Acyclovir for herpes simplex or herpes zoster or Valganciclovir for cytomegalovirus (CMV)] with variable durations (12, 18, and 24 months).[31,32] These have been shown to effectively control inflammation and intraocular pressure (IOP). In these long-term periods, it is necessary to monitor the patient's renal function and complete blood count due to the nephrotoxicity and cytopenias associated with antiviral use.[33]

NON-GRANULOMATOUS ANTERIOR UVEITIS

Case Presentation

Personal Data

- Female, 40 years old
- No systemic disease history.
- No drugs were used.

History of Present Illness

Bilateral blurred vision, eye redness, eye pain, light sensitivity, and dark floating spots for 1 week.

Physical Examination

The patient presented with a best-corrected visual acuity (BCVA) of 20/100 in OU, normal IOP, anterior chamber inflammation with posterior synechiae development, spillover of cells into the vitreous, and cystoid macular edema **(Table 1 and Fig. 4)**.

Differential Diagnosis

In cases of AU, testing for HLA-B27 can aid in narrowing the differential diagnosis. However, HLA-B27 results should be used as a reference rather than a definitive criterion. For instance, patients with spondyloarthropathy, inflammatory bowel disease, and psoriatic arthritis are generally HLA-B27 positive, yet there are instances of HLA-B27 negative cases. Conversely, conditions such as juvenile idiopathic arthritis, systemic vasculitis, and collagen vascular diseases, such as systemic lupus erythematosus and scleroderma, typically test negative for HLA-B27, although there can be HLA-B27-positive presentations.[34,35]

TABLE 1: Physical examination of a patient having non-granulomatous anterior uveitis.

OD	*Parameter*	*OS*
20/100	BCVA	20/100
14 mm Hg	IOP	16 mm Hg
Moderate diffuse hyperemia	Conjunctiva	Moderate diffuse hyperemia
Clear, dusty keratic precipitates and fibrin nets all over the cornea	Cornea	Clear, dusty keratic precipitates and fibrin nets all over the cornea
No hypopyon ACC 2+	Anterior chamber	No hypopyon ACC 2+
Posterior synechiae at CH12 and CH3	Iris	Posterior synechiae at CH12 and CH3
Retropupillary pigment and nuclear sclerosis	Lens	Retropupillary pigment and nuclear sclerosis
Anterior vitreous cells and haze	Vitreous	Anterior vitreous cells and haze
Cystoid macular edema	Fundus	Cystoid macular edema

(ACC: anterior chamber cellularity; BCVA: best-corrected visual acuity; CH: clock hour; IOP: intraocular pressure)

Source: Uveitis Webinar - Grand Round 1. International Uveitis Study Group (IUSG). 2025. https://youtu.be/zjP2f03Lqms?si=IoNshiovs2Ew2tuJ.

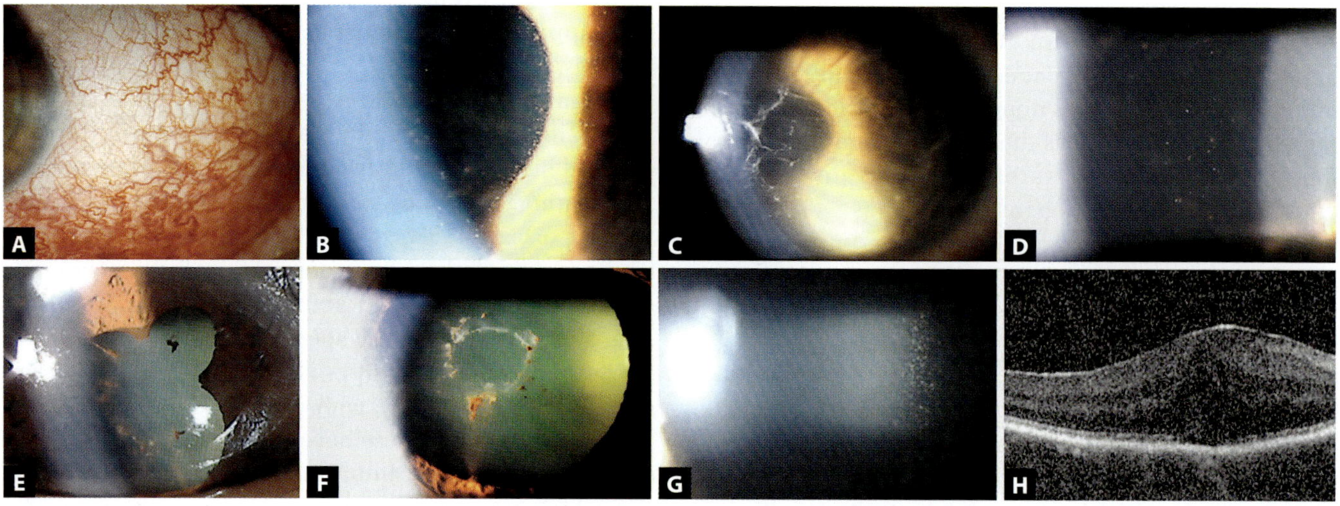

Figs. 4A to H: Non-granulomatous anterior uveitis: (A) Moderate conjunctival hyperemia in the OS; (B) Diffuse dusty keratic precipitates in the OS; (C) Fibrin deposits in the anterior chamber in the OS; (D) Anterior chamber cellularity 2+ in the OS; (E) Posterior synechiae at clock hours 12 and 3 in the OD; (F) pigment on the intensive lens capsule and nuclear sclerosis in the OD; (G) Inflammatory cells in the anterior vitreous (behind the lens) of the OD; (H) Macular edema in the OD. (OD: right eye, OS: left eye).

Source: Uveitis Webinar - Grand Round 1. International Uveitis Study Group (IUSG). 2025. https://youtu.be/zjP2f03Lqms?si=IoNshiovs2Ew2tuJ.[4]

Treatment

- Topical 1% prednisolone acetate, applied every hour for 3–5 days, followed by a gradual tapering
- 2.5% hydrocortisone ointment, applied nightly for 1 week
- 0.5% atropine, twice a day

The patient improved and did not require further consultation.

If the patient presents with a protracted course (chronic or recurrent according to the SUN criteria), systemic corticosteroids **(Table 2)** and immunomodulatory therapy may be indicated.

Corticosteroid-sparing immunosuppressants that could be prescribed for recalcitrant cases include methotrexate, mycophenolate, azathioprine, tacrolimus, interferon-α-2a, cyclosporine, and TNF inhibitors. Use of any of these should be done in consultation with a rheumatologist if additional expertise needed.[4]

In the case of increased IOP, topical hypotensive eye drops, such as beta-blockers, carbonic anhydrase inhibitors (including systemic options), α-mimetics, and prostaglandin derivates, would be indicated. However, it is important to note that the risk of macular edema is particularly associated with the use of prostaglandin derivatives, relegating this class to second or third-line status. Miotics such as pilocarpine are contraindicated due to disruption of the aqueous humor barrier and the risk of posterior synechiae formation.[4]

If the patient presents with new, pronounced posterior synechiae, one treatment option could be a subconjunctival injection of atropine 1%, novocaine 2%, suprarenin (1/1,000) or phenylephrine 0.5%, procaine 1%, and homatropine 0.4%, if the synechiae fail to break open with atropine drops.[4]

TABLE 2: Oral corticosteroid reduction scheme.[36]

Prednisolone doses (daily in mg)	***Reduction (every 1–2 weeks)***
>40 mg	Reduction by 10–20 mg
40–20 mg	Reduction by 5–10 mg
20–10 mg	Reduction by 2.5–5 mg
10–0 mg	Reduction by 1–2.5 mg
High doses are used to achieve suppression of inflammation (induction treatment), while lower doses are used to maintain suppression (maintenance treatment).	

Source: Uveitis Webinar - Grand Round 1. International Uveitis Study Group (IUSG). 2025. https://youtu.be/zjP2f03Lqms?si=IoNshiovs2Ew2tuJ.

Discussion

- It is crucial to note that for the diagnosis of AU, both the anterior and posterior chambers should be examined using a dilated fundus examination to assess for the primary location of the inflammation. This principle is important to understand, as even though AU can lead to retinal complications, it is still classified as "AU" if the main site of inflammation is the anterior chamber.[21]
- Regarding non-granulomatous AU, several factors must be considered, including:
  - *HLA-B27:* Approximately 50% of patients with non-granulomatous AU worldwide are HLA-B27 positive. Although the specific pathophysiologic mechanisms of this association are not entirely clear, it is known that this high frequency of positivity is not observed in cases of granulomatous AU. This highlights the importance of making the correct anatomic and etiologic diagnosis of the uveitis.[4] According to the SUN criteria, acute AU is defined as follows:[21]
    - Sudden onset
    - Limited duration (<3 months)
    - *Recurrent course:* Repeated episodes sometime occur, separated by periods of inactivity of >3 months

    Whenever we encounter a patient with non-granulomatous AU with these characteristics, it is important to request an HLA-B27 to identify the most probable diagnosis and guide treatment.[4]
  - *Presence of a prodromal period:* Another characteristic of HLA-B27-positive patients is the prodromal period of ocular discomfort different from photophobia or foreign body sensation, indicating that the patient will soon have a uveitis flare. However, at the time of the slit-lamp examination, no signs of inflammation are observed in the prodromal phase. Some studies with experimental uveitis models in mice have observed that, before the clinical signs of uveitis, there is cellular migration to the iris and vasculature that increase over time until the clinical signs appear after 3 days.[37] This cellular migration could explain these prodromal symptoms in patients with non-granulomatous AU **(Fig. 5)**.

    Experimental studies of uveitis in mouse models have demonstrated cellular migration in the vasculature and iris following the injection of green fluorescent protein (GFP) + R14-spec pathogen into the anterior chamber, which only becomes clinically evident on the third day post injection.[37]

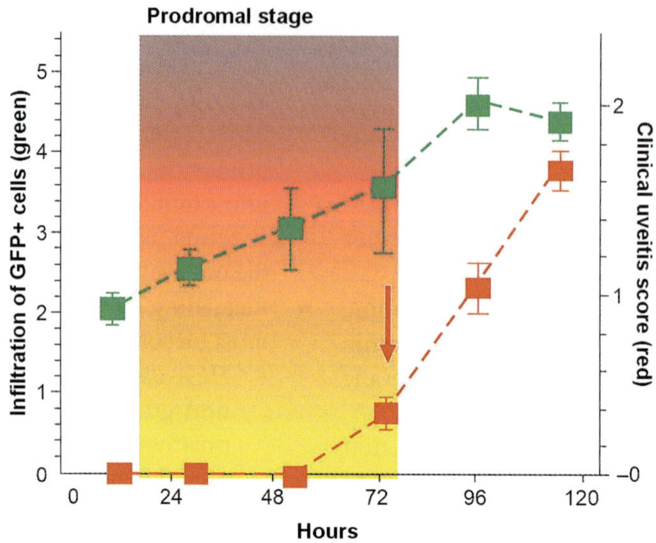

Fig. 5: Cellular migration before clinical signs of uveitis. (GFP: green fluorescent protein)
Source: Uveitis Webinar - Grand Round 1. International Uveitis Study Group (IUSG). 2025. https://youtu.be/zjP2f03Lqms?si=IoNshiovs2Ew2tuJ.

- *Laterality of relapses:* Although the literature describes alternating characteristics, this does not occur in every patient. Generally, the eye that flares first will develop more subsequent attacks.[4]
- *Associated systemic diseases:* The typical presentation of non-granulomatous AU (sudden onset, limited duration, and single recurrent course) occurs in 50% of patients with HLA-B27+ and ankylosing spondylitis.[21] The presence of other systemic diseases, such as inflammatory bowel disease, reactive arthritis, and psoriasis, alters the clinical picture, with these characteristics manifesting in only 15–30% of cases. The latter set of systemic diseases more often have bilateral involvement, chronicity of AU, and more frequent complications in the posterior segment. Intermediate uveitis or retinal vasculitis can occur in a number of cases, even when it may appear to be isolated non-granulomatous AU. A careful examination, along with ancillary imaging studies, should be done to rule out posterior segment inflammation (anterior + intermediate uveitis or panuveitis).[4]

ANTERIOR UVEITIS WITH ELEVATED IOP

Case Presentation

Personal Data

- Male, 57 years old
- Long-standing glaucoma in the right eye (OD)
- Bimatoprost eye drop (one drop/daily) and dexamethasone (three drops/daily) (OD)

History of Present Illness

The patient was referred for a mild anterior chamber reaction in the right eye with the presence of long-standing glaucoma; there were no other complaints.

Physical Examination

The patient presented with a visual acuity of 20/40 in OD and 20/25 in OS, high IOP in OD, no anterior chamber cells but with small keratic precipitates, mild corneal edema, and a cup–disc ratio of 0.95 in OD **(Table 3 and Fig. 6)**.

Ancillary Test

Optic nerve optical coherence tomography (OCT) documented a marked decrease in the right eye's temporal retinal nerve fiber layer thickness, which corresponded to a nasal scotoma in the right eye on visual field testing **(Fig. 7)**.

Differential Diagnosis

Anterior chamber tap: Antibody index testing, also known as the Goldmann-Whitmer Coefficient, for CMV was positive **(Fig. 8)**. Intraocular antibody index is a diagnostic test to confirm intraocular production of antibodies for a specific microorganism, allowing for a more targeted and effective treatment. A value >3 indicates a positive result.

TABLE 3: Physical examination of a patient having anterior uveitis with elevated IOP.

OD	***Parameter***	***OS***
20/40	BCVA	20/25
32 mm Hg	IOP	15 mm Hg
Quiet	Conjunctiva	Quiet
Small, non-pigmented keratic precipitates with mild corneal edema	Cornea	Clear
• No hypopyon • ACC: 0+ • Wide open angle	Anterior chamber	• No hypopyon • ACC: 0+C • Wide open angle
Unremarkable	Iris	Unremarkable
Clear	Lens	Clear
Unremarkable	Vitreous	Unremarkable
Optic nerve head with a sharp margin, pale, CDR 0.95, macula with pigment change, and retina attached	Fundus	Optic nerve head with a sharp margin, normal CDR, macula with pigment change, and retina attached

(ACC: anterior chamber cellularity; BCVA: best-corrected visual acuity; CDR: cup–disc ratio; IOP: intraocular pressure)
Source: Uveitis Webinar - Grand Round 1. International Uveitis Study Group (IUSG). 2025. https://youtu.be/zjP2f03Lqms?si=loNshiovs2Ew2tuJ.

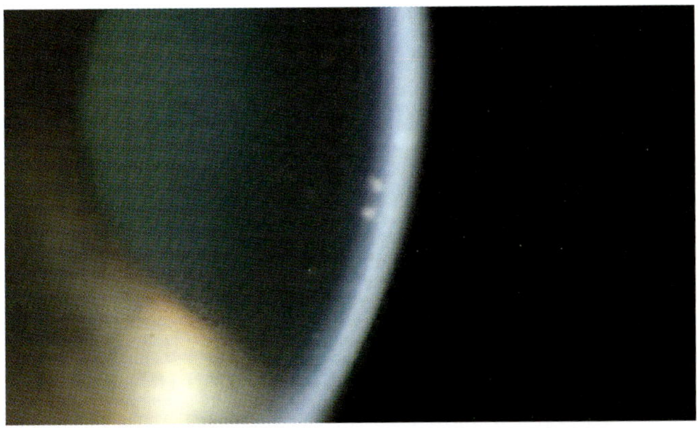

Fig. 6: Small, non-pigmented keratic, coin-shaped precipitates are seen on the corneal enothelium of the right eye. Mild corneal edema is also noted.
Source: Uveitis Webinar - Grand Round 1. International Uveitis Study Group (IUSG). 2025. https://youtu.be/zjP2f03Lqms?si=loNshiovs2Ew2tuJ.[4]

Final diagnosis: Posner–Schlossman syndrome due to CMV (CMV hypertensive anterior uveitis).

Treatment

- Valganciclovir 900 mg twice a day for 2 weeks then 450 mg twice a day thereafter
- Dexamethasone eye drops 1x daily
- Bimatoprost/timolol eye drops 1x daily
- Brinzolamide/brimonidine eye drops 2x daily

Course

One year after valganciclovir therapy, an elevated IOP reoccurred, requiring combined cataract surgery with trabeculectomy. After several months, a new inflammatory episode occurred with the IOP exceeding 20 mm Hg. The patient underwent a cyclodestructive procedure (cyclophotocoagulation). Since then, the patient has remained stable using preservative-free apraclonidine and dorzolamide eye drops.

Discussion

- Acute, unilateral AU with elevated IOP is generally secondary to an infectious process, with viruses from the Herpesviridae family being the most implicated pathogens. However, ocular tuberculosis or toxoplasmosis should also be considered, as well as autoimmune diseases, such as sarcoidosis.[4,38] Hence, it is important to perform a complete slit lamp and dilated fundus examination, in addition to a review of systemic symptoms.[4,38]
- Among all herpes viruses, those of the alpha family, which are herpes simplex virus types 1 and 2 (HSV-1, HSV-2) and the varicella-zoster virus (VZV), are the most common.[39] Once these viruses cause a primary infection, they persist in the neural ganglia and can reactivate. Other less common viruses are those of the beta family (CMV) and the gamma family [Epstein-Barr

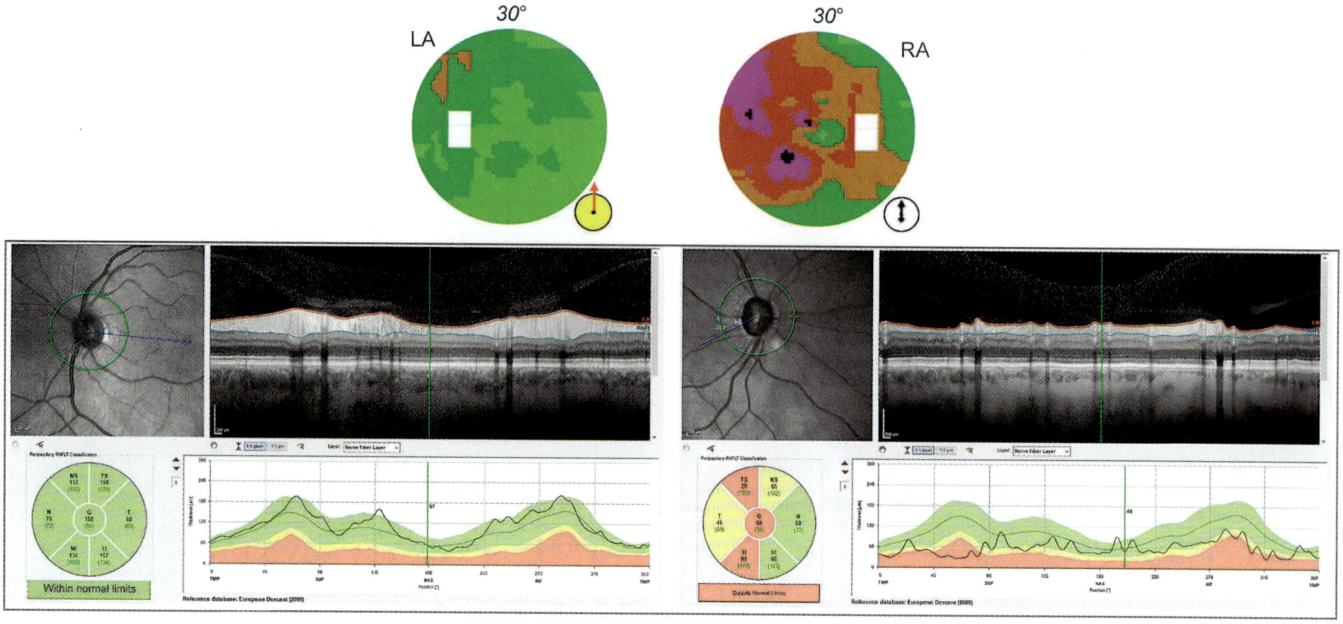

Fig. 7: OCT scans of the optic nerves show a normal nerve fiber layer thickness in the left eye (left, bottom) compared with temporal thinning seen in the right eye (right, bottom). The nerve fiber layer loss in the right eye corresponds to a nasal scotoma on Octopus visual field testing (right, superior) in the setting of high IOPs. The visual field is grossly normal in the left eye (superior, left).. (OCT: optical coherence tomography; IOP: intraocular pressure)
Source: Uveitis Webinar - Grand Round 1. International Uveitis Study Group (IUSG). 2025. https://youtu.be/zjP2f03Lqms?si=loNshiovs2Ew2tuJ.

$$\frac{\text{Titer of antibody in aqueous}}{\text{Titer of antibody in serum}} \times \frac{\text{Concentration of serum globulins}}{\text{Concentration of aqueous globulins}}$$

>3: Diagnostic of intraocular antibody production

Fig. 8: Intraocular antibody index testing protocol, which is also known as the Goldmann-Witmer Coefiicient. Results >3 indicate pathogen-specific antibody production in the aqueous humor.

virus (EBV)].[4,38] In Asia, an increased frequency of AU due to the rubella virus also has been reported, specifically in Fuchs' uveitis syndrome **(Fig. 9)**.[4,38]

- There are clinical characteristics that can help differentiate which virus might be involved. However, definitive viral characterization is only possible through PCR.[4,38] Some of these characteristics are as follows:
  - Diffuse and stellate KPs are characteristic of Fuchs' uveitis syndrome and are often mid-sized.
  - Varicella-zoster virus tends to cause a more severe presentation [greater degree of inflammation, with significant iris atrophy and necrosis, hypopyon, hyphema, synechiae, higher IOP (30–40 mm Hg), and anterior vitreous inflammation]. Additionally, the dermatitis caused by VZV is more extensive and follows the entire dermatome innervated by the ophthalmic branch of the trigeminal nerve (V1).
  - Herpes simplex virus tends to behave very similarly to VZV but with less severity.
  - Cytomegalovirus generates greater damage to the corneal endothelium compared to HSV and VZV, so it is advisable to perform specular or confocal microscopy before glaucoma or cataract surgeries.[40]
  - Varicella-zoster virus, in addition to ocular involvement, causes a post-infectious pain syndrome known as trigeminal neuralgia, which causes severe pain along the entire course of V1. The resulting severe pain is a significant cause of suicide in people over 70 years old.[39]
  - Certain demographic and personal factors can also increase the risk of herpes zoster infection:[42]
    - *Age:* The incidence of VZV is higher in people over 80 years old (10–11 × 1,000 persons) compared to patients aged 20–29 years (1–2 × 1,000 persons).
    - *Immunodeficiencies:* Patients with HIV have a higher incidence of VZV (30–50 × 1,000 persons) than patients with active malignancies (25–40 × 1,000 persons).

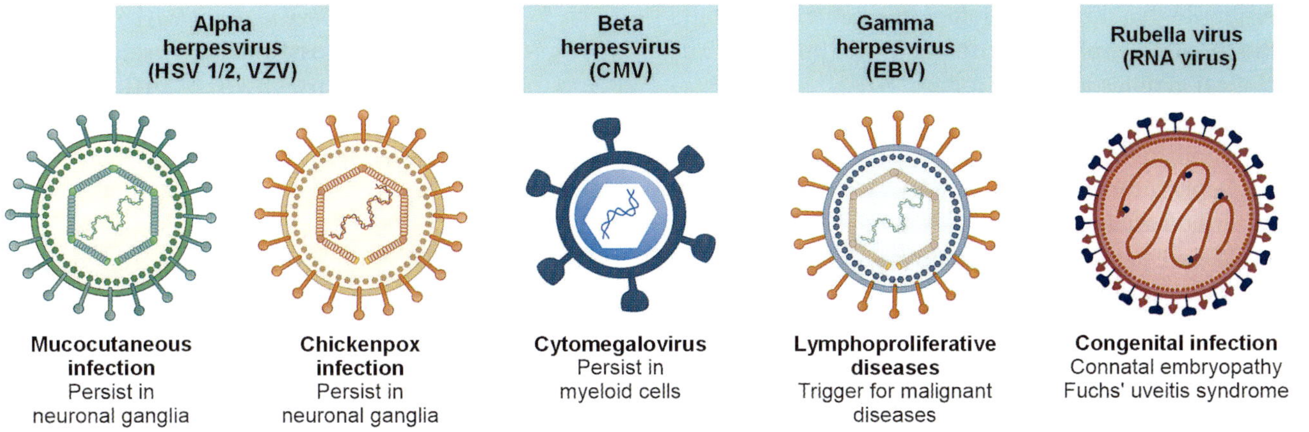

Fig. 9: Viruses associated with acute anterior uveitis with elevated intraocular pressure. (CMV: cytomegalovirus; EBV: Epstein-Barr virus; HSV: herpes simplex virus; VZV: varicella-zoster virus)
Source: Presented by Uwe Pleyer in the uveitis rounds of the International Uveitis Study Group (IUSG);[40] Adapted from Robert Koch Institute.[41]

- Furthermore, the risk of VZV can increase due to immunosuppression secondary to common medications in patients with uveitis, such as disease-modifying anti-rheumatic drugs (incidence of 5.6 × 1,000 persons), TNF inhibitors (incidence of 11.1 × 1,000 persons), and Janus kinase (JAK) inhibitors (15 × 1,000 persons).[4,42] Therefore, patients starting an immunosuppressive agent should be vaccinated against VZV before initiating therapy.[4,42]
- *Fuchs' uveitis syndrome:* In the context of acute, unilateral AU with an elevated IOP, another important differential diagnosis to consider is Fuchs' uveitis syndrome. It is often under diagnosed given a lack of all clinical findings. The initially described heterochromia is only present in one-third of the patients, leading to misclassification as intermediate uveitis or panuveitis. The initial description by Ernst Fuchs in 1906 included:
  - Mild unilateral AU (90%)
  - Bilateral in 10% of cases
  - Fine and disseminated keratic precipitates (80–100%)
  - Heterochromia due to iris atrophy (35%)
  - Absence of synechiae (100%)
  - Vitreous haze without cystoid macular edema (80%)
  - Cataracts (20–50%)
  - Ocular hypertension (20–50%)
- In 2021, the SUN Working Group updated the diagnostic criteria for Fuchs' uveitis syndrome **(Fig. 10)**. However, these criteria have limitations as they exclude the 10% of patients with a bilateral presentation and do not associate the syndrome with any specific etiological agent. In a case-control study of 63 patients with Fuchs' uveitis syndrome, up to 100% of cases had an intraocular antibody index for rubella virus; conversely, none of the controls were positive.[43] Therefore, performing an intraocular antibody index to assess for rubella virus is valuable whenever possible in these patients.[4]

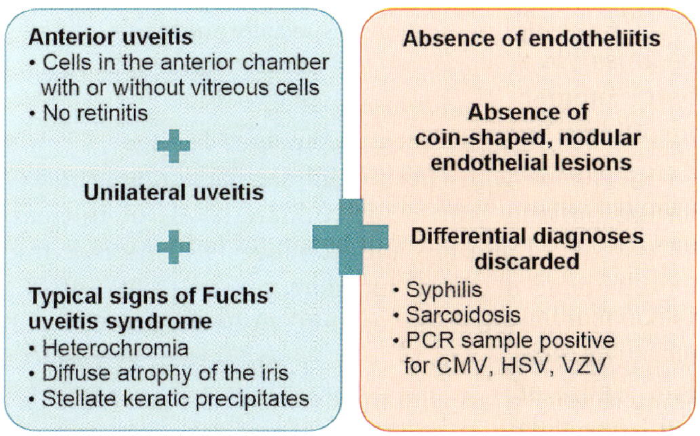

Fig. 10: SUN criteria for Fuchs' uveitis syndrome published in 2021.[44]
(CMV: cytomegalovirus; HSV: herpes simplex virus; PCR: polymerase chain reaction; SUN: Standardization of Uveitis Nomenclature; VZV: varicella-zoster virus)
Source: Presented at the International Uveitis Study Group (IUSG) uveitis rounds by Uwe Pleyer;[4] Adapted from the Standardization of Uveitis Nomenclature (SUN) Working Group.[44]

- *Posner–Schlossman syndrome:*[45,46] This syndrome was first described in 1948 as a glaucomatocyclitic crisis. It is proposed that the main etiological mechanism behind the disease is trabeculitis due to a viral infection. The clinical manifestations include:

- Recurrent episodes of AU, mostly unilateral, with significantly increased IOP
- Open anterior chamber angle
- Endothelial precipitates
- Diffuse to sectoral iris atrophy
- No posterior synechiae
- Mild anterior chamber reaction
- Ranges from asymptomatic to causing severe pain
- An average duration of 2 weeks duration
- Attacks occur spontaneously
- *Etiology:* CMV in the Western world and rubella in Asia.

It must be clear that this syndrome is not a benign entity, as often described in the literature. On the contrary, due to its high risk of recurrence and progression, it poses a high risk of complications, especially among:[47,48]

- Elderly patients
- Immunocompromised patients
- Patients with prior glaucomatous damage
- Patients with a positive intraocular antibody index

For patients with acute, unilateral AU of unclear etiology, there are additional tests to narrow the differential diagnosis, including:

- Polymerase chain reaction (70–80% sensitivity and specificity >95%)
- Intraocular antibody index
- Corneal sample if keratitis is present. The sample is obtained by gently scraping the corneal surface with a swab or small spatula to collect cells and infectious material for laboratory analysis.

Serologic testing for the herpes viruses is less useful given the high percentage of seropositivity in most populations. However, a negative result is useful for ruling out other diagnoses. Additionally, while a negative PCR result largely rules out CMV AU, the diagnosis should be reconsidered if the clinical course increases the post-test probability of the diagnosis.[43,49]

Recently, the role of OCT-angiography (OCT-A) in the early detection of glaucomatous damage in patients with AU and elevated IOP has been highlighted, as well as evidence that the use of valganciclovir has positive effects on the retinal vascular density.[50]

- A three pronged approach should be taken in the treatment of patients with AU and elevated IOP:[4]

1. *Inflammation control with topical corticosteroids:*
   a. Topical corticosteroids are useful to reduce trabecular meshwork inflammation, consequently lowering IOP.
   b. Prednisolone acetate 1%, not dexamethasone or fluorometholone, must be used given the better anterior chamber penetration.
   c. Corticosteroids should be used sparingly.
   d. No risk of IOP elevation and cataract formation has been observed with dosing of one drop per day or less.[23]
2. *IOP control*: Topical therapy with/without oral therapy should be the first-line treatment, and in refractory cases, glaucoma surgery.
3. *Antiviral therapy:*
   a. *HSV I-II:* Acyclovir 400 mg orally five times daily for 2 weeks and then 400 mg two to three times daily.
   b. *Varicella-zoster virus:* Acyclovir 800 mg orally five times daily for 2 weeks and then 400 mg two to three times daily.
      i. In case of acyclovir resistance, valacyclovir 1 g three times a day and then 500 mg twice a day.
   c. *Cytomegalovirus:* Valganciclovir 900 mg orally twice a day for two weeks and then 450 mg twice a day. Topical valganciclovir gel is used three to five times daily when available (see questions and answers at the end of the chapter).

GRANULOMATOUS ANTERIOR UVEITIS

Case Presentation

Personal Data

- Female, 42 years old
- Urinary tract infection 1-month ago that resolved after treatment with an antibiotic by her general physician.
- She then developed hypopigmented skin lesions treated with an unknown ointment prescribed by her doctor.
- Serologic testing showed a blood count with leukocytosis (18,000 cells/mm^3) and an elevated erythrocyte sedimentation rate (62 mm/h).
- The rest of the laboratory results were normal (Manatoux test, syphilis, and HIV serologies).

History of Present Illness

Left eye pain of insidious onset and gradually progressive eye redness for 1 month.

Physical Examination

The patient presented with a BCVA of 20/20 in the OD and 20/30 in the OS. The slit-lamp examination in the OD was unremarkable. However, the OS showed granulomatous KPs and anterior chamber cells 1+ with iris atrophy and vitreous cells. Fundoscopy was normal at baseline. However, during follow-up, the patient developed 2+ vitreous haze **(Table 4 and Fig. 11)**.

Differential Diagnosis

Two differential diagnoses were considered: (1) Viral AU versus (2) drug-induced uveitis secondary to fluoroquinolone use **(Table 5)**.

Another probable diagnosis was Vogt–Koyanagi–Harada (VKH) syndrome due to hypopigmented skin lesions. However, the patient did not present with other signs suggestive of VKH, such as prodromal symptoms

TABLE 4: Physical examination of patient having granulomatous anterior uveitis.

OD	*Parameter*	*OS*
20/20	BCVA	20/30
12 mm Hg	IOP	38 mm Hg
Quiet	Conjunctiva	Moderate-to-severe hyperemia
Unremarkable	Cornea	Granulomatous keratic precipitates
• No hypopyon • ACC: 0+ • Wide open angle	Anterior chamber	• No hypopyon • ACC: 1+ • Gonioscopy with peripheral anterior synechiae in the inferior quadrant, the rest of the angle was open
Unremarkable	Iris	Iris atrophy
Clear	Lens	Clear
Unremarkable	Vitreous	Unremarkable
Unremarkable	Fundus	Unremarkable

(ACC: anterior chamber cellularity; BCVA: best-corrected visual acuity; IOP: intraocular pressure)
Source: Uveitis Webinar - Grand Round 1. International Uveitis Study Group (IUSG). 2025. https://youtu.be/zjP2f03Lqms?si=IoNshiovs2Ew2tuJ.

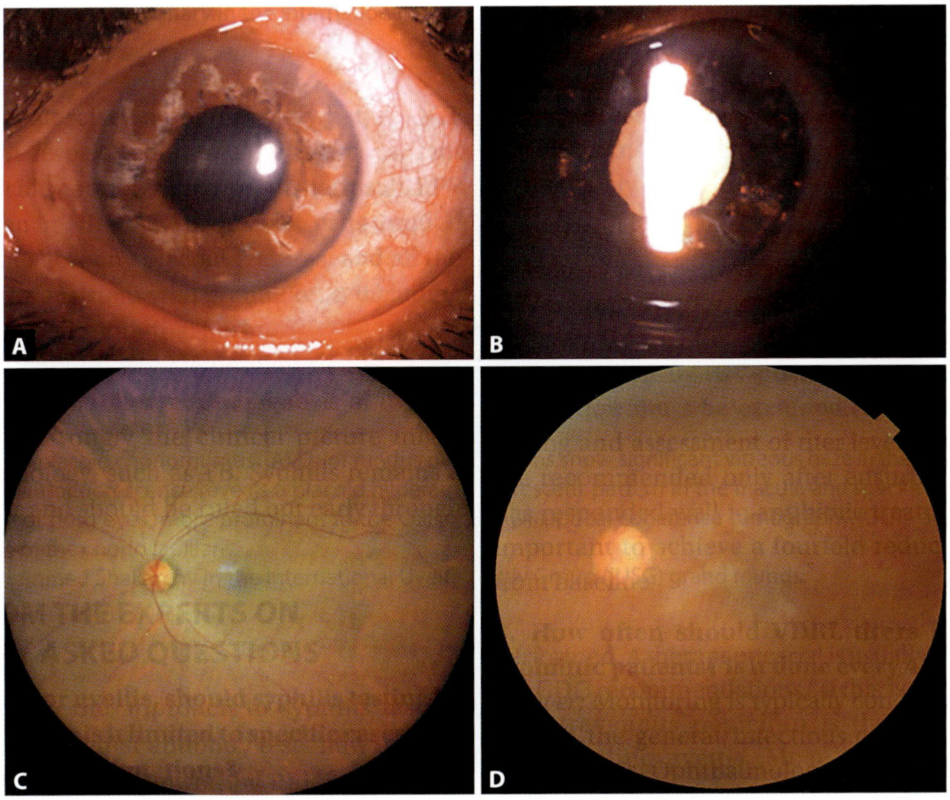

Figs. 11A to D: Anterior segment photographs and fundoscopy at baseline and during follow-up. Left eye with (A) moderate-to-severe hyperemia and iris atrophy. (B) Transillumination defects and (C) normal fundus (before the onset of uveitis), later followed by (D) glaucomatous damage and 2+ vitreous haze.
Source: Uveitis Webinar - Grand Round 1. International Uveitis Study Group (IUSG). 2025. https://youtu.be/zjP2f03Lqms?si=IoNshiovs2Ew2tuJ.

TABLE 5: Differential diagnosis of granulomatous anterior uveitis case.

Viral anterior uveitis	***Drug-induced uveitis (fluoroquinolone-induced)***
In favor	*In favor*
Unilateral	History of intake of oral antibiotic intake for UTI treatment 1 month before symptoms
Elevated IOP	History of skin lesions following antibiotic usage
Endothelial-pigmented granulomatous KPs	Pigment dispersion
Iris atrophy with transillumination defects	Iris atrophy with transillumination defects including anterior lamellar atrophy
	Posterior and peripheral anterior synechiae
Against	*Against*
No history of blistering skin rash over the forehead	Unilateral
No history or evidence of keratitis	Inflammation persisted despite stopping the antibiotic

(IOP: intraocular pressure; KPs: keratic precipitates; UTI: urinary tract infection)
Source: Uveitis Webinar - Grand Round 1. International Uveitis Study Group (IUSG). 2025. https://youtu.be/zjP2f03Lqms?si=IoNshiovs2Ew2tuJ.

of meningismus or bilateral serous retinal detachments. Additionally, symptoms and signs persisted after fluoroquinolone discontinuation. Therefore, viral AU was considered more likely.

Treatment

- Valacyclovir 1,000 mg orally three times a day for 15 days
- Dexamethasone eye drops four times a day for 7 days in the left eye with weekly decrements
- Dorzolamide + Timolol eye drops twice daily in the left eye
- Acetazolamide 250 mg orally twice a day for 3 days

Course

During the next year, the patient experienced recurrent episodes of AU despite medical management. Due to financial constraints, the patient did not maintain her required treatment with oral valacyclovir, and the visual acuity in the left eye dropped from 20/30 to 20/80. Additionally, the patient developed a posterior subcapsular cataract and optic nerve damage (cup-disc ratio of 0.8 with bayonetting of vessels and thinning of the neuroretinal rim). The aqueous chamber tap in the left eye was negative for HSV, VZV, and CMV. A laser peripheral iridotomy was performed due to a partial pupillary block.

Despite the negative result of the aqueous chamber tap and given the recurrence of uveitis after discontinuation of the fluoroquinolone with elevation of the IOP, valacyclovir was started again. After controlling the inflammation, the patient underwent trabeculectomy and phacoemulsification with placement of a posterior chamber intraocular lens (PCIOL) to control the IOP.

Final Diagnosis

Idiopathic granulomatous anterior uveitis (viral suspected).

Discussion

- This case is intriguing because, not all acute, unilateral AU cases with elevated IOP are viral. Perhaps with metagenomic studies, more viruses associated with the development of uveitis can be identified. However, many cases remain idiopathic. Granulomatous AU tends to be very severe and has multiple etiologies. Nevertheless, four main etiologies should be remembered **(Figs. 12A to H)**:[4]
  1. *Tuberculosis:* Typically, it presents with granulomas in the anterior chamber and high peripheral anterior synechiae, sometimes with a hypopyon. Systemically, the patient may have pulmonary involvement in a small number of cases, which is not necessary to make the diagnosis. It is usually bilateral. Tuberculosis testing will be positive (10 × 10 mm or larger induration for the Mantoux test in immunocompetent patients or a positive Quantiferon gamma release assay).[4] An online calculator helping aid treatment decisions for ocular tuberculosis is available.[51]
  2. *Sarcoidosis:* Also presents with granulomas associated with predominantly hilar lymphadenopathy.[4]
  3. *Mycotic:* Commonly occurs after plant-related traumas, especially among people working in agriculture and diabetic patients. There are many species that vary by geographic area, with *Cladosporium* being particularly dominant in India. Viral coinfection is commonly found in aspirates from these eyes.[4]

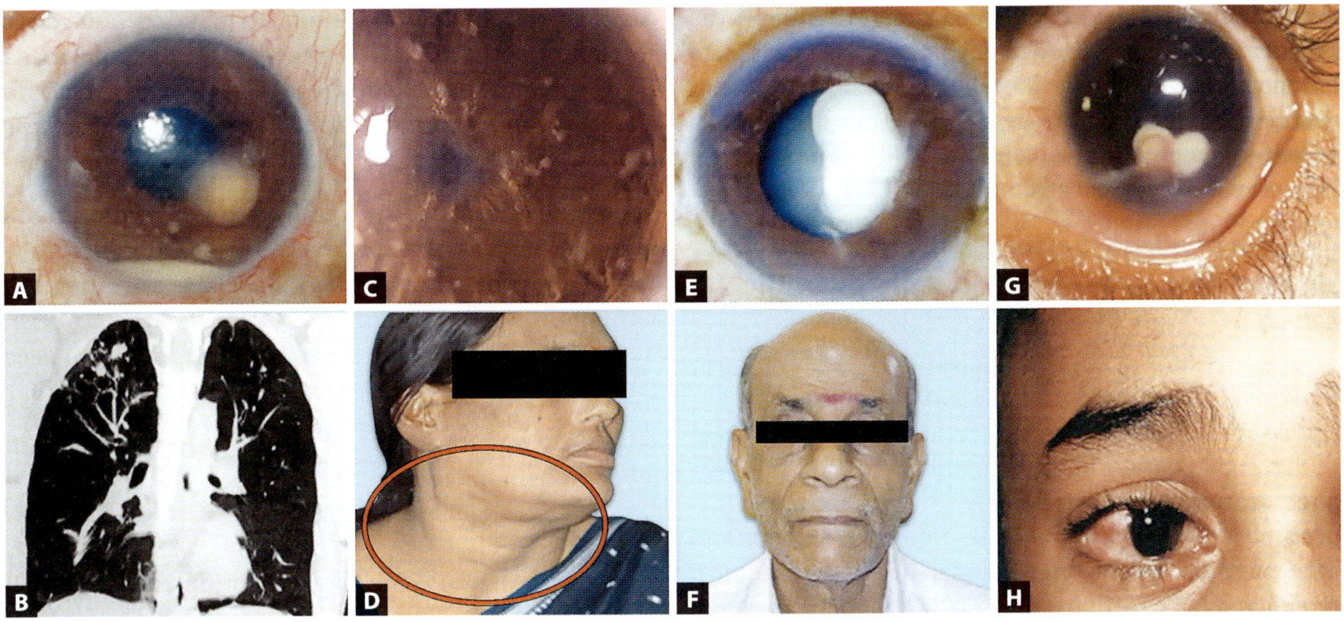

Figs. 12A to H: Common causes of granulomatous anterior uveitis: (A) A slit lamp photograph showing anterior, granulomatous uveitis secondary to ocular tuberculosis with grade 1 hypopyon; (B) Pulmonary nodules secondary to sarcoidosis, as seen in a coronal chest CT image; the patient additionally presented with (C) iris nodules and 360 degrees of synechiae and (D) bilateral neck lymphadenopathy; (E) Granuloma formation in the anterior chamber due to *Cladosporium* with (F) an infection of the skin above the nasal bridge; (G) Anterior chamber granuloma formation with (H) the presence of a conjunctival granuloma secondary to trematode infection.
Source: Uveitis Webinar - Grand Round 1. International Uveitis Study Group (IUSG). 2025. https://youtu.be/zjP2f03Lqms?si=IoNshiovs2Ew2tuJ.

4. *Parasitic:* In a region of southern India, several cases of granulomatous AU with a solitary granuloma in the conjunctiva have been reported. Rathinam et al., reported through field research that cases were associated with bathing in local ponds. After culturing 40 samples, three tested positive for trematode particles. Subsequently, larvae from the river water were collected. DNA found in the larvae matched the particles in the conjunctival samples confirming trematode infection as the cause of the granulomas. These patients were initially treated with antituberculous therapy with partial improvement; however, aspiration for those with larger granulomas showed improved patient outcomes.[52,53] As with this example, there are multiple microorganisms that can cause granulomatous inflammation, including schistosomiasis in Africa and in parts of the Americas. Recently, trematode infections have also been identified in other regions such as Brazil, Egypt, Madagascar, and various Asian islands. This makes it an important diagnosis to consider in patients with granulomatous AU with conjunctival granulomas without evident *Mycobacterium tuberculosis* infection.[52,53]

- Other causes of granulomatous uveitis include VKH disease, sympathetic ophthalmia, syphilis, toxoplasmosis, bacterial infections, neoplasms, drug reactions, ocular trauma, or it can even be idiopathic.

PEARLS FROM THE EXPERTS ON FREQUENTLY ASKED QUESTIONS

Non-granulomatous Anterior Uveitis

1. Are there known triggering factors for HLA-B27 uveitis attacks?

Answer: No specific triggering factors have been identified. An increase in anterior acute uveitis relapses in early spring has been noted, but the role of seasonality remains unclear. Other factors, such as pregnancy, have been associated with a reduced number of relapses.[54]

2. Does trauma play a role in relapses of recurrent anterior uveitis?

Answer: It is possible, but such occurrences are rare.

3. Is tropicamide suitable for patients who cannot tolerate the blurred vision caused by atropine?

Answer: Yes, it is an acceptable mydriatic agent; however, it requires a more frequent dosing of three times per day.

4. Regarding the use of topical NSAIDs for reducing the recurrence rates in HLA-B27 AU, what is the efficacy compared to other treatments?

Answer: Topical NSAIDs are generally not used due to limited efficacy and potential harm to the ocular surface. When suppressive dosing is required, topical or oral corticosteroids are preferred. As mentioned previously, non-corticosteroid immunosuppressive agents are another alternative in patients requiring longterm, non-corticosteroid suppressive dosing.

5. Is it advisable to perform fluorescein angiography in patients with AU and cystoid macular edema?

Answer: Fluorescein angiography is of little to no indication in this context. Cystoid macular edema is not a frequent complication in patients with AU, but it can occur. It is generally better to thoroughly examine the patient and reassess the primary site of inflammation.[21] It is important to remember that complications do not change the diagnosis of AU if the primary site of inflammation is the anterior chamber. OCT assesses anatomic structures (thickening of the macula or the presence of cysts), whereas fluorescein angiography assesses retinal vasculature physiology (detecting leakage). Treatment is needed in cases where leakage produces anatomical thickening.[55]

Anterior Uveitis with Elevated Intraocular Pressure

1. What are the indications to perform a diagnostic paracentesis in suspected viral AU cases?

Answer: All cases with clinical features indicative of viral AU warrant paracentesis, if possible.

2. Is ganciclovir ointment recommended for CMV AU?

Answer: In Asia, a 2% valganciclovir ointment effectively treats AU caused by CMV. However, the maximum concentration available in the Western world is 1.5%. Therefore, oral treatment with valganciclovir 900 mg BID for 2 weeks, followed by 450 mg BID orally twice daily for at least 2 weeks, is always preferred. Longer-term treatment is often necessary to avoid recurrences. Costs and adverse effects need to be considered.

Topical treatment could be especially useful in patients whose viral load was very low on quantitative PCR, but again the ointment is not widely available.

3. Is the combination of topical and systemic carbonic anhydrase inhibitors recommended in hypertensive AU cases?

Answer: This combination can be used, but always combine IOP lowering medications with antiviral treatment.

4. In cases of viral AU resembling CMV with negative PCR results, is the administration of valganciclovir recommended despite the negative results?

Answer: The decision should be based on the individual case.

5. Is the use of a prostaglandin analog contraindicated due to the fact that it might increase inflammation?

Answer: Its use is not an absolute contraindication in patients with AU with an elevated IOP. Prostaglandin analogs are potent topical medications for lowering raised IOP in patients with uveitis and are not associated with an increased risk of cystoid macular edema or AU.[56] However, it should be used with caution in cases of viral uveitis, as reactivation has been reported. Thus, it can be used but is not first-line.[57]

6. In CMV AU, are corticosteroids initiated before PCR results or is treatment limited to ganciclovir?

Answer: Treatment approaches vary. Topical steroids are often started even before the diagnosis of CMV AU with ganciclovir added upon confirmation with PCR testing.

7. What is the recommended duration for antiviral treatment in patients with Posner–Schlossman syndrome?

Answer: The duration of treatment should be tailored to the individual case. It is recommended for at least 6 months. Some literature suggests continuing for 2 years; however, this can be very costly and not always feasible. Additionally, the risk of adverse effects, such as leukopenia, increases over time, so one aims to maintain the valganciclovir treatment if it is beneficial and safe.

8. Is there a recommendation for more sensitive and specific detection of a microorganism in uveitis cases?

Answer: Combining the use of PCR with the Goldmann–Witmer coefficient allows for the detection of more cases than using either of these methods alone. PCR can detect DNA days before antibodies are formed, whereas the Goldmann–Witmer coefficient tends to be positive when PCR is negative due to infection control through antibody formation. This combination approach is valid for both viral infections and infections caused by toxoplasmosis or tuberculosis.

9. Is there a risk that patients with a history of viral AU may subsequently develop acute retinal necrosis?

Answer: While it is not the most frequent occurrence, there are cases of patients with a history of AU who end up with the more severe presentation of retinal necrosis. This can be explained by the fact that herpetic viruses remain dormant in the body and can reactivate under certain specific circumstances such as stress, immunosuppression, or with increasing age and its associated state of immunosuppression or cellular quiescence.

10. Does a negative PCR result completely rule out an infection?

Answer: No, a positive PCR result confirms the diagnosis, but a negative result does not entirely rule out the infection. If clinical indications suggest an infectious etiology, empirical treatment should be administered and the patient's response should be observed.

11. How frequently is monitoring renal function in patients undergoing anti-CMV treatment recommended?

Answer: It is important to conduct an initial assessment to determine if medication dose adjustment is necessary. The first test should be ordered between 4 and 6 weeks after initiation and repeated every 2–3 months. Additionally, it is important to remember that leukopenia is a more common side effect than renal damage, so it is crucial to request both renal function tests and a complete blood count.

Granulomatous Anterior Uveitis

1. In the case of the patient with leukocytosis and an elevated erythrocyte sedimentation rate, would you still consider herpes viral infection as a cause?

Answer: In this particular case, leukocytosis may be attributed to urinary tract infection. However, for situations without any evident factor associated with leukocytosis, it may be prudent to repeat the PCR from the anterior chamber, especially since CMV and rubella can sometimes yield false negatives.

2. What tests are typically conducted for Lyme disease?

Answer: The Centers for Disease Control and Prevention (CDC) testing algorithm for Lyme disease involves an initial enzyme-linked immunosorbent assay (ELISA) test followed by a confirmatory Western blot, regardless of whether the area where the patient lives is endemic or non-endemic. In non-endemic areas, greater emphasis is placed on confirming positive ELISA results with a Western blot due to the higher risk of false positives when pre-test probability is low.

3. For parasitic uveitis, is there any effective systemic treatment available?

Answer: There is no systemic parasitic treatment for this condition because, it typically involves a dead parasite or larva in the anterior chamber. Therefore, the best option is surgical removal.

FINAL WRAP-UP

In Conclusion

- *In non-granulomatous AU*, patients often experience a prodrome, even when cells may not be visible on the slit-lamp examination. Advise the patients to have their topical corticosteroid accessible for immediate use at the onset of prodromal symptoms. Additionally, HLA-B27 testing can be a useful tool in narrowing the differential diagnosis. However, HLA-B27 results should not delay diagnosis or treatment, as the management approach is very similar regardless of the result. Topical treatments are the cornerstone of therapy, with immunosuppression being added only when necessary. It is also important to evaluate the entire eye, including the posterior segment, as the presence of posterior involvement affects the decision whether to administer systemic immunosuppression or biologic therapy.
- *In AU with elevated IOP*, a viral infection should be the primary diagnostic suspicion, but not the only one. PCR and the Goldmann–Witmer coefficient are recommended tests to confirm the diagnosis. Nevertheless, empiric treatment should be initiated immediately if these tests are unavailable. Repeating an aqueous tap to evaluate the response to treatment is not recommended. Clinical resolution of inflammation should be considered an indicator of a positive response. Currently, there is no definitive evidence to guide the duration of treatment to prevent recurrences; treatment duration could vary from 6 months to 2 years. The approach should be to advocate for the longest possible duration that does not pose risks or cause adverse effects. Additionally, topical valganciclovir is not widely used, but it has shown promising results for CMV AU.
- *In granulomatous AU,* tuberculosis and sarcoidosis are the most common diagnoses. However, it is crucial to also rule out fungal and parasitic infections, as the causative microorganism can vary depending on the geographical region. Additionally, less frequent cases, such as drug-induced uveitis, can present as granulomatous uveitis.

REFERENCES

1. Päivönsalo-Hietanen T, Vaahtoranta-Lehtonen H, Tuominen J, Saari KM. Uveitis survey at the University Eye Clinic in Turku. Acta Ophthalmologica. 1994;72(4):505-12.
2. Rothova A, Buitenhuis HJ, Meenken C, Brinkman CJ, Linssen A, Alberts C, et al. Uveitis and systemic disease. Br J Ophthalmol. 1992;76(3):137-41.
3. Rodriguez A, Calonge M, Pedroza-Seres M, Akova YA, Messmer EM, D'Amico DJ. Referral patterns of uveitis in a tertiary eye care center. Arch Ophthalmol. 1996;114(5):593-9.
4. Uveitis Webinar - Grand Round 1. International Uveitis Study Group (IUSG). 2024. https://www.youtube.com/watch?v=zjP2f03Lqms&t=22s.
5. Sobrin L, Pistilli M, Dreger K, Kothari S, Khachatryan N, Artornsombudh P, et al. Factors predictive of remission of chronic anterior uveitis. Ophthalmology. 2020;127(6):826-34.
6. García-Aparicio Á, García De Yébenes MJ, Otón T, Muñoz-Fernández S. Prevalence and incidence of uveitis: a systematic review and meta-analysis. Ophthal Epidemiol. 2021;28(6):461-8.
7. Tsirouki T, Dastiridou A, Symeonidis C, Tounakaki O, Brazitikou I, Kalogeropoulos C, et al. A focus on the epidemiology of uveitis. Ocul Immunol Inflamm. 2018;26(1):2-16.
8. Wakabayashi T, Morimura Y, Miyamoto Y, Okada AA. Changing patterns of intraocular inflammatory disease in Japan. Ocul Immunol Inflamm. 2003;11(4):277-86.
9. Polanía D, Reyes-Guanes J, Rojas-Carabali W, Pardo-Pizza D, Barraquer-Lopez D, Cifuentes-González C, et al. A new look into uveitis in Colombia: changes in distribution patterns and clinical characteristics over the last 25 years. Graefes Arch Clin Exp Ophthalmol. 2023;261(2):561-73.
10. Luca C, Raffaella A, Sylvia M, Valentina M, Fabiana V, Marco C, et al. Changes in patterns of uveitis at a tertiary referral center in Northern Italy: analysis of 990 consecutive cases. Int Ophthalmol. 2018;38(1):133-42.
11. Shirahama S, Kaburaki T, Nakahara H, Tanaka R, Takamoto M, Fujino Y, et al. Epidemiology of uveitis (2013–2015) and changes in the patterns of uveitis (2004–2015) in the central Tokyo area: a retrospective study. BMC Ophthalmol. 2018;18(1):189.
12. De-la-Torre A, López-Castillo CA, Rueda JC, Mantilla RD, Gómez-Marín JE, Anaya J. Clinical patterns of uveitis in two ophthalmology centres in Bogota, Colombia. Clin Exp Ophthalmol. 2009;37(5):458-66.
13. Baharani A, Reddy P. RR. Leptospiral uveitis: case series and review of literature. Ocul Immunol Inflamm. 2024;32(8):1760-8.
14. Chen EJ, Bin Ismail MA, Mi H, Ho SL, Lim WK, Teoh SC, et al. Ocular autoimmune systemic inflammatory infectious study (oasis)—report 1: epidemiology and classification. Ocul Immunol Inflamm. 2018;26(5):732-46.
15. Lin P, Suhler EB, Rosenbaum JT. The future of uveitis treatment. Ophthalmology. 2014;121(1):365-76.
16. De Parisot A, Kodjikian L, Errera MH, Sedira N, Heron E, Pérard L, et al. Randomized controlled trial evaluating a standardized strategy for uveitis etiologic diagnosis (ULISSE). Am J Ophthal. 2017;178:176-85.
17. Sève P, Cacoub P, Bodaghi B, Trad S, Sellam J, Bellocq D, et al. Uveitis: diagnostic work-up. A literature review and recommendations from an expert committee. Autoimmun Rev. 2017;16(12):1254-64.
18. Hwang DK, Hung JH, Chang YC, Chen CL, Chen SN, Cheng CK, et al. Step-wise diagnostic approach for patients with uveitis—experts consensus in Taiwan. J Microbiol Immunol Infect. 2022;55(4):573-80.
19. Whitcup SM, Sen HN. Whitcup and Nussenblatt's Uveitis: Fundamentals and Clinical Practice, 5th edition. London: Elsevier; 2022.
20. Foster CS, Vitale AT. Diagnosis and Treatment of Uveitis, 2nd edition. New Delhi: Jaypee Brothers Medical (P) Pvt. Ltd.; 2013. p 1290.
21. Jabs DA, Nussenblatt RB, Rosenbaum JT. Standardization of uveitis nomenclature for reporting clinical data. Results of the First International Workshop. Am J Ophthalmol. 2005;140(3):509-16.
22. Zierhut M, Pavesio C, Ohno S, Orefice F, Rao NA. Intraocular Inflammation. Berlin, Heidelberg: Springer; 2016.
23. Papaliodis GN, Rosner BA, Dreger KA, Fitzgerald TD, Artornsombudh P, Kothari S, et al. Incidence of and risk factors for cataract in anterior uveitis. Am J Ophthal. 2023;254:221-32.
24. Radwan AE, Arcinue CA, Yang P, Artornsombudh P, Abu Al-Fadl EM, Foster CS. Bromfenac alone or with single intravitreal injection of bevacizumab or triamcinolone acetonide for treatment of uveitic macular edema. Graefes Arch Clin Exp Ophthalmol. 2013;251(7):1801-6.
25. Hariprasad S, Akduman L, Clever JA, Ober M, Recchia FM, Mieler WF. Treatment of cystoid macular edema with the new-generation NSAID nepafenac 0.1%. Clin Ophthalmol.. 2009;3:147-54.
26. Jabs DA, Rosenbaum JT, Foster CS, Holland GN, Jaffe GJ, Louie JS, et al. Guidelines for the use of immunosuppressive drugs in patients with ocular inflammatory disorders: recommendations of an expert panel. Am J Ophthal. 2000;130(4):492-513.
27. Rathinam SR, Gonzales JA, Thundikandy R, Kanakath A, Murugan SB, Vedhanayaki R, et al. Effect of corticosteroid-sparing treatment with mycophenolate mofetil vs. methotrexate on inflammation in patients with uveitis: a randomized clinical trial. JAMA. 2019;322(10):936-45.
28. Al-khersan H, Fowler BJ, Clauss KD, Kunkler AL, Yannuzzi NA, Patel NA, et al. Cost-utility analysis of mycophenolate

mofetil versus methotrexate for noninfectious uveitis. Ophthalmol Retina. 2021;5(12):1281-2.
29. Eurelings LEM, Missotten TOAR, van Velthoven MEJ, van Daele PLA, van Laar JAM, van Hagen PM, et al. Long-term follow-up of patients with uveitis treated with adalimumab: response rates and reasons for discontinuation of therapy. Am J Ophthal. 2022;240:194-204.
30. Ramanan AV, Dick AD, Jones AP, McKay A, Williamson PR, Compeyrot-Lacassagne S, et al. Adalimumab plus methotrexate for uveitis in juvenile idiopathic arthritis. N Engl J Med. 2017;376(17):1637-46.
31. Rodriguez A, Power WJ, Neves RA, Foster CS. Recurrence rate of herpetic uveitis in patients on long-term oral acyclovir. Doc Ophthalmol. 1995;90(4):331-40.
32. Wong VW, Chan CK, Leung DY, Lai TY. Long-term results of oral valganciclovir for treatment of anterior segment inflammation secondary to cytomegalovirus infection. Clin Ophthalmol. 2012;6:595-600.
33. Lee EJ, Jang HN, Cho HS, Bae E, Lee TW, Chang SH, et al. The incidence, risk factors, and clinical outcomes of acute kidney injury (staged using the RIFLE classification) associated with intravenous acyclovir administration. Renal Failure. 2018;40(1):687-92.
34. Deodhar A, Gill T, Magrey M. Human leukocyte antigen B27-negative axial spondyloarthritis: what do we know? ACR Open Rheumatol. 2023;5(7):333-44.
35. Zhang S, Wang Y, Peng L, Su J, Zeng X, Li M, et al. Comparison of clinical features in hla-b27 positive and negative patients with axial spondyloarthritis: results from a cohort of 4,131 patients. Front Med. 2020;7:609562.
36. Kempen JH, Altaweel MM, Holbrook JT, Jabs DA, Louis TA, Sugar EA, et al. Randomized comparison of systemic anti-inflammatory therapy versus fluocinolone acetonide implant for intermediate, posterior, and panuveitis: the multicenter uveitis steroid treatment trial. Ophthalmology. 2011;118(10):1916-26.
37. Thurau SR, Mempel TR, Flügel A, Diedrichs-Möhring M, Krombach F, Kawakami N, et al. The fate of autoreactive, GFP+ T cells in rat models of uveitis analyzed by intravital fluorescence microscopy and FACS. Int Immunol. 2004;16(11):1573-82.
38. Ahmad F, Deshmukh N, Webel A, Johnson S, Suleiman A, Mohan RR, et al. Viral infections and pathogenesis of glaucoma: a comprehensive review. Clin Microbiol Rev. 2023;36(4):e00057-23.
39. Yawn BP, Lindsay AC, Yousefi M, Wang C. Risk of, and risk factors for, vasculopathy associated with acute herpes zoster. J Stroke Cerebrovasc Dis. 2023;32(2):106891.
40. Thng ZX, Putera I, Testi I, Chan K, Westcott M, Chee SP, et al. The infectious uveitis treatment algorithm network (titan) report 1—global current practice patterns for the management of herpes simplex virus and varicella zoster virus anterior uveitis. Eye. 2024;38(1):61-7.
41. Robert Koch Institut. (2018). Public Health—Health for all. [online] Available from https://www.rki.de/EN/Home/home_node.html. [Last accessed February, 2025].
42. Kim BS, Maverakis E, Alexanian C, Wang JZ, Raychaudhuri SP. Incidence, clinical features, management, and prevention of herpes zoster in patients receiving antitumor necrosis factor therapy: a clinical review. J Cutan Med Surg. 2020;24(3):278-84.
43. Ruokonen PC, Metzner S, Ücer A, Torun N, Hofmann J, Pleyer U. Intraocular antibody synthesis against rubella virus and other microorganisms in Fuchs' heterochromic cyclitis. Graefes Arch Clin Exp Ophthalmol. 2010;248(4):565-71.
44. Standardization of Uveitis Nomenclature (SUN) Working Group. Classification criteria for fuchs uveitis syndrome. Am J Ophthal. 2021;228:262-7.
45. Posner A, Schlossman A. Syndrome of unilateral recurrent attacks of glaucoma with cyclitic symptoms. Arch Ophthal. 1948;39(4):517-35.
46. van Boxtel LAA, van Der Lelij A, van Der Meer J, Los LI. Cytomegalovirus as a cause of anterior uveitis in immunocompetent patients. Ophthalmology. 2007;114(7):1358-62.
47. Lenglinger M, Schick T, Pohlmann D, Pleyer U. Cytomegalovirus-positive Posner-Schlossman syndrome: impact on corneal endothelial cell loss and retinal nerve fiber layer thinning. Am J Ophthal. 2022;237:290-8.
48. Joseph DM, Lim LL, Samalia PD, Wells JM, McCluskey PJ, Paul E, et al. Long-term outcome and prognostic indicators in Posner-Schlossman syndrome. Clin Exp Ophthalmol. 2023;51(8):781-9.
49. Pohlmann D, Schlickeiser S, Metzner S, Lenglinger M, Winterhalter S, Pleyer U. Different composition of intraocular immune mediators in Posner-Schlossman-Syndrome and Fuchs' uveitis. PLoS ONE. 2018;13(6):e0199301.
50. Hülse P, Reitemeyer E, Rübsam A, Pleyer U, Maier AKB. Cytomegalovirus-positive Posner-Schlossman syndrome: to compare differences in retinal vessel area density between the affected and non-affected eye using optical coherence tomography angiography. Graefes Arch Clin Exp Ophthalmol. 2023;261(11):3263-74.
51. Agrawal R, Ludi Z, Betzler BK, Testi I, Mahajan S, Rousellot A, et al. The collaborative ocular tuberculosis study (COTS) calculator—a consensus-based decision tool for initiating antitubercular therapy in ocular tuberculosis. Eye. 2023;37(7):1416-23.
52. Rathinam SR, Usha KR, Rao NA. Presumed trematode-induced granulomatous anterior uveitis: a newly recognized cause of intraocular inflammation in children from South India. Am J Ophthal. 2002;133(6):773-9.
53. Rathinam S, Fritsche TR, Srinivasan M, Vijayalakshmi P, Read RW, Gautom R, et al. An outbreak of trematode-induced granulomas of the conjunctiva. Ophthalmology. 2001;108(7):1223-9.

54. Verhagen FH, Braakenburg AM, Kremer T, Drylewicz J, Rothova A, de Boer JH. Reduced number of relapses of human leucocyte antigen-B27-associated uveitis during pregnancy. Acta Ophthalmol. 2017;95(8): e798-9.
55. Kempen JH, Sugar EA, Jaffe GJ, Acharya NR, Dunn JP, Elner SG, et al. Fluorescein angiography versus optical coherence tomography for diagnosis of uveitic macular edema. Ophthalmology. 2013;120(9):1852-9.
56. Chang JH, McCluskey P, Missotten T, Ferrante P, Jalaludin B, Lightman S. Use of ocular hypotensive prostaglandin analogues in patients with uveitis: does their use increase anterior uveitis and cystoid macular oedema? Br J Ophthal. 2008;92(7):916-21.
57. Babu K, Murthy GJ. Cytomegalovirus anterior uveitis in immunocompetent individuals following topical prostaglandin analogues. J Ophthalmic Inflamm Infect. 2013;3(1):55.

CHAPTER 2

Intermediate Uveitis

John H Kempen, Jyotirmay Biswas, François Willermain, Alejandro Fonollosa, Anshukita, Aurélie Le, Jose Manuel Cachero Rodríguez, Germán Mejía-Salgado, Meghan Berkenstock, Vishali Gupta, Alejandra de-la-Torre

INTRODUCTION[1]

Intermediate uveitis (IU) typically is a bilateral chronic inflammatory disease of insidious onset with an estimated incidence of 1.4–2.0/100,000 persons and a prevalence of 5.9/100,000 persons.[2] It is characterized by inflammation seen primarily in the vitreous, presenting as vitreous cells and haze **(Fig. 1)**, snowballs, snowbanking **(Fig. 2)**, and/or peripheral retinal vessel sheathing. Systemic diseases such as multiple sclerosis (MS) and sarcoidosis have been related to IU, as well as some infectious diseases. However, systemic disease associations are less common than with other forms of uveitis.[3] Cystoid macular edema (CME) commonly occurs in IU, but is considered a complication of the inflammation of IU rather than part of the primary disease.[4]

Pars planitis is a large subset of IU in which pars plana exudates and vitreous snowballs are typically seen but are not associated with systemic or infectious diseases. It has an insidious onset, a persisting duration >3 months, and a chronic course with a high incidence of relapse if suppressive therapy is stopped. The Standardization of Uveitis Nomenclature (SUN) Working Group classification criteria for pars planitis can be found in **Figure 1**.[3]

According to the SUN Working Group, a combined form of "anterior and intermediate uveitis", with features of both, but no chorioretinal lesions, makes up a subset of intermediate uveitis.[4] This form of uveitis tends to be less indolent than classic intermediate uveitis. If it is a combined case of anterior and intermediate uveitis, symptoms of both usually will be present. Some consider combined anterior and intermediate uveitis, a separate disease pattern from typical intermediate uveitis.

PRACTICAL TIPS IN THE MANAGEMENT OF INTERMEDIATE UVEITIS[1]

Typical Symptoms of Intermediate Uveitis

- Floaters (as a result of inflammatory cells and/or debris in the vitreous)
- Blurred or cloudy vision (usually reflecting cloudy vitreous media or macular edema)

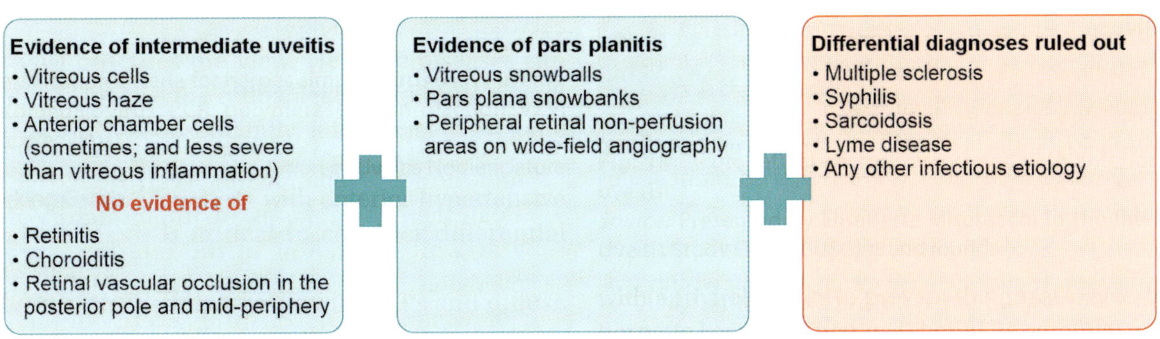

Fig. 1: Classification criteria for pars planitis.
Source: Modified from Standardization of Uveitis Nomenclature (SUN) Working Group.[4]

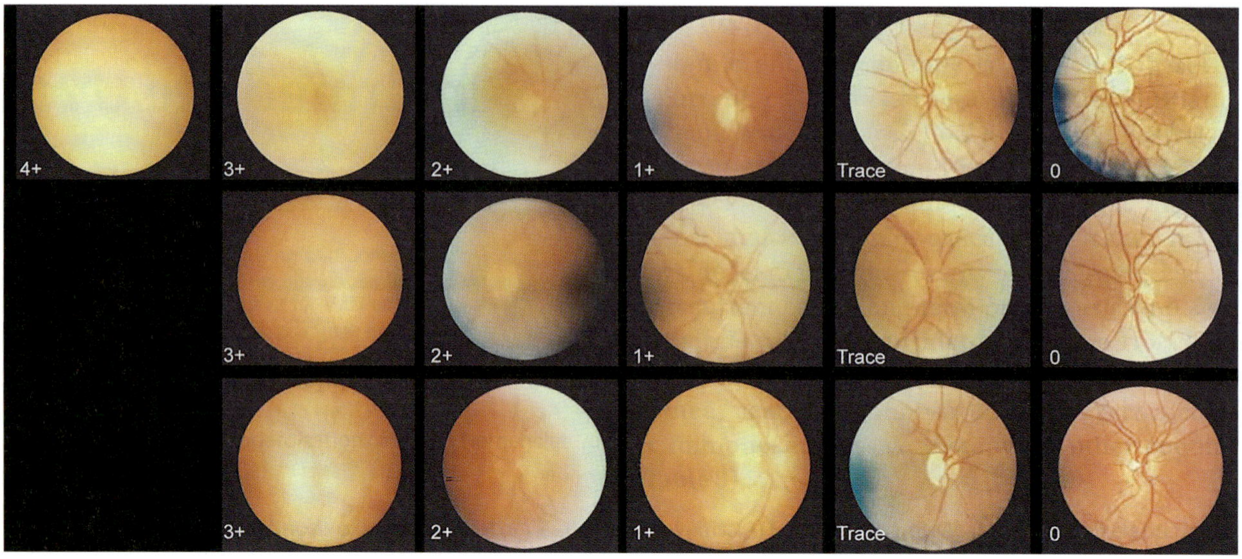

Fig. 2: Grading scale for vitreous haze. Representative standard images. Grade 4: Dense opacity obscuring optic nerve head. Grade 3: Optic nerve visible, borders blurred, and no retinal vessels seen. Grade 2: Significant blurring of the optic nerve and retinal vessels but still visible. Grade 1: Few opacities and mild blurring of the optic nerve and retinal vessels. Trace (0.5+): Trace. Grade 0: Clear.
Source: Reprint from Ophthalmology, 1986; 93(7):984-8, with permission.

- Visual loss in patients with retinal detachment, vitreous hemorrhage, and severe or chronic CME[3]
- Pain and photophobia are uncommon because the iris and ciliary muscles are not primarily involved.

Signs

- In intermediate-only uveitis, anterior chamber cellular reaction is usually mild, with more cells and inflammatory material behind the lens. Anterior chamber cells might result from "spillover" from the vitreous chamber.
- Intraocular pressure is usually within limits; trabeculitis or ciliary body inflammation leading to an increase in the intraocular pressure are absent.
- Gonioscopy may reveal cellular aggregates in the angle without an anterior chamber reaction.
- The incidence of cataract formation increases over time but is not present in the majority of cases within the first few years after diagnosis.[5,6]
- Vitreous cells and haze are typically present in cases of active IU. Vitreous haze is graded by different scales **(Fig. 2)**:[7,8]
  - Grading is done according to the approach endorsed by the SUN Working Group, which was developed at the National Eye Institute.[4,7]
  - A reading center-based grading method has also been proposed and used in clinical research.[9]

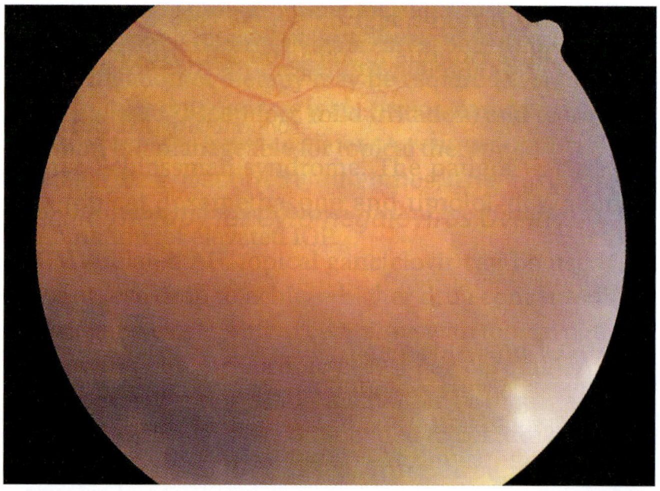

Fig. 3: Snowballs, as seen inferiorly and temporally in this fundus photograph, are a typical sign of intermediate uveitis and can aggregate to form a "string of pearls."
Source: Presented by John Kempen in the International Uveitis Study Group (IUSG) grand rounds.[1]

- Focal vitreous opacities, also called "snowballs", indicate active inflammation **(Fig. 3)**.[10,11]
- Coalescent aggregates of inflammatory debris of gray-white or yellow in the inferior vitreous base overlying the pars plana and anterior retina, also called "snowbanking", reflects the severity of the disease.[3] Snowbanking may evolve into a fibrotic area that does not disappear with control of the inflammation.

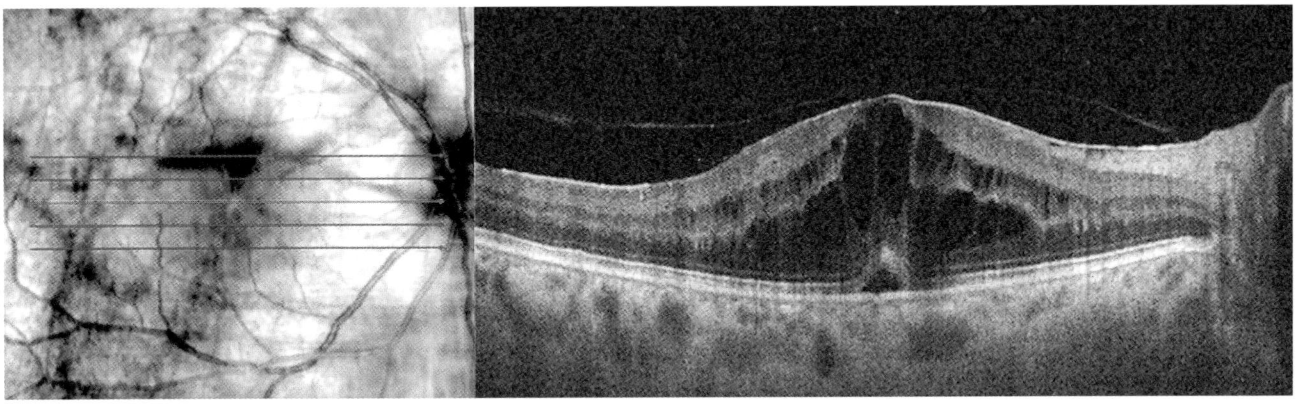

Fig. 4: Optical coherence tomography (OCT) of a right eye with cystoid macular edema showing multiple, intraretinal cystic spaces in the outer and inner nuclear layers with hyperreflective dots in the vitreous.
Source: Presented by John Kempen in the International Uveitis Study Group (IUSG) grand rounds.[1]

- Vascular sheathing in the periphery may include diffuse capillary leakage on fluorescein angiogram.[12]

Complications

- *Cystoid macular edema* is the most common complication seen in IU.[9] CME is well characterized by optical coherence tomography (OCT) as macular thickening (an anatomic definition of macular edema) and also by fluorescein angiography that can often demonstrate extensive leakage (a physiologic indicator of macular pathology and cause of macular thickening) **(Fig. 4)**. Macular leakage on angiography can occur in the absence of macular thickening due to compensatory removal of excess fluid or conversely, when excess fluid is not removed after the leakage stops only thickening may be present.[13]
- *Disc swelling:* Chronic disc swelling can lead to adjacent juxtapapillary choroidal neovascularization.[14]
- *Epiretinal membrane (ERM):* An ERM may, in turn, lead to CME. OCT is an important imaging modality that differentiates tractional from non-tractional macular edema. However, attempts to treat CME associated an ERM via medical management should be undertaken prior to membrane peeling as improvement can occur without surgical intervention.
- *Peripheral retinal neovascularization* secondary to retinal ischemia.[10,11] Typical treatments such as scatter photocoagulation may be required.[15]
- *Retinoschisis* is one of the rarer complications that can develop. It usually will be static and does not reach the posterior pole. However, in some cases, it can progress. Cases of posterior pole involvement have been reported mainly in children, usually beginning inferiorly, with an absolute scotoma in the area of schisis.[16,17] If the schisis approaches the macula, it may result in noticeable vision loss. There are no proven ways to stop progression, but control of the adjacent inflammation may help.

Clinical Course

In most cases, the IU course tends to be chronic with an overall low incidence of remission quiescence without anti-inflammatory treatment for at least 3 months.[4] The incidence of remission in a retrospective cohort study of 849 eyes with IU was 8.6/1,000 eye-years **(Fig. 5)**.[18] Factors that predicted remission included prior pars plana vitrectomy (PPV) [hazard ratio (HR) vs. no PPV = 2.39; 95% confidence interval (CI), 1.42–4.00], diagnosis of IU in the last year (HR vs. diagnosis >5 years ago = 3.82; 95% CI, 1.91–7.63), age >45 years (HR vs. age <45 years = 1.79; 95% CI, 1.04–2.49), and Hispanic race/ethnicity (HR vs. White race = 2.81; 95% CI 1.23–6.41). The presence of systemic disease, laterality, and smoking status was not associated with differential incidences.[18]

Principles of Treatment[1]

Management of IU should be based on the cause of inflammation. If an infectious etiology is identified, treatment should target the specific pathogen. Before initiating immunomodulatory agents, infections, malignancies, and multiple sclerosis should be ruled out. Ruling out tuberculosis and MS is especially important before treating with antitumor necrosis factor (TNF) inhibitors, that may worsen these conditions.

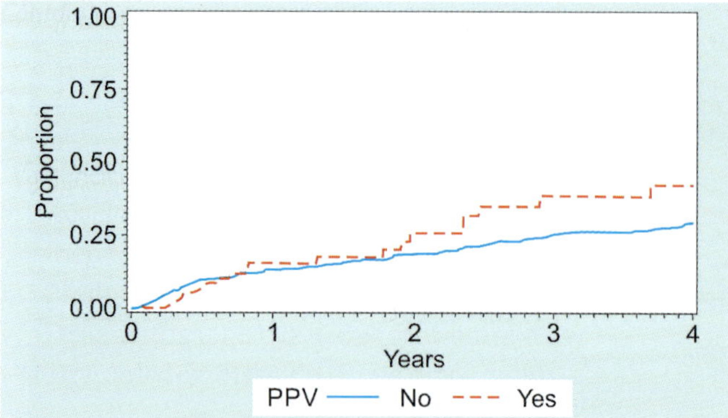

Fig. 5: Kaplan–Meier incidence of remission of intermediate uveitis (IU) over time in patients who have undergone or have not had a pars plana vitrectomy (PPV). Patients with IU who underwent a PPV present a higher incidence of remission during follow-up.
Source: Reprinted from Am J Ophthalmol. 2016;164:110-7, with permission.

Mild vitreous inflammation with few cells and with minimal or no symptoms/visual impairment may be observed without treatment. Begin treatment if there is reduced vision or structural complications, such as macular edema, ERM, and others (see Complications above). It has been reported that 25–35% of patients with pars planitis have a mild form of the disease with no complications and do not require treatment, as these patients can maintain good vision over at least 10 years of follow-up.[2]

When treatment is required, oral corticosteroids and immunomodulatory therapy (most commonly antimetabolites and biologic drugs) are the mainstay of treatment. As the vitreous is the main site of inflammation, corticosteroid eye drops have poor penetration. Long-lasting corticosteroid injections or implants are preferred if local treatment is required, most commonly with macular edema.[19] Local therapy is more attractive for unilateral or asymmetric cases with the absence of a systemic disease. It can also be used as an adjunct to systemic therapy (e.g., to treat macular edema or to "induce" control of the inflammation). It is also recommended when there are contraindications or intolerances to systemic therapy. In bilateral cases, systemic therapy becomes more attractive, although it is also a reasonable treatment approach for unilateral involvement since the dose can be adjusted with the development of side effects.

Surgical approaches may be necessary to manage complications (e.g., ERM peeling) or difficult-to-treat cases. Cryoretinopexy and scatter panretinal photocoagulation (PRP) have been reported to reduce peripheral retinovascular leakage[16] and are associated with higher remission of vitreous cells or CME.[20,21] Nevertheless, these therapies are controversial and medical therapy should be the primary treatment to reduce inflammation. PRP may be an easier procedure with fewer complications and less pain than cryoretinopexy. Vitrectomy has been proposed as an alternative that may be used when there is no response to local therapy with injections, cryotherapy, or laser.[22] Still, it is rarely used by those taking a medical approach to managing IU.

The following case examples illustrate the approach to patients with IU, and the discussion section aims to help the reader understand the thought process of experts when evaluating a patient. However, the cases do not cover the entire disease spectrum of IU and are being presented to give reader an overall idea about approaching these patients.

PARS PLANITIS[1]

Case Presentation

Personal Data

- Female, 9 years old
- No treatment was used previously.

History of Present Illness

Blurred vision and floaters in the left eye.

Physical Examination

The patient presented with a visual acuity (VA) of 20/30 in the OD and 20/50 in the OS, with a quiet conjunctiva, 0.5+ cells in the anterior chamber, and 1+ vitreous cells in both eyes. Moreover, snowballs and snowbanks were observed in the inferior vitreous cavity in both eyes, as well as a vasoproliferative tumor (VPT) in the inferior temporal area of the OS **(Table 1)**.

Optical coherence tomography showed CME in both eyes **(Figs. 6A and B)**. Fundus fluorescein angiography was not performed.

Laboratory tests were within normal parameters [complete blood count (CBC), erythrocyte sedimentation rate (ESR), C-reactive protein (CRP), Human Immunodeficiency Virus (HIV), *Toxoplasma* serology, *Borrelia* serology, syphilis, and purified protein derivative (PPD)]. The patient was diagnosed with pars planitis, an idiopathic, chronic, and relapsing form of IU with inflammatory exudates seen in the vitreous, commonly presenting in

TABLE 1: Physical examination of patient having pars planitis.

OD	Parameters	OS
20/30	BCVA	20/50
Within normal limits	IOP	Within normal limits
Normal	Conjunctiva	Normal
Mutton-fat KP	Cornea	Pigmented KP
0.5+	Anterior chamber cells	0.5+
Clear	Lens	Clear
Vitreous cells 1+	Vitreous	Vitreous cells 1+
Snowballs and snowbanks	Fundus	Snowballs, snowbanks, and vasoproliferative tumor

(BCVA: best-corrected visual acuity; IOP: intraocular pressure; KP: keratic precipitate)

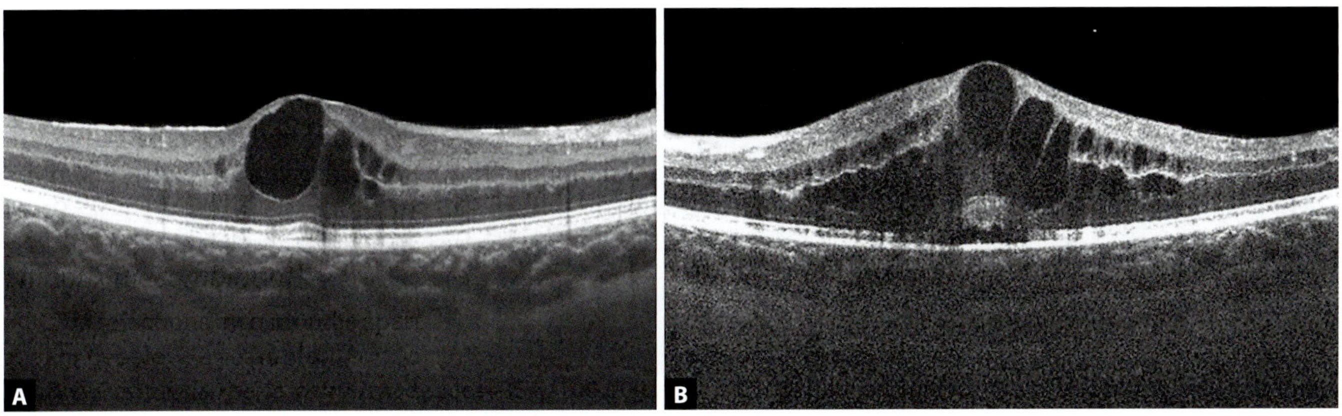

Figs. 6A and B: Initial macular optical coherence tomography (OCT). (A) Cystoid macular edema was seen in the OD; (B) Cystoid macular edema was also observed in the OS.
Source: Presented by Jose Manuel Cachero in the International Uveitis Study Group (IUSG) grand rounds.[1]

childhood or younger adulthood. Treatment was initiated with oral corticosteroids (prednisone 30 mg with tapering doses) resulting in improved edema and VA **(Figs. 7A and B)**. Peri- or intraocular depot therapy could also be used, but would have to be applied bilaterally with a risk of local side effects of treatment in this young child.

Five months after the start of treatment, with the patient on prednisone 5 mg, vitritis and recurrence of CME with decreased VA in the left eye were observed. No inflammation in the anterior chamber was observed. Subsequently, a peribulbar triamcinolone injection was applied in OS and treatment for amblyopia was started. A month later, residual microcysts in the OS remained, so an intravitreal dexamethasone implant was performed. We decided to initiate immunosuppressive therapy. Both methotrexate (MTX) alone and the combination of adalimumab plus MTX were ineffective. Hence, intravenous tocilizumab (TCZ) 350 mg every 4 weeks was started, which achieved macular edema resolution after the third dose. After 1 year of monotherapy with TCZ, it was adjusted to 350 mg every 6 weeks, but CME in the left eye reappeared, which obligated us to give TCZ again every 4 weeks **(Figs. 8A to G)**. After 2 years of disease control and amblyopia treatment for the left eye, the VA was 20/20 in the right eye and 20/50 in the left eye. In the latter, there were many vitreous opacities, so a PPV was performed with an intravitreal dexamethasone implant.

During the vitrectomy, endolaser was applied to the feeder vessels of the VPT, which was also treated by means of cryotherapy. Follow-up showed control of inflammation, an improvement in VA (20/20), and no recurrence of CME in the left eye **(Fig. 9)**. TCZ was continued at the initial dose (350 mg every 4 weeks) for the following 6 months.

At that moment, since monthly visits to receive intravenous TCZ treatment were difficult to fulfill for the patient, subcutaneous TCZ 162 mg/week was initiated.

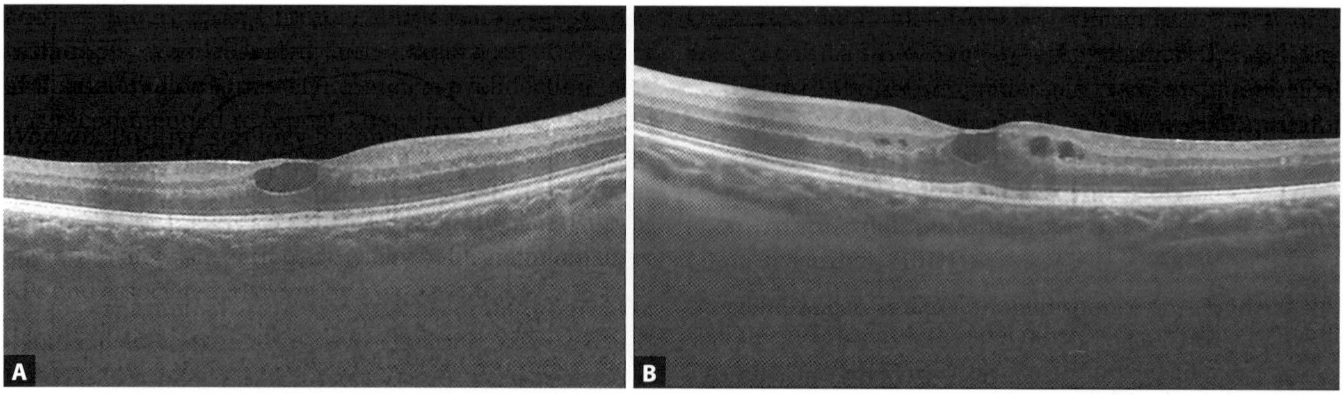

Figs. 7A and B: Macular OCTs after oral corticosteroid treatment. Follow-up macular OCT showed a reduction of CME in both eyes. (CME: cystoid macular edema; OCT: optical coherence tomography)

Source: Presented by Jose Manuel Cachero in the International Uveitis Study Group (IUSG) grand rounds.[1]

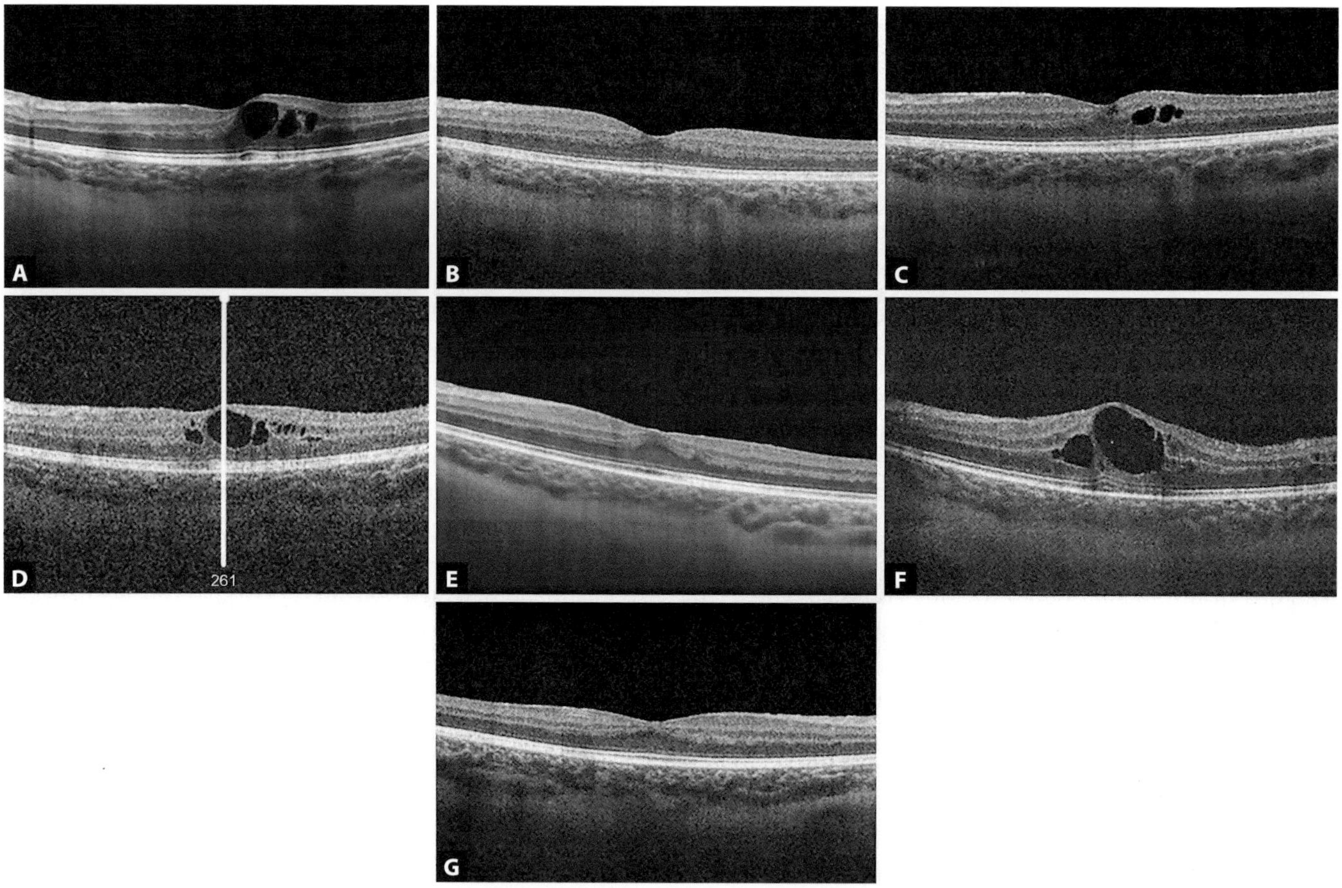

Figs. 8A to G: Macular OCT follow-up of CME evolution with various treatment regimen: (A) September 2013, prednisone 5 mg; (B) October 2013, prednisone + MTX 12.5 mg; (C) January 2014, prednisone + MTX 12.5 mg + ADA 0.8 mL/2 weeks; (D) April 2014, MTX 17.5 mg + ADA 0.8 mL/2 weeks; (E) October 2014, prednisone + MTX 17.5 mg + TCZ 350 mg/4 weeks; (F) December 2015, TCZ 350 mg/6 weeks; (G) March 2016, TCZ 350 mg/4 weeks. (ADA: adalimumab; CME: cystoid macular edema; MTX: methotrexate; OCT: optical coherence tomography; TCZ: tocilizumab)

Source: Presented by Jose Manuel Cachero in the International Uveitis Study Group (IUSG) grand rounds.[1]

MTX 10 mg weekly and prednisolone 5 mg were also added because, we expected the subcutaneous administration to be less effective. This regimen was maintained for 1 year due to psychosocial constraints, which included illicit drug use and pregnancy. Local treatment was a better option; hence, an intravitreal fluocinolone acetonide implant was administered in both eyes with a good response. Systemic immunosuppressive medications were progressively withdrawn.

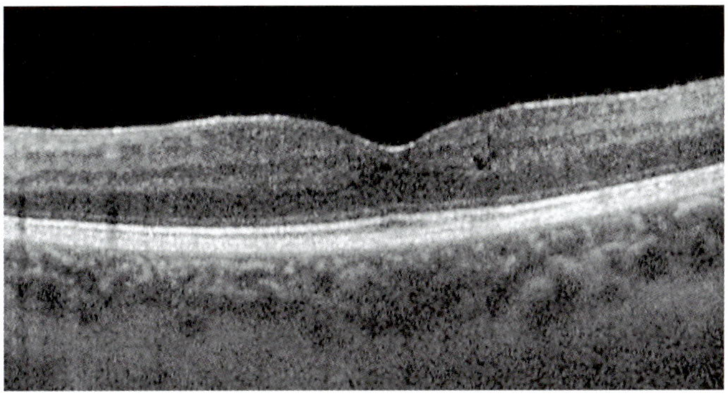

Fig. 9: Macular optical coherence tomography (OCT) post-surgery OS (performed in September 2019). OS CME improvement with evidence of residual microcyst.
Source: Presented by Jose Manuel Cachero in the International Uveitis Study Group (IUSG) grand rounds.[1]

Five months after the intravitreal fluocinolone injections and while being off systemic immunosuppressive agents, the patient underwent cataract surgery in OS with an improvement to 20/25 vision (before surgery, VA 20/50). The macular OCT remained stable for the following 12 months in both eyes **(Figs. 10A to D)**.

Last Follow-up (Performed in February 2020) Ocular Examination (Table 2)

TABLE 2: Ocular examination of patient having pars planitis.

OD	Parameters	OS
20/25	BCVA	20/25
20 mm Hg	IOP	21 mm Hg
Normal	Conjunctiva	Normal
No KP	Cornea	Pigmented KP
No cells	Anterior chamber	No cells
Posterior subcapsular cataract	Lens	Pseudophakia
No inflammation	Vitreous	No inflammation
Stable	Fundus	Stable

(BCVA: best-corrected visual acuity; IOP: intraocular pressure; KP: keratic precipitate)

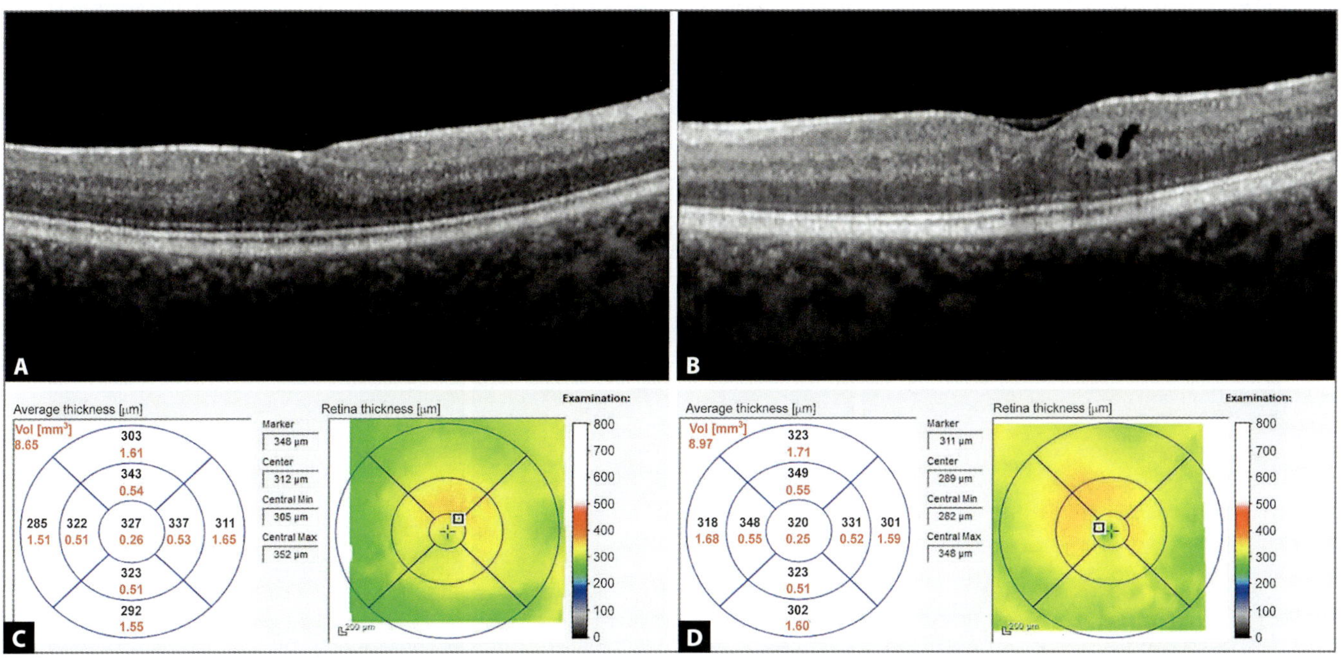

Figs. 10A to D: Macular OCTs peformed at the last follow-up in February 2020. (A and C) Improvement in CME in OD; (B and D) Presence of residual microcysts in the OS. (CME: cystoid macular edema; OCT: optical coherence tomography)
Source: Presented by Jose Manuel Cachero in the International Uveitis Study Group (IUSG) grand rounds.[1]

Discussion[1]

Some points must be highlighted from this case:

- It is important to establish the diagnosis of pars planitis based on the SUN criteria.[4]
- Most pediatric uveitis cases are idiopathic, but they can also be associated with systemic diseases such as juvenile idiopathic arthritis (JIA), tubulointerstitial nephritis and uveitis (TINU), and Behçet disease, each of which might evolve into a broader uveitis syndrome over time. Therefore, these children need to be investigated for these conditions before the disease is labeled idiopathic.[23]
- Multimodal imaging techniques are of great value due to challenges with cooperation in clinical examination (**Figs. 11A to E**). Ultrawide-field fluorescein angiography reveals mild-to-moderate peripheral vascular leakage and can be used as a tool to monitor response to therapy. In this case, fluorescein angiography was not performed, so we cannot be sure if the patient presented with peripheral vascular leakage, which is a frequent sign of pars planitis, as stated in the introduction.
- Treatment of pediatric uveitis is crucial, considering that approximately 25–40% of the cases may develop vision loss, and up to 25% may progress to legal blindness.[4,10,11]
- Management is a controversial topic, as some experts describe pars planitis as a benign disease requiring treatment only in cases with poor VA (<0.5) or with complications such as CME.[24] Conversely, other authors suggest considering pars planitis as a severe, chronic disease necessitating treatment in all cases, except those who are asymptomatic with good VA (20/20), very few cells, and snowballs.[25,26] When treatment is considered, assuming chronicity, long-term immunosuppressive therapy often is required. However, it is reasonable to try a course of corticosteroids or periocular triamcinolone injection in unilateral cases.[25,26] Some agents reported to be well

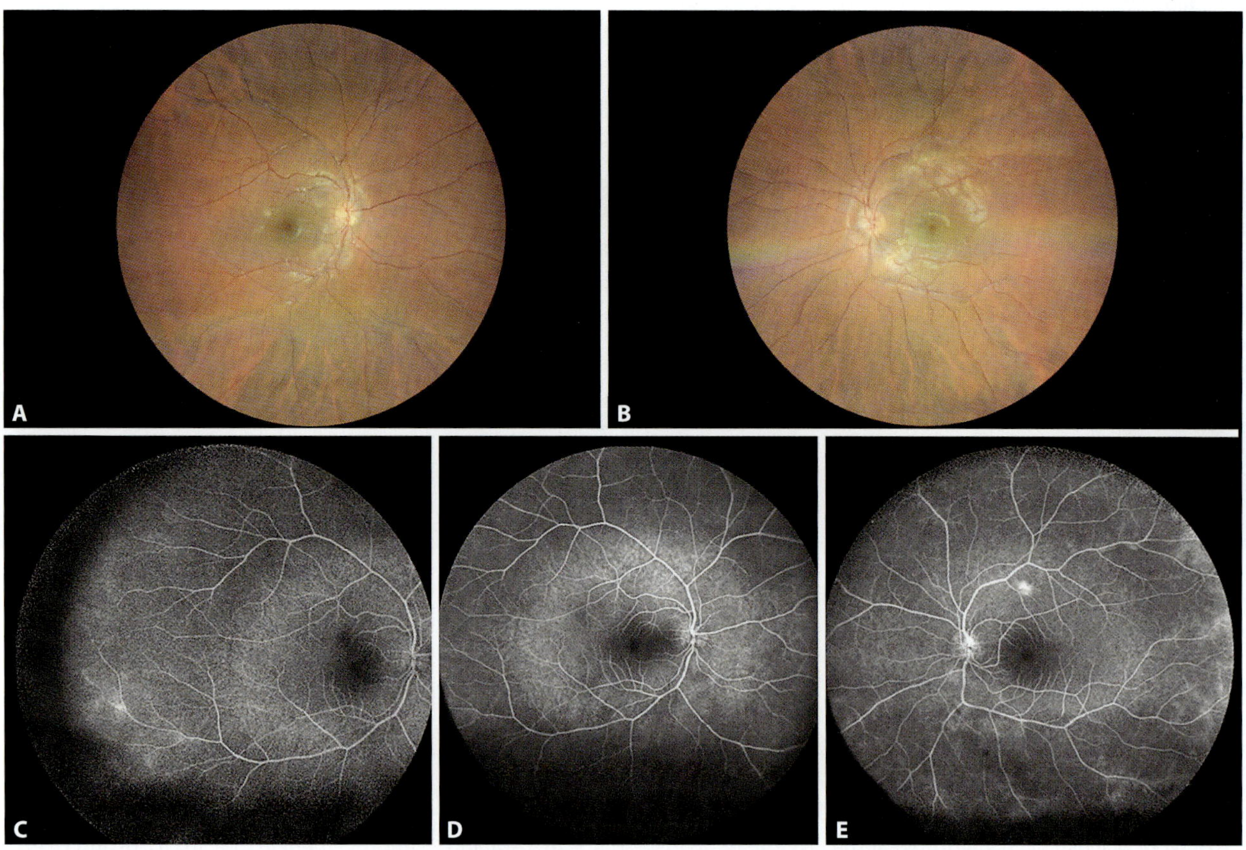

Figs. 11A to E: Multimodal imaging of a patient with pars planitis. (A) Right eye and (B) left eye wide-field color fundus photographs showing a clear vitreous cavity; however, wide-field fluorescein angiography shows peripheral leakage.
Source: Presented by Alex Fonollosa in the International Uveitis Study Group (IUSG) grand rounds.[1]

tolerated in children are MTX, mycophenolate mofetil (MMF), azathioprine, and cyclosporine.[25] Anti-TNF-α agents can be used as a third-line therapy in patients not responsive to traditional, non-biologic, with the concern about the possibility of developing MS. Finally, the fourth step of treatment includes surgery, such as PPV, cryotherapy, and laser photocoagulation. Some argue that cryotherapy should be avoided as it has been reported to aggravate blood-ocular barrier disruption. It may also hypothetically accelerate the incidence of retinal detachment by inducing vitreous contraction leaving laser photocoagulation as the preferred treatment.[26]

ANTERIOR + INTERMEDIATE UVEITIS ASSOCIATED WITH SARCOIDOSIS[1]

Case Presentation

Personal Data

- Male, 36 years old
- No systemic disease
- *Previous treatment:* Prednisolone acetate 1% and bromfenac 0.09% eye drops

History of Present Illness

The patient presented for a second opinion consultation with a 3-month; history of floaters, hyperemia, and decreased VA in both eyes and a diagnosis of granulomatous uveitis.

Physical Examination

The patient presented with a VA of 20/20 in the OU; in addition, both eyes presented with pigmented keratic precipitates, anterior chamber cells, posterior synechiae, and vitreous cells **(Figs. 12 to 14 and Table 3)**.

An anterior segment OCT was performed, identifying iris nodules extending into the angle in both eyes **(Figs. 14A and B)**.

Based on the findings, bilateral, granulomatous anterior and IU was diagnosed. Subsequently, ancillary tests were ordered: CBC, liver function testing (LFT), renal function testing (RFT), HLA-B27, angiotensin-converting

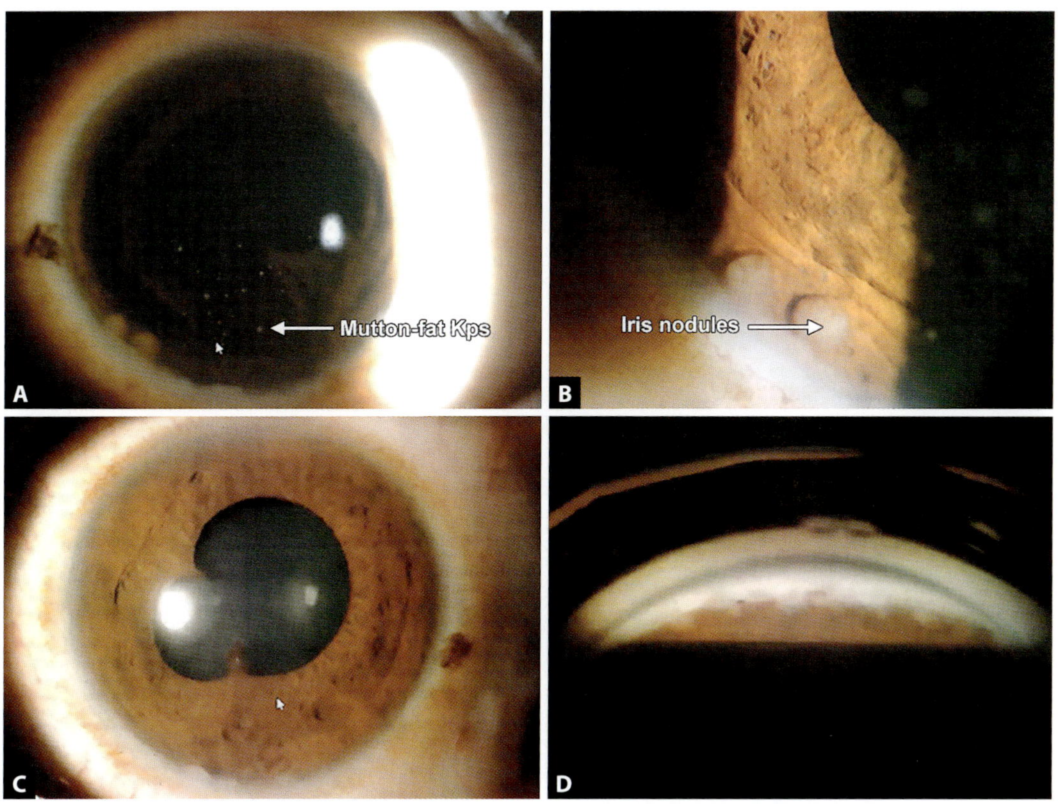

Figs. 12A to D: Slit-lamp examination: (A) Mutton-fat keratic precipitates (KP) in OD; (B) Iris nodules in OD; (C) Pigmented deposition on the lens anterior capsule with posterior synechiae is OS; (D) Peripheral iris nodules in OS on gonioscopy.
Source: Presented by Anshukita in the International Uveitis Study Group (IUSG) grand rounds.[1]

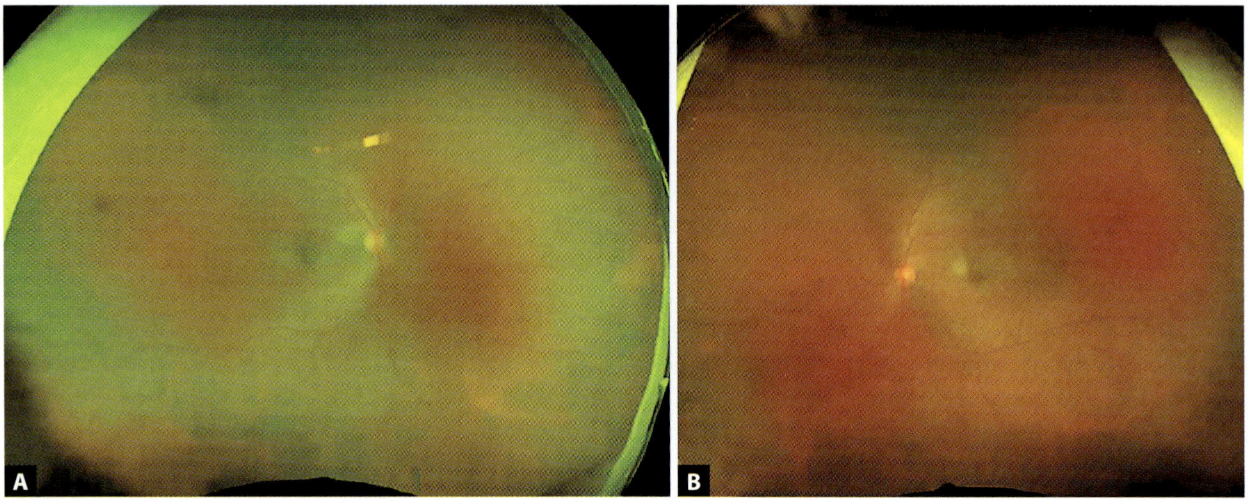

Figs. 13A and B: Fundus examination findings: (A) Peripheral vitreous with opacities are seen in OD. The macula and optic disc are within normal limits; (B) Vitreous haze with mild disc and macular edema are seen in the OS.
Source: Presented by Anshukita in the International Uveitis Study Group (IUSG) grand rounds.[1]

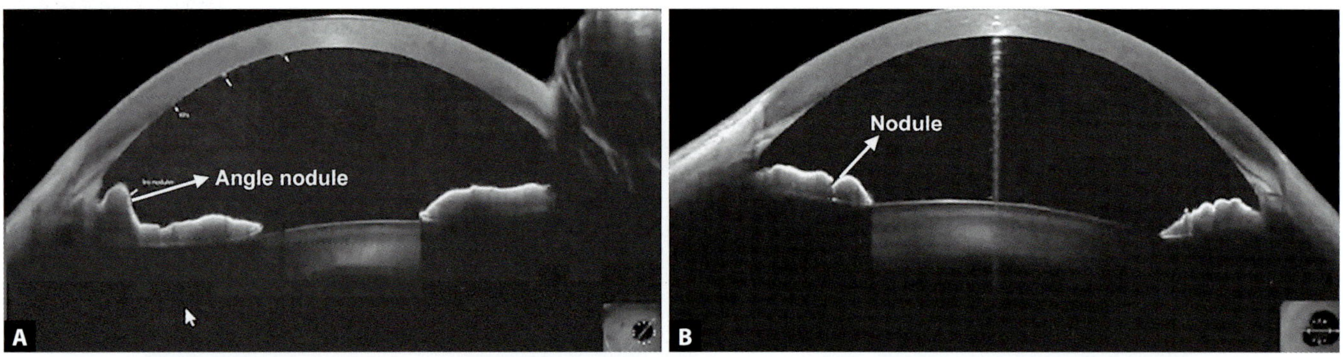

Figs. 14A and B: Anterior segment optical coherence tomography findings. (A) Angle iris nodules in OD; (B) Iris nodules OS.
Source: Presented by Anshukita in the International Uveitis Study Group (IUSG) grand rounds.[1]

TABLE 3: Physical examination of patient having anterior + intermediate uveitis associated with sarcoidosis.

OD	***Parameters***	***OS***
20/20	BCVA	20/20
16 mm Hg	IOP	18 mm Hg
Normal	Conjunctiva	Normal
Mutton-fat KP	Cornea	Pigmented KP over the endothelium
ACC: 1+, Van Herick grading 4	Anterior chamber	ACC: 0.5+, Van Herick grading 4
Broad-based posterior synechiae at 4–7 o'clock and peripheral iris nodules at 8 o'clock	Iris	Broad-based posterior synechiae at 10 and 7 o'clock and inferior peripheral anterior synechiae at 5–7 o'clock
Clear	Lens	Clear
Vitreous cells 1+	Vitreous	Vitreous cells 0.5+
Peripheral vitreous opacities; macula, and disc within normal parameters	Fundus	Vitreous haze, macula, and disc within normal parameters

(ACC: anterior chamber cellularity; BCVA: best-corrected visual acuity; IOP: intraocular pressure; KP: keratic precipitate) enzyme (ACE), Mantoux skin test, and anterior chamber polymerase chain reaction (PCR). All were within normal parameters, except for high ACE level (56.3 μL). High-resolution computed tomography (HRCT) of the chest revealed bilateral mediastinal lymphadenopathy with patchy peripheral parenchyma infiltrates and a few thing, plate-like areas of atelectasis in the right lung **(Fig. 15)**. Mantoux skin test and PCR from the aqueous humor ruled out tuberculosis.

Final Diagnosis

Presumed sarcoidosis-related uveitis was diagnosed based on the revised criteria from of the International Workshop on Ocular Sarcoidosis (IWOS) 2019 **(Fig. 16)**.[27] The patient had bilateral anterior and intermediate uveitis per the SUN criteria with mutton-fat keratic precipitates (KP), bilateral iris and angle nodules, and bilateral hilar lymphadenopathy.

Treatment

- Topical treatment for this case consisted of prednisolone acetate 1% eye drops in both eyes (OU) six times a day and homatropine eye drops in OU two times a day.
- For systemic treatment, oral prednisolone 40 mg was given once daily with a weekly tapering scheme, along with calcium carbonate 500 mg two times daily, pantoprazole 40 mg daily, and MMF 1000 mg, two tablets two times daily.
- One month after the initiation of the treatment, the patient's slit-lamp examination showed an improvement compared to previous findings, with a resolution of cells, KPs, and nodules **(Figs. 17A to F)**.

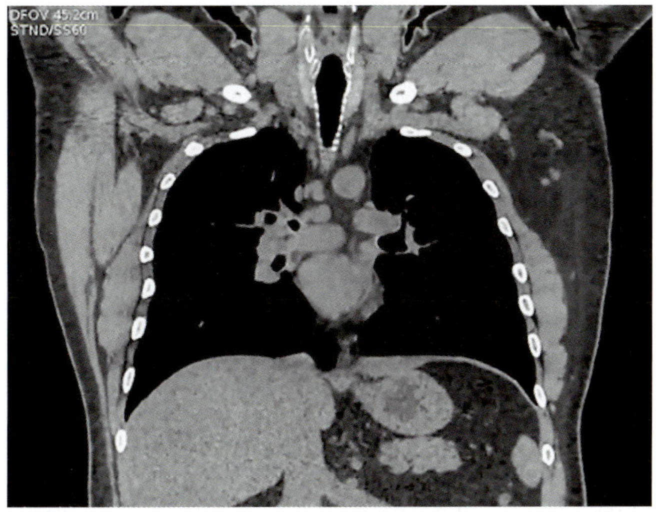

Fig. 15: High-resolution computed tomography (HRCT) of the chest. Bilateral mediastinal lymphadenopathy, patchy peripheral parenchyma infiltrates, and a few thin, plate-like areas of atelectasis are seen in the right lung.
Source: Presented by Anshukita in the International Uveitis Study Group (IUSG) grand rounds.[1]

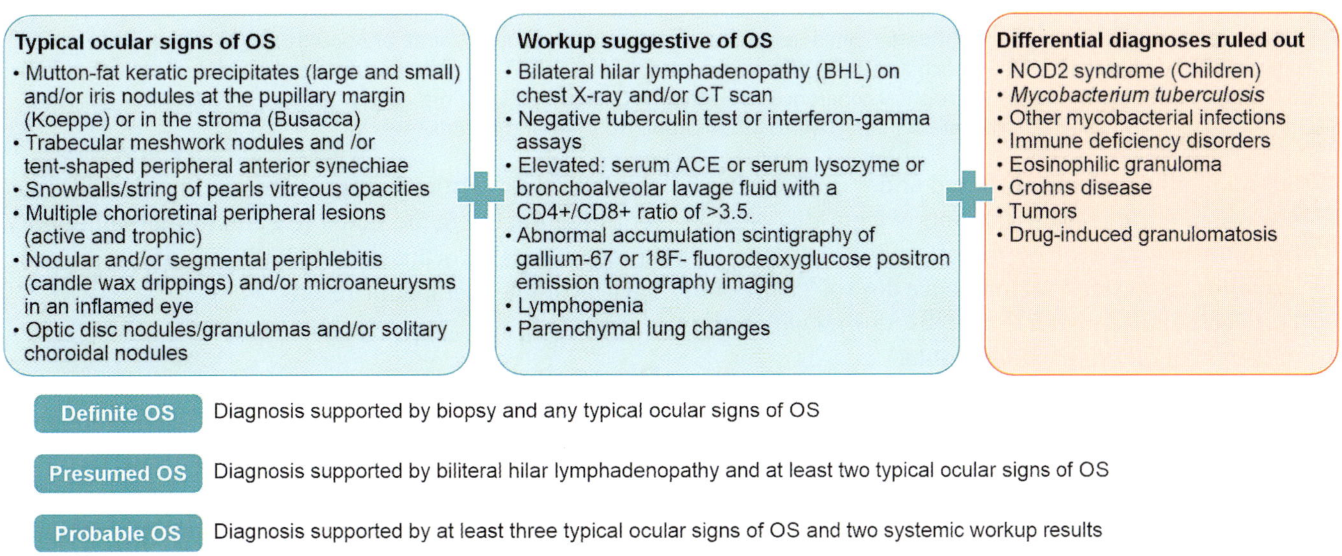

Fig. 16: Revised criteria of the International Workshop on Ocular Sarcoidosis (IWOS) 2019. (ACE: angiotensin-converting enzyme; CT: computed tomography; OS: ocular sarcoidosis)
Source: Adapted from Mochizuki et al.[27]

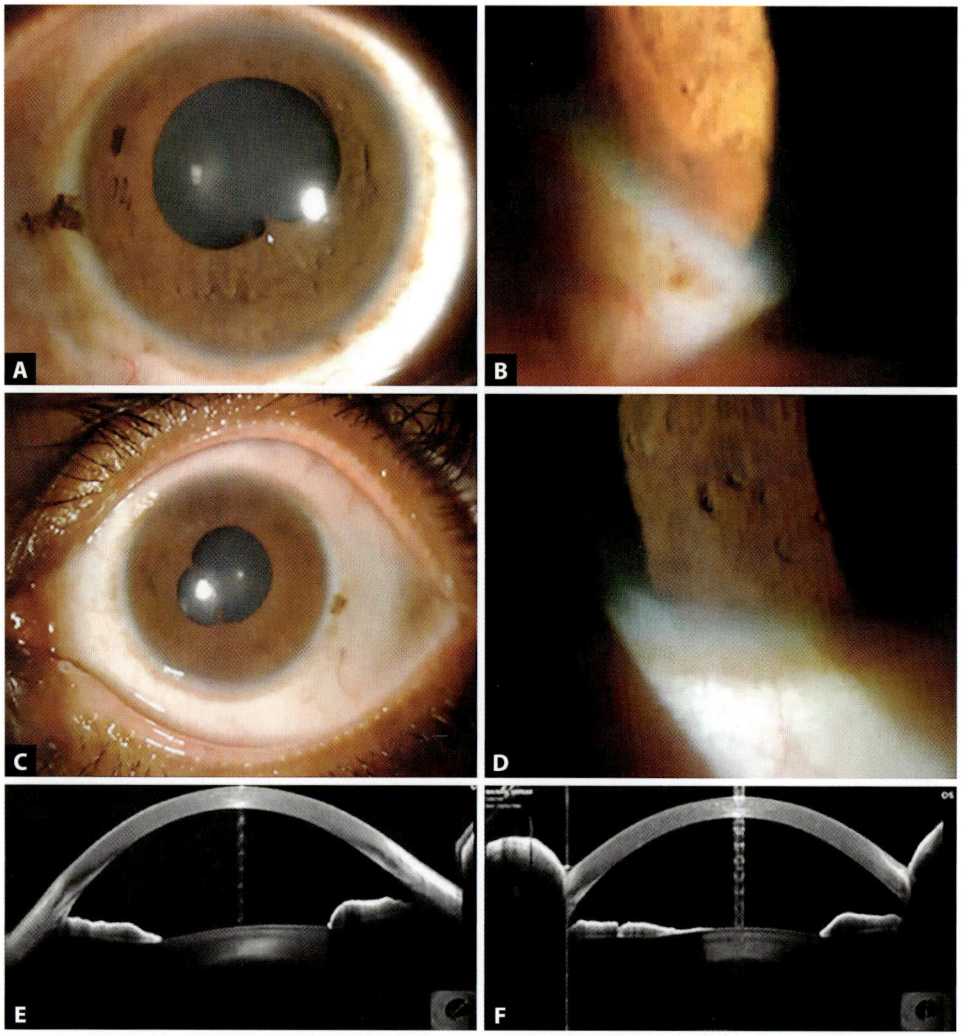

Figs. 17A to F: Slit-lamp findings 1 month after initial treatment. (A) OD with no mutton-fat KP or nodules; (B) OD with no nodules; (C) OS with no KP and improvement of synechiae; (D) OS with no nodules; (E and F) OCT OU with no evidence of nodules in the trabecular meshwork. (KP: keratic precipitate; OCT: optical coherence tomography; OS: left eye; OD: right eye)
Source: Presented by Anshukita in the International Uveitis Study Group (IUSG) grand rounds.[1]

- Subsequently, the patient started and was maintained on a regimen of MMF 1000 mg twice a day with a maintenance dose of 7.5 mg of prednisone daily for 3 months, alongside a maintenance dose of 7.5 mg oral corticosteroids daily for 3 months, during which the patient's condition remained stable.

In conclusion, sarcoidosis frequently presents as an IU. However, it can manifest as anterior (most frequently), posterior, or panuveitis. In this case, it was predominantly an anterior and IU. When granulomatous uveitis is noted on examination, the diagnosis of sarcoidosis needs to be ruled out through a systemic evaluation to assess for additional organ system involvement. Diagnosis must be prompt with early initiation of systemic management, particularly if clinically important extraocular findings requiring treatment are noted (e.g., abnormal pulmonary function tests). Corticosteroids and immunomodulators have favorable therapeutic results.

Discussion[1]

- Sarcoidosis is a chronic, multisystemic, granulomatous disease that creates a robust cellular immune response versus a variety of self and non-self-antigens with a genetic basis. A non-caseating granuloma upon biopsy of affected tissues is the gold-standard diagnosis. However, the diagnosis of ocular sarcoidosis is often based on clinic-radiological features.

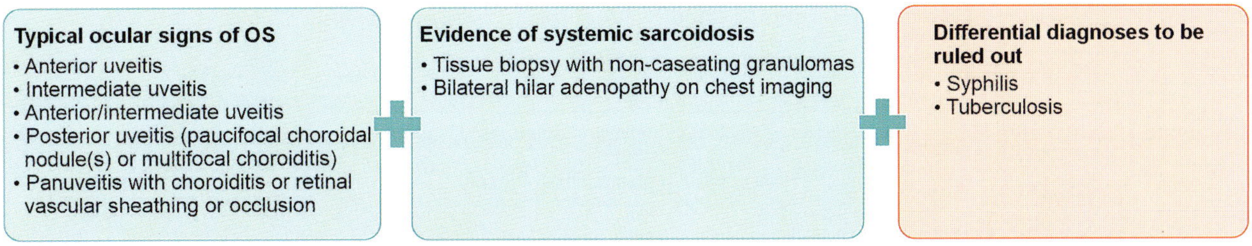

Fig. 18: SUN classification criteria for sarcoidosis-associated uveitis. (SUN: Standardization of Uveitis Nomenclature; OS: ocular sarcoidosis)
Source: Modified from the Standardization of Uveitis Nomenclature (SUN) Working Group.[30]

- Pulmonary disease is the most commonly affected site in 85–95% of cases with bilateral hilar adenopathy frequently seen on chest imaging. Other organs potentially affected by the disease are the liver, spleen, lymph nodes, skin, central nervous system (CNS), and the eye (10–55%), where uveitis is the most frequent presentation (20–30%).[28,29]
- The SUN group recently completed a classification criteria for sarcoidosis **(Fig. 18)**, in addition to the IWOS group criteria. Sarcoidosis is linked with various types of uveitis, with anterior uveitis being the most common worldwide (65–70%), followed by IU, posterior, panuveitis, and even choroiditis.[30]
- Sarcoid is an important cause of IU. In a retrospective cross-sectional study of 362 subjects with definite or presumed sarcoid uveitis, IU with snowballs accounted for 46.4% of the cases. Other common findings of this disease were CME, vitreous opacities, ERM, optic neuritis, and glaucoma.[31] Sarcoidosis accounted for 21.6% of IU in a tertiary eye care center in South India[32] with a mean age of 42.14 ± 11.31 years, female preponderance, and a bilateral presentation. Decreased vision was the most common ocular finding in all the patients (100%), followed by floaters (30%), redness (12.2%), and pain (8.1%). Ocular findings included anterior chamber cells and flare (22.4%), posterior synechiae (20.4%), small and/or mutton-fat KP (14.2%), iris nodules (only in one patient), and trabecular meshwork precipitates (in four patients). Vitreous exudates were seen in 18.3% and snowball opacities in 10.2% of the patients.[32] The most common complications seen were glaucoma (27.5%), ERM (20.4%), cataract formation (17.2%), CME (6%), choroidal neovascular membrane (in one eye), retinal neovascularization (three patients), and the presence of a pars plana membrane (1%).[32]
- The most common tests for diagnosing sarcoidosis include chest imaging and ACE serum levels. Additionally, infectious diseases must be ruled out before making a diagnosis of sarcoidosis.[30] The specificity of the use of ACE serum levels was questioned in a single-center, retrospective study of 755 patients,[33] as it can be a non-specific marker of lung inflammation and might be suppressed by the use of ACE inhibitors for hypertension or other indications. In this study, elevated ACE levels were noted in 76% of the presumed sarcoidosis-associated uveitis cases [odds ratio (OR) 3.603 ($p < 0.002$)]. Likewise, elevated ACE levels were found in 46% of cases with tubercular uveitis (OR 1.19, $p < 0.002$). The study concluded that high ACE levels associated with lymphopenia did not significantly distinguish between sarcoidosis-associated uveitis (17%) and tubercular uveitis (9.7%).[33] Chest imaging may be preferable, as the sensitivity and specificity are relatively favorable and findings indicate a possible biopsy site to provide a histologic diagnosis. *It is to be remembered that Bacillus Calmette-Guérin (BCG) vaccination may cause a false-positive Mantoux reaction.* The algorithm for diagnosing sarcoidosis is depicted in **Flowchart 1**.

Regarding treatment, local or systemic corticosteroid therapy is the preferred management for sarcoidosis-associated uveitis. In cases of refractory disease, immunosuppressives or biological treatment is sometimes used **(Flowchart 2)**. The treatment decision must be based not only on symptomatology but also on the best corrected visual acuities and the presence of ocular complications.[28]

In a cross-sectional study, MMF has been reported to be safe and efficient in treating IU. It reduced vitreous haze in 80% of the cases in the first year of treatment, with corticosteroid withdrawal being successful in 85%. VA improved in 56% of the eyes, and none of the patients developed serious systemic complications.

In summary, sarcoid-related IU is an important potential cause of IU, which responds well to anti-inflammatory therapy with systemic corticosteroids, supplemented by

Flowchart 1: Diagnostic algorithm for suspected ocular sarcoidosis.[28]

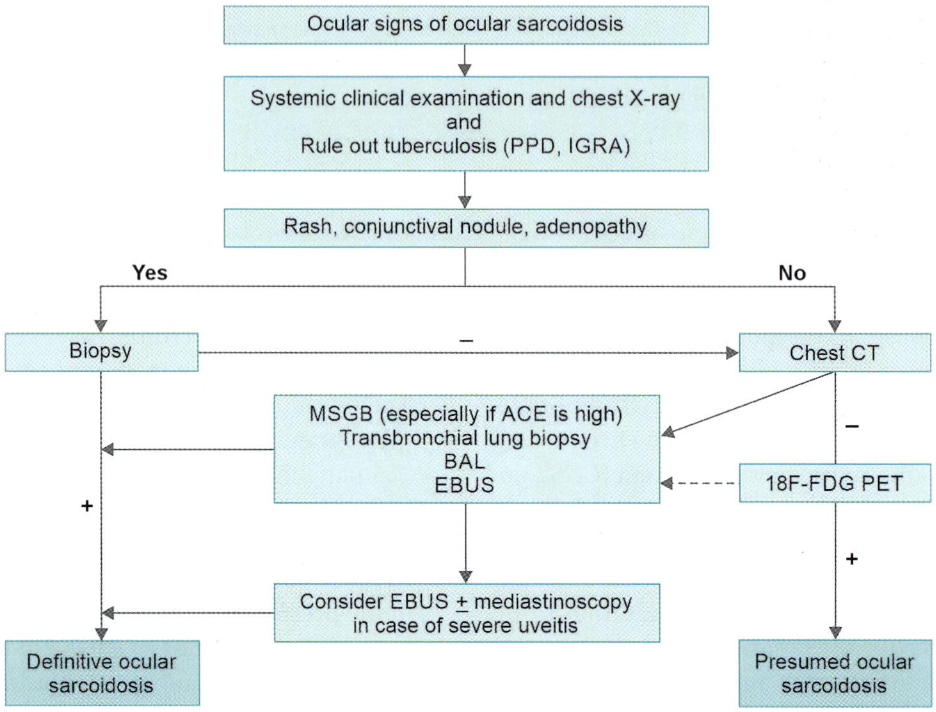

(ACE: angiotensin-converting enzyme; BAL: bronchoalveolar lavage; CT: computed tomography; EBUS: endobronchial ultrasound; IGRA: interferon gamma release assay; MSGB: minor salivary gland biopsy; 18F-FDG PET: 18-fluorodeoxyglucose positron emission tomography; PPD: purified protein derivative) Chest CT has a higher X-ray exposure than a simple chest X-ray and is more expensive but may be a more sensitive test.[34] Local conditions may guide which test is preferable in a given setting.
Source: Adapted from Giorgiutti et al.[28]

topical corticosteroids and/or immunosuppressive drugs when needed. It offers a chance to make a potentially life-changing diagnosis when important systemic complications are present.

INTERMEDIATE UVEITIS ASSOCIATED WITH MULTIPLE SCLEROSIS

Case Presentation

Personal Data

- Male, 27 years old
- History of an intracranial infection at 10 years of age
- No previous treatment

History of Present Illness

A 3-day history of blurred vision in the right eye.

Physical Examination (Fig. 19)

The patient presented with a VA of 20/60 in the OD and 20/25 in the OS, with no cells in the anterior chamber. Fundus examination showed vitreous haze 1+, snowballs, snowbanking, retinal vasculitis, and hemorrhages in both eyes **(Table 4)**.

The dense vitreous haze did not allow for a detailed examination of the retinal periphery. A fluorescein angiogram **(Figs. 20A and B)**, indocyanine green angiogram **(Figs. 21A and B)**, and an OCT of the retina **(Figs. 22A and B)** were performed to assess for ischemic areas and the cause of the retinal hemorrhages.

Laboratory testing was normal or negative, including a CBC, ESR, CRP, syphilis serologies, interferon gamma release assay (IGRA), Lyme titers, HIV, Bartonella, toxoplasmosis, herpes simplex virus, varicella-zoster virus, ACE and lysozyme, RFT, and chest X-ray. An MRI of the brain showed lesions in the white matter, suggestive of demyelinating disease **(Fig. 23)**. Subsequently, a positive Lhermitte's sign was found on neurologic examination (sudden, electrical shock-like sensation running down the back and into the limbs, often triggered by bending the neck forward), high immunoglobulin G (IgG) index, and oligoclonal bands in the cerebrospinal fluid.

Flowchart 2: Algorithm of management of sarcoidosis-associated uveitis depending on anatomical location.[35]

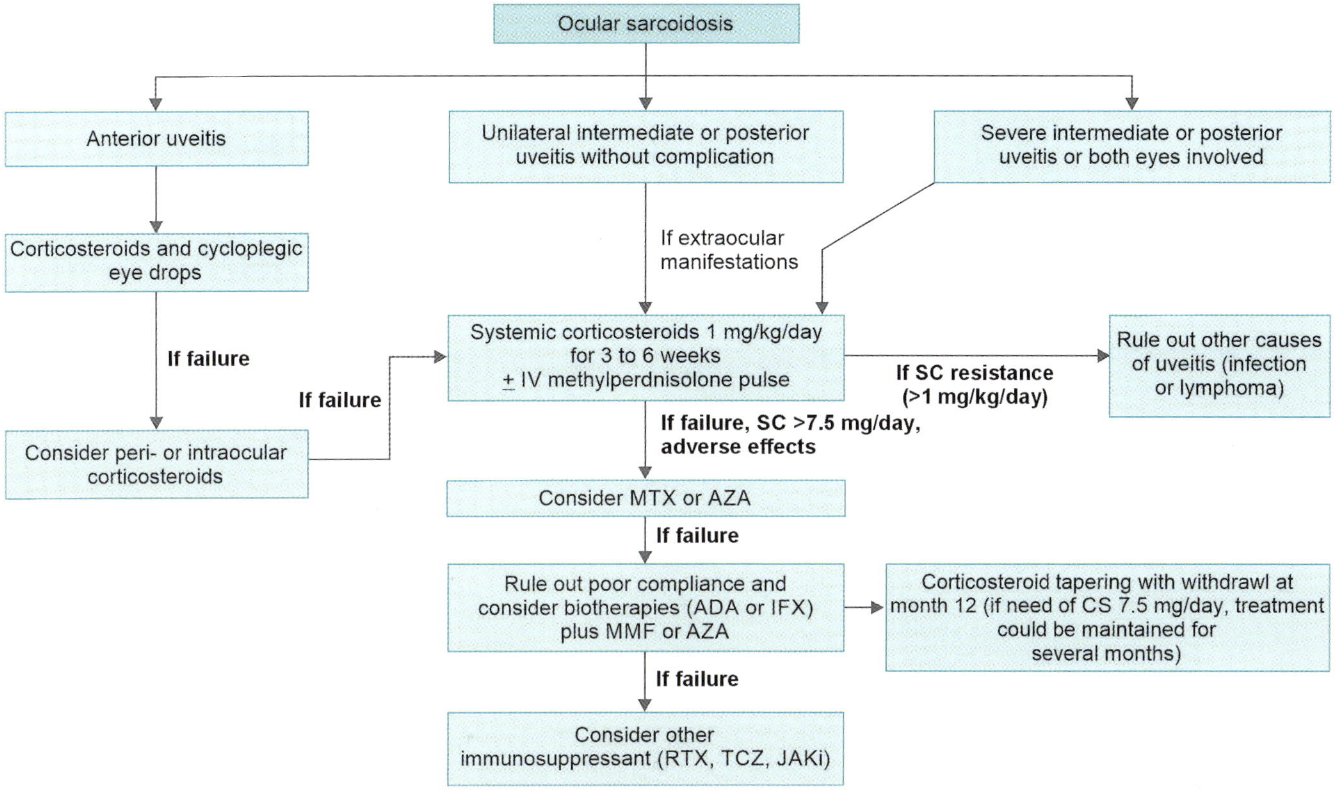

(ADA: adalimumab; AZA: azathioprine; IV: intravenous; IFX: infliximab; JAKi: Janus kinase inhibitor; MMF: mycophenolate mofetil; MTX: methotrexate; RTX: rituximab; SC: systemic corticosteroids; TCZ: tocilizumab)
Source: Adapted from Sève et al.[35]

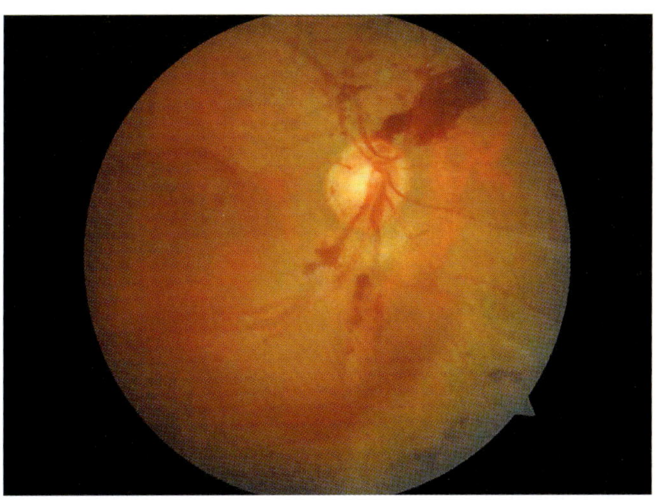

Fig. 19: A Color fundus photograph of the right eye. Vitreous and retinal hemorrhages can be seen at the superior nasal quadrant.
Source: Presented by Aurélie Le in the International Uveitis Study Group (IUSG) grand rounds.[2]

The patient was diagnosed with IU associated with MS based on the vitreous as the primary site of inflammation, the presence of peripheral vasculitis, and ischemic retinal complications. Some uveitis specialists may consider retinal vascular occlusion a reason to classify this case as a posterior uveitis. However, others consider vascular occlusions a complication of the peripheral vascular involvement that may occur with IU. This discussion

TABLE 4: Physical examination of patient having intermediate uveitis associated with multiple sclerosis.

OD	***Parameters***	***OS***
20/60	Best-corrected visual acuity (BCVA)	20/25
Clear	Cornea	Clear
No cells	Anterior chamber	No cells
Clear	Lens	Clear
Vitreous haze 2+	Vitreous	Vitreous haze 1+
Vitreous and retinal hemorrhage and vasculitis at the periphery	Fundus	Vasculitis at the periphery

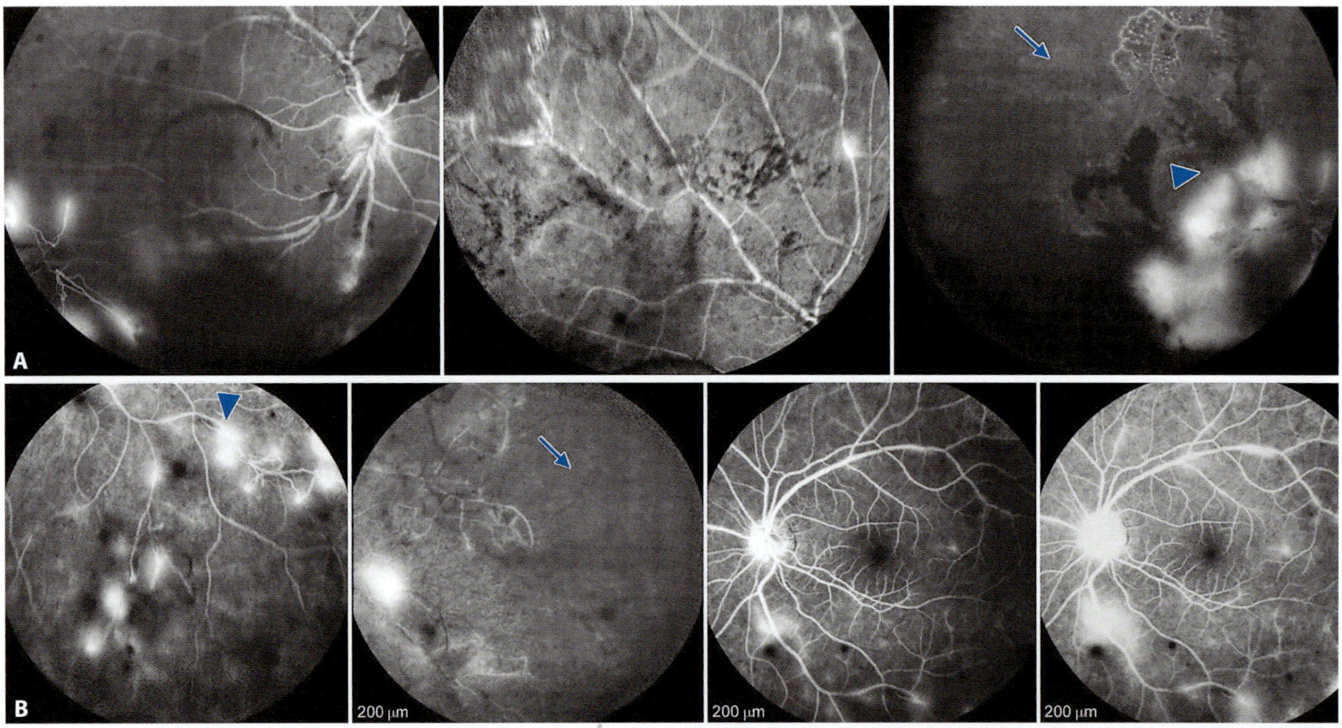

Figs. 20A and B: Fluorescein angiography showing intermediate and late phase images of the right (A) and left eye (B). Note the large ischemic areas (blue arrows) and several areas of neovascularization (blue arrowheads).
Source: Presented by Aurélie Le in the International Uveitis Study Group (IUSG) grand rounds.[1]

centers on difficulties with the term "retinal vasculitis" as to whether retinal vascular occlusion and retinal vascular sheathing fundamentally differ and belong to different forms of uveitis—which hopefully will be settled by greater consensus in due course.

The patient was started on topical, intraocular, and systemic treatment, including:

- *Topical treatment:*
  - Prednisolone, 1% eye drops once every hour
- *Intraocular treatment:*
  - Medical:
    - Corticosteroid intravitreal injections in both eyes (dexamethasone)
    - Anti-vascular endothelial growth factor (VEGF) injections in both eyes (bevacizumab) for neovascularization
  - Surgical:
    - Laser retinal photocoagulation was applied to retinal ischemic areas in both eyes.
- *Systemic treatment:*
  - Oral methylprednisolone 60 mg/day with slow tapering, until 8 mg/day

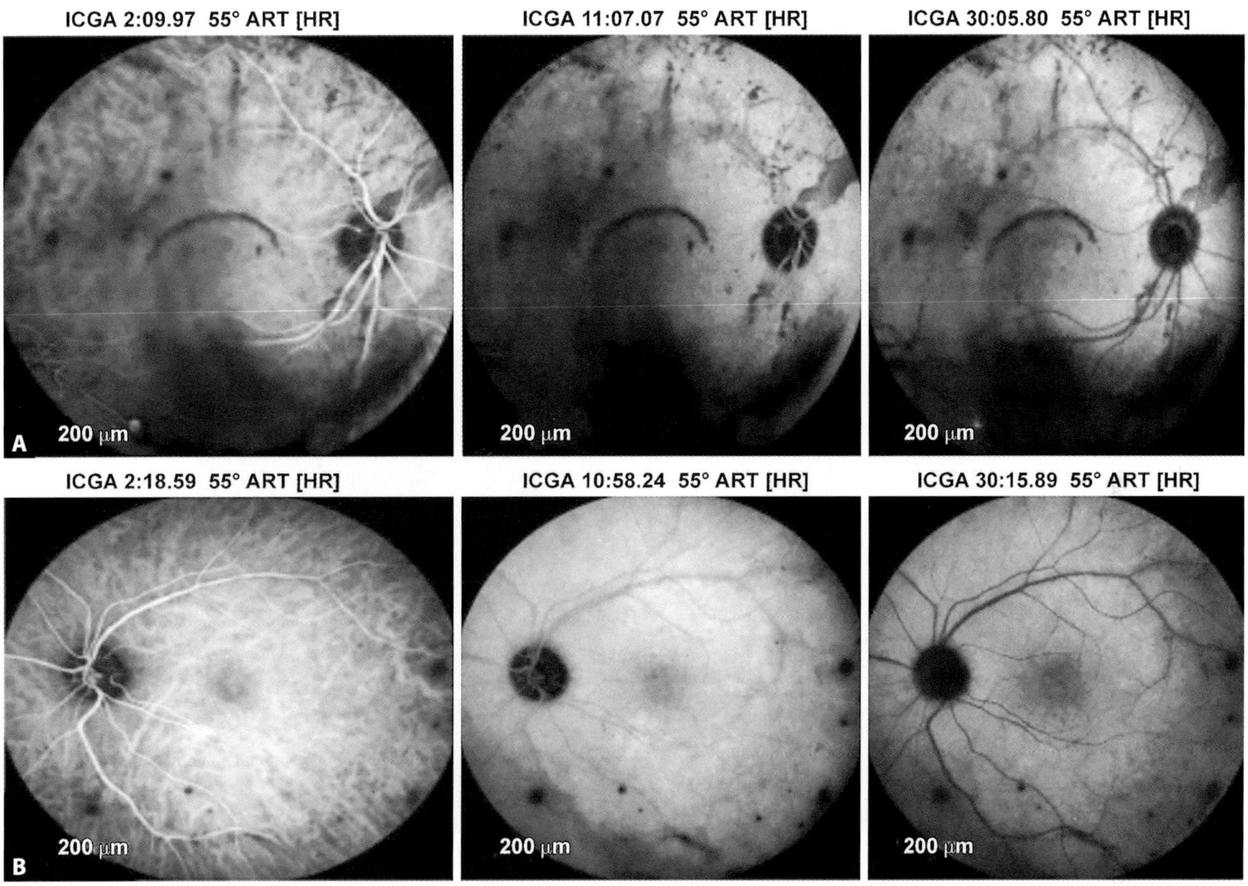

Figs. 21A and B: Indocyanine green angiography showing intermediate and late phase images of the right (A) and left eye (B). Hypocyanescent lesions correspond to blocking from blood in the vitreous. No choroidal lesions were found.
Source: Presented by Aurélie Le in the International Uveitis Study Group (IUSG) grand rounds.[1]

- Immunomodulatory therapy, starting with MTX 15 mg/week, which was then changed to MMF 1.5 g/day
- Interferon beta was not well tolerated and was replaced by ocrelizumab (humanized anti-CD20 monoclonal antibody).

Ophthalmologic follow-up showed improved VA in both eyes (20/20 OU), and imaging follow-up showed a resolution of the vitritis and vasculitis.

Discussion[1]

- Multiple sclerosis is the most prevalent chronic inflammatory disease of the CNS, affecting more than 2 million people worldwide, mostly middle-aged adults especially in temperate regions.[36,37] It is characterized by focal areas of demyelination, inflammation, and glial reaction with recurrent neurological attacks that are separated by space and time. Female sex, HLA-DR15, higher altitudes, smoking, Epstein-Barr virus (EBV), and obesity are some factors that have been related to the autoimmune reaction against the myelin-derived peptide.[36] Environmental factors play an important role in the development of autoimmune diseases. Some may trigger clonal activation of autoreactive lymphocytes in genetically susceptible patients, leading to disease development.[38]
- The clinical manifestations of MS can be partially reversible episodes of neurological impairment, such as monocular visual loss due to optic neuritis, double vision due to brainstem lesions, limb weakness or sensory loss secondary to transverse myelitis, and ataxia due to cerebellar lesions.[36,39] Neurological signs and symptoms may precede ocular inflammation in 50% of cases. Moreover, ocular inflammation (including optic neuritis) as the initial presentation accounts for 40% of cases, with the remaining 10% experiencing concomitant neurological and ocular symptoms.[40]

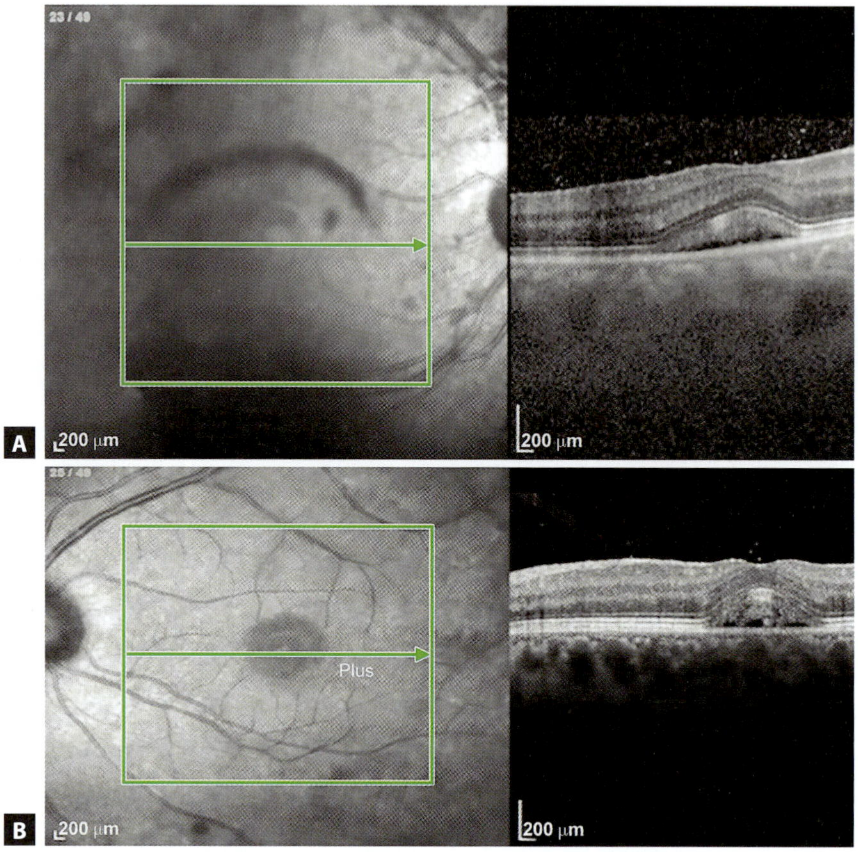

Figs. 22A and B: Optical coherence tomography (OCT) images of the right eye (A) and the left eye (B) showing serous retinal detachments under both foveas and the presence of vitreous cells.
Source: Presented by Aurélie Le in the International Uveitis Study Group (IUSG) grand rounds.[1]

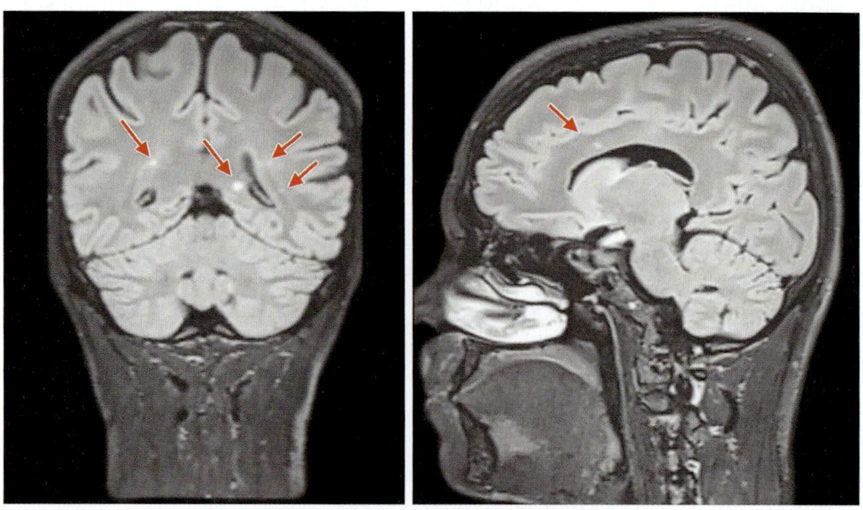

Fig. 23: Brain magnetic resonance imaging (MRI) findings. Brain MRI T2/flair: Presence of multiple non-enhancing, demyelinating lesions of the periventricular white matter (pointed with red arrows) consistent with an inflammatory demyelinating disease.
Source: Presented by Aurélie Le in the International Uveitis Study Group (IUSG) grand rounds.[1]

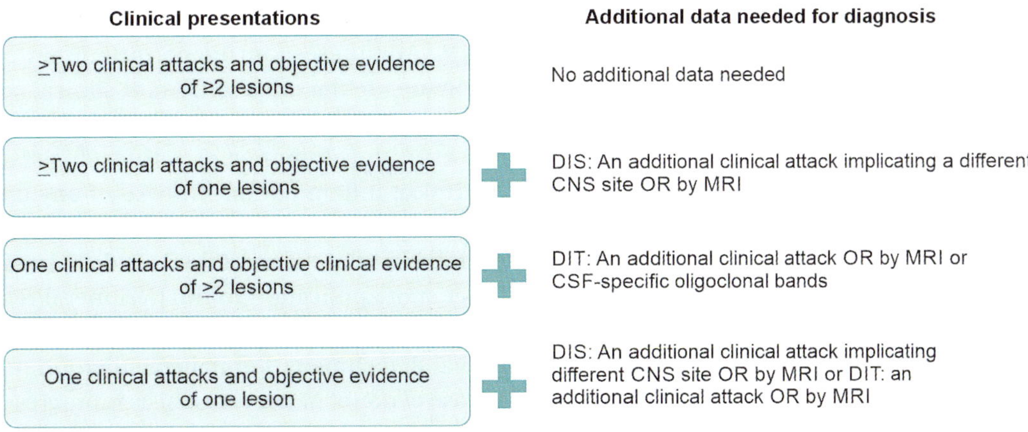

Fig. 24: McDonald MS diagnostic criteria 2017.

a. DIS by MRI: New lesions on follow-up imaging or both gadolinium-enhancing and non-enhancing lesions on a single MRI.
b. DIT by MRI: ≥One symptomatic or asymptomatic lesion in ≥two areas, including cortical/juxtacortical, periventricular, infratentorial, or spinal.

(CNS: central nervous system; CSF: cerebrospinal fluid; DIS: disseminated in space; DIT: disseminated in time; MRI: magnetic resonance imaging)
Source: Adapted from Thompson et al.[43]

- Concerning ocular involvement, uveitis and optic neuritis are prevalent. Patients with MS face a 10-fold increased risk of developing uveitis compared to the general population. Additionally, MS is diagnosed in 1–14% of patients with uveitis, most commonly presenting as IU in 52% of cases, followed by anterior uveitis in 23%.[40] Optic neuritis is observed in 30–50% of MS patients, typically presented as painful vision loss with optic disc swelling.[41]
- The diagnosis of MS is primarily based on the 2017 McDonald criteria **(Fig. 24)**, which integrates clinical and radiological evidence with the ruling out of alternate infectious and non-infectious causes of uveitis.[42] Brain MRI is the most important imaging for suspected MS.

It is important to note that for the management of cases with MS and uveitis, not only treatments directed at the inflammatory activity of the CNS, but also those specific to ocular inflammation should be considered. We should also consider the possibility of adverse effects or benefits from both treatments.

- Both MS and uveitis necessitate immunomodulatory therapy. Common medications for uveitis include methotrexate, azathioprine, MMF, and anti-TNF agents; others include TCZ and interferon alpha. Some of these treatments are also effective for managing MS. However, anti-TNF therapy and TCZ (anti-IL-6) have been linked to demyelination and are, therefore, not recommended for MS patients. Conversely, specific treatments employed for MS, such as fingolimod, have been associated with ocular complications, including CME. The impact of other therapies for MS, such as glatiramer acetate, teriflunomide, cladribine, and natalizumab, on ocular inflammation have not been extensively studied and warrant further investigation **(Table 5)**.[1] Therefore, treating uveitis associated with MS must be interdisciplinary between ophthalmologists and neurologists.[37,44-46]

TABLE 5: Treatment for multiple sclerosis (MS) and non-infectious uveitis.

Are non-infectious uveitis systemic treatments efficient in MS?	
MS	*Non-infectious uveitis*
√	Systemic corticosteroids
√	Azathioprine and MMF
X	Anti-TNF
X	Tocilizumab
IFN-β preferred	IFN-α
Are MS treatment efficient in non-infectious uveitis?	
MS	*Non-infectious uveitis*
IFN-β	IFN-α preferred
Glatiramer	?*
Teriflonomide	?*
Cladribine	?*
Natalizumab	?*
Dimethyl fumarate	?*
S1P receptors modulators	Fingolimod-associated CME reported
Anti-CD52 (alemtuzumab)	√
Anti-CD20	√

(√: indicated; X: contraindicated; ?*: unknown, further studies are required; CME: cystoid macular edema; IFN: interferon; MMF: mycophenolate mofetil; TNF: tumor necrosis factor)

PEARLS FROM THE EXPERTS ON FREQUENTLY ASKED QUESTIONS

1. What parameters determine that a patient with mild IU need not be treated?

Answer: Some consider that it is imperative to treat all patients who present with IU, regardless of the level of inflammation, to prevent progression toward a chronic phase and avoid developing severe complications that could compromise VA. Others argue that patients who show mild clinical findings, retain normal vision, and report minimal symptoms may be observed. However, in this view, therapeutic intervention is required in those cases where a decrease in VA, CME, ERM formation, or other significant ocular findings are present. The main goal should be to prevent and/or reverse the spread of these complications. The decision to treat or not treat can be made taking into consideration the age of the patients, laterality, duration of the inflammation, VA, and the presence or absence of complications. The risk–benefit ratio of treatment versus observation should be discussed with the patient and the decision made by mutual consent. For example, a 30-year-old woman with a VA of 20/20 in both eyes, mild vitreous inflammation, no inflammation in the anterior chamber, and no complications, such as CME and ERM can be observed. As one would avoid immunosuppressive therapy, especially if she would like to conceive. However, these patients should be kept under close observation with regular follow-up.

2. Can treatment of IU with systemic corticosteroid monotherapy lead to remission?

Answer: As IU is a chronic disease that often relapses with the withdrawal of suppressive treatment, the patient requires a long-acting therapy. Although corticosteroid management reduces inflammation, it is a short-term therapy; a relapse may occur when medication is stopped or reduced. Thus, treatment with immunosuppressive agents is considered the gold standard as it can be administered on long-term basis. Intermediate-term use of low-dose corticosteroids (7.5 mg/day or less prednisone or a bioequivalent) can be considered for suppressive therapy, particularly in low-income scenarios; however, this approach is *relatively* contraindicated among children because of potential growth side effects.

3. What is the treatment approach for inferior retinoschisis associated with pars planitis that is quiescent with immunosuppressive treatment?

Answer: Retinoschisis is an uncommon complication of IU. Adequate control of inflammation and strict follow-up are the most important clinical considerations. Retinoschisis, per se, does not require any intervention; however, development of retinoschisis suggests poor control of inflammation. In case of any doubt between retinal detachment and retinoschisis, one can either try peripheral OCT (if available) or do a laser uptake test. Laser spot application to the peripheral retina will show blanching in cases of retinoschisis and no change with a retinal detachment. Retinal consultation may be needed in case of doubt or if retinoschisis is progressing.

4. Is there a role for anti-VEGF in the treatment of vasoproliferative tumors (VPTs) secondary to IU?

Answer: The primary treatment must be immunosuppressive agents for inflammation control. If the vasoproliferative lesion is causing complications or seems likely to cause them, treatment such as laser photocoagulation of the tumor or possibly anti-VEGF therapy could be considered. However, intravitreal anti-VEGF injections can lead to VPT contraction and the development of a retinal detachment. If laser photocoagulation is being considered, one should be mindful to use laser burn settings that are low power and long duration.

5. Should TNF-α inhibitors be avoided in the treatment of IU?

Answer: Demyelinating diagnoses have been associated with the use of TNF-α inhibitors. Since MS is associated with IU, we should be careful not to increase the risk by prescribing TNF-α inhibitors unless the intraocular inflammation cannot be controlled with other treatments. It is important to rule out MS before initiating anti-TNF therapy if treatment is deemed necessary.

6. In the case of a patient diagnosed with sarcoid IU, with a VA of 20/20 in both eyes, mild vitreous involvement, and without any ocular complications or macular edema, is the recommendation of a systemic treatment combining oral corticosteroids with an immunomodulatory agent based on the diagnosis of sarcoidosis alone? Is the intent to treat to prevent ocular complications? Or should the treatment approach be to observation?

Answer: The answer to this question can vary significantly between specialists. The decision to administer treatment primarily depends on the presence/extent of extraocular manifestations in the scenario presented. When eye disease occurs in isolation, you may not need an intervention. Typically, a diagnosis of sarcoidosis implies systemic involvement, which would warrant treatment in many, if not most, cases.

7. How prevalent is sarcoidosis as a cause of IU in children?

Answer: Sarcoidosis is infrequently observed as a cause of IU in children. It is important to consider that ACE levels are typically elevated in the pediatric population. Thus, the diagnosis should not solely rely on this parameter. Childhood sarcoidosis is more commonly manifested as multifocal choroiditis rather than IU. Childhood sarcoidosis would also need to be differentiated from Blau syndrome.

8. Are VPTs common in cases of IU, and does extensive fibrosis present a high risk?

Answer: VPTs are indeed common in patients with a delayed diagnosis of IU and suboptimal management, which results in this complication due to poor inflammation control.

9. In recent years, some cases of IU have been linked to HLA-B27. Should HLA-B27 be included in the initial workup for IU in patients with no history of back pain or digestive symptoms?

Answer: This association has not been widely observed, and, thus, routine inclusion of HLA-B27 in the initial workup for IU has not been commonly adopted. Testing for HLA-B27 may be considered if there are clinical symptoms or signs suggestive of spondylarthritis and anterior uveitis in overlapping anterior and IU cases.

10. Given the significant anterior component of inflammation, can sarcoidosis manifest solely as IU?

Answer: While the IWOS criteria have identified sarcoidosis primarily through anterior or posterior findings, isolated IU is possible (though uncommon). Sarcoidosis should be considered if chest imaging is highly suspicious, categorizing the condition as sarcoid-related IU. Pathological confirmation in a scenario with suspicious chest imaging is desirable to provide a definitive diagnosis.

11. Is a neurology consultation recommended for patients with IU without neurological symptoms?

Answer: A neurology consultation is not generally recommended in the absence of neurological symptoms. However, it is indicated in cases presenting neurological signs or symptoms. Alternatively, it should be considered when initiating treatment with a TNF inhibitor after poor response to prior immunosuppressive agents.

12. In MS, which form of retinal vasculitis is more common: occlusive or non-occlusive?

Answer: Non-occlusive forms of retinal vasculitis are more commonly observed in patients with MS.

FINAL WRAP-UP

In conclusion:

- *Intermediate uveitis* is often (~80%) a bilateral chronic disease of insidious onset, which presents mainly as a vitreous inflammation OR with vitreous haze, snowballs, and snowbanking. The most common complications seen, in patients independent of the case of IU, are CME, disc edema, ERM, and peripheral retinal neovascularization. The low remission rate increases in patients with a previous PPV, diagnosis of IU in the last year, who are greater than 45 years of age, and are of a Hispanic race.[13]
- *In uveitis associated with sarcoidosis*, the anterior chamber is the most commonly affected location, although IU is also possible. The diagnosis can be made using the IWOS or SUN diagnostic criteria. The disease can present with decreased VA and floaters and the presence of mutton fat KPs, trabecular meshwork nodules, snowballs, and posterior/anterior synechiae. However, a biopsy demonstrating non-caseating granulomas is the gold standard for diagnosis. Chest imaging showing hilar lymphadenopathy and a high ACE level must be associated with a negative tuberculosis test, as the two diseases can have similar findings. Treatment must be directed to improving VA and decreasing or preventing structural complications. A systemic treatment approach is preferred due to the potential for multisystem involvement.
- *Multiple sclerosis* is the most common systemic disease associated with IU, at least in temperate regions; the diagnosis is made using the McDonald criteria which combines clinical, neurological, and radiological findings. Common symptoms of IU associated with MS are floaters, decreased VA, pain, and photophobia with signs such as snowballs, snowbanking, macular edema, and periphlebitis. Optic neuritis is one of the first and most common clinical manifestations of MS. When having a middle-aged patient with neurological symptoms and IU, before treatment is initiated, an MRI of the brain must be ordered to rule out MS. TNF-α inhibitors may cause demyelination and fingolimod can cause CME in patients with MS. Interdisciplinary management with the neurology service is crucial.

Systemic corticosteroids, MMF, azathioprine, anti-CD25, and anti-CD20 agents have proven value in treating both diseases.

- *Pars planitis* is an idiopathic IU seen in children, manifesting as floaters and decreased VA. The SUN criteria specify pars planitis is diagnosed in the absence of an infectious or systemic disease with the presence of vitritis and either snowballs, snowbanking, or the absence of posterior pole occlusive retinal vasculitis. Management is typically with systemic or local therapy; eye drops do not adequately reach the posterior segment to treat this condition alone. However, as clinical progression is severe and not self-limited, treatment with peri- or intraocular corticosteroids should be added to systemic therapies in cases of continued macular edema. If systemic therapy is contraindicated or incompletely effective, local therapies and surgical interventions may be necessary adjuncts.

REFERENCES

1. Uveitis Webinar - Grand Round 02. International Uveitis Study Group (IUSG). 2024. https://www.youtube.com/watch?v=zjP2f03Lqms&t=22s.
2. Moura-Coelho N. (2023). Intermediate Uveitis. Available from https://eyewiki.aao.org/Intermediate_Uveitis. [Last accessed February, 2025].
3. Davis JL. Intermediate uveitis. In: Albert DM, Miller JW, Azar DT, Young LH (Eds). Albert and Jakobiec's Principles and Practice of Ophthalmology. Cham: Springer International Publishing; 2022. pp. 4161-91.
4. Standardization of uveitis nomenclature for reporting clinical data. Results of the First International Workshop. Am J Ophthalmol. 2005;140(3):509-16.
5. Minkus CL, Pistilli M, Dreger KA, Fitzgerald TD, Payal AR, Begum H, et al. Risk of cataract in intermediate uveitis. Am J Ophthalmol. 2021;229:200-9.
6. Vidovic-Valentincic N, Kraut A, Hawlina M, Stunf S, Rothova A. Intermediate uveitis: long-term course and visual outcome. Br J Ophthalmol. 2009;93(4):477-80.
7. Nussenblatt RB, Palestine AG, Chan CC, Roberge F. Standardization of vitreal inflammatory activity in intermediate and posterior uveitis. Ophthalmology. 1985;92(4):467-71.
8. Davis JL, Madow B, Cornett J, Stratton R, Hess D, Porciatti V, et al. Scale for photographic grading of vitreous haze in uveitis. Am J Ophthalmol. 2010;150(5):637-41.e1.
9. Madow B, Galor A, Feuer WJ, Altaweel MM, Davis JL. Validation of a photographic vitreous haze grading technique for clinical trials in uveitis. Am J Ophthalmol. 2011;152(2):170-6.e1.
10. Arellanes-García L, Navarro-López LP, Recillas-Gispert C. Pars planitis in the Mexican Mestizo population: ocular findings, treatment, and visual outcome. Ocul Immunol Inflamm. 2003;11(1):53-60.
11. Prieto JF, Dios E, Gutierrez JM, Mayo A, Calonge M, Herreras JM. Pars planitis: epidemiology, treatment, and association with multiple sclerosis. Ocul Immunol Inflamm. 2001;9(2):93-102.
12. Berker N, Sen E, Elgin U, Atilgan CU, Dursun E, Yilmazbas P. Analysis of clinical features and visual outcomes of pars planitis. Int Ophthalmol. 2018;38(2):727-36.
13. Kempen JH, Sugar EA, Jaffe GJ, Acharya NR, Dunn JP, Elner SG, et al. Fluorescein angiography versus optical coherence tomography for diagnosis of uveitic macular edema. Ophthalmology. 2013;120(9):1852-9.
14. Mehta S, Hariharan L, Ho AC, Kempen JH. Peripapillary choroidal neovascularization in pars planitis. J Ophthalmic Inflamm Infect. 2013;3(1):13.
15. Gupta S, Shah DN, Joshi SN, Aryal M, Puri LR. Patterns of macular edema in uveitis as diagnosed by optical coherence tomography in tertiary eye center. Nepal J Ophthalmol. 2018;10(1):39-46.
16. Pichi F, Srivastava SK, Nucci P, Baynes K, Neri P, Lowder CY. Peripheral retinoschisis in intermediate uveitis. Retina. 2017;37(11):2167-74.
17. Malalis JF, Bhat P, Shapiro M, Goldstein DA. Retinoschisis in pars planitis. Ocul Immunol Inflamm. 2017;25(3):344-8.
18. Kempen JH, Gewaily DY, Newcomb CW, Liesegang TL, Kaçmaz RO, Levy-Clarke GA, et al. Remission of intermediate uveitis: incidence and predictive factors. Am J Ophthalmol. 2016;164:110-7.e2.
19. Jonas JB. Intravitreal triamcinolone acetonide: a change in a paradigm. Ophthalmic Res. 2006;38(4):218-45.
20. Sohn EH, Chaon BC, Jabs DA, Folk JC. Peripheral cryoablation for treatment of active pars planitis: long-term outcomes of a retrospective study. Am J Ophthalmol. 2016;162:35-42.e2.
21. Pulido JS, Mieler WF, Walton D, Kuhn E, Postel E, Hartz A, et al. Results of peripheral laser photocoagulation in pars planitis. Trans Am Ophthalmol Soc. 1998;96:127-37.
22. Kaplan HJ. Surgical treatment of intermediate uveitis. In: Böke WRF, Manthey KF, Nussenblatt RB (Eds). Developments in Ophthalmology. Basel: Karger; 1991. pp. 185-9.
23. Diala FGI, McCarthy K, Chen JL, Tsui E. Multimodal imaging in pediatric uveitis. Ophthalmol Eye Dis. 2021;13:251584142110592.
24. Dutta LC, Dutta NK. Modern Ophthalmology, 3rd edition. New Delhi: Jaypee Brothers Medical (P) Pvt. Ltd.; 2005.
25. Ozdal P, Berker N, Tugal-Tutkun I. Pars planitis: epidemiology, clinical characteristics, management and visual prognosis. J Ophthalmic Vis Res. 2015;10(4):469.
26. Foster CS, Vitale AT. Diagnosis and Treatment of Uveitis, 2nd edition. New Delhi: Jaypec Brothers Medical (P) Pvt. Ltd.; 2013. p. 1290.

27. Mochizuki M, Smith JR, Takase H, Kaburaki T, Acharya NR, Rao NA. Revised criteria of International Workshop on Ocular Sarcoidosis (IWOS) for the diagnosis of ocular sarcoidosis. Br J Ophthalmol. 2019;103(10):1418-22.
28. Giorgiutti S, Jacquot R, El Jammal T, Bert A, Jamilloux Y, Kodjikian L, et al. Sarcoidosis-related uveitis: a review. J Clin Med. 2023;12(9):3194.
29. Bodaghi B, Touitou V, Fardeau C, Chapelon C, LeHoang P. Ocular sarcoidosis. La Presse Médicale. 2012;41(6):e349-54.
30. Classification criteria for sarcoidosis-associated uveitis. Am J Ophthalmol. 2021;228:220-30.
31. Ness T, Boehringer D, Heinzelmann S. Intermediate uveitis: pattern of etiology, complications, treatment and outcome in a tertiary academic center. Orphanet J Rare Dis. 2017;12(1):81.
32. Ramdoss J, Jain A, Thejesvi GN, Biswas J. Prevalence, clinical profile, investigations, and visual outcome of sarcoid intermediate uveitis in a tertiary eye care center in South India. Indian J Ophthalmol. 2022;70(7):2454-7.
33. Elango N, Ramdoss J, Udayakumar J, Bavaskar SH, Ranganathan P, Subramaniam Rajesh B, et al. Diagnostic efficacy of elevated serum angiotensin-converting enzyme and lymphopenia between presumed sarcoid uveitis and presumed tubercular uveitis. Int Ophthalmol. 2023;43(10):3651-7.
34. Kaiser PK, Lowder CY, Sullivan P, Sanislo SR, Kosmorsky GS, Meziane MA, et al. Chest computerized tomography in the evaluation of uveitis in elderly women. Am J Ophthalmol. 2002;133(4):499-505.
35. Sève P, Jamilloux Y, Tilikete C, Gerfaud-Valentin M, Kodjikian L, El Jammal T. Ocular sarcoidosis. Semin Respir Crit Care Med. 2020;41(5):673-88.
36. Reich DS, Lucchinetti CF, Calabresi PA. Multiple sclerosis. N Engl J Med. 2018;378(2):169-80.
37. Abraham A, Nicholson L, Dick A, Rice C, Atan D. Intermediate uveitis associated with MS: diagnosis, clinical features, pathogenic mechanisms, and recommendations for management. Neurol Neuroimmunol Neuroinflamm. 2021;8(1):e909.
38. Fathman CG, Soares L, Chan SM, Utz PJ. An array of possibilities for the study of autoimmunity. Nature. 2005;435(7042):605-11.
39. Brownlee WJ, Hardy TA, Fazekas F, Miller DH. Diagnosis of multiple sclerosis: progress and challenges. Lancet. 2017;389(10076):1336-46.
40. Brézin AP. (2010). Les Uvéites. Available from https://linkinghub.elsevier.com/retrieve/pii/C20110094516. [Last accessed February, 2025].
41. Frohman EM, Frohman TC, Zee DS, McColl R, Galetta S. The neuro-ophthalmology of multiple sclerosis. Lancet Neurol. 2005;4(2):111-21.
42. Grumet P, Kodjikian L, de Parisot A, Errera MH, Sedira N, Heron E, et al. Contribution of diagnostic tests for the etiological assessment of uveitis, data from the ULISSE study (uveitis: clinical and medicoeconomic evaluation of a standardized strategy of the etiological diagnosis). Autoimmun Rev. 2018;17(4):331-43.
43. Thompson AJ, Banwell BL, Barkhof F, Carroll WM, Coetzee T, Comi G, et al. Diagnosis of multiple sclerosis: 2017 revisions of the McDonald criteria. Lancet Neurol. 2018;17(2):162-73.
44. Dick AD, Rosenbaum JT, Al-Dhibi HA, Belfort R, Brézin AP, Chee SP, et al. Guidance on noncorticosteroid systemic immunomodulatory therapy in noninfectious uveitis. Ophthalmology. 2018;125(5):757-73.
45. Velazquez-Villoria D, Macia-Badia C, Segura-García A, Pastor-Idoate SP, Arcos-Algaba G, Velez-Escola L, et al. Eficacia del tratamiento inmunomodulador con interferón-β o acetato de glatirámero en las uveítis asociadas a esclerosis múltiple. Archivos de la Sociedad Española de Oftalmología. 2017;92(6):273-9.
46. Hedayatfar A, Falavarjani KG, Soheilian M, Elmi Sadr N, Modarres M, Parvaresh MM, et al. Mycophenolate mofetil for the treatment of multiple sclerosis-associated uveitis. Ocul Immunol Inflamm. 2017;25(3):308-14.

CHAPTER

3 Posterior Uveitis

Carlos Pavesio, Katerina Lazari, Sofia Androudi, Charlotte van Meerwijk, Marc de Smet, Araniko Pandey, Janet Davis, Germán Mejía-Salgado, Meghan Berkenstock, Vishali Gupta, John H Kempen, Alejandra de-la-Torre

INTRODUCTION[1]

Posterior uveitis is a term that denotes the primary site of inflammation is the choroid or the retina.[2] It represents 15–30% of the total uveitis cases worldwide, outnumbered only by anterior uveitis, and accounting for around 50% of all cases.[3] Inflammation in posterior uveitis can result in focal, multifocal, or diffuse choroiditis. Alternatively, it can also manifest as chorioretinitis, retinochoroiditis, retinitis, neuroretinitis, or retinal vasculitis. It could be secondary to infectious, non-infectious, or malignant processes; therefore, its diagnosis and treatment are challenging and complex.[1]

PRACTICAL TIPS IN THE MANAGEMENT OF POSTERIOR UVEITIS[1]

Diagnosis in posterior uveitis. How to test? What to order?

When facing a patient with uveitis, it is crucial to consider the patient's whole clinical picture to make the diagnosis, including social history, initial symptoms, and signs, as well as a full slit-lamp and fundoscopic examination. These initial clinical findings provide a foundational understanding of the disease's natural course without any intervention, providing valuable information for the diagnosis. Additionally, the history and clinical examination (ocular and systemic) will guide further investigations needed to obtain the diagnosis.[1,4]

The rationale behind ancillary tests lies primarily in the need to rule out infectious diseases or potential masquerades. While lymphoma ranks high on the list of concerns, various other masquerades warrant exclusion.[5] The main objective of investigative measures in uveitis is to avoid mismanagement. Administering antibiotics to a non-infectious process inadvertently delays appropriate treatment. Conversely, immunosuppression in the context of an infectious disease could lead to a catastrophic outcomes.[6] Moreover, the overlook of malignancies could lead to severe consequences, including death.

A comprehensive diagnostic approach is recommended for all patients presenting with uveitis. However, some uveitis specialists suggest that initial testing may be unnecessary in specific instances, such as the first episode of mild, non-granulomatous, acute anterior uveitis in otherwise healthy individuals.[1] Furthermore, diagnostic testing may be redundant in cases where the etiology of uveitis has been previously established. For example:

- A patient with acute anterior uveitis, a known history of ankylosing spondylitis, and human leukocyte antigen (HLA)-B27 positivity may not require further testing.
- A patient with unilateral hypertensive uveitis and atrophic iritis suggests a viral etiology.
- A patient presenting with panuveitis and a history of trauma in the contralateral eye is likely experiencing sympathetic ophthalmia.
- A patient displaying retinochoroidal scars with satellite lesions is indicative of ocular toxoplasmosis.

Diagnostic testing should be targeted and based on a comprehensive evaluation, including a thorough review of the patient's medical history, systemic signs and symptoms, and ocular manifestations. Structured questionnaires assessing each of these clinical endpoints can guide the clinician in deciding the necessity and extent of diagnostic testing.[7]

A practical approach to diagnostic assessment in uveitis involves pattern-based learning, which entails recognizing uveitis entities associated with specific clinical features such as dermatological or neurological manifestations, hypopyon, ischemia, or retinal vasculitis to narrow the probable diagnoses. For instance, dermatological manifestations can limit the differential diagnoses to conditions such as syphilis, systemic lupus erythematosus (SLE), varicella, Vogt–Koyanagi–Harada (VKH) syndrome, psoriasis, Lyme disease, sarcoidosis, and Behçet's disease. Notably, a phenomenon emerging in recent literature is the association between ocular inflammation and tattoos, underscoring the need to consider external factors in assessing ocular inflammation.[1,8]

In posterior uveitis, classic signs guide the differential diagnosis, such as retinal scars in ocular toxoplasmosis, Dalen–Fuchs nodules in VKH syndrome or sympathetic ophthalmia, a macular star in *Bartonella*-associated neuroretinitis and a posterior granuloma with vitreous bands with toxocariasis **(Figs. 1A to F)**. When evaluating retinal vasculitis, determining the type of vessel involved is critical. Collagen diseases, SLE, and Susac syndrome predominantly affect arteries, whereas Behçet disease, ocular toxoplasmosis, acute retinal necrosis, tuberculosis, and syphilis can involve both arteries and veins. Exclusive venous involvement is particularly seen in multiple sclerosis or sarcoidosis.[1,9]

Drug-induced uveitis is another important consideration, although relatively uncommon. A thorough inquiry into the patient's medication history can unveil potential correlations between the drug regimen and ocular manifestations. Systemic medications such as cidofovir, used as a treatment for cytomegalovirus (CMV) retinitis, can pose serious complications to the eye, including hypotony. It is essential to be mindful of drugs such as rifabutin, bisphosphonates, and antitumor necrosis factor (TNF) inhibitors, as they are increasingly associated with the development of non-infectious uveitis particularly etanercept.[10] Furthermore, intraocular medications such as triamcinolone acetonide and antivascular endothelial growth factor (VEGF) therapies can induce inflammation, emphasizing the need to avoid injecting inflamed eyes. Additionally, certain topical medications such as metipranolol, betaxolol, and brimonidine can

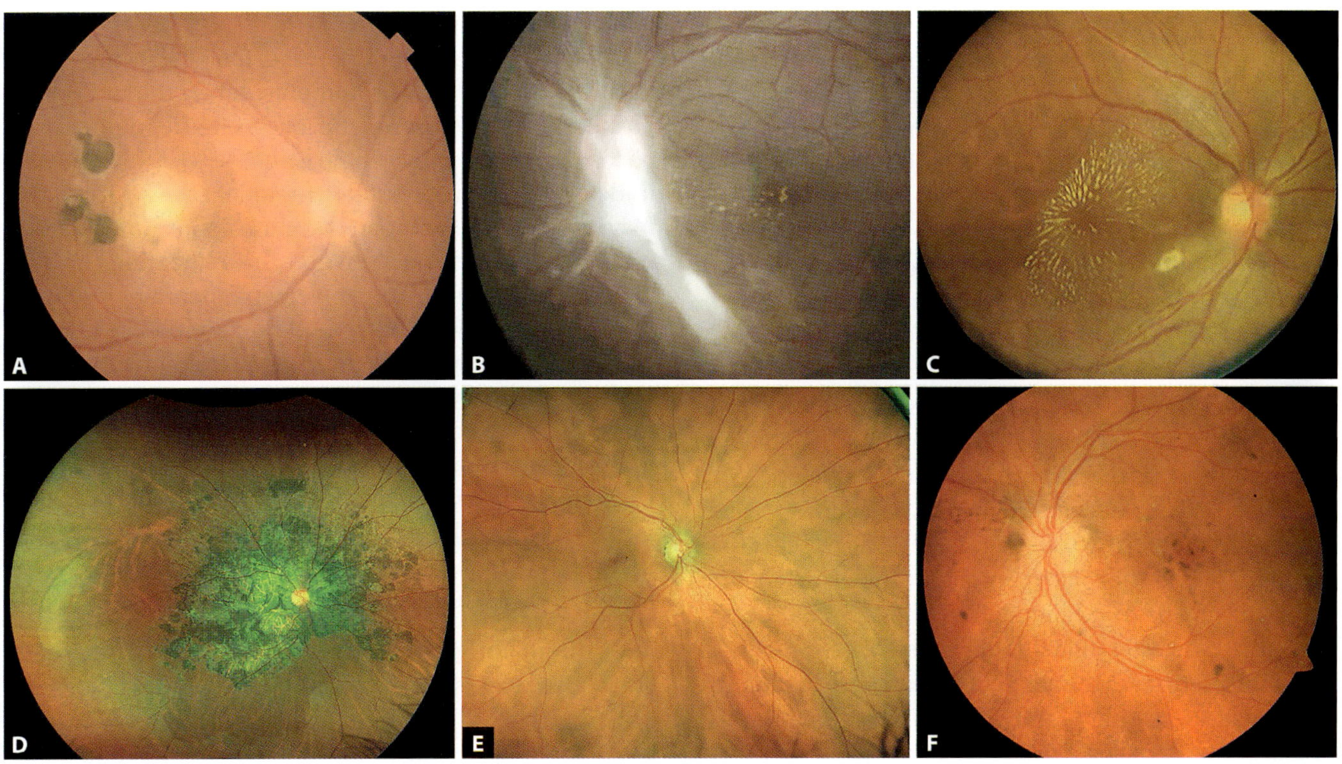

Figs. 1A to F: Clinical picture of fundus in common uveitis etiologies. (A) Retinal scars surrounded by satellite macular yellow-white lesions indicative of ocular toxoplasmosis; (B) Fibrotic band characteristic of *Toxocara canis* infection; (C) Macular star, a hallmark of neuroretinitis, is frequently associated with *Bartonella henselae* infections; (D) Serpiginous choroiditis showcasing areas of white subretinal fibrosis; (E) Birdshot chorioretinopathy with the classic yellow, ovoid spots clustered in the posterior pole; (F) Pigment migration, a chronic feature of Vogt–Koyanagi–Harada syndrome (sunset glow).

TABLE 1: The Naranjo criteria for establishing the association between a medication and an adverse reaction.

Criteria	*Yes*	*No*	*Do not know*
Have there been previous conclusive reports on this reaction?	+1	0	0
Did the adverse event appear after the suspected drug was administered?	+2	−1	0
Did the adverse reaction improve when the drug was discontinued or a specific antagonist was administered?	+1	0	0
Did the adverse reaction reappear when the drug was readministered?	+2	−1	0
Are there alternative causes (other than the drug) that could, on their own, have caused the reaction?	−1	+2	0
Did the reaction reappear when a placebo was given?	−1	+1	0
Was the drug detected in the blood (or other fluids) in concentrations known to be toxic?	+1	0	0
Was the reaction more severe when the dose was increased or less severe when the dose was decreased?	+1	0	0
Did the patient react similarly to the same or similar drugs in any previous exposure?	+1	0	0
Did any objective evidence confirm the adverse event?	+1	0	0
Total score: 0–13 (definitive: 9–13, probable: 5–8, possible: 1–4, doubtful: 0)			

Source: Presented and taken from Carlos Pavesio[1] in the International Uveitis Study Group (IUSG) grand rounds; Adapted from Naranjo et al.[11]

also induce the onset of uveitis and should be used cautiously.[10] Establishing an association between drug use and uveitis can be aided by the use of the Naranjo criteria **(Table 1),** which helps determine the probability of such an association based on a 13 point questionnaire. This approach can assist in assessing the likelihood of the association being definite, probable, possible, or doubtful.[11]

Regarding vaccines, amidst the heightened awareness surrounding the COVID-19 pandemic, it is imperative to acknowledge potential associations between vaccination and ocular inflammation.[12] While reports have emerged, suggesting a link between the hepatitis B vaccination and uveitis, similar associations have also been noted with other vaccines including the human papillomavirus (HPV), influenza, measles, mumps, and rubella (MMR), varicella, Bacillus Calmette-Guérin (BCG), and COVID-19.[13] However, it is crucial to weigh the benefits against the risks, and if there is no absolute contraindication, vaccinations should always be recommended.

Further investigation should cease once a diagnosis is established, and the clinical picture is satisfactorily addressed. Retesting is warranted if there are changes in disease patterns or if test results are incongruent with clinical judgment.[1] In complex cases where the diagnosis remains elusive or multiple pathologies are suspected, a biopsy may be necessary to elucidate the underlying cause. This is particularly critical in scenarios such as suspected lymphoma, where biopsy confirms the diagnosis and aids in excluding systemic involvement, emphasizing the importance of comprehensive evaluation and tailored management strategies.[14]

Furthermore, the importance of imaging techniques in facilitating the diagnosis and elucidating the underlying pathophysiology cannot be overstated. Angiography, particularly with indocyanine green (ICG), is instrumental in detecting covert or subtle choroidal abnormalities that may not be clinically apparent. In the context of vasculitis, imaging modalities are pivotal in delineating the type and severity of vascular involvement, including detection of occlusions **(Figs. 2A to C)**. For example, in birdshot chorioretinopathy (BCR), imaging documents the extent of disease activity and differentiates between active and inactive lesions across the choroid and retinal vessels. Wide-field imaging stands out for its capacity to provide a panretinal assessment for critical details that conventional photography might miss. Therefore, integrating advanced imaging techniques is essential for a thorough evaluation and precise diagnosis in cases of uveitis.

Treatment in posterior uveitis; How to manage infectious uveitis versus non-infectious?

In both cases, the treatment objectives are the following:

- To identify the cause and control active inflammation
- To prevent recurrent episodes
- To prevent loss of visual function
- To prevent and treat complications such as cystoid macular edema (CME), cataracts, and glaucoma
- To avoid collateral damage as much as possible

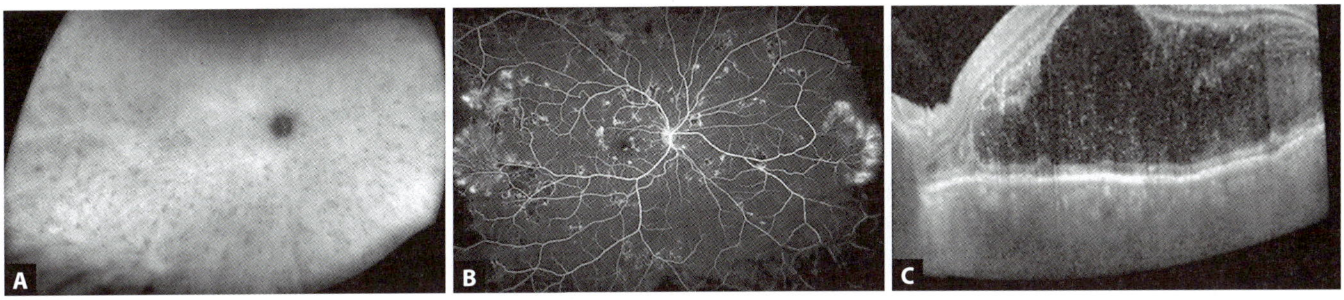

Figs. 2A to C: Multimodal imaging in posterior uveitis. (A) Diffuse choroiditis in birdshot chorioretinopathy, highlighted by indocyanine green angiography; (B) Tubercular choroiditis with peripheral neovascularization, revealed through fluorescein angiography; (C) Serous retinal detachment characteristic of Vogt–Koyanagi–Harada disease.
Source: Presented and taken from Carlos Pavesio in the International Uveitis Study Group (IUSG) grand rounds.[1]

Some factors affecting treatment decisions include:

- Location, severity, and duration of the inflammation
- Evaluation of visual acuity (VA) and the prospect of reversibility
- Laterality of the disease
- Presence of a concurrent systemic disease that requires immunosuppression
- General health of the patient
- Potential drug-related adverse events and interactions
- Secondary effects of treatment on comorbid conditions
- Patient compliance

In infectious uveitis, appropriate treatment with antimicrobial therapy is essential to ensure adequate clinical resolution. For cases of viral retinitis, corticosteroid use is only considered after 24 hours after initiation of local and systemic therapy, and for toxoplasmosis, 24–48 hours following initiation of antibiotic therapy.[15] However, for other infections, such as syphilis or TB, corticosteroid therapy may be initiated alongside antimicrobial treatment with close clinical monitoring. It is crucial to refrain from using corticosteroids in fungal infections and to remain vigilant for immune recovery reactions associated with previous infectious processes.[16]

For non-infectious uveitis, treatment strategies are tailored based on the location and severity of the uveitis while considering the patient's overall health and age. Local corticosteroids, particularly topical for anterior disease and intravitreal injections for posterior involvement, are primary options. Systemic therapy with corticosteroids may be necessary in some instances along with immunosuppressants and biologics. Compliance with treatment regimens is critical for successful management.[17]

Local therapy is indicated in unilateral or asymmetric cases where the eye itself is the sole reason for treatment. It can be used as an adjunctive therapy or when there are contraindications or intolerances to systemic treatment.

TABLE 2: Immunosuppressants.

Class of treatment	***Examples***
Corticosteroids	• Dexamethasone • Triamcinolone acetonide • Fluocinolone acetonide • Prednisolone (methylprednisolone sodium)
T-cell inhibitors	• Cyclosporine • Tacrolimus • Voclosporin
Alkylating agents	• Cyclophosphamide • Chlorambucil
Antimetabolites	• Azathioprine • Methotrexate • Mycophenolate mofetil
Biologic antitumor necrosis factor (TNF) agents	• Infliximab • Adalimumab • Etanercept • Certolizumab • Golimumab
Other biologic agents	• Daclizumab • Rituximab • Abatacept • Tocilizumab

Source: Presented and taken from Carlos Pavesio[1] in the International Uveitis Study Group (IUSG) grand rounds; Adapted from Durrani et al.[18] and Denniston et al.[19]

Additionally, local treatment is particularly pertinent for certain uveitis entities, such as intermediate uveitis and retinal vasculitis. The available options for local treatment include topical (drops), periocular injections (subconjunctival, sub-Tenon's, orbital floor), intraocular injections (intravitreal), and intraocular slow-release devices (dexamethasone—Ozurdex® and fluocinolone acetonide—Retisert®, Iluvien®).[17]

In terms of systemic therapy options, several alternatives are available for consideration **(Table 2)**. Initially, oral corticosteroids are often prescribed, followed by antimetabolites and T-cell modulators. However, there is a growing preference for biologics due to their increasing effectiveness and fewer side effects than traditional medications, such as alkylating agents, which are now rarely used. It is crucial to administer corticosteroids at adequate doses to achieve the desired outcomes, avoiding low doses that may not be effective, and considering intravenous administration for acute presentations. Immunosuppressive agents are valuable for achieving control of the uveitis, particularly when corticosteroids alone are insufficient; however, side effects may limit use and require expert monitoring. Biologic therapies, including adalimumab, are gaining popularity and proving useful across various medical specialties, including ophthalmology. Although the experience with biologics in ophthalmology is still limited, they offer promising benefits.[1]

When managing choroidal neovascularization-associated inflammation, combining anti-VEGF and corticosteroid therapy prevents recurrences without requiring a loading regimen. Patient preferences and quality-of-life considerations should guide treatment decisions, emphasizing a balanced approach that considers the condition's diagnosis, anatomic location, and severity. Combining different treatment approaches may offer better control with fewer side effects.

INFECTIOUS POSTERIOR UVEITIS[1]

Case Presentation

Personal Data

- Female, 57 years old.
- Previous history of diabetes, a recent fungal genital infection, and a urologic procedure to remove renal calculi 1 month prior. At the presentation, the patient was wearing a J-stent urinary catheter.

History of Present Illness

The patient was referred for a second opinion with a diagnosis of severe posterior uveitis in both eyes (OU).

Physical Examination (Table 3 and Fig. 3)

TABLE 3: Physical examination of the patient having infectious posterior uveitis.

OD	*Parameter*	*OS*
Counting fingers	BCVA	Counting fingers
15 mm Hg	IOP	17 mm Hg
Normal	Conjunctiva	Normal
Mutton-fat KP	Cornea	Pigments KP over the endothelium
ACC: 0.5+, open angle	Anterior chamber	ACC: 0.5+, open angle
Normal	Iris	Normal
Clear	Lens	Clear
Vitreous cells 3+, white fluffy masses, and a "string of pearls"	Vitreous	Vitreous cells 3+, white fluffy masses, and a "string of pearls"
Normal	Fundus	Vitreous haze

(ACC: anterior chamber cellularity; BCVA: best-corrected visual acuity; IOP: intraocular pressure; KP: keratic precipitate)

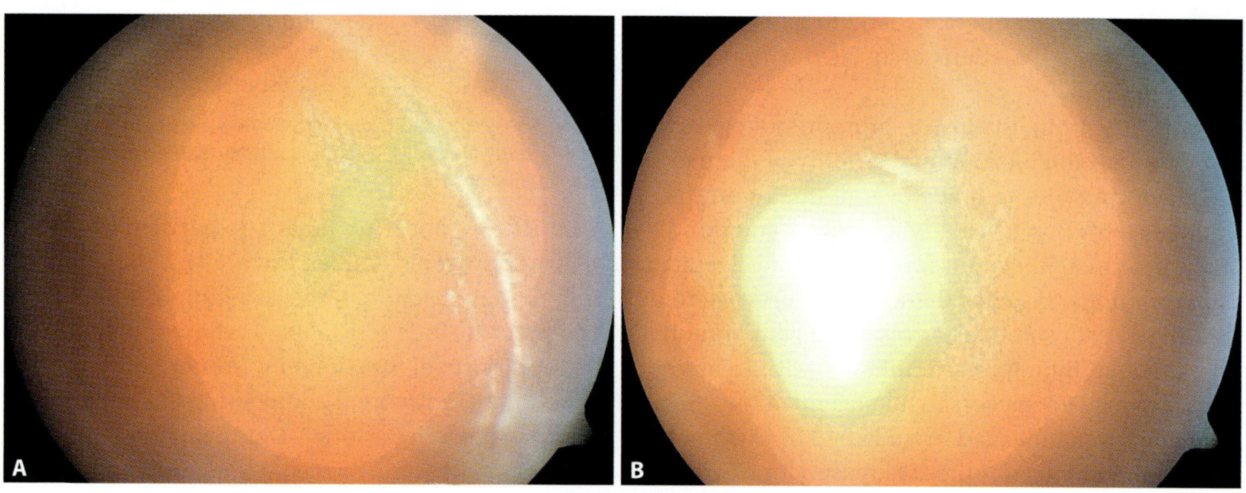

Figs. 3A and B: Initial clinical picture of intense vitreous haze in the right (A) and left (B) eye.
Source: Presented by Katerina Lazari in the International Uveitis Study Group (IUSG) grand rounds.[1]

Suspected Diagnosis

Fungal endophthalmitis.

Treatment

Immediate action was taken, including blood and urine cultures, catheter removal for culture, and initiation of intravenous fluconazole. Bilateral pars plana core vitrectomy and intravitreal injection of amphotericin B were also performed within the first 24 hours.

Following surgery, both urine and catheter cultures were positive for *Candida albicans*, confirming the fungal source. However, vitreous cultures were negative for fungi. Post core vitrectomy, the foci of inflammation remained active in both eyes **(Figs. 4A and B)**. Optical coherence tomography (OCT) revealed a focal macular lesion with subsequent posterior shadow in the right eye **(Fig. 4C)** and focal traction with a retinal detachment in the left eye **(Fig. 4D)**. Therefore, the patient underwent a second pars plana vitrectomy (PPV) with intraocular administration of amphotericin B. Additionally, silicone oil was placed in the left eye to prevent further retinal detachment. Retinal anatomy improved in both eyes with residual hyperreflective zones in the ellipsoid layer **(Figs. 4E and F)**.

Following the second PPV, the patient received four additional bilateral intraocular injections of amphotericin B and systemic fluconazole administration. This treatment regimen improved the retinal architecture, culminating in a final VA of 20/200 OU **(Fig. 5A and B)**.

Case Presentation

Personal Data

- Female, 60 years old.
- Previous history of chronic pancreatitis, chronic obstructive pulmonary disease, and hypertension. Additionally, the patient recently underwent an embolectomy in the right lower leg with post-operative bleeding. She also received pembrolizumab, paclitaxel and carboplatin chemotherapies for squamous cell lung carcinoma.

History of Present Illness

Two months after the embolectomy, the patient reported a decreased VA in the right eye. Elsewhere, the patient was diagnosed with branch retinal vein occlusion with macular edema. One month later, the patient developed moderate vitritis and presented to our clinic for a second opinion.

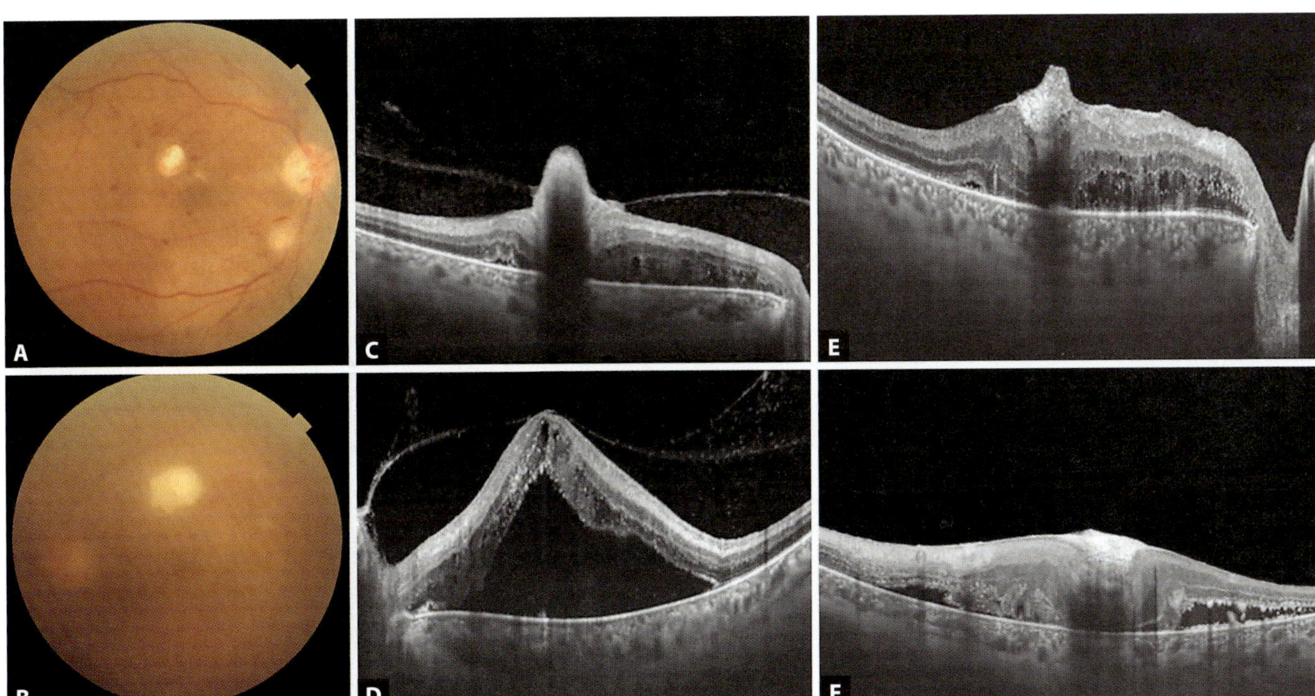

Figs. 4A to F: Follow-up. Funduscopy of the right eye (A) and left eye (B) after the first PPV with corresponding OCT images (C and D). Retinal thickness and architecture improvement after the second PPV (E and F). (OCT: optical coherence tomography; PPV: pars plana vitrectomy)

Source: Presented by Katerina Lazari in the International Uveitis Study Group (IUSG) grand rounds.[1]

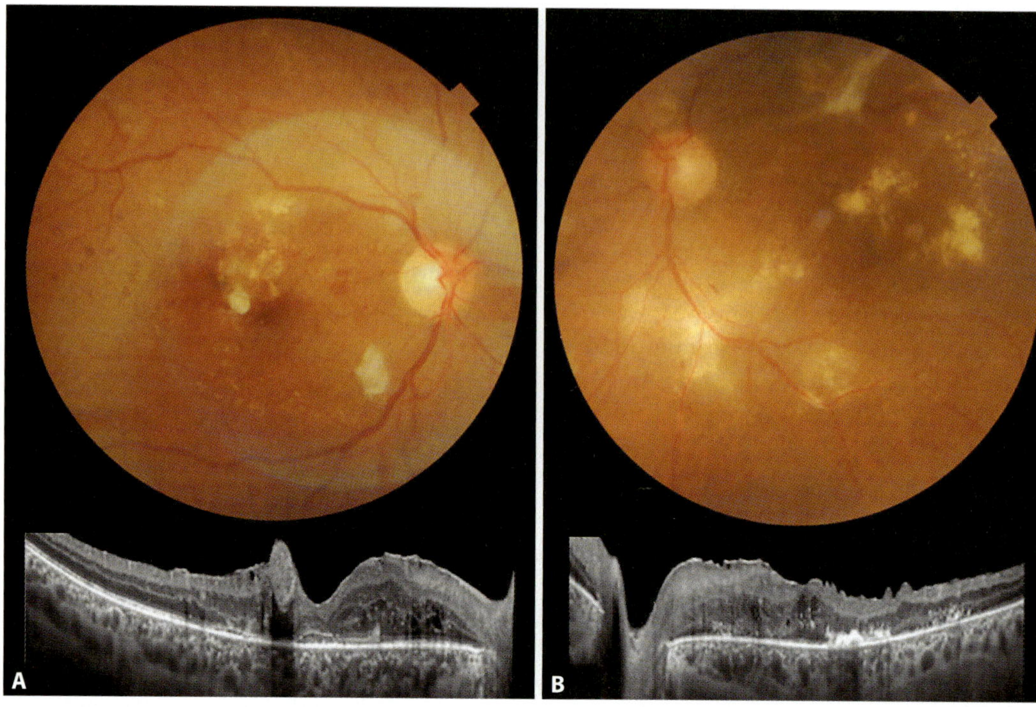

Figs. 5A and B: Color fundus photos of both eyes taken at the final follow-up for fungal posterior uveitis in the right (A) and left (B) eye. *Source:* Presented by Katerina Lazari in the International Uveitis Study Group (IUSG) grand rounds.[1]

Physical Examination (Table 4 and Fig. 6)

TABLE 4: Physical examination of the patient having infectious posterior uveitis.

OD	*Parameter*	*OS*
Counting fingers	BCVA	20/20
15 mm Hg	IOP	15 mm Hg
Normal	Conjunctiva	Normal
Clear	Cornea	Clear
ACC: 1+, open angle	Anterior chamber	ACC: 0+, open angle
Normal	Iris	Normal
Clear	Lens	Clear
Vitreous cells 3+	Vitreous	Normal
Macular cotton–wool-like spots	Fundus	Normal

(ACC: anterior chamber cellularity; BCVA: best-corrected visual acuity; IOP: intraocular pressure)

Suspected Diagnosis

Infectious posterior uveitis.

Management

Infectious etiologies were assessed via polymerase chain reaction (PCR), Goldmann–Witmer coefficient, and serologic tests for herpes simplex virus (HSV), varicella-zoster virus (VZV), CMV, rubella, and *Toxoplasma gondii*, along with a chest X-ray. All of which were negative or normal. Subsequently, the patient was started on oral corticosteroids at 30 mg/day. Despite this treatment, the lesions persisted and progressed, raising the suspicion for an infectious etiology. A diagnostic and therapeutic PPV was then performed, identifying *Candida albicans* hyphae. As a result, the patient was treated with one intravitreal injection of amphotericin B and systemic fluconazole for 8 weeks. No systemic focus of infection was identified, as blood and urine cultures were negative. Although the infection was controlled, vision did not improve due to the central location of the lesion.

Case Presentation

Personal Data

- Male, 69 years old

History of Present Illness

The patient recently returned from Gran Canaria, Spain, where he felt tired, had reduced appetite, and subsequently experienced loss of vision in the left eye.

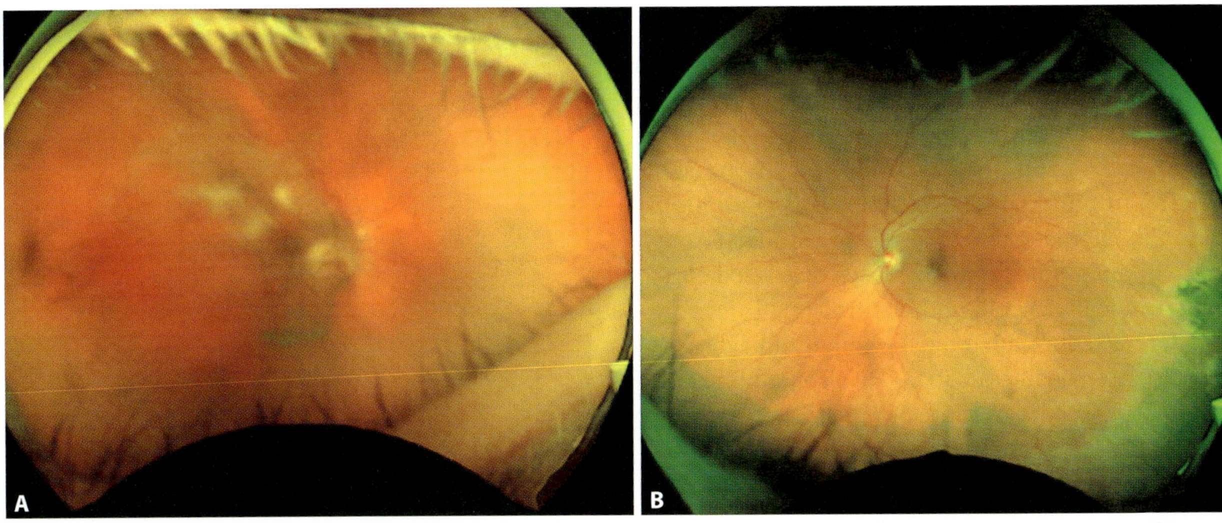

Figs. 6A and B: Initial clinical picture. (A) Vitreous haze and macular cotton–wool-like spots in the posterior pole of the right eye; (B) Fundoscopy was normal in the left eye.
Source: Presented by Charlotte van Meerwijk in the International Uveitis Study Group (IUSG) grand rounds.[1]

Physical Examination (Table 5 and Fig. 7)

TABLE 5: Physical examination of the patient having infectious posterior uveitis.

OD	Parameter	OS
20/25	BCVA	Light perception
15 mm Hg	IOP	17 mm Hg
Normal	Conjunctiva	Normal
Clear	Cornea	Clear
No cells, open angle	Anterior chamber	Fibrin in the anterior chamber
Normal	Iris	Normal
Clear	Lens	Moderate cataract
Normal	Vitreous	Vitreous cells 4+
Normal	Fundus	Multiple hemorrhages with extensive vascular sheathing

(ACC: anterior chamber cellularity; BCVA: best-corrected visual acuity; IOP: intraocular pressure)

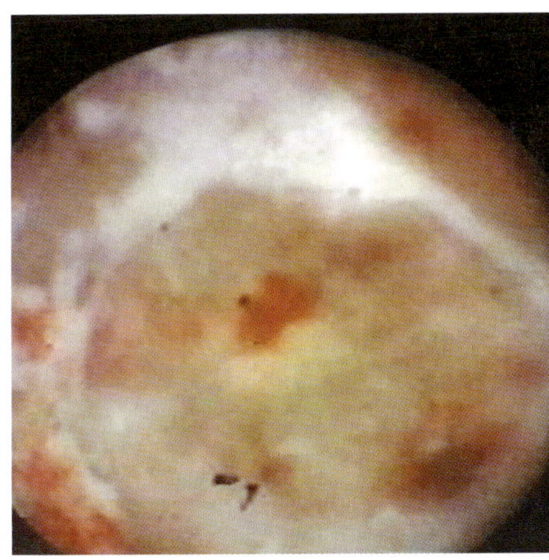

Fig. 7: Initial clinical picture. Fundoscopy of the left eye revealed intense vitritis, multiple intraretinal hemorrhages, and extensive vascular sheathing.
Source: Presented by Charlotte van Meerwijk in the International Uveitis Study Group (IUSG) grand rounds.[1]

Suspected Diagnosis

Infectious posterior uveitis.

Management

A diagnostic and therapeutic PPV was performed and a vitreous sample was sent for Giemsa staining, culture, and pathological examination. In addition, treatment was initiated with an intravitreal injection of ceftazidime, vancomycin, and intravenous fluoroquinolones.

After the first day of treatment, the patient reported reduced discomfort. By the second day, the hypopyon and inflammation had decreased noticeably. Microbiological analysis eventually identified *Streptococcus milleri* as the causative agent. Although the bacteria was susceptible to the antibiotic treatments, the vision did not improve due to the central location of the lesion.

Discussion

Endophthalmitis is classified into two types: (1) exogenous and (2) endogenous. Exogenous endophthalmitis originates from an external source, such as keratitis, trauma, or intraocular surgery, and typically presents unilaterally. In contrast, endogenous endophthalmitis arises from the hematogenous spread of pathogens, often leading to bilateral infection. The cases discussed earlier exemplify endogenous endophthalmitis.[1]

Endogenous endophthalmitis, whether of bacterial or fungal in origin, constitutes up to 20% of all endophthalmitis cases. Fungal infections are more prevalent, accounting for 11.1–17.54% of cases,[20] particularly in tropical climates,[21] with *Candida* species being the most common etiology. *Aspergillus* infections are frequently linked to trauma or surgical interventions and are known to cause severe inflammation, whereas *Fusarium* endophthalmitis usually develops after keratitis.[21] Regarding bacterial infections, methicillin-resistant *Staphylococcus aureus* and *Escherichia coli* are among the most frequent pathogens.[22]

Key risk factors for endogenous endophthalmitis include diabetes mellitus, which affects approximately 50% of patients; cancer, which affects 12–33%; and intravenous drug use, which affects 8–43% of cases.[22] Patients with fungal endophthalmitis, particularly those caused by mold species, often have histories of iatrogenic immunosuppression, organ transplantation, or the presence of an indwelling venous line.[23]

Additional factors associated with endogenous endophthalmitis include:[24,25]

- Human immunodeficiency virus (HIV) and other immunosuppressive diseases
- Broad-spectrum antibiotic therapy
- Corticosteroid therapy and other immunosuppressive therapies
- Gastrointestinal trauma or surgery
- Intravenous hyperalimentation
- Indwelling intravenous catheters
- Neutropenia
- Renal insufficiency
- Recent hospitalization
- Organ transplant
- Hemodialysis
- Pregnancy, abortion, and postpartum state
- Lung disease (specific to *Aspergillus*)

Pathogens commonly reach the eye via the hematogenous route, predominantly target the choroid due to its high blood flow, often leading to chorioretinitis.

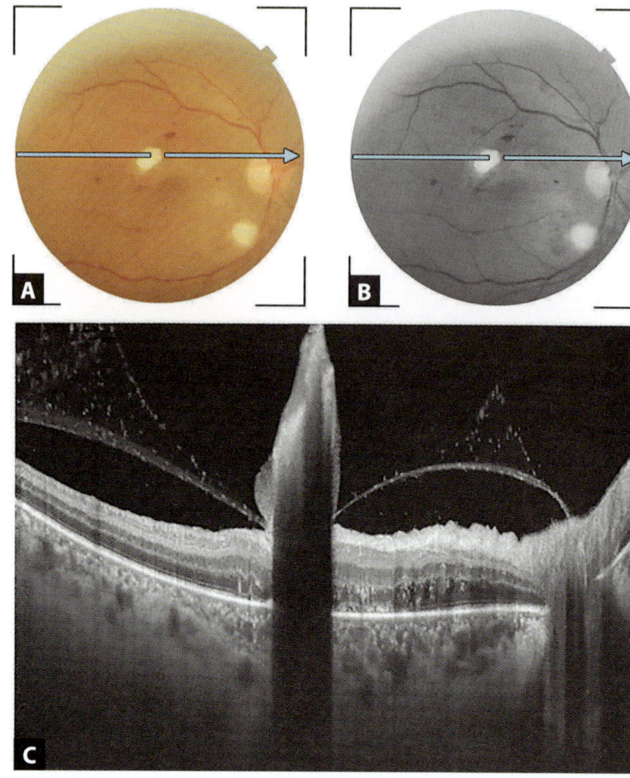

Figs. 8A to C: A color fundus photo of a right eye showing a macular, yellow-white. Yellow-white fluffy lesion (A) with the accompanying red-free image (B). On optical coherence tomography (C), spread of the infection into the vitreous produces an appearance of "puff ball abscesses."
Source: Presented by Katerina Lazari in the International Uveitis Study Group (IUSG) grand rounds.[1]

Subsequently, the infection may progress to involve the retina and vitreous leading to the appearance of intravitreal "puff ball abscesses" **(Figs. 8A to C)**. Predisposing factors for endogenous fungal endophthalmitis include immunosuppression, intravenous drug abuse, bacterial sepsis, systemic antibiotics, recent hospitalization, recent trauma or major surgery including invasive urologic procedures, urinary tract infections, diabetes, and indwelling catheters.[26] The dysfunction of the blood-retinal barrier caused by diabetes, along with elevated urine glucose levels, creates an environment conducive to microbial growth. Urologic procedures predispose patients to fungal endophthalmitis due to the spread of urinary tract infections, mechanical trauma from the procedure itself, and catheter-related fungal invasion.[27]

Symptoms of endogenous fungal endophthalmitis typically include vision loss and floaters, with less frequent ocular pain and redness than seen in cases of bacterial endophthalmitis. Ophthalmoscopic examination

TABLE 6: Clinical differences between bacterial and fungal endophthalmitis.

Characteristics	*Bacterial endophthalmitis*	*Fungal endophthalmitis*
Frequency and disease association	More frequent. Most cases are from post-cataract surgery and bleb associated	Less common; however, it accounts for the leading cause of endogenous endophthalmitis cases, fungal is relatively more common in tropical locations
Time course	Rapidly progressive (days)	Indolent (weeks)
Characteristic lesions	Diffuse intraocular inflammation and subretinal abscess can also occur	Clumped appearance of intraocular inflammation, choroidal mass projecting into the vitreous chamber, chorioretinal creamy-white or "string of pearls" lesions in *Candida* species

Source: Presented by Katerina Lazari in the International Uveitis Study Group (IUSG) grand rounds;[1] Adapted from Haseeb et al.[28]

reveals characteristic features such as white lesions in the posterior pole, vitreous inflammation with "string of pearls" exudates, papilledema, and in advanced cases, intravitreal "puff ball" abscesses.[28] **Table 6** shows clinical differences between fungal and bacterial endophthalmitis.

Diagnostic confirmation of endogenous fungal endophthalmitis relies on clinical suspicion supported by blood, urine, and vitreous cultures. Multimodal imaging aids in diagnosis and monitoring, with findings such as hypofluorescence on fluorescein angiography and hyperreflective lesions on OCT **(Figs. 9A to F)**. Culture-negative cases are not uncommon; therefore, the culture must be kept for at least 4–6 weeks to ensure that slow-growing or fastidious fungal organisms are not missed. PCR testing is a rapid and highly sensitive to quickly differentiate between bacterial and fungal infections.[29]

Remarkably, 50% of cases of endogenous fungal endophthalmitis cases are initially misdiagnosed as non-infectious uveitis, leading to the administration of corticosteroids with clinical progression. Therefore, conducting a comprehensive systematic history before establishing a diagnosis of non-infectious uveitis is crucial. Particular attention should be paid to a history of fever or recent invasive procedures, which are pivotal to differentiate between infectious and non-infectious etiologies. Accurate diagnosis leads to initiation of appropriate treatment in a timely manner.

According to the Infectious Disease Society of America guidelines, the treatment for endogenous fungal endophthalmitis typically involves systemic antifungal therapy with intravitreal injections indicated in cases of macular threatening lesions or significant vitritis. For vitreous involvement, intravitreal administration of amphotericin or voriconazole is recommended. Liposomal amphotericin is preferred for the involvement of the macula because, of the extended half-life in the vitreous humor.[30] It is crucial to meticulously prepare the intravitreal anti-fungal compounded drug to prevent toxicity, ensuring the solution remains colorless; any color change indicates that the solution should be discarded to avoid damaging the eye. A vitrectomy may be required for extensive vitreous involvement or to drain a subretinal abscess.[31] Systemic antifungal treatment should continue for at least 4–6 weeks, guided resolution of the lesions. In cases where the infection is resistant, intravitreal injections may be repeated every 72 hours.

In managing bacterial endophthalmitis, empirical antibiotic therapy often includes intravitreal injections of vancomycin (1 mg/0.1 cm^3) and ceftazidime (2.25 mg/0.1 cm^3). It is essential to be aware that an initial exacerbation of inflammation may occur following the administration of intravitreal ceftazidime, a phenomenon attributed to its beta-lactam properties. Despite this, a reduction in pain can be a useful clinical sign indicating the effectiveness of the treatment. The early initiation of systemic antibiotics is also crucial, with ceftazidime being a preferred option due to its broad-spectrum activity against prevalent pathogens. Adhering to proper dosing and administration guidelines is essential to maximize therapeutic success and minimize the risk of adverse effects.[32]

Concerning prognosis, endogenous endophthalmitis generally has a worse prognosis and outcome than exogenous endophthalmitis due to compromised host immunity, the initial involvement of the posterior segment, and more aggressive pathogens.

In conclusion, endophthalmitis is a medical emergency in which rapid diagnosis and treatment are crucial to preserving vision. *Candida* species are the predominant pathogens in endogenous endophthalmitis. A multidisciplinary approach involving ophthalmologists and infectious disease specialists is essential for optimal management. Diagnosis of fungal endogenous endophthalmitis is primarily clinical and can be challenging

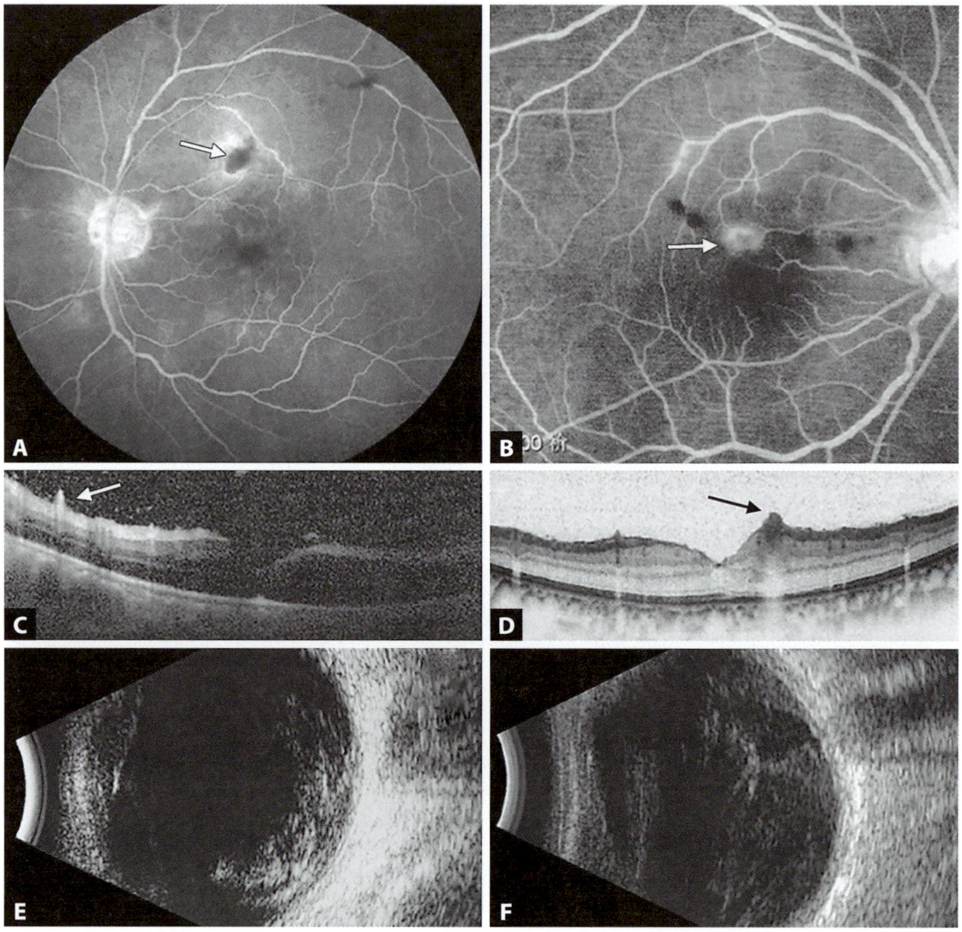

Figs. 9A to F: Multimodal imaging findings in a case of fungal endophthalmitis. On fluorescein angiography, there is notable hypofluorescence of the retinal exudates, encircled by hyperfluorescence due to capillary leakage (white arrows) (A and B). Optical coherence tomography (OCT) images reveal hyperreflectivity of the lesions, indicating their distinct optical properties (white and black arrows) (C and D). Finally, ultrasound B-scans show significant vitreous opacities and show the lesions as echogenic spots located near the retina. The diffuse inflammation shows the extent of the infection within the ocular structures (E and F).
Source: Presented by Katerina Lazari in the International Uveitis Study Group (IUSG) grand rounds.[1]

due to an asymptomatic presentation, particularly in the early stages of the disease. Blood cultures may yield negative results, but characteristic clinical findings suggestive of fungal endophthalmitis warrant prompt antifungal treatment, even without positive blood cultures.

NON-INFECTIOUS POSTERIOR UVEITIS[1]

Case Presentation

Personal Data

- Female, 37 years old.
- The patient was already on an oral prednisone regimen of 30 mg, which had been tapered down to 10 mg, accompanied by mycophenolate 500 mg BID by the time of her presentation.

History of Present Illness

Floaters and difficulty driving at night in the last 2 months.

Physical Examination (Table 7 and Figs. 10A to D)

The macular OCT showed perifoveal loss and disruption of the outer retinal layer, accompanied by the deposition of hyperreflective material in the retinal pigment epithelium (RPE), along with hyperreflectivity of the core capillaries in both eyes **(Fig. 11)**. Moreover, fluorescein angiography displayed significant venous leakage, sparing the arteries, and leakage of the optic nerve in both the early and late phases **(Figs. 12A to H)**. ICG angiography revealed diffuse hypofluorescent, small, round lesions in the macula and periphery, consistent with bilateral involvement **(Figs. 13A to H)**.

TABLE 7: Physical examination of the patient having non-infectious posterior uveitis.

OD	***Parameter***	***OS***
20/20	BCVA	20/20
12 mm Hg	IOP	13 mm Hg
White and quiet	Conjunctiva	White and quiet
Clear, no KPs	Cornea	Clear, no KPs
No cells or flare	Anterior chamber	No cells or flare
Round, flat, no nodules, and no posterior synechiae	Iris	Round, flat, no nodules, and no posterior synechiae
Clear	Lens	Clear
Vitreous cells 1+	Vitreous	No vitreous cells, no haze
Normal disc, CD ratio 0.2, blunted reflex and macular pigmentary changes, normal vascular trajectory, and no sheathing. Faint oval- to spindle-shaped, yellow choroidal lesions in the periphery	Fundus	Normal disc, CD ratio 0.2, blunted reflex and macular pigmentary changes, normal vascular trajectory, and no sheathing. Faint oval- to spindle-shaped, yellow choroidal lesions in the periphery

(BCVA: best-corrected visual acuity; CD ratio: cup–disc ratio; KP: keratic precipitate; IOP: intraocular pressure)

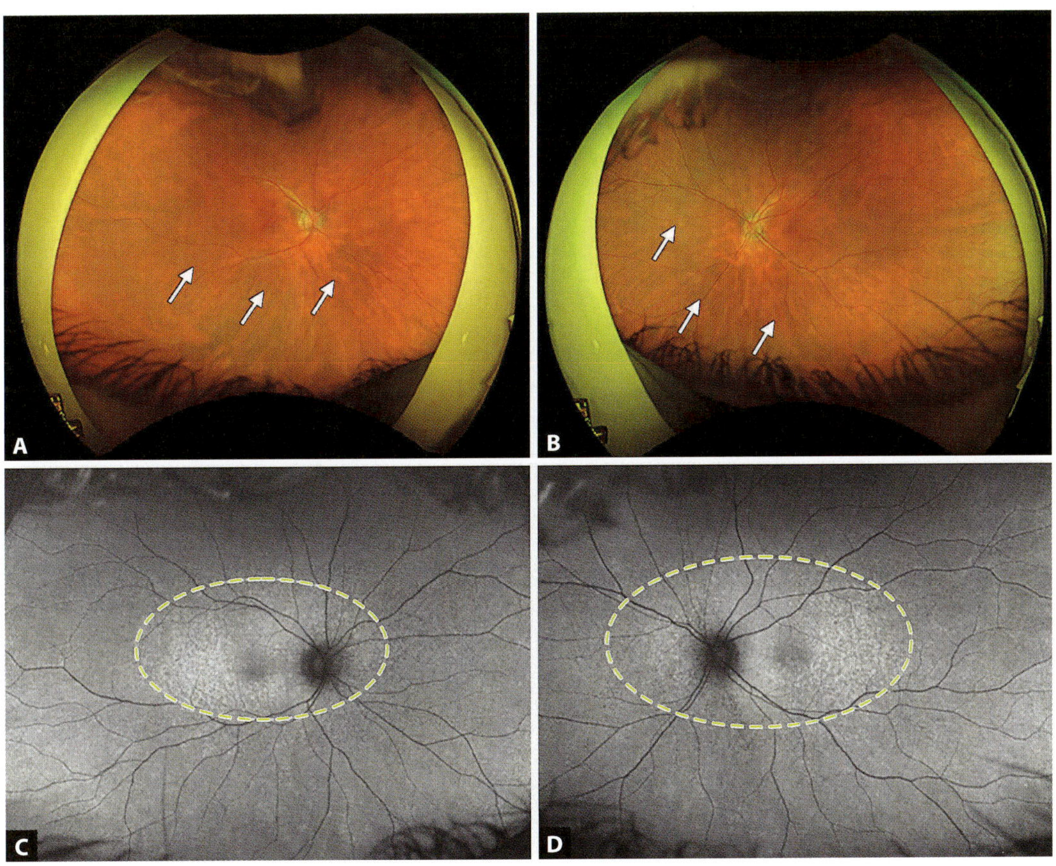

Figs. 10A to D: The initial clinical presentation of a case of non-infectious posterior uveitis. (A and B) Fundoscopy imaging: Faint oval- to spindle-shaped, yellow choroidal lesions in the periphery of both eyes; (C and D) Fundus autofluorescence: Evidencing a distinct perifoveal mixed pattern of hyper- and hypoautofluorescence with granularity in both eyes.
Source: Presented by Araniko Pandey in the International Uveitis Study Group (IUSG) grand rounds.[1]

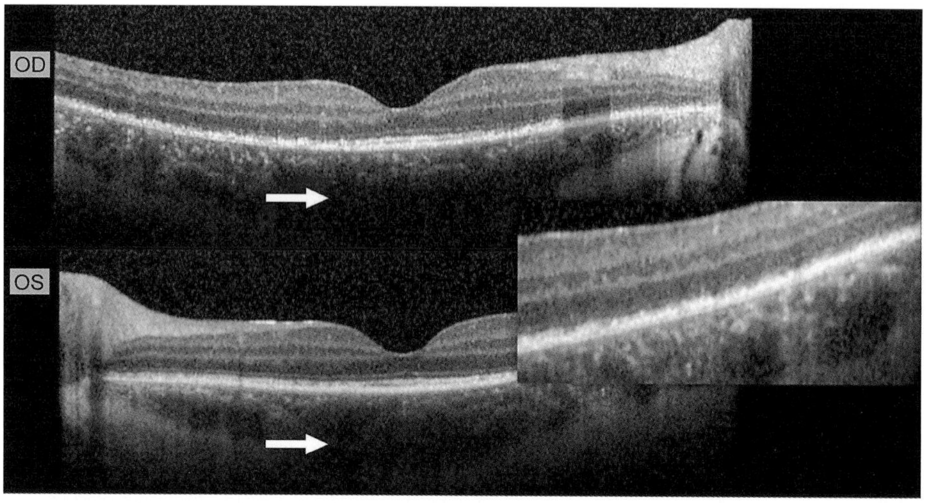

Fig. 11: Initial optical coherence tomography (OCT) findings in the non-infectious posterior uveitis case. Disruption and perifoveal loss of the outer retinal layer with hyperreflective deposits in the retinal pigment epithelium (image to the right). Hyporreflectivity of the choriocapillaris (white arrows).
Source: Presented by Araniko Pandey in the International Uveitis Study Group (IUSG) grand rounds.[1]

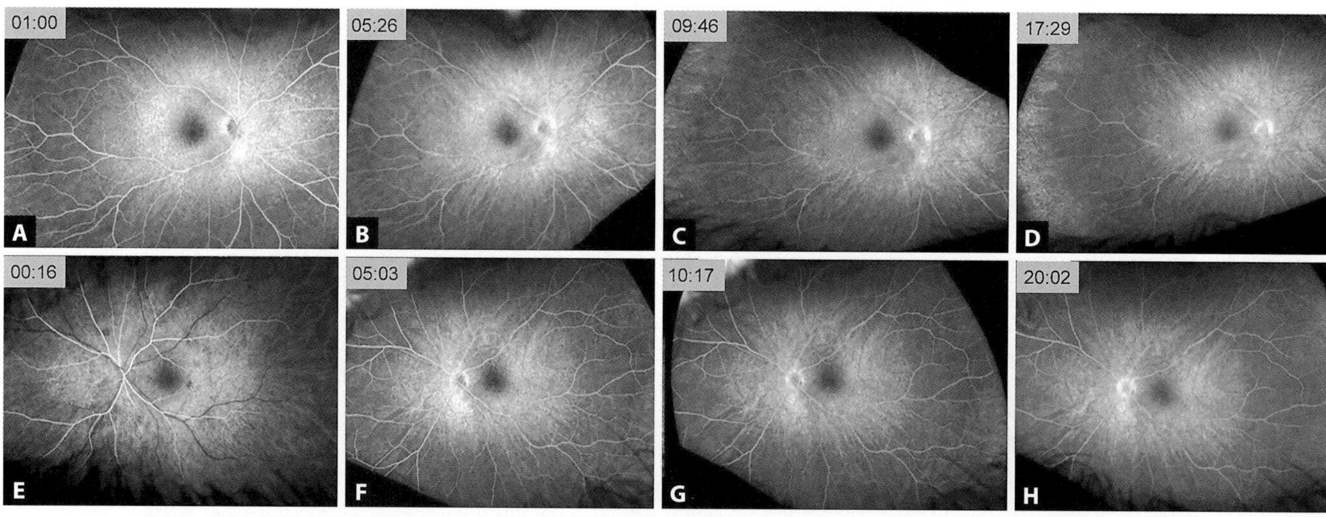

Figs. 12A to H: Initial fluorescein angiography findings in the non-infectious posterior uveitis case. There was significant venous leakage, sparing the arteries and leakage of the optic nerve in both the early and late phases in the right (A to D) and left (E to H) eye.
Source: Presented by Araniko Pandey in the International Uveitis Study Group (IUSG) grand rounds.[1]

Suspected Diagnosis

Birdshot chorioretinopathy (BCR): The patient underwent a comprehensive uveitis laboratory workup, including erythrocyte sedimentation rate, comprehensive metabolic panel, and complete blood count, all of which were within normal limits. Tests for syphilis, tuberculosis, HIV, toxoplasmosis, Lyme disease, angiotensin-converting enzyme, lupus anticoagulant, vasculitis panel, and HLA-B27 and HLA-B51 were negative. However, the presence of the HLA-A29 antigen was notably positive, leading to a diagnosis of BCR. As a result, the dosage of mycophenolate was increased to 1 gram twice daily with a recommendation to taper off prednisone.

Subsequently, the patient reported anxiety as a side effect, necessitating a psychiatric consultation. At the follow-up visit a month later, she was managing well on mycophenolate, and the dosage was further increased to the optimal level of 1.5 gram twice daily.

During subsequent visits, the patient showed a worsening of the vitritis, prompting the recommendation for implantation of an intravitreal dexamethasone implant. Due to financial constraints, she instead opted to continue oral prednisone 30 mg daily with the mycophenolate while continuing psychiatric follow-up. Improvement in vitritis was noted after 2 months, and she was asked to taper the prednisone to 5 mg over the next 6 weeks. However, persistent leakage of the large vessels and birdshot lesions continued to worsen despite improving vitritis during the following 2 months. Consequently, her prednisone dosage was increased again to 30 mg daily, then gradually tapered to 7.5 mg daily over the next 2 months, with ongoing mycophenolate therapy. Furthermore, adalimumab was prescribed and the patient remains under follow-up **(Fig. 14)**.

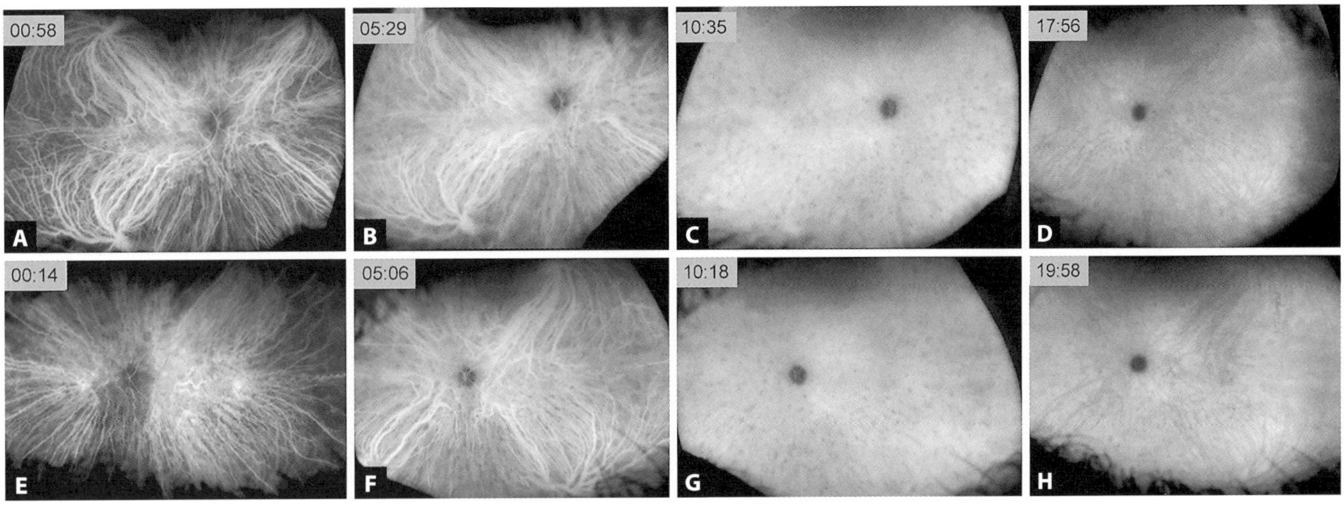

Figs. 13A to H: Initial indocyanine green angiography findings in a non-infectious posterior uveitis case. There were diffuse hyperfluorescent lesions and small round lesions in the macula and periphery in the right (A to D) and left (E to H) eye.
Source: Presented by Araniko Pandey in the International Uveitis Study Group (IUSG) grand rounds.[1]

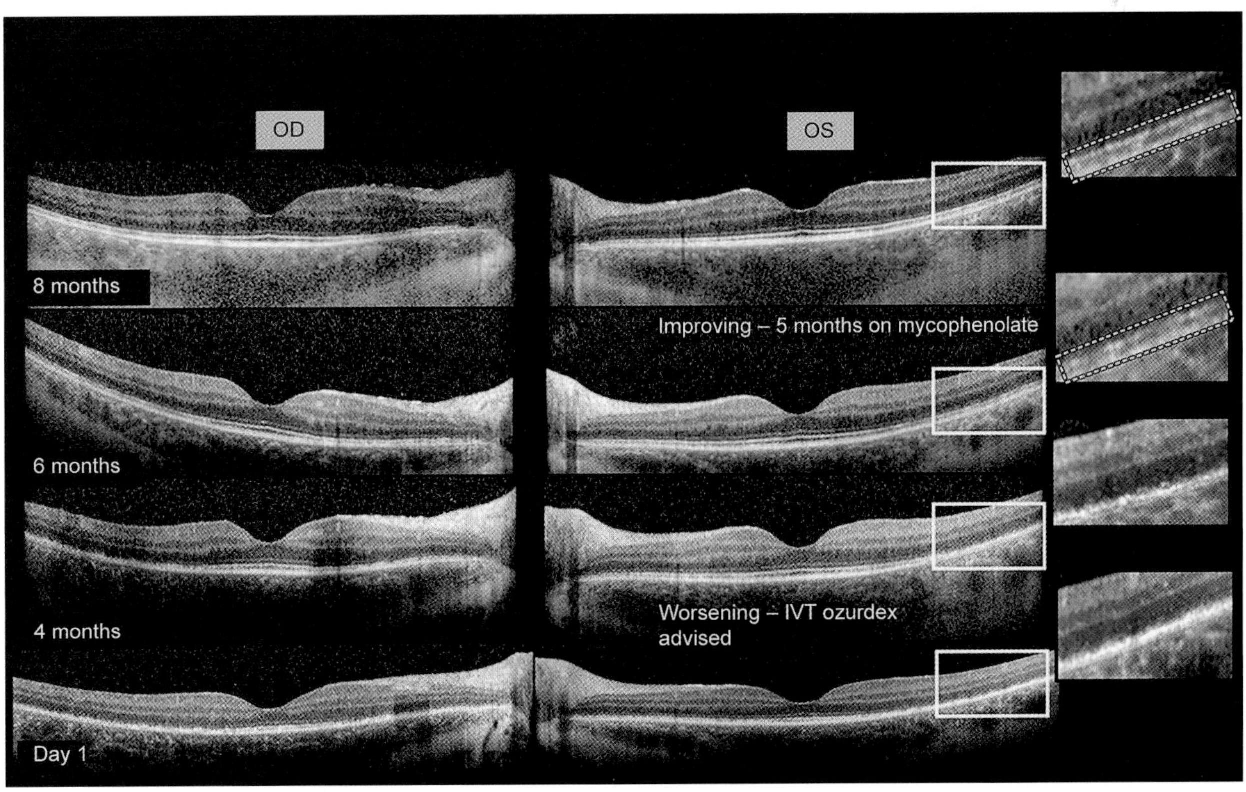

Fig. 14: Optical coherence tomography (OCT) findings during follow-up. Outer retinal changes serve as a biomarker during the follow-up of patients with birdshot chorioretinopathy.
Source: Presented by Araniko Pandey in the International Uveitis Study Group (IUSG) grand rounds.[1]

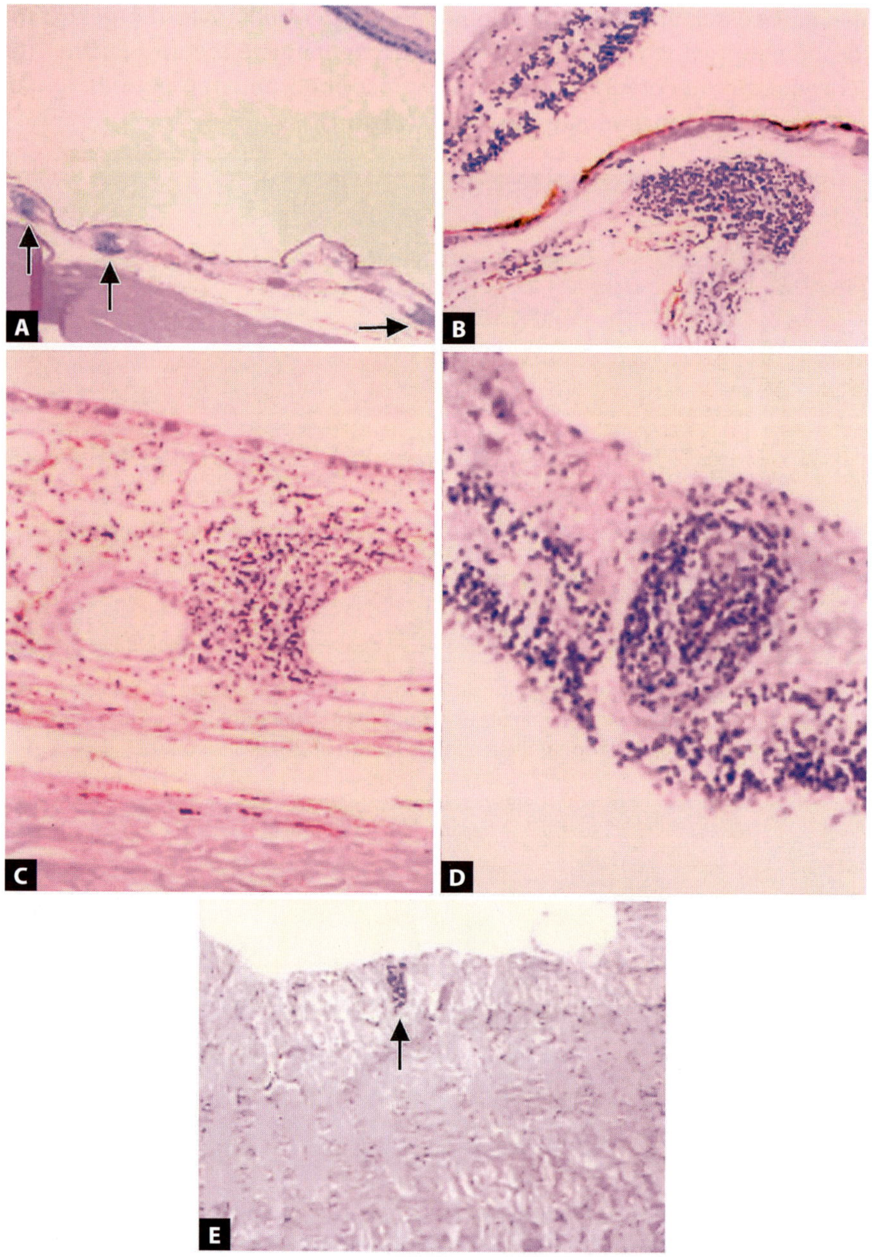

Figs. 15A to E: Histopathological findings in birdshot chorioretinopathy. (A) Choroidal lymphocytic infiltrates; (B) Choriocapillaris not involved; (C) Choroidal lymphocytes abutting choroidal vessels; (D) Focal retinal vasculitis; (E) Lymphocytic infiltrate in the prelaminar optic nerve.
Source: Adapted from Gaudio;[34] Presented by Janet L Davis in the International Uveitis Study Group (IUSG) grand rounds.[1]

Discussion

Birdshot chorioretinopathy is a rare, chronic, bilateral posterior uveitis characterized by a distinct clinical phenotype and a strong association with HLA-A29. It predominantly affects middle-aged individuals, with a higher prevalence in females than males.[1,33]

This particular case is concerning due to the patient's young age at onset, severe form of the disease, and acute nature of the presentation. Typically, younger patients experience more aggressive forms of the disease, while older adults tend to present with milder symptoms. Acute onset also tends to correlate with a worse clinical prognosis.[1,33]

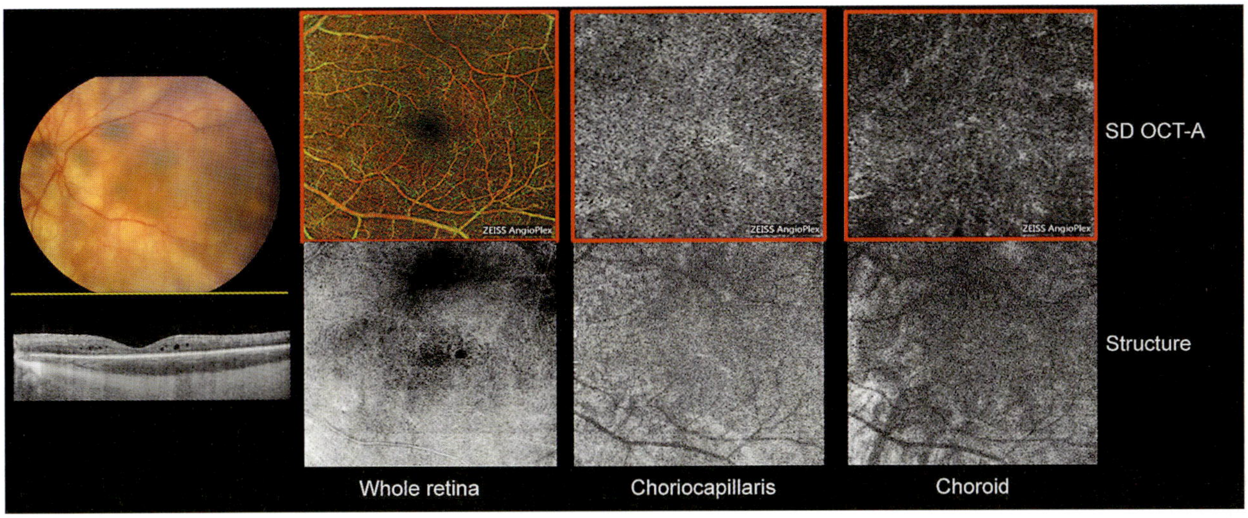

Fig. 16: Optical coherence tomography (OCT) angiography findings in birdshot chorioretinopathy. The structural slab evidenced a compromised vascular integrity throughout the portion of the retina that was scanned. Notably, the macular edema appears chronic in nature. Hyporeflectivity in the choroid is observable, with corresponding flow voids evident on the spectral-domain OCT and structural scans.
Source: Presented by Janet L Davis in the International Uveitis Study Group (IUSG) grand rounds.[1]

Birdshot chorioretinopathy is generally a lifelong condition requiring systemic therapy, though spontaneous remission can occur. Additionally, prolonged treatment may lead to a period of drug-free remission. Treatment typically involves systemic immunosuppression, as BCR is considered an autoimmune disorder. However, using a dexamethasone implant is beneficial for short-term induction at treatment onset with a fluocinolone implant being effective for long-term management.[1,33]

There has been an ongoing debate about whether BCR is primarily a retinal or choroidal disease. Most experts now agree that it is predominantly a choroidal disease, hence the term "chorioretinopathy." Meanwhile, retinal vasculitis damage is more of a consequence of the choroidal inflammatory process. Histopathological evidence **(Figs. 15A to E)** and OCT angiography **(Fig. 16)** support this consensus, showing that the choroid is the primary site of pathological changes in BCR; therefore, choroidal alterations are a critical factor in the prognosis of the disease.

Angiography is a pivotal imaging modality for the follow-up of BCR, utilized primarily to monitor disease progression during treatment. Over the long term, treatment tends to stabilize the leakage observed in fluorescein angiography, indicative of retinal repair, which often aligns with improvements in the visual field. Conversely, ICG angiography usually remains active, displaying numerous lesions even when patients are asymptomatic **(Fig. 17A and B)**. Fundus photography is valuable for tracking progressive choroidal disease, revealing increased spots and streaks observable during fundoscopy **(Figs. 18A and B)**.[1,33]

In the chronic stages of BCR, fundoscopic examination reveals degenerative hallmarks, including optic nerve atrophy, vascular attenuation, and pigmentary changes. While fundus fluorescein angiography and ICG remain crucial for precisely controlling active disease, their utility diminishes in advanced stages where scarring predominates over active inflammation. For comprehensive monitoring across all stages of BCR, a combination of imaging modalities is essential. Color fundus photography is valuable for detecting choroidal depigmentation, while visual field testing is important for assessing the decline in visual function due to retinal damage. Although OCT and autofluorescence (AF) are pivotal in identifying progressive, full-thickness choroidal atrophy and ongoing RPE damage in severely affected eyes, they should not be the sole tools for monitoring. These methods are more reflective of the extent of irreversible damage rather than the disease's active progression. Therefore, to ensure a comprehensive assessment, OCT and AF should be used in conjunction with color fundus and visual field testing to monitor the disease effectively at any stage **(Figs. 19A to F)**.

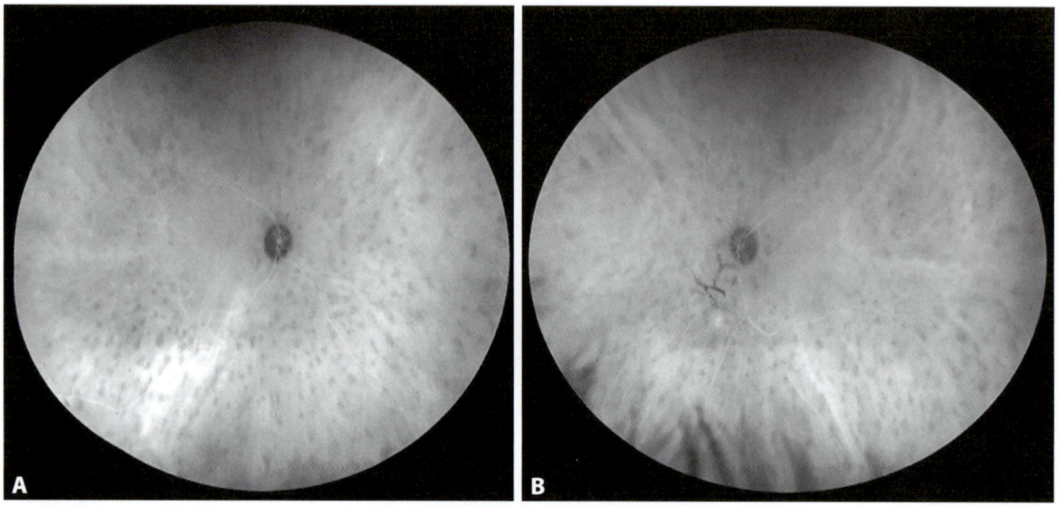

Fig. 17A and B: Indocyanine green angiography findings during treatment. Persistent hyperfluorescent lesions in indocyanine green angiography in the right (A) and left eye (B) of a patient with birdshot chorioretinopathy (BCR) with structural stabilization and visual improvement after 9 months of immunosuppressive treatment, including oral corticosteroids, immunosuppressive drugs, and biologics.
Source: Presented by Janet L Davis in the International Uveitis Study Group (IUSG) grand rounds.[1]

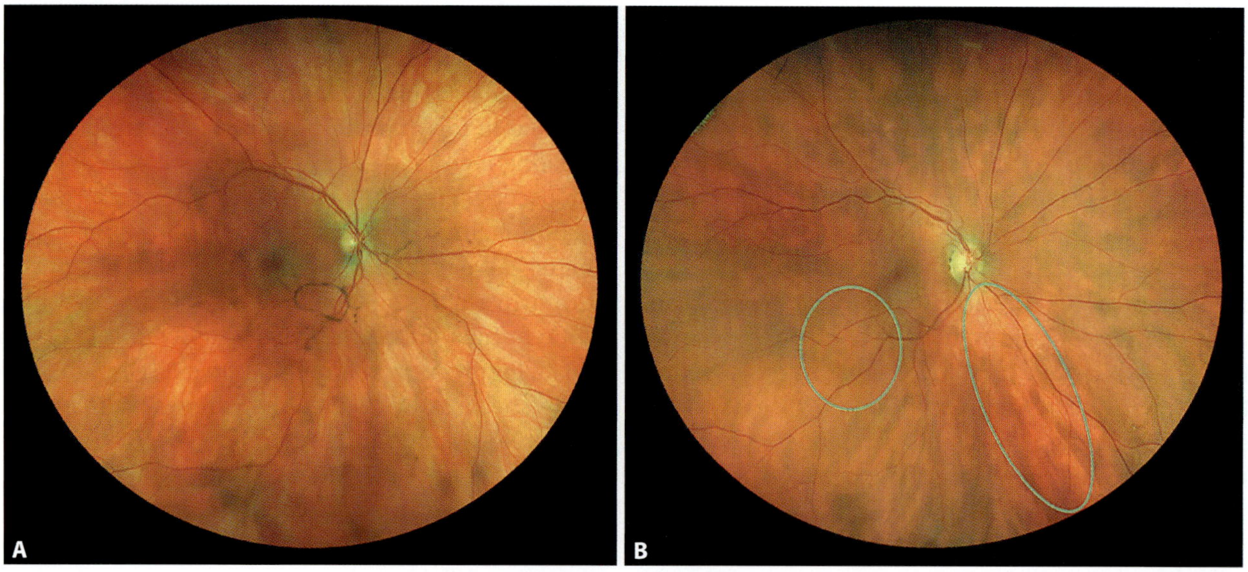

Figs. 18A and B: Fundoscopy progression of birdshot chorioretinopathy. (A) Baseline and (B) 9 months later, new retinal atrophic spots and streaks are evident, requiring escalation of immunosuppressive therapy.
Source: Presented by Janet L Davis in the International Uveitis Study Group (IUSG) grand rounds.[1]

GENERAL DISCUSSION AND CONTROVERSIES ON POSTERIOR UVEITIS

For infectious uveitis cases

1. Can corticosteroids be used in fungal endophthalmitis?
Answer: It is crucial to exercise caution when considering corticosteroid therapy in cases of suspected fungal endophthalmitis. Corticosteroids, particularly injected intravitreally, can exacerbate the condition by suppressing the immune response, which is necessary for clearing the fungal infection. While topical corticosteroids may be used cautiously in cases where antifungal treatment has been initiated and with close supervision, intravitreal steroid injections should be avoided entirely.

In cases of anterior segment inflammation, such as autoimmune or herpetic keratitis, topical corticosteroids

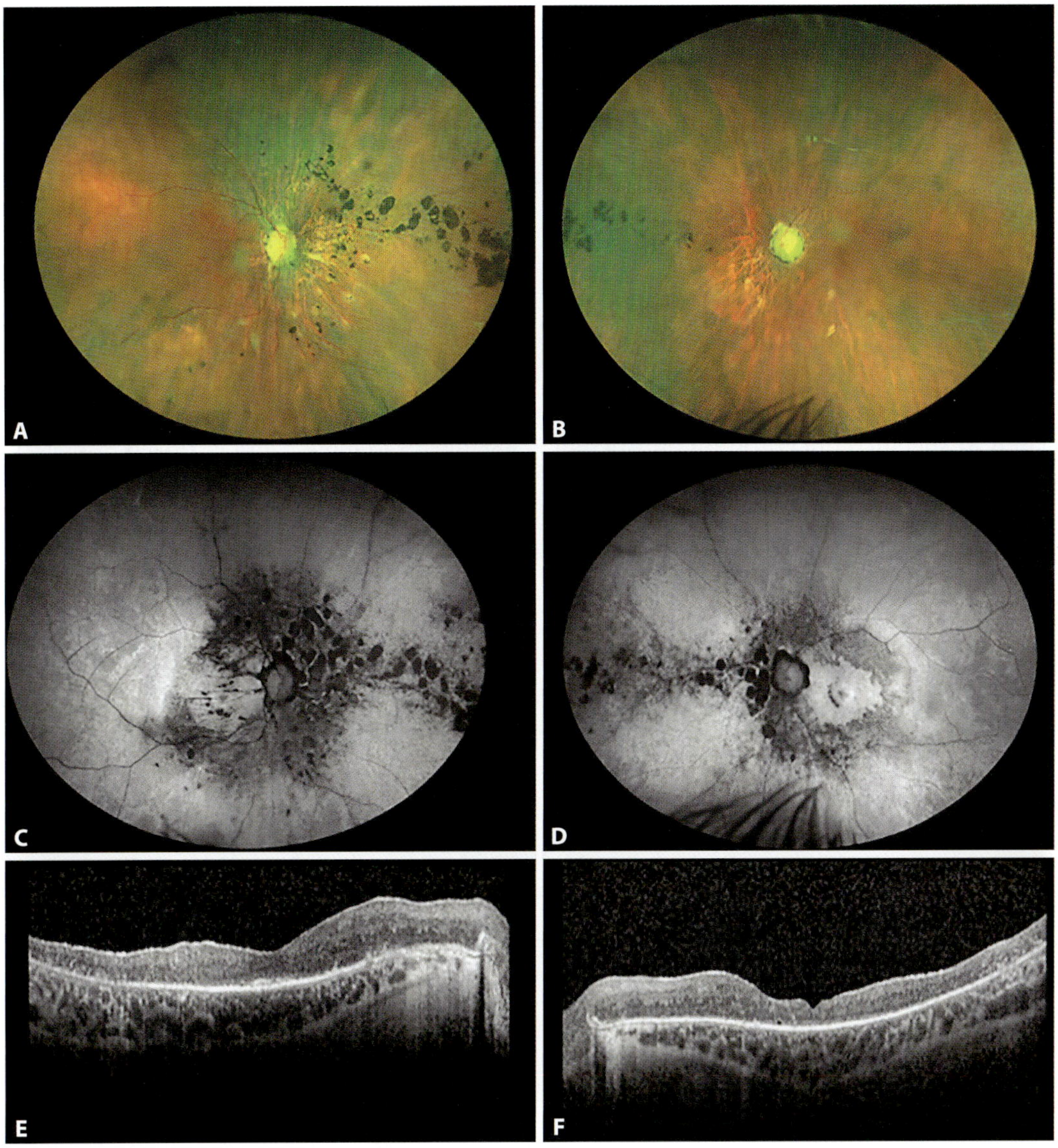

Figs. 19A to F: Clinical picture of birdshot chorioretinopathy in a chronic stage. (A and B) Fundoscopy findings: Optic nerve atrophy, vascular attenuation, and pigmentary changes; (C and D) Autofluorescence: RPE damage; (E and F) OCT findings such as progressive choroidal atrophy, reduced width of the ellipsoid zone (E), disorganization of the inner retinal layers (DRIL), and increased luminal area in the choroid (F). (OCT: optical coherence tomography; RPE: retinal pigment epithelium)
Source: Presented by Janet L Davis in the International Uveitis Study Group (IUSG) grand rounds.[1]

may be utilized alongside appropriate antifungal or antiviral therapy to mitigate inflammation. However, in cases of posterior uveitis involving fungal infection, the risks of exacerbating the infection outweigh the potential benefits of corticosteroid therapy.

It is important to emphasize that the primary approach to managing fungal endophthalmitis involves halting fungal replication to allow the immune system to clear the infection. Blocking the immune response with corticosteroids can impede this process, leading to further complications. Therefore, using corticosteroids in such cases should be approached with extreme caution, and consultation with an ophthalmologist specializing in the treatment of infectious diseases is advisable to ensure optimal management strategies.

2. How should a more severe recurrence of previously treated posterior uveitis be approached?

Answer: In addressing a recurrence of posterior uveitis that is more severe than previous episodes, it is essential to reassess the patient to confirm the initial diagnosis and exclude the possibility of a masquerade syndrome or missed infectious etiology. For infectious uveitis, such as tuberculosis, the recurrence could suggest incomplete initial treatment. For non-infectious uveitis, such as VKH, recurrences can happen despite comprehensive treatment. It is crucial to adapt the treatment based on the individual's response and previous interventions, perhaps extending the duration or escalating the therapy, to prevent further recurrences.

3. Can you discuss in detail the preparation of intravitreal antifungal injections and the volume for concurrent administration with vancomycin?
Answer: To avoid toxicity, intravitreal antifungal agents must be prepared at specific concentrations for ocular use. For voriconazole, a typical preparation involves 100 µg in a 0.1-mL volume. Fluconazole is prepared at 200 µg/mL for intravitreal administration. When combined with vancomycin, the total injection volume typically should not exceed 0.1 mL. In the absence of vitritis, systemic antifungals are preferred. Intravitreal amphotericin B or voriconazole should be considered in cases with vitreous involvement, and dosing should be aligned with the severity of the infection.

4. What is the role of systemic antifungals in treating endogenous fungal infections?
Answer: Systemic antifungals are critical in treating endogenous fungal infections to address potential fungemia and prevent dissemination to other body parts. Negative blood and urine cultures do not definitively rule out endophthalmitis; thus, the clinical context and presentation should guide the treatment approach.

5. What is the advised duration for treating patients with systemic antifungal medication?
Answer: The recommended duration of systemic antifungal treatment typically spans 6–8 weeks. However, if the infection recurs, the treatment may need to be extended or repeated.

6. Are there reasons to avoid a complete vitrectomy with posterior hyaloid removal?
Answer: Full vitrectomy with posterior hyaloid removal can pose risks, particularly if the underlying retina is compromised or necrotic. It may lead to iatrogenic retinal breaks. Therefore, a core vitrectomy is generally preferred as the initial procedure to mitigate such risks.

7. Is screening for endophthalmitis in an unconscious intensive care unit patient with clinical sepsis necessary?
Answer: Yes, screening for endophthalmitis, particularly for *Candida* endophthalmitis, is mandatory in patients who have experienced fungemia. Guidelines recommend ocular screening 1 month after the event to identify and treat potential involvement.

8. What is the justification for conducting fundoscopic examinations in asymptomatic patients with systemic candidemia, and what is the recommended timing for these examinations?
Answer: Fundoscopic examinations in patients with systemic candidemia, even when asymptomatic, are akin to a low-risk, high-value diagnostic test. These examinations can reveal ocular involvement necessitating specific intervention. Some studies support the high positive predictive value of this approach. Examinations should be conducted promptly, ideally within a day or two of the suspicion or diagnosis of candidemia.

9. After PPV for endophthalmitis, if there is a need to repeat intravitreal antibiotic or antifungal injections, should the dosage be full or half, given the vitrectomized state of the eye?
Answer: In a vitrectomized eye, a half dose of intravitreal antibiotics or antifungals is usually sufficient due to the altered pharmacokinetics in the absence of the vitreous body.

10. Is intravitreal voriconazole or amphotericin B preferred to treat fungal endophthalmitis?
Answer: Both voriconazole and amphotericin B are options for treating fungal endophthalmitis. Amphotericin B is known for its longer half-life, which may be advantageous. However, due to its potential toxicity, it requires careful preparation to avoid complications.

For non-infectious uveitis cases

1. What is the optimal imaging modality for monitoring the progression of birdshot chorioretinitis at different stages of the disease?
Answer: The best imaging modality for birdshot chorioretinitis varies depending on the stage of the disease. Initially, ICG angiography is invaluable for diagnosing and monitoring choroidal inflammation. If ICG is not accessible, OCT angiography can serve as an alternative, though it may not provide the same level of detail regarding choroidal blood flow. Standard OCT scans can also identify structural changes in the choroid indicative of disease progression. During acute phases, fluorescein angiography, in conjunction with ICG, is critical for comprehensive assessment. Fundus photography is beneficial for monitoring disease control, and in advanced stages, fundus AF helps identify areas

of atrophy. While treatment options become limited in later stages, adapting imaging techniques to the resources available and the individual patient's condition is essential for ongoing management.

2. Is electrophysiology a reliable method for monitoring birdshot chorioretinitis?

Answer: Electrophysiology, particularly electroretinography (ERG), is a significant tool for assessing retinal function in birdshot chorioretinitis, especially in the early and active stages of the disease. ERG can detect retinal dysfunction, such as negative B-wave amplitudes, which indicates disease activity and can guide the treatment response. As the disease progresses and more permanent retinal changes occur, ERG may become less sensitive. The 30-Hz flicker implicit time in the ERG is a sensitive marker for retinal activity and can reflect treatment efficacy. Visual field testing is also crucial throughout the disease, offering a functional measure of the patient's vision and response to therapy. Although electrooculography (EOG) is less informative for birdshot chorioretinitis, integrating ERG and visual field testing with clinical evaluation and imaging findings provides a comprehensive approach to disease management.

3. In the absence of Ozurdex, would intravitreous triamcinolone be considered in BCR?

Answer: In scenarios where Ozurdex is unavailable, intravitreous triamcinolone may be used cautiously to quickly control inflammation. However, in diseases such as BCR, it is treated with systemic immunosuppression, generally starting with high doses of disease-modifying antirheumatic drugs (DMARDs) for long-term management.

4. Are there cases of birdshot chorioretinitis in children?

Answer: Birdshot chorioretinitis predominantly affects middle-aged individuals and is uncommon in children. Cases in pediatric populations are rare and warrant a thorough investigation to confirm the diagnosis and rule out other uveitis conditions that may present with similar clinical features.

FINAL WRAP-UP

In conclusion:

- *Infectious posterior uveitis*, including endogenous endophthalmitis, is frequently associated with systemic health issues, such as diabetes or intravenous catheter use, which can serve as essential diagnostic indicators. Nonetheless, the absence of these indicators does not preclude the possibility of an infectious etiology. Clinicians should be cautious about delaying treatment based solely on negative cultures, as the clinical presentation can sufficiently indicate a severe infectious process. Rapid and appropriate intervention prevents irreversible ocular damage and preserves vision. Hence, a thorough assessment remains essential in managing infectious posterior uveitis.
- *For non-infectious posterior uveitis*, recurrence can be a significant challenge, even after intensive initial treatment. The variability in presentation and severity necessitates long-term follow-up and a high degree of clinical vigilance. In such cases, it is essential to thoroughly exclude infectious causes before proceeding with corticosteroid therapy. The treatment regimen should be carefully tailored, incorporating systemic therapies and considering intravitreal interventions when necessary. Given the potential for varied clinical manifestations, a detailed patient history and comprehensive examination are critical. Tailoring treatment to individual patient needs, considering regional disease prevalence and patient-specific factors, ensures the best possible outcomes. Remaining vigilant and adjusting management plans based on disease activity and patient response are essential in achieving long-term control and preventing complications.

REFERENCES

1. Uveitis Webinar - IIUSG Grand Round 03 (09-March 2024). https://youtu.be/32lloUwMqmA?si=a8SnVSy81tE06BN0.
2. Jabs DA, Nussenblatt RB, Rosenbaum JT; Standardization of Uveitis Nomenclature (SUN) Working Group. Standardization of uveitis nomenclature for reporting clinical data. Results of the First International Workshop. Am J Ophthal. 2005;140(3):509-16.
3. Tsirouki T, Dastiridou A, Symeonidis C, Tounakaki O, Brazitikou I, Kalogeropoulos C, et al. A focus on the epidemiology of uveitis. Ocul Immunol Inflamm. 2018;26(1):2-16.
4. Uy HS, Yu-Keh E, Chan PS. Posterior uveitis. In: Nguyen QD, Rodrigues EB, Farah ME, Mieler WF, Do DV (Eds). Developments in Ophthalmology. Basel: Karger; 2016. pp. 163-6.
5. Tabbara KF. Clinical diagnosis of posterior uveitis. Int Ophthalmol Clin. 1995;35(3):1-19.
6. Lee JH, Agarwal A, Mahendradas P, Lee CS, Gupta V, Pavesio CE, et al. Viral posterior uveitis. Surv Ophthalmol. 2017;62(4):404-5.

7. Jabs DA, Busingye J. Approach to the diagnosis of the uveitides. Am J Ophthalmol. 2013;156(2):228-36.
8. Peterson AS, Patterson AW. Case series: tattoo-associated uveitis. Optom Vis Sci. 2022;99(4):383-8.
9. Kassem A, Dahabra L, Abou Yassine A, Assaad M, Muhammad M, El-Sayegh D. Association between sarcoidosis and risk of venous thromboembolism: a retrospective chart review. Cureus. 2022;14(5):e25520.
10. Paez-Escamilla M, Caplash S, Kalra G, Odden J, Price D, Marroquin OC, et al. Challenges in posterior uveitis—tips and tricks for the retina specialist. J Ophthal Inflamm Infect. 2023;13(1):35.
11. Naranjo CA, Busto U, Sellers EM, Sandor P, Ruiz I, Roberts EA, et al. A method for estimating the probability of adverse drug reactions. Clin Pharmacol Ther. 1981;30(2):239-45.
12. Habot-Wilner Z, Neri P, Okada AA, Agrawal R, Xin Le N, Cohen S, et al. COVID vaccine-associated uveitis. Ocul Immunol Inflamm. 2023 ;31(6):1198-205.
13. Cunningham ET, Moorthy RS. Vaccine-associated posterior uveitis. Retin Cases Brief Rep. 2022;16(1):1-4.
14. Guex-Crosier Y. Uveitis masquerade syndrome and orbital lymphoma: two challenging diagnosis. Klin Monatsbl Augenheilkd. 2014;231(4):303.
15. Gomez-Marin JE, de-la-Torre A. Ocular Disease due to *Toxoplasma gondii*. In: Gomez-Marin JE, de-la-Torre A (Eds). Toxoplasma Gondii, 3rd edition. London: Elsevier; 2020. pp. 229-91.
16. Nussenblatt RB, Palestine AG, Chan CC, Roberge F. Standardization of vitreal inflammatory activity in intermediate and posterior uveitis. Ophthalmology. 1985;92(4):467-71.
17. Couret C, Ducloyer JB, Touhami S, Angioi-Duprez K, Rougier MB, Labalette P, et al. Treatment of noninfectious intermediate uveitis, posterior uveitis, or panuveitis. J F Ophtalmol. 2020;43(4):341-61.
18. Durrani OM, Tehrani NN, Marr JE, Moradi P, Stavrou P, Murray PI. Degree, duration, and causes of visual loss in uveitis. Br J Ophthal. 2004;88(9):1159-62.
19. Denniston AK, Barry RJ, Nguyen QD, Lee RW, Murray PI. Pharmacotherapy for uveitis: current management and emerging therapy. Clin Ophthalmol. 2014;1891-911.
20. Sharma S, Padhi TR, Basu S, Kar S, Roy A, Das T. Endophthalmitis patients seen in a tertiary eye care centre in Odisha: a clinico-microbiological analysis. Indian J Med Res. 2014;139(1):91-8.
21. Durand ML. Bacterial and fungal endophthalmitis. Clin Microbiol Rev. 2017;30(3):597-613.
22. Budoff G, Thangamathesvaran L, Zarbin MA, Bhagat N. Bacterial endogenous endophthalmitis in bacteremic inpatients. Ophthalmol Retina. 2019;3(11):971-8.
23. Sridhar J, Flynn HW, Kuriyan AE, Miller D, Albini T. Endogenous fungal endophthalmitis: risk factors, clinical features, and treatment outcomes in mold and yeast infections. J Ophthal Inflamm Infect. 2013;3(1):60.
24. Klotz SA, Penn CC, Negvesky GJ, Butrus SI. Fungal and parasitic infections of the eye. Clin Microbiol Rev. 2000;13(4):662-85.
25. Sadiq MA, Hassan M, Agarwal A, Sarwar S, Toufeeq S, Soliman MK, et al. Endogenous endophthalmitis: diagnosis, management, and prognosis. J Ophthal Inflamm Infect. 2015;5(1):32.
26. Uppuluri A, Zarbin MA, Budoff G, Bhagat N. Risk factors for endogenous endophthalmitis in hospitalized patients with candida fungemia. Ophthalmol Retina. 2021;5(7):687-95.
27. Lou B, Sun Y, Lin J, Yuan Z, He L, Long C, et al. Clinical features of endogenous endophthalmitis secondary to minimally invasive upper urinary tract calculus removal. Ocul Immunol Inflamm. 2022;30(1):104-10.
28. Haseeb AA, Elhusseiny AM, Siddiqui MZ, Ahmad KT, Sallam AB. Fungal endophthalmitis: a comprehensive review. J Fungi. 2021;7(11):996.
29. Sallam A, Lynn W, McCluskey P, Lightman S. Endogenous Candida endophthalmitis. Expert Rev Anti-infect Ther. 2006;4(4):675-85.
30. Riddell J, Comer GM, Kauffman CA. Treatment of endogenous fungal endophthalmitis: focus on new antifungal agents. Clin Infect Dis. 2011;52(5):648-53.
31. Samiy N, D'Amico DJ. Endogenous fungal endophthalmitis. Int Ophthalmol Clin. 1996;36(3):147-62.
32. Danielescu C, Anton N, Stanca HT, Munteanu M. Endogenous endophthalmitis: a review of case series published between 2011 and 2020. J Ophthal. 2020;2020:8869590
33. Bousquet E, Duraffour P, Debillon L, Somisetty S, Monnet D, Brézin AP. Birdshot chorioretinopathy: a review. J Clin Med. 2022;11(16):4772.
34. Gaudio PA. Histopathology of birdshot retinochoroidopathy. Br J Ophthal. 2002;86(12):1439-41.

CHAPTER 4

Panuveitis

Reema Bansal, Lucia Sobrin, Jie Sun, Ariel Schlaen, Agustina Nieddu, Sapna Gangaputra, Russel Dinh, Germán Mejía-Salgado, Meghan Berkenstock, John H Kempen, Alejandra de-la-Torre, Vishali Gupta

INTRODUCTION[1]

Panuveitis is characterized by inflammation involving all eye segments, including the anterior chamber, vitreous chamber, retina, and/or choroid. This condition can be limited to the eye or be part of a systemic condition. The causative factors of panuveitis are diverse, ranging from infectious agents, which often cause unilateral symptoms, to noninfectious systemic diseases more commonly associated with bilateral eye involvement.[2,3] Additionally, masquerade syndromes can mimic the presentation of panuveitis, making diagnosis and treatment challenging. **Flowchart 1** shows a differential diagnosis of the primary etiology of panuveitis.

The clue toward possible etiology may come from the phenotypic presentation combined with history and systemic findings. For instance, vitiligo is commonly associated with chronic Vogt–Koyanagi–Harada (VKH) disease, while a history of eye surgeries or trauma to the contralateral eye frequently accompanies sympathetic ophthalmia (SO). Additionally, characteristic imaging features, such as the "fern pattern," are linked with Behçet's disease **(Figs. 1A to C)**. This chapter explores essential diagnostic and therapeutic strategies to ensure precise diagnosis and effective treatment.

PRACTICAL TIPS IN THE MANAGEMENT OF PANUVEITIS[1]

Based on the clinical examination, systemic history, and findings, it is recommended to make the differential diagnosis of panuveitis. Tailored imaging studies and laboratory tests can be advised based on the diseases listed in differential diagnosis. For instance, in suspected ocular tuberculosis, it is prudent to obtain the following tests: Fundus fluorescein angiography (FFA), indocyanine green angiography (ICGA), tuberculin skin test (TST), contrast-enhanced computed tomography (CECT), and interferon gamma release assay (IGRA). In contrast, a presumed diagnosis of birdshot chorioretinopathy (BSCR) necessitates a different focus, where HLA-A29 testing, alongside ICGA, takes precedence. The epidemiological context and the patient's clinical presentation are important in differential diagnoses.[5] **Table 1** delineates the recommended imaging and laboratory investigations aligned with specific clinical suspicions in panuveitis. This chapter will cover clinical cases with panuveitis. Conditions such as ocular toxoplasmosis and ocular tuberculosis causing predominantly posterior uveitis shall be discussed in other chapters.

To effectively manage various forms of panuveitis, it is essential to consider individual patient factors, severity of the disease, and available treatment modalities to optimize outcomes and prevent recurrences.[6]

Tubercular Panuveitis

Treatment for tubercular panuveitis begins with topical corticosteroids and cycloplegics. Oral prednisolone is prescribed at a dosage of 0.5–1 mg/kg/day and is tapered depending upon the clinical response, usually decreased by 5 mg every week. Antituberculosis therapy (ATT) is initiated after assessing baseline liver function and involves a four-drug regimen for 9 months.[1,3]

Flowchart 1: Clinical approach to the patient with panuveitis.[4]

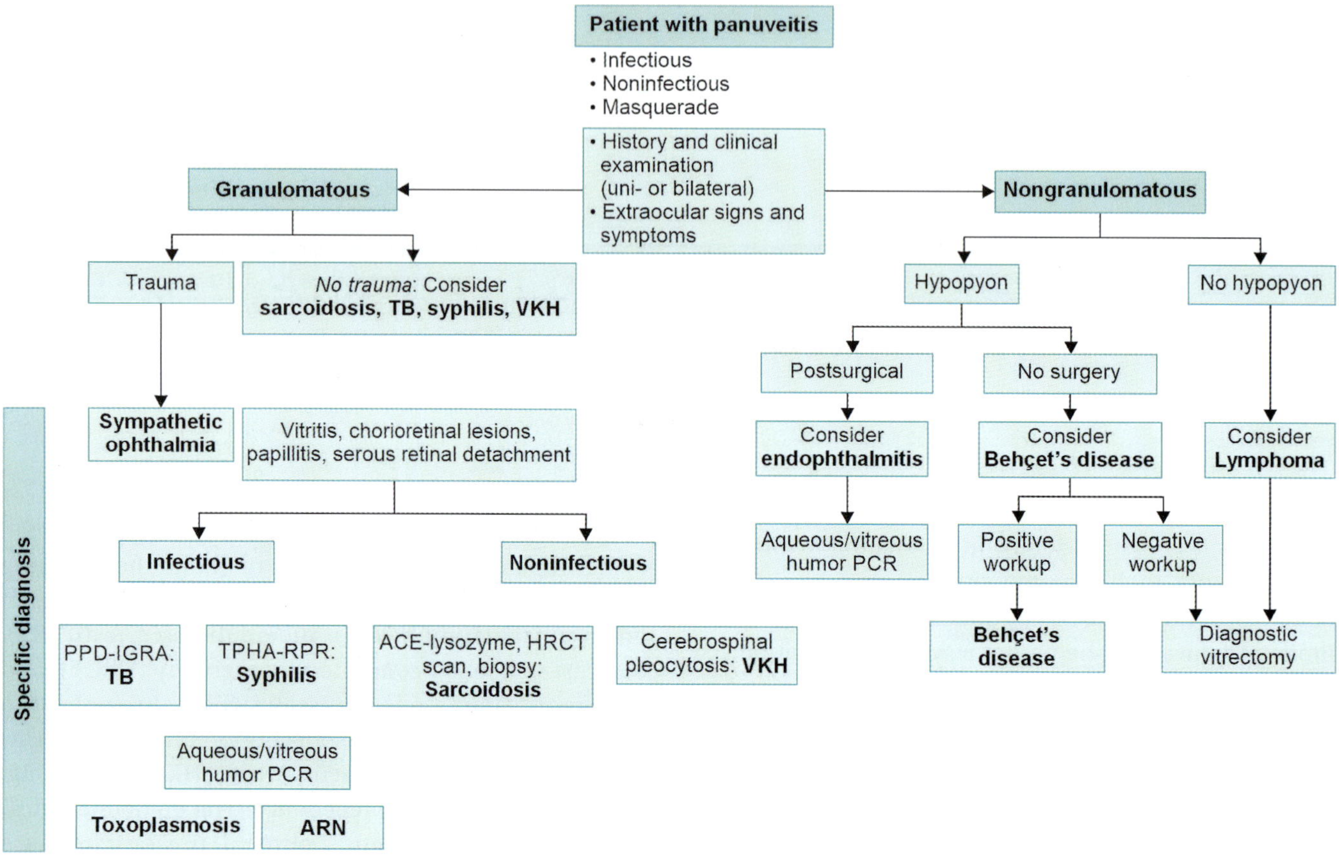

(ACE: angiotensin-converting enzyme; ARN: acute retinal necrosis; HRCT: high-resolution computed tomography; IGRA: interferon gamma release assay; PCR: polymerase chain reaction; PPD: purified protein derivative; RPR: rapid plasma reagin; TB: tuberculosis; TPHA: *Treponema pallidum* hemagglutination assay; VKH: Vogt–Koyanagi–Harada)

Source: Modified from Cimino et al.[4]

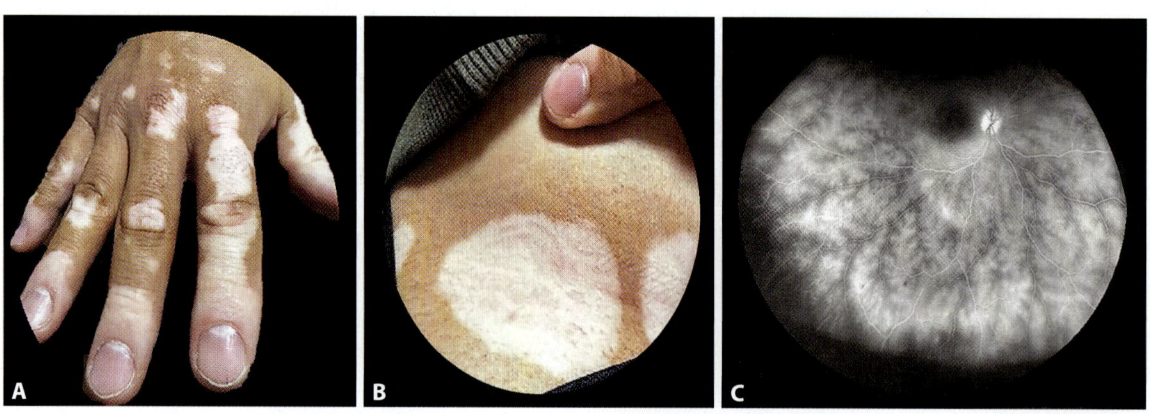

Figs. 1A to C: Typical clinical patterns of panuveitis diagnoses: (A and B) Vitiligo in right hand and torso suggestive of Vogt–Koyanagi–Harada disease; (C) Fern pattern in fundus fluorescein angiography suggestive of Behçet's disease.

TABLE 1: Differential diagnoses in a patient with panuveitis.[1]

Clinical diagnosis	*Ancillary investigations (retinal imaging)*	*Laboratory investigations*	*Additional test*
Infectious panuveitis			
Ocular tuberculosis	FFA and ICGA	TST, CECT chest, IGRA, and TPHA	PCR
Ocular toxoplasmosis	OCT and fundus photography	Serum IgG, IgM	PCR
Viral (HSV/VZV)	Fundus photography	Serum IgG, IgM, and HIV	PCR
Viral (CMV)	Fundus photography	HIV, immune status, and CD4	PCR
Syphilis	AF, OCT, and fundus photography	TPHA and VDRL	Dermatology assessment
Noninfectious panuveitis			
VKH disease	FFA, OCT, and ICGA		CBC, RFT, and LFT
Sympathetic ophthalmia	FFA, OCT, and ICGA		CBC, RFT, and LFT
Behçet's disease	FFA and OCT		HLA-B51 and rheumatology assessment
Sarcoidosis	FFA, OCT, and ICGA	TST, CECT, and chest biopsy	
Birdshot chorioretinopathy	FFA and ICGA	HLA-A29	
Masquerades			
PVRL	OCT, AF, and FFA	Vitreous biopsy, cytology IL-10: IL-16 and MYD88 gene mutation	MRI brain
Choroidal metastasis	OCT, AF, and FFA	PET-CT	

(AF: autofluorescence; CBC: complete blood count; CECT: contrast-enhanced computed tomography; FFA: fundus fluorescein angiography; HLA: human leukocyte antigen; HIV: human immunodeficiency virus; ICGA: indocyanine green angiography; IgG: immunoglobulin G; IgM: immunoglobulin M; IGRA: interferon gamma release assay; LFT: liver function test; MRI: magnetic resonance imaging; OCT: optical coherence tomography; PCR: polymerase chain reaction; PET-CT: positron emission tomography-computed tomography; PVRL: primary vitreoretinal lymphoma; RFT: renal function test, TPHA: Treponema pallidum hemagglutination; TST: tuberculin skin test; VDRL: Venereal Disease Research Laboratory; VKH: Vogt–Koyanagi–Harada)

First-line four (ATT) includes:

1. Isoniazid: 5 mg/kg/day
2. Rifampicin: 450 mg/day for individuals weighing ≤50 kg or 600 mg/day for those >50 kg
3. Ethambutol: 15 mg/kg/day
4. Pyrazinamide: 25–30 mg/kg/day

The detailed combination for tubercular uveitis is found in Chapter 7.

Toxoplasmic Panuveitis

First-line therapy for ocular toxoplasmosis includes triple therapy with pyrimethamine, sulfadiazine, and folinic acid. Other therapies for ocular toxoplasmosis include trimethoprim and sulfamethoxazole, azithromycin, clindamycin (oral or intravitreal injections), and steroids that should be used in combination with antiparasitic/antibiotic therapy.[7,8] Doses and route of administration for ocular toxoplasmosis are detailed in Chapter 6.

Viral Retinitis[9,10]

The treatment of viral retinitis includes antiviral drugs, corticosteroids, and, in some cases, antiplatelet drugs. Chapter 10 provides detailed treatment schemes for viral retinitis.

Syphilitic Panuveitis

Ocular syphilis must be managed similarly to neurosyphilis, with the standard treatment regimen, as given in **Table 2**.

Aqueous crystalline penicillin G is administered intravenously with a total daily dose of 18–24 million units. This dosage is divided and given every 4 hours or by continuous infusion over 10–14 days. Other therapies

TABLE 2: Treatment for noninfectious panuveitis.[1]

Diagnosis	Systemic steroids	Immunosuppressive therapy	Adjunct treatment
Sarcoidosis	• Oral prednisolone 0.5–1.0 mg/kg/day • Tapered over 8–10 weeks	• Methotrexate	
VKH disease	• IVMP 1,000 mg/day (3–5 days) • Oral prednisolone 1.0–1.5 mg/kg/day	• Azathioprine 2.0–2.5 mg/kg/day (tapered and stopped over 2–3 years) • MMF may be an alternative to azathioprine	• Calcium supplements • CBC/LFT 4–6 weekly
Sympathetic ophthalmia	• IVMP 1,000 mg/day (3–5 days) • Oral prednisolone 1.0–1.5 mg/kg/day	• Azathioprine 2.0–2.5 mg/kg/day (tapered and stopped over 2–3 years) • MMF may be an alternative to azathioprine	• Calcium supplements • CBC/LFT 4–6 weekly
Behçet's disease	• Oral prednisolone 0.5–1.0 mg/kg/day	• Azathioprine 2.0–2.5 mg/kg/day (tapered and stopped over 2–3 years) • Cyclosporine 3–5 mg/kg/day (tapered and stopped over 2–3 years) • Biological therapy, including anti-TNF-alpha inhibitors, has become the first-line therapy over immunosuppressants such as cyclosporine • Other biological drugs: Anti-IL-1	• Calcium supplements • CBC/LFT 4–6 weekly • BP monitoring daily

(BP: blood pressure; CBC: complete blood count; IL: interleukin; IVMP: intravenous methylprednisolone; LFT: liver function test; MMF: mycophenolate mofetil; VKH: Vogt–Koyanagi–Harada)

include procaine penicillin G and ceftriaxone. Detailed doses and schemes are found in Chapter 8.

SYMPATHETIC OPHTHALMIA

Case Presentation

Personal Data

- Male, 67 years old
- *Past medical history:* Hyperlipidemia
- *Past ophthalmic history:* Rhegmatogenous retinal detachment in the right eye
- Past surgical history of the right eye includes:
  - The patient developed cataracts, rubeosis iridis, hyphema, proliferative vitreoretinopathy (PVR), and recurrent retinal detachment after the initial vitrectomy and retinal detachment repair.
  - Procedures performed include cataract extraction with intraocular lens (IOL) implantation, multiple pars plana vitrectomies, membrane peeling, one intravitreal injection of avastin, and 13 intravitreal injections of methotrexate.

History of Present Illness

Blurred vision and floaters in the left eye over several months.

Physical Examination

The patient presents with visual acuity (VA) of counting fingers in OD and 20/30 in OS, 1+ anterior chamber cells, disc edema in OU, and yellow choroidal lesions in the nasal peripapillary area in OS **(Fig. 2 and Table 3)**.

Based on the clinical suspicion and history of surgical intervention in the right eye, the most plausible diagnosis is SO. However, comprehensive differential diagnoses include VKH disease, sarcoidosis-related uveitis, idiopathic multifocal choroiditis, BSCR, infectious uveitis, and primary vitreoretinal lymphoma. The workup included multimodal imaging with the left eye showing disc hyperfluorescence in the late phase of fluorescein angiogram and hypocyanescence of nasal peripapillary lesions on ICG **(Figs. 3 and 4)**. Optical coherence tomography (OCT) of the left eye showed nasal retinal thickening and intraretinal fluid without obvious choroidal thickening. His chest X-ray was normal, and her complete blood count was normal. Serum angiotensin-converting enzyme levels were elevated at 80 μg/L (normal 9-67 μg/L). Additionally, the patient tested positive for HLA-A29. Other tests, including lysozyme levels, erythrocyte sedimentation rate (ESR), C-reactive protein (CRP), rapid plasma reagin, fluorescent treponemal antibody-absorption, QuantiFERON-TB Gold, and Lyme Western blot, had normal or nonreactive results.

TABLE 3: Physical examination of the patient having sympathetic ophthalmia.

OD	*Parameters*	*OS*
Counting fingers	BCVA	20/30
4 mm Hg	IOP	36 mm Hg
White and quiet	Conjunctiva	White and quiet
Clear, no KPs	Cornea	Clear, no KPs
ACC: 1+, open angle	Anterior chamber	ACC: 1+, open angle
No nodules, no posterior synechiae	Iris	No nodules, no posterior synechiae
Significant disc edema, inferior retina scars with laser	Fundus	Vitreous haze, disc edema, snowballs, and nummular yellow choroidal lesions in nasal peripapillary area

(ACC: anterior chamber cellularity; BCVA: best-corrected visual acuity; IOP: intraocular pressure; KPs: keratic precipitates)

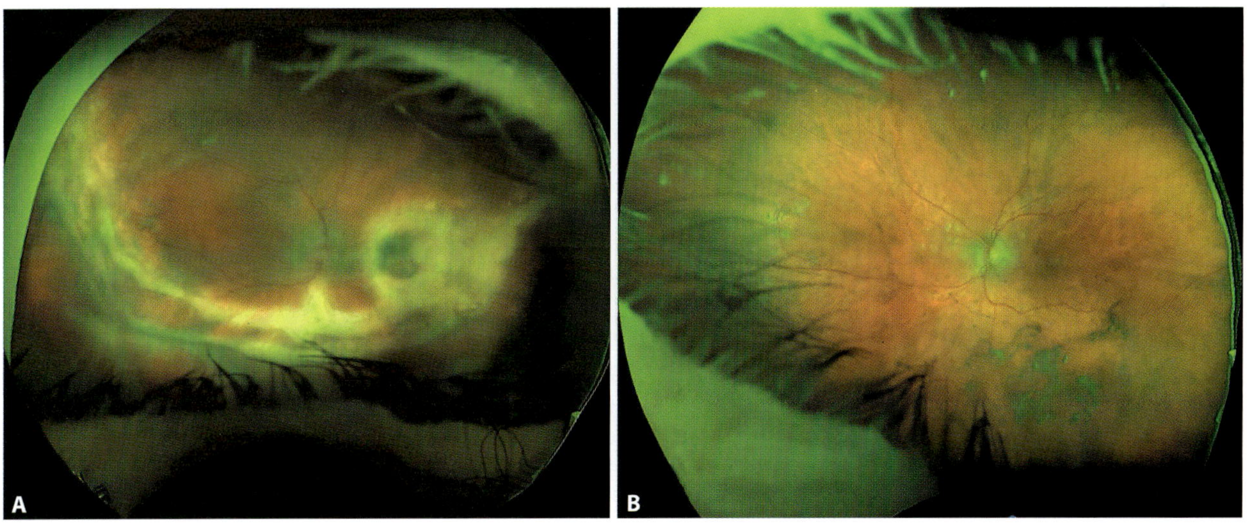

Figs. 2A and B: Fundus photography findings: (A) Right eye with significant disc edema and inferior retina scars with laser; (B) Left eye with vitreous haze, disc edema, and nummular yellow choroidal lesions in nasal peripapillary area.

Initial management with topical corticosteroids and ocular hypotensive drops improved the intraocular pressure (IOP) of the left eye and anterior chamber inflammation in both eyes. Once infectious etiologies were ruled out, oral prednisone was initiated at 60 mg daily with a 9-week tapering regimen. This improved visual acuity from 20/40 to 20/25 and reduced vitreous haze in the left eye. However, vitreous cells persisted.

One month after the prednisone taper, the patient's visual acuity deteriorated alongside increased vitreous haze and the emergence of more yellow chorioretinal lesions. He was referred from the retina service to the uveitis service. Given the normal laboratory results and the patient's extensive history of ocular surgeries, SO was considered as the primary diagnosis. Treatment was initiated with a daily regimen of oral prednisone at 60 mg with a slow taper, alongside biweekly subcutaneous injections of adalimumab at 40 mg. This therapeutic approach was accompanied by continued use of topical steroids and ocular hypotensive drops. This led to an improvement in the left eye's visual acuity from 20/50 to 20/30. During follow-up, there was a notable resolution in disc edema and vitreous haze. Moreover, the subretinal hyperreflective material significantly improved **(Figs. 5A to D)**.

Discussion

Sympathetic ophthalmia was first documented by William McKenzie in 1840 as a bilateral granulomatous panuveitis. It was primarily observed following penetrating ocular

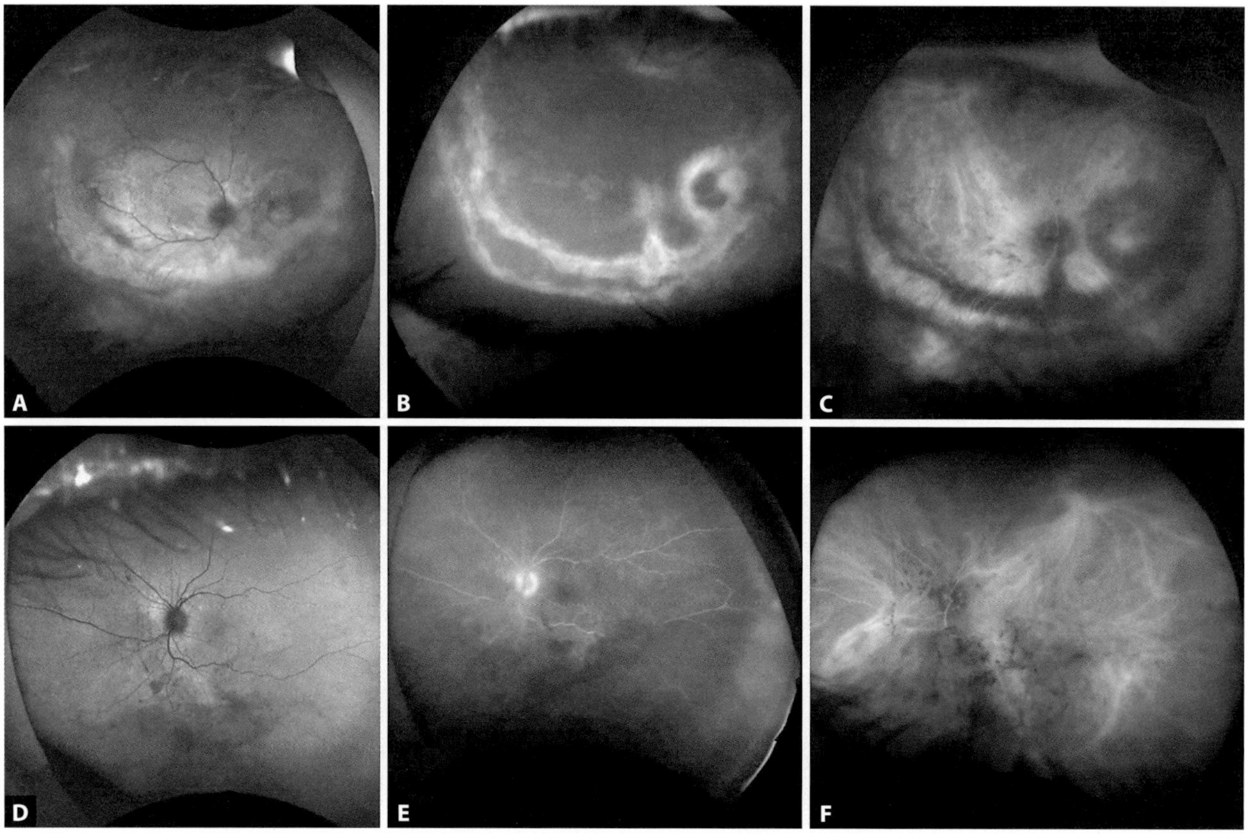

Figs. 3A to F: Fundus autofluorescence, fundus fluorescein angiography, and indocyanine green angiography findings at baseline: (A to C) The right eye demonstrates (A) areas of hyperautofluorescence and hypoautofluorescence at the relaxing retinectomy margin, (B) late-phase optic disc and macular leakage, and (C) late-phase hypocyanescence of peripapillary spots; (D to F) The left eye demonstrates (D) vitreous debris and a few peripapillary hyperautofluorescence lesions, (E) leakage from optic disc and peripapillary lesions with shadowing from vitreous debris, and (F) late-phase hypocyanescence of nasal peripapillary spots.

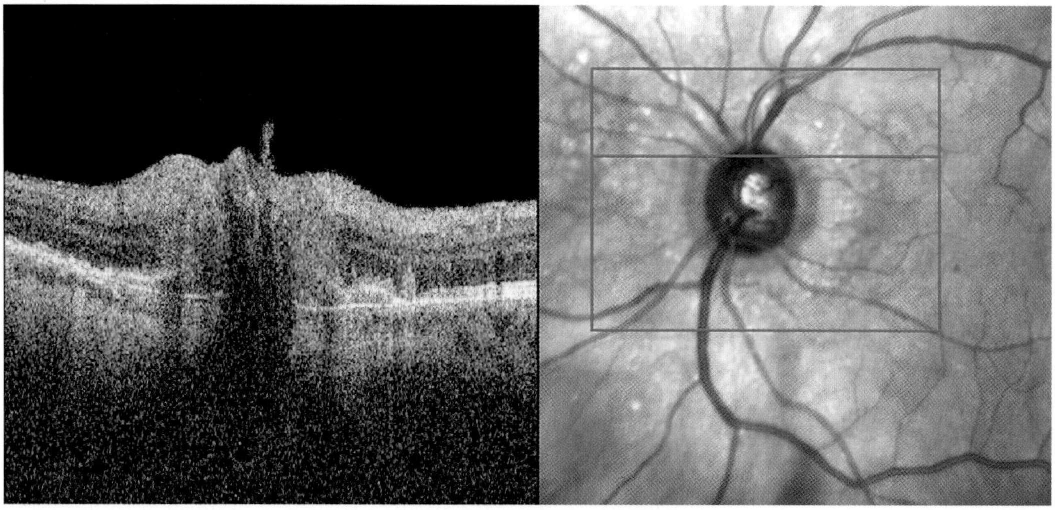

Fig. 4: Optical coherence tomography findings of the left eye. The left eye demonstrates peripapillary subretinal hyperreflective material.

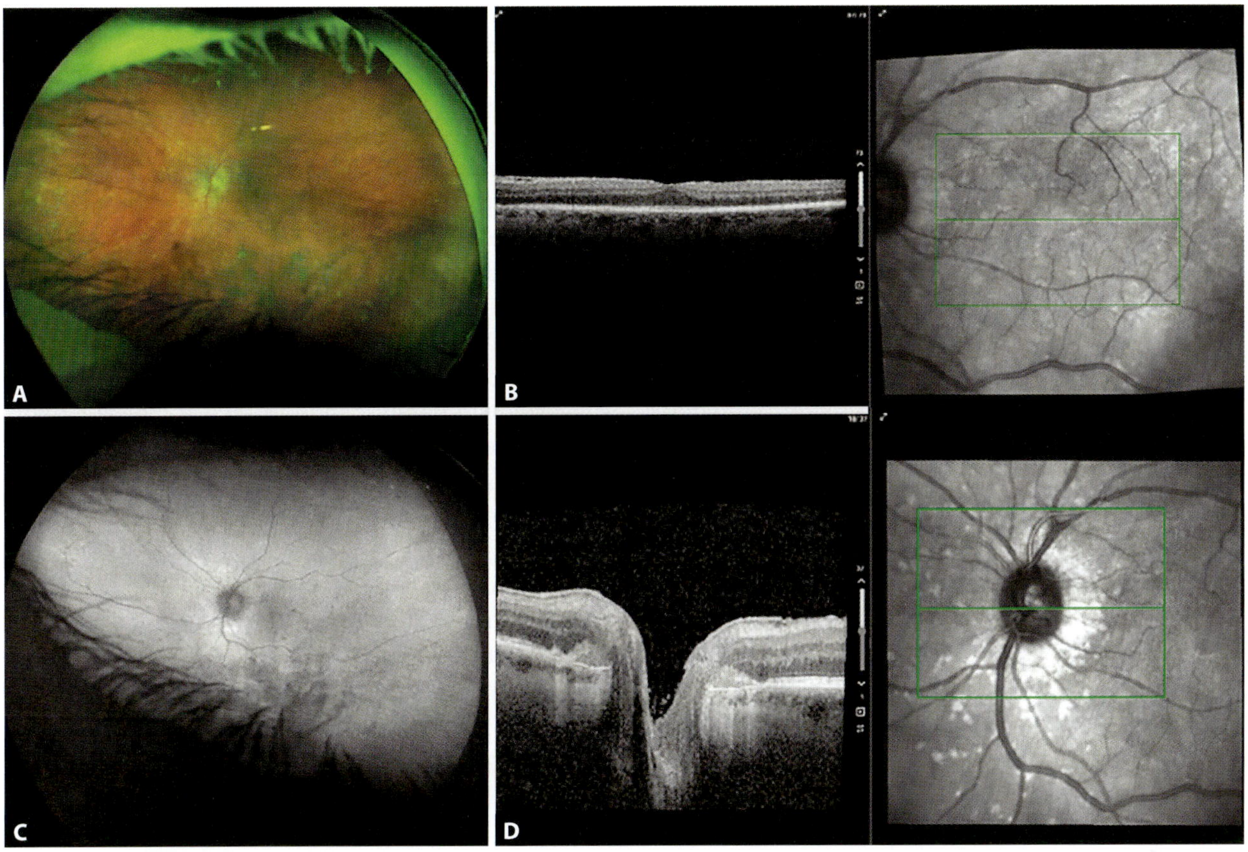

Figs. 5A to D: Multimodal imaging at final follow-up. Improvements in the left eye were noted across several parameters. (A) There was a reduction in the vitreous haze and stable diffuse scattered choroidal lesions; (B) Nasal subretinal hyperreflective lesions identified on optical coherence tomography (OCT) diminished; (C) Hyperautofluorescent lesions showed regression; (D) Optic disc thickening was improved, along with a decrease in subretinal hyperreflective material.
Source: Presented by Jie Sun in the International Uveitis Study Group (IUSG) grand rounds.[1]

trauma, where the affected eye was termed the "exciting eye," and the unaffected contralateral eye was termed the "sympathizing eye." Most cases manifest within the initial year postinjury.

Epidemiology

Sympathetic ophthalmia accounts for merely 1–2% of all uveitis cases. The primary risk factors include ocular trauma and ocular surgeries. An analysis of Japan's national database reported that the incidence after trauma is 0.073%, whereas after vitrectomy, it diminishes to 0.016%.[11] Despite the high frequency of vitrectomies globally, the overall incidence of SO remains higher posttrauma. In the United States, the IRIS database records a prevalence of 0.0207% after traumatic incidents and 0.0124% following ocular surgeries.[12] The higher incidence posttrauma is attributed to heightened antigen exposure compared to well-executed surgeries.[12]

Pathophysiology

The precise pathogenesis of SO remains elusive. It is believed to involve an autoimmune response by T-cell lymphocytes to ocular antigens from the retinal pigment epithelium (RPE) or choroid that are not usually exposed to the immune system. The immune system's recognition of these antigens could trigger an inflammatory reaction.[13]

Clinical Manifestations

Early disease signs include near-vision loss from ciliary body edema, along with common panuveitis symptoms such as light sensitivity, discomfort, floaters, flashing lights, and visual distortions. Differentiating SO from VKH syndrome can be challenging, but a history of trauma or surgery is a distinguishing factor. Occasionally, SO may present with extraocular manifestations such as those seen in VKH syndrome, such as cerebrospinal fluid pleocytosis, auditory disturbances, alopecia, poliosis, and vitiligo. Therefore, these do not rule out SO.[13]

Characteristic findings in the anterior segment may include granulomatous keratic precipitates (KPs), iris thickening from lymphocytic infiltration, and/or posterior synechiae formation. In the posterior segment, vitritis and Dalen-Fuchs nodules—pigmented epithelioid cell clusters between the RPE and Bruch's membrane—are typically present.[14]

Multimodal Imaging

Imaging plays a crucial role in diagnosing panuveitis. In fundus autofluorescence, a hyperautofluorescence signal suggests a metabolically active RPE and a hypoautofluorescence signal indicates RPE loss or blockage. Fluorescein angiography reveals multifocal early hyperfluorescence with late pooling in areas of serous retinal detachment, if present, although their occurrence can vary. ICGA might demonstrate hypocyanescent spots corresponding to Dalen-Fuchs nodules.[14,15]

Diagnosis

Diagnosis is primarily based on clinical presentation, especially a history of trauma or surgeries, and supported by imaging results. The principal differential diagnosis is VKH syndrome, which shares many clinical features with SO. Other potential causes of granulomatous uveitis, such as sarcoidosis, tuberculosis, and syphilis, should also be considered based on clinical context.

Birdshot chorioretinopathy was considered a possible diagnosis by the referring retinal physicians due to the patient's positive HLA-A29. Yet, clinical characteristics suggested a different condition. BSCR typically manifests as posterior uveitis, though anterior segment inflammation and KPs may occur in rare cases. Despite a strong association with HLA-A29, this alone is not definitive for BSCR diagnosis, given its prevalence in the general US population (7%). ICGA is essential for differentiating BSCR, as it has more extensive and numerous hypocyanescent lesions than SO **(Figs. 6A to D)**.[16,17] In BSCR, fluorescein angiography may show optic disc hyperfluorescence akin

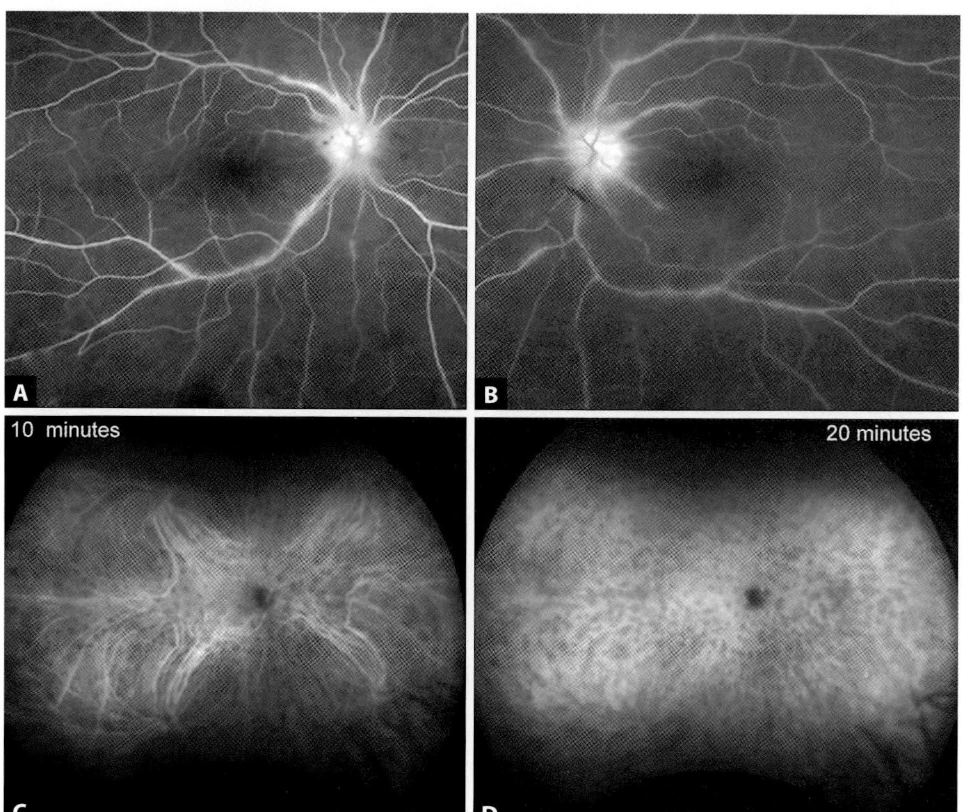

Figs. 6A to D: Typical imaging pattern of birdshot chorioretinopathy: (A and B) Contiguous, perineural retinal vascular leakage and along the arcades; (C and D) Diffuse choroidal lesions at 10–20 minutes.
Source: Presented by Lucia Sobrin in the International Uveitis Study Group (IUSG) grand rounds.[1]

to SO, but retinal vasculitis is more prominent, often with leakage extending from the optic nerve along the arcades.

Treatment

Standard treatment involves administering high-dose systemic corticosteroids (initially pulses of methylprednisolone followed by oral steroids that are gradually tapered off), complemented by the commencement of immunomodulatory therapy (IMT). IMT is usually indicated in patients with SO to decrease the need for and side effects caused by prolonged systemic corticosteroid use. The duration of IMT depends on the severity of the disease. Some patients may continue to experience ongoing vitreous and chorioretinal inflammation, requiring long-term treatment with IMT. When IMT fails to control inflammation, biologics can be used.

The question frequently posed is whether prompt enucleation of the traumatized eye could have circumvented the development of SO. It is generally suggested that enucleation within the first 2 weeks postinjury might reduce the risk of this complication. However, one study documented that the interval between trauma and the onset of SO could be as short as 5 days, casting doubt on the absolute preventive value of early enucleation.[17] Currently, although the benefit of early enucleation is recognized, ensuring meticulous wound closure is given more priority.[14,18]

After a traumatic eye injury, the decision to proceed with enucleation to decrease the risk for SO requires careful deliberation, ensuring it is reserved for eyes with no light perception and no potential for visual recovery. Given the availability of effective IMTs for the rare occurrence of SO, enucleation should be considered carefully.[17]

Recurrence

Patients with SO should be monitored regularly based on the severity of the disease and their response to treatment. Recurrence of the disease can be indicated by several symptoms, including cellular activity in the anterior chamber, decreased visual acuity, and signs of inflammation in the posterior segment, such as the appearance of new choroidal lesions (Dalen–Fuchs nodules), serous retinal detachments, and optic nerve edema. Regular monitoring for these symptoms and signs with clinical assessments and multimodal imaging is essential to ensure timely intervention and management.[13]

SARCOID PANUVEITIS[1]

Case Presentation

Personal Data

- Female, 50 years old
- *Systemic diseases:* Poorly controlled hypercholesterolemia; the last cholesterol measurement was 278 mg/dL
- No current medication
- History of corticosteroid high responder
- *Past ophthalmic history:* Phakic posterior chamber intraocular lens implanted in the left eye 12 years ago
- Three months earlier, a palpable right submandibular lymph node was noted. A node ultrasound revealed inflammatory changes, and a subsequent fine-needle aspiration biopsy confirmed nonnecrotizing granulomatous inflammation. Notably, a chest CT scan at this time did not demonstrate any pathological findings.

History of Present Illness

Over the past several months, the patient has experienced a progressive decline in visual acuity accompanied by photopsia, predominantly in the right eye.

Physical Examination

See **Figure 7** and **Table 4**.

Differential Diagnosis

Various differential diagnoses were considered, including ocular sarcoidosis, SO stemming from ocular surgery two decades earlier, ocular tuberculosis, ocular syphilis, and granulomatosis with polyangiitis—the latter primarily considered for its systemic manifestations rather than for ocular involvement.

A thorough diagnostic workup was undertaken to rule out specific diagnoses and as part of the screening process before administering immunosuppressants, including a purified protein derivative (PPD) test and serological testing for syphilis, hepatitis, Chagas disease, and ultrawide-field FFA **(Figs. 8A and B)**. All test results were normal except for the lymph node biopsy, which suggested a sarcoidosis etiology based on granulomatous inflammation.

Treatment

- Topical prednisolone acetate 1% is to be applied every 3 hours in both eyes.

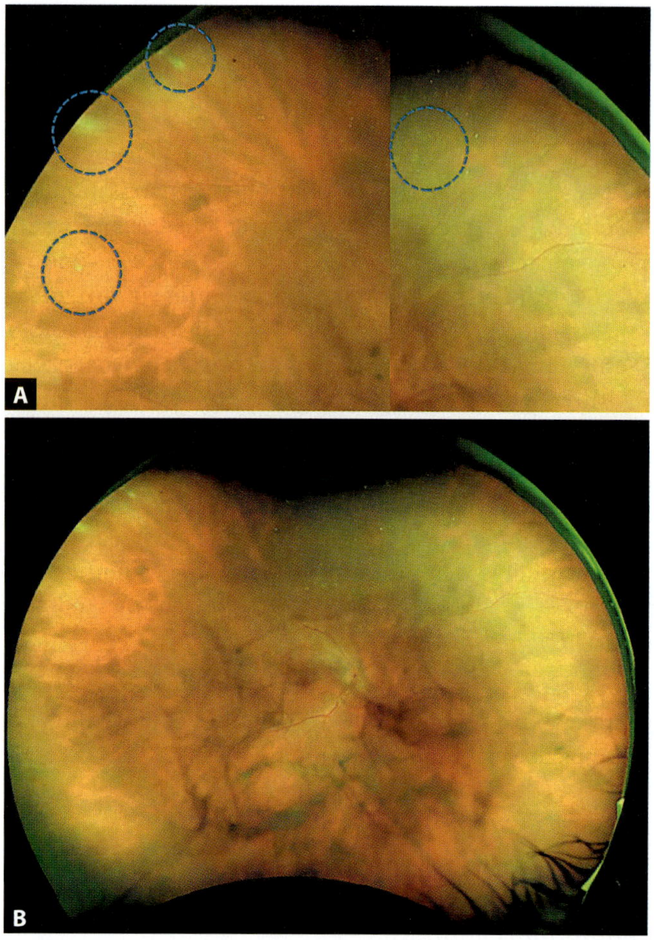

Figs. 7A and B: Ultrawide-field fundus photographs of the right eye at the initial examination: (A) Multifocal choroiditis in the periphery (blue circles); (B) Right eye with disc edema and 2+ vitreous haze.

- Oral prednisone at a daily dose of 60 mg
- Methotrexate at 20 mg/week

Follow-up

Upon the recurrence of symptoms following the tapering of steroids, the therapeutic regimen was revised to increase the methotrexate dosage to 25 mg/week and introduce biweekly adalimumab injections at 40 mg. Additionally, dexamethasone intraocular implants were applied in both eyes to achieve remission.

After 9 months, best-corrected visual acuity (BCVA) improved from 20/60 to 20/30. Papillitis and vasculitis improved, but atrophic lesions induced by multifocal choroiditis persisted. OCT scans revealed a small epiretinal membrane in the right eye, while the left eye showed no abnormalities.

Final Diagnosis

Sarcoid panuveitis was ultimately diagnosed. Tissue biopsy was instrumental in reaching this conclusion. The role of ultrawide fluorescein angiography was crucial in assessing the posterior segment and monitoring treatment efficacy. It facilitated the decision to escalate immunosuppressive treatment, which proved beneficial in achieving a positive outcome for this patient.

Discussion

Sarcoidosis is a multisystem disorder predominantly affecting the lungs, with ocular involvement observed in 13–79% of patients.[19] The risk of ocular involvement is

TABLE 4: Physical examination of the patient having sarcoid panuveitis.

OD	*Parameters*	*OS*
20/60	BCVA	20/30
17 mm Hg	IOP	17 mm Hg
White and quiet	Conjunctiva	White and quiet
Fine KPs	Cornea	Clear, no KPs
ACC: 1+, flare: 0.5+	Anterior chamber	ACC: 1+, flare: 0.5+
Koeppe nodule at 7-hour meridian, no synechiae	Iris	Phakic IOL, iridotomies at 11- and 7-hour meridian, and posterior synechiae between 11 and 12 hours
Clear	Lens	Clear
3+ cells, 2+ vitreous haze	Vitreous	1+ cells
Multifocal choroiditis	Fundus	Multifocal choroiditis

(ACC: anterior chamber cellularity; BCVA: best-corrected visual acuity; IOL: intraocular lens; IOP: intraocular pressure; KPs: keratic precipitates)

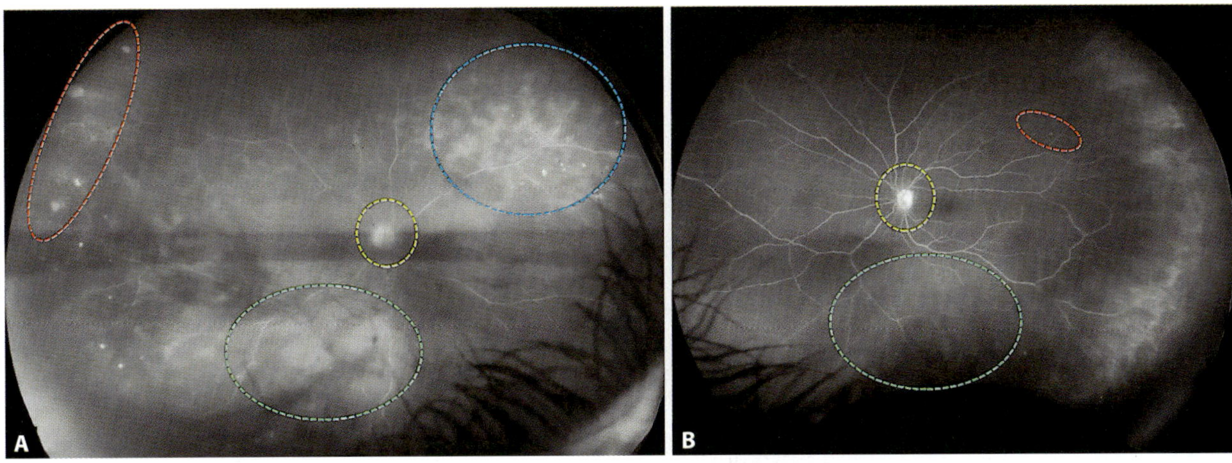

Figs. 8A and B: Ultrawide-field fundus fluorescein angiography at the initial examination: (A) Right eye: Evidencing multifocal hyperfluorescence stain pattern in the superior temporal retina due to multifocal choroiditis (red circle), fern pattern in the superior nasal retina due to diffuse capillary leakage (blue circle), optic disc hyperfluorescence suggesting papillitis (yellow circle), and diffuse hyperfluorescence in inferior retina suggestive of retinal edema (green circle); (B) Left eye: Evidencing optic disc hyperfluorescence suggestive of papillitis (yellow circle), multifocal hyperfluorescent staining pattern due to multifocal choroiditis (red circle), and diffuse hyperfluorescence in the inferior retina indicative of retinal edema (green circle).

notably higher among female patients and individuals of African-American descent. The disease typically presents in a bimodal age distribution, with peaks between 20–30 and 50–60 years.[20]

Globally, sarcoidosis accounts for 10% of all uveitis cases. In 30–40% of these cases, ocular symptoms may be the first manifestation of the disease.[19,20] Uveitis is the most common ocular complication, affecting approximately 80% of patients with OS. This form of uveitis is usually bilateral and follows a chronic course in about 90% of cases. Panuveitis accounts for 22–38% of all sarcoid-related uveitis cases.[19,20]

Diagnostic Criteria

The International Workshop on Ocular Sarcoidosis (IWOS)[21] and the Standardization of Uveitis Nomenclature (SUN)[22] have established sets of criteria for the diagnosis of OS. The SUN guidelines incorporate characteristic ocular signs aligned with sarcoidosis **(Figs. 9 and 10)** and evidence of systemic involvement, such as a corroborating tissue biopsy or definitive chest imaging. The IWOS criteria classify definite, presumed, and probable OS based on ocular findings, bilateral hilar lymphadenopathy, and biopsy. Both criteria are found in Chapter 2.

The key goals in managing OS are to achieve remission and mitigate inflammation. For anterior segment inflammation, topical corticosteroids, mainly prednisolone acetate 1% or difluprednate 0.05%, are administered with mydriatics such as atropine 1% or cyclopentolate 0.5%.[20] In cases involving the posterior segment, therapeutic options extend to oral corticosteroids—prednisone at a daily intake of 1 mg/kg or 60 mg/day—and regional steroid injections. Periocular delivery of triamcinolone acetonide at 20–40 mg/1 mL, intravitreal administration of triamcinolone acetonide in doses of 2–4 mg, or dexamethasone implants of 0.7 mg serve as alternative interventions.[20,23]

Immunosuppressants are introduced for persistent forms of OS, with methotrexate often leading as the first-line immunosuppressive therapy. Other alternative immunosuppressants such as azathioprine and mycophenolate mofetil can be used in cases of intolerance or hepatic damage due to methotrexate. When methotrexate fails to control inflammation, antitumor necrosis factor (TNF) inhibitors such as adalimumab or infliximab are preferred. As a third-line option, biologics with other mechanisms of action, such as interleukin-6 receptor (IL-6r) inhibition or anti-CD20, might be alternatives.[20,24-26]

In the present clinical case, adalimumab was introduced as a second-line option after a partial response to methotrexate. When the disease failed to respond at 20 mg of methotrexate weekly, it was considered that a dose of 25 mg weekly of methotrexate would not be sufficient for the patient. Therefore, adalimumab was added to achieve sustained control of inflammation. Currently, the patient is still on adalimumab. Corticosteroid-free

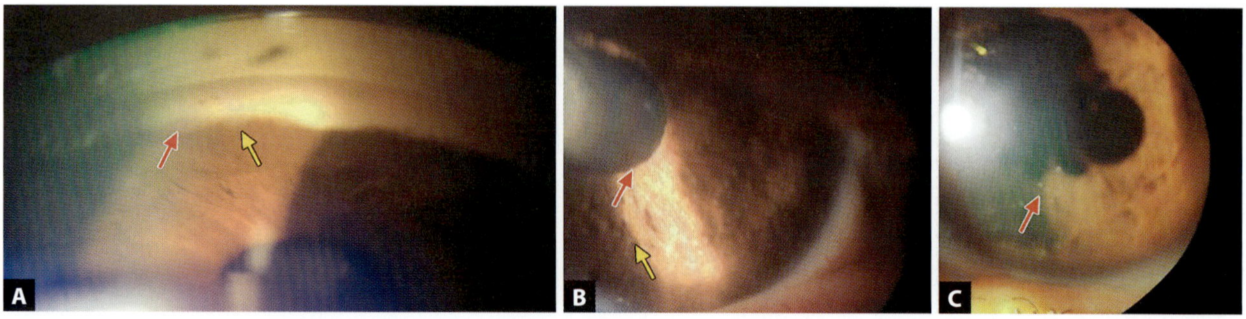

Figs. 9A to C: Typical ocular signs of sarcoidosis in the anterior segment: (A) Berlin nodule (red arrow) with tent-shaped anterior synechiae (yellow arrow); (B) Koeppe (red arrow) and Busacca nodules (yellow arrow); (C) Granulomatous keratic precipitates (KPs) (red arrow).

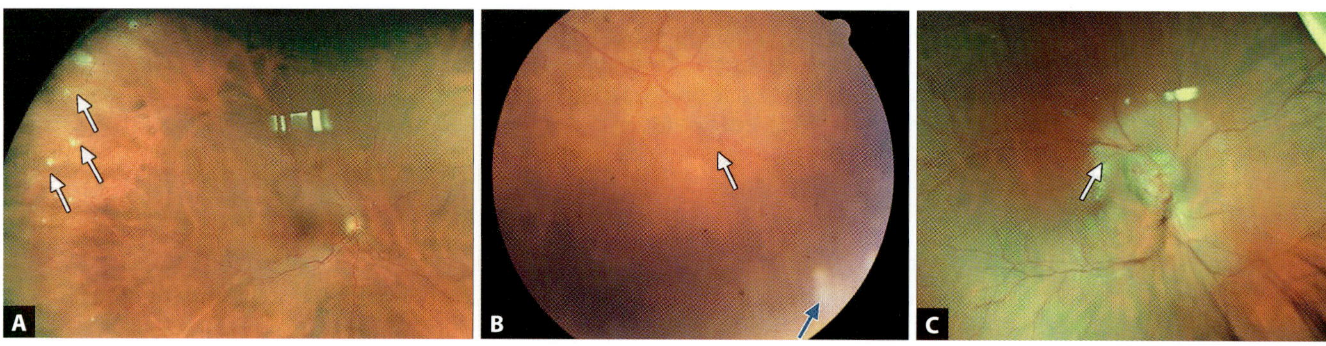

Figs. 10A to C: Typical ocular signs of sarcoidosis in the posterior segment: (A) Right eye with small yellowish lesions at periphery indicative of multifocal choroiditis (white arrows); (B) Segmental periphlebitis at the inferotemporal arcade (white arrow) with snowballs in a string of pearls appearance (blue arrow); (C) Optic disc swelling suggestive of sarcoid granuloma (white arrow).
Source: Presented by Ariel Schlaen in the International Uveitis Study Group (IUSG) grand rounds.[1]

remission must last at least 2 years before considering the tapering and eventual withdrawal of the immunosuppressant medication.

VOGT–KOYANAGI–HARADA SYNDROME[1]

Case Presentation

Personal Data

- Female, 13 years old
- *Family history:* Mother with multiple sclerosis

History of Present Illness

She had a 1-week history of blurred vision, redness, and pain in both eyes, which led to her visit to the emergency room. Before the onset of these ocular symptoms, she experienced persistent headaches, fevers, and malaise for 3 weeks. These headaches, primarily located behind the eyes and accompanied by aching sensations, were only mildly alleviated with paracetamol and promethazine. Additionally, she reported a recent onset of floaters and photophobia. The external exam was normal at presentation, with no poliosis or vitiligo.

Physical Examination

The patient presents with a VA of 20/60 in OD and 20/70 in OS, red eyes, no KPs, 1+ of anterior chamber cells, edematous and hyperemic optic disc, and multiple serous retinal detachment in OU **(Fig. 11 and Table 5)**.

Multimodal imaging, including fundus autofluorescence, OCT, and AGF, was performed, evidencing septate retinal detachment, optic disc hyperfluorescence, and spots of choroidal leakage in the macula of the right eye consistent with VKH disease activity **(Figs. 12A to D)**.

Workup

A comprehensive diagnostic evaluation was conducted, including tests for tuberculosis, Lyme disease, syphilis, meningitis, cryptococcus, and human immunodeficiency virus (HIV). In addition, a neurologic workup for optic

TABLE 5: Physical examination of the patient having Vogt–Koyanagi–Harada syndrome.

OD	***Parameters***	***OS***
20/60	BCVA	20/70
1+ injection, blanches fully with phenylephrine	Conjunctiva	1+ injection, blanches fully with phenylephrine
Clear, no KPs	Cornea	Clear, no KPs
ACC: 1+	Anterior chamber	ACC: 1+
Normal, no transillumination defects	Iris	Normal, no transillumination defects
Clear	Lens	Clear
0.5+ cells	Vitreous	0.5+ cells
Edematous and hyperemic optic nerves, multiple serous retinal detachments, normal vessels, and normal periphery	Fundus	Edematous and hyperemic optic nerves, multiple serous retinal detachments, normal vessels, and normal periphery

(ACC: anterior chamber cellularity; BCVA: best-corrected visual acuity; KPs: keratic precipitates).

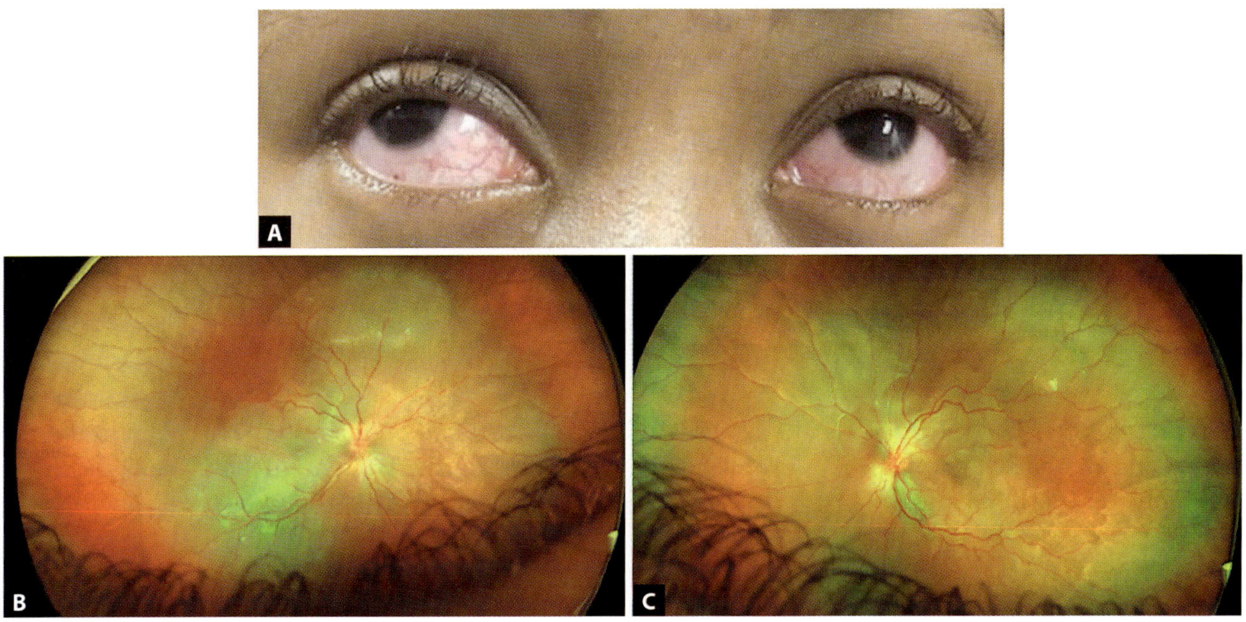

Figs. 11A to C: External examination and fundoscopy at baseline: (A) 1+ conjunctival injection in both eyes that blanch fully with phenylephrine; (B and C) Edematous and hyperemic optic nerves with multiple serous retinal detachments.
Source: Presented by Russel Dinh in the International Uveitis Study Group (IUSG) grand rounds.[1]

head edema was performed, including a lumbar puncture to check the cerebrospinal fluid (CSF) for cytomegalovirus, herpes simplex virus I-II, varicella-zoster virus, and cryptococcus. The patient also underwent a chest X-ray [posteroanterior (PA) and lateral views], tests for HLA-B27, and inflammatory markers such as ESR/CRP.

Final Diagnosis

Vogt–Koyanagi–Harada syndrome was diagnosed based on clinical and multimodal imaging of the eyes.

Treatment and Follow-up

The initial treatment approach for the patient began with the administration of 1 gram of methylprednisolone in the emergency room. This was quickly followed by a regimen of 60 mg of oral prednisone daily. After 1 week, the treatment plan was expanded to include 25 mg of methotrexate weekly while continuing the 60 mg daily dose of prednisone. The prednisolone dosage was gradually tapered, with the medication being completely discontinued after 15 months. The methotrexate dosage

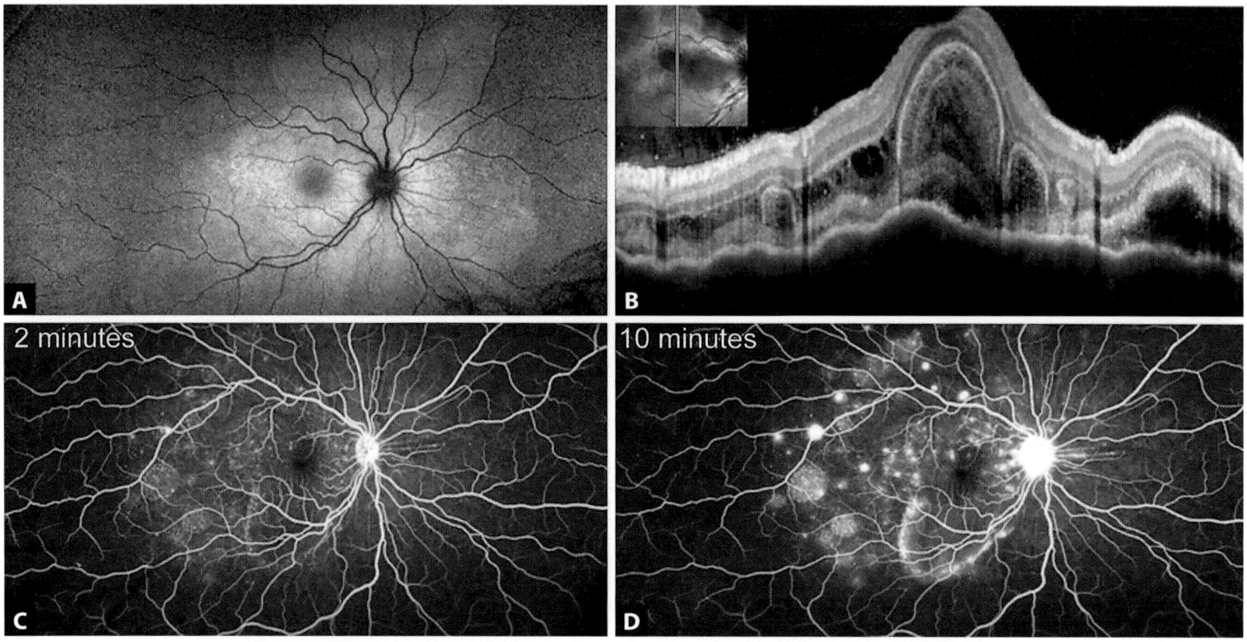

Figs. 12A to D: Multimodal imaging: (A) Fundus autofluorescence imaging displays a hyperautofluorescent signal surrounding the optic disc and extending toward the macula, indicating active inflammation and serous retinal detachment; (B) Optical coherence tomography (OCT) reveals significant serous retinal detachment with a dome-shaped elevation and hyperreflective septae within the subretinal fluid. The ellipsoid zone is also disrupted; (C) Early-phase fluorescein angiography at 2 minutes shows multiple pinpoint hyperfluorescent spots indicative of choroidal leakage and dye pooling in the subretinal space around the optic disc; (D) Late-phase fluorescein angiography at 10 minutes demonstrates diffuse hyperfluorescence, late staining of the optic disc, and persistent leakage spots and pooling.
Source: Presented by Russel Dinh in the International Uveitis Study Group (IUSG) grand rounds.[1]

was also reduced, starting with a taper to 15 mg weekly, then 10 mg, and eventually discontinued entirely achieving 20/20 in both eyes **(Figs. 13A and B)**.

Discussion

There are several classification criteria for VKH syndrome, one of which is the SUN classification criteria[27] **(Fig. 14)**, which delineates the early and late stages. Early diagnosis is crucial and requires observation of either retinal detachment or panuveitis, accompanied by neurological symptoms. Additionally, differentiating VKH from similar syndromes such as SO is essential, particularly by excluding any history of penetrating ocular trauma or prior vitreoretinal surgery.[28]

Epidemiology

Vogt–Koyanagi–Harada predominantly occurs in East Asia, Southeast Asia, and the Middle East, where it is one of the most common uveitic conditions.[29] Despite recent literature indicating a universal susceptibility across all races, a notable predisposition is linked to the human leukocyte antigen (HLA) genotype. The disease typically affects individuals aged 24–40 years, who often experience more severe manifestations.[30]

Pathogenesis

The precise etiology of VKH remains elusive, though it is mediated by T cells and primarily affects melanocytes. This association suggests a predisposition in individuals with darker-pigmented skin. The inflammation mainly involves the choroidal stroma. While fluorescein angiography is commonly used, ICGA is particularly effective in identifying choroidal involvement. Choroidal depigmentation following chronic inflammation contributes to the classic sunset-glow fundus appearance.[28]

Imaging

Multimodal imaging is vital for diagnosing panuveitis associated with VKH. Pathognomonic signs and retinal detachments can be clinically observed and documented

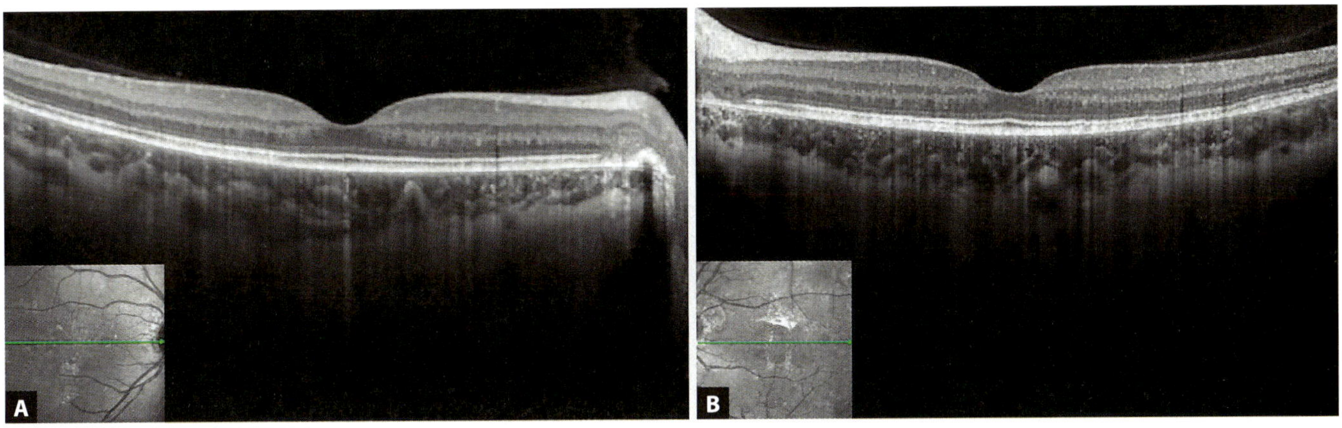

Figs. 13A and B: Optical coherence tomography (OCT) after treatment: (A) The right eye demonstrates a resolved serous retinal detachment, restoring the retina to its normal anatomical configuration; (B) OCT of the left eye also shows resolution of serous retinal detachment with normalized retinal architecture.
Source: Presented by Russel Dinh in the International Uveitis Study Group (IUSG) grand rounds.[1]

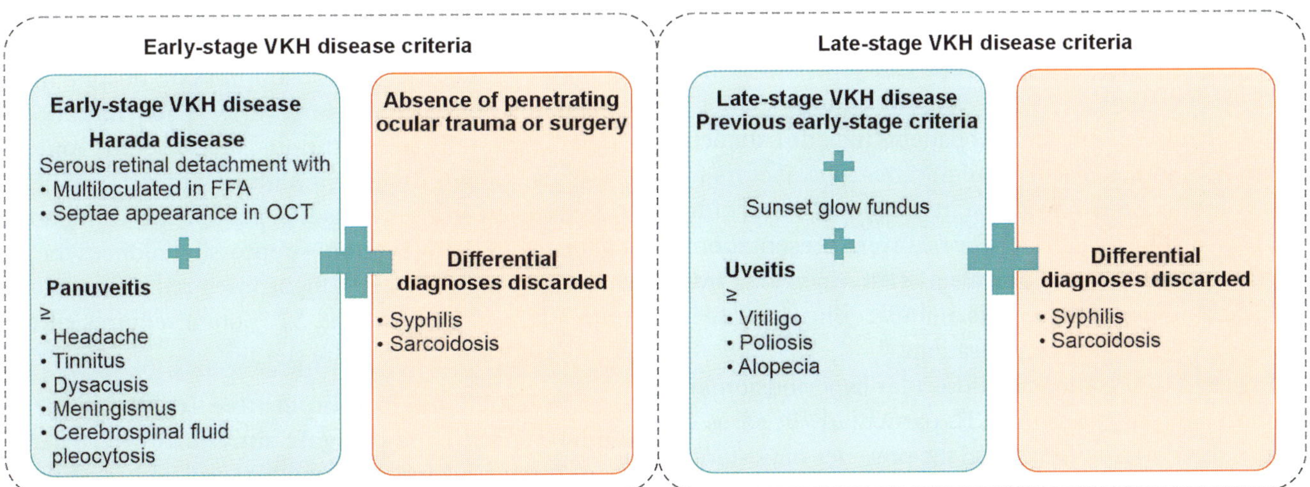

Fig. 14: Classification criteria for Vogt–Koyanagi–Harada (VKH) disease by SUN.[21] (FFA: fundus fluorescein angiography; OCT: optical coherence tomography; SUN: Standardization of Uveitis Nomenclature)
Source: Modified from Standardized Uveitis Nomenclature.[27]

using wide-angle color fundus photography. OCT imaging highlights specific features such as bacillary and septal detachments. Enhanced depth imaging (EDI) OCT reveals choroidal thickening, and ICGA emphasizes choroidal thickening, which are crucial for monitoring the disease's progression and treatment efficacy.[31]

Course

A comprehensive study in Japan reviewed VKH cases from the early stages to assess the treatment response. Findings showed that treatment exclusively with corticosteroids resulted in higher rates of chronicity (61%) and sunset glow fundus (53%) compared to a combination of corticosteroids with immunosuppressive therapy (2% chronicity, 17% sunset glow fundus).[18,30] This underscores the importance of early and aggressive treatment, including high-dose oral prednisone and possibly IV methylprednisolone, complemented by a gradual taper of steroids with a steroid-sparing agent.

Recurrence

The high risk of recurrences necessitates long-term monitoring. ICGA, when available, is advised every 6 weeks for 6 months, then every 2–3 months.[30] Recurrences could present with anterior segment inflammation. Therefore, a slit-lamp examination and dilated fundoscopy in every follow-up visit are mandatory.[28] Geographic variations in the incidence of recurrences have been noted in studies, underscoring the importance of individualized patient monitoring to identify those at risk. Regular monitoring enables healthcare providers to detect and manage recurrences promptly, optimizing patient outcomes.[1]

Management

Vogt–Koyanagi–Harada responds well to prompt and aggressive treatment. Initial management typically involves IV methylprednisolone followed by high-dose oral corticosteroids, with early initiation of immunosuppressive therapy. Continuous monitoring for recurrences and complications such as anterior uveitis and glaucoma is essential for long-term management.[28]

Complications

Frequent complications in VKH patients include cataracts, glaucoma, and neovascular membranes. Risk factors for these complications have been identified as being older than 16 years, having chronic or recurrent presentations, and the presence of mutton-fat KPs. However, IMT significantly reduces these risks, underscoring its value in managing VKH-related complications.[32]

Angle-closure glaucoma and ocular hypertension are common complications in VKH, particularly in cases of chronic or recurrent disease and the presence of posterior synechiae.[33] Regularly monitoring these patients for IOP elevation is crucial to detect early signs of glaucoma development, ideally annually. Prompt detection is essential as changes in cup–disc ratio can occur abruptly, necessitating timely intervention to prevent vision loss from glaucoma.[34]

Immunotherapy-induced Vogt–Koyanagi–Harada

The increasing use of immunotherapy for malignant melanoma has led to a rise in cases of associated uveitis, particularly panuveitis. While spontaneous resolution may occur after several treatment infusions, unresolved cases may necessitate collaboration between ophthalmologists and oncologists for potential treatment adjustments. Despite reports of a potential HLA association, conclusive evidence is lacking.[1]

COVID-19 Vaccination

Recent reports indicate a recurrence of VKH following COVID-19 vaccination worldwide. Symptoms typically manifest 1–2 weeks after the first vaccine dose, sometimes after the second, with prompt treatment response and favorable visual prognosis. While a genetic predisposition linked to HLA-DR4 has been suggested, scientific evidence remains limited. Hence, clinicians are advised to inquire about recent COVID-19 vaccination and immunotherapy during VKH patient evaluations.[35]

GENERAL DISCUSSION AND CONTROVERSIES IN PANUVEITIS[1]

1. Should early immunosuppression be indicated in noninfectious panuveitis and other forms of uveitis?

Answer: Recently, there has been a shift toward initiating immunosuppressive therapy earlier in treatment, departing from traditional practices. New data suggest better outcomes with early immunosuppression despite initial expectations based on case severity. Early initiation is crucial, especially in conditions such as VKH and SO, which are known to carry a high risk of recurrence. As these drugs have a slow onset of action, early initiation is advantageous. Early immunosuppression reduces the risk of chronicity in VKH. While high-dose prednisone initially suffices for some conditions, VKH often requires chronic immunosuppression to spare steroids.

2. Is specific imaging imperative in all scenarios, and how should one navigate situations where access to sophisticated imaging equipment and facilities is limited?

Answer: Clinical evaluation is essential and critical for establishing a diagnosis in most cases. However, imaging tools such as OCT and FFA help improve the certainty of a definitive diagnosis. An early referral to specialized uveitis centers is recommended in atypical cases or those showing poor response to initial therapy.

Smartphone-based fundus photography and affordable handheld OCT devices can aid diagnostic assessments in resource-limited settings. Continuous education and resourceful use of available technologies are essential for improving uveitis treatment and emphasizing the importance of clinical expertise in guiding treatment decisions.

3. Would a positive IgM with the typical features of ocular toxoplasmosis be considered diagnostic? If not,

what alternative diagnostic approaches do you suggest besides relying solely on immunoglobulins?

Answer: Diagnosing ocular toxoplasmosis primarily relies on clinical presentation, with characteristic retinochoroidal lesions being key indicators. While serological confirmation with immunoglobulin G (IgG) and immunoglobulin M (IgM) antibodies is desirable, Ig testing has limited value due to the high prevalence of positive results. A positive IgM may be helpful, but negative results are typically more informative for ruling out toxoplasmosis. In atypical cases where diagnosis is uncertain, polymerase chain reaction (PCR) testing can be helpful. IgM indicates a recent infection, while IgG remains positive as a memory antibody for life. Additional insights into the diagnosis of toxoplasmosis will be provided in subsequent chapters.

4. Considering the similarities between SO and VKH, are HLA-DR4 and HLA-DR1 tests recommended to differentiate these conditions?

Answer: Testing HLA is not possible for all patients. The primary difference between SO and VKH is the history of trauma or ocular surgery.

5. When should you start oral steroids in tuberculosis (TB) and how long should it take?

Answer: The initiation of oral steroids will depend upon the phenotype of ocular TB. In serpiginous-like choroiditis and retinal vasculitis, the disease is primarily immune driven and in such scenarios, oral corticosteroids may be initiated, especially if the lesions are involving or threatening the fovea and specific ATT added when test results are available. However, in cases with large tuberculomas and abscess-like appearance, one should avoid the use of corticosteroids and initiate ATT. Oral steroids are initiated promptly upon diagnosing TB panuveitis, with the administration of antitubercular therapy after conducting a baseline liver function test.

6. Is there any guide or literature that shows the start times of corticosteroids and the duration of their use in infectious uveitis?

Answer: There are no guidelines. However, oral steroids usually start 24–48 hours after antibiotics or antivirals are started in toxoplasmosis and viral panuveitis. Duration is tailored according to clinical response.

7. Is there any alternative/biologics treatments for neuro-Behçet's disease?

Answer: Mycophenolate mofetil and adalimumab.

8. How often do you see SO with a thin choroid on OCT?

Answer: Acute SO has a very thick choroid. A thin choroid is usually seen in the convalescent phase of VKH and SO.

9. Does systemic steroid use before the diagnostic investigation affect the results of infectious screening? Should you ask to stop steroids before doing screening tests? How long is free steroid necessary?

Answer: Usually, systemic steroids should not be started until the infectious etiologies have been ruled out.

10. Are there diseases resembling VKH, such as those that occur in many cases after checkpoint inhibitor therapy and large tattoos?

Answer: Yes, obtaining a full medical history in all patients with uveitis is important, especially in the era of the increasing use of checkpoint inhibitors and tattoos.

11. Very often, patients come under steroid treatment without evidence of infection being ruled out yet. In that case, what advice can I get?

Answer: It is crucial to rule out infectious uveitis. It is very risky to treat with steroids without excluding infection. Educating physicians about this point is crucial. If a patient presents with this situation, you should perform the workup for infectious uveitis.

12. Could we use interferon alpha-2a for VKH syndrome?

Answer: No, antimetabolites are typically used for VKH syndrome, with escalation to biologics if further immunosuppression is required.

13. Where are the most common locations of snowballs in ocular sarcoidosis?

Answer: Typically, they are at an inferior location due to gravity. If they are abundant, they may be elsewhere.

14. Segmental nonocclusive vasculitis is a typical sign of sarcoidosis. Does this mean that occlusive retinal vasculitis can be a negative key sign?

Answer: No, occlusive vasculitis may occur in ocular sarcoidosis. Indeed, it is part of the SUN working group's classification criteria.

15. Do Dalen-Fuchs nodules differ in SO, VKH, and sarcoid uveitis?

Answer: No, they look the same. Sunset glow fundus is an additional finding in VKH or SO.

16. How to monitor glaucoma by retinal nerve fiber layer (RNFL) evaluation?

Answer: Repeat RNFL OCT every 3–4 months to assess the thinning of the RNFL layer.

FINAL WRAP-UP

In conclusion, rates of visual impairment are higher with panuveitis compared with other anatomic locations. Etiologies can include both infectious and noninfectious and masquerade syndromes. Clinical differentiation is facilitated by the unilateral predominance of infectious uveitis presentations, in contrast to bilateral involvement, which is more indicative of noninfectious etiologies. Accurately diagnosing and managing panuveitis requires a multidisciplinary approach, that integrates various investigative modalities, including retinal imaging and laboratory analyses.

REFERENCES

1. Uveitis Course - IUSG Grand Round 04. (13th April 2024). https://youtu.be/xyO8H6UZeng?si=cGz7OMV2j5e1lzUf.
2. Heiligenhaus A, Rothaus K, Pleyer U. Entwicklung von Klassifikationskriterien für Uveitiden von der Standardization of Uveitis Nomenclature (SUN) Working Group. Ophthalmologe. 2021;118(9):913-8.
3. Agrawal R, Testi I, Bodaghi B, Barisani-Asenbauer T, McCluskey P, Agarwal A, et al. Collaborative ocular tuberculosis study consensus guidelines on the management of tubercular uveitis—report 2. Ophthalmology. 2021;128(2):277-87.
4. Cimino L. Algorithm for workup of panuveitis. In: Gupta V, Nguyen QD, LeHoang P, Herbort CP (Eds). The Uveitis Atlas. New Delhi: Springer; 2016. pp. 1-23.
5. Tsirouki T, Dastiridou A, Symeonidis C, Tounakaki O, Brazitikou I, Kalogeropoulos C, et al. A focus on the epidemiology of uveitis. Ocul Immunol Inflamm. 2018;26(1):2-16.
6. Bansal R, Gupta V, Gupta A. Current approach in the diagnosis and management of panuveitis. Indian J Ophthalmol. 2010;58(1):45.
7. Soheilian M, Ramezani A, Azimzadeh A, Sadoughi MM, Dehghan MH, Shahghadami R, et al. Randomized trial of intravitreal clindamycin and dexamethasone versus pyrimethamine, sulfadiazine, and prednisolone in treatment of ocular toxoplasmosis. Ophthalmology. 2011;118(1):134-41.
8. de-la-Torre A, Stanford M, Curi A, Jaffe GJ, Gomez-Marin JE. Therapy for ocular toxoplasmosis. Ocul Immunol Inflamm. 2011;19(5):314-20.
9. Powell B, Wang D, Llop S, Rosen RB. Management strategies of acute retinal necrosis: current perspectives. Clin Ophthalmol. 2020;14:1931-43.
10. Rangel CM, Restrepo-Arango M, Mejía-Salgado G, Gómez-Rocha MA, Gómez Velasco M, García MF, et al. Acute retinal necrosis: experience in a reference center in Santander-Colombia. Ocul Immunol Inflamm. 2024 ;32(7):1342-50.
11. Hashimoto Y, Yamana H, Iwagami M, Ono S, Takeuchi Y, Michihata N, et al. Ocular adverse events after coronavirus disease 2019 mRNA vaccination: matched cohort and self-controlled case series studies using a large database. Ophthalmology. 2023;130(3):256-64.
12. Hall N, Douglas VP, Ivanov A, Ross C, Elze T, Kempen JH, et al. The epidemiology and risk factors for the progression of sympathetic ophthalmia in the United States: an IRIS registry analysis. Am J Ophthalmol. 2024;258:208-16.
13. Parchand S, Agrawal D, Ayyadurai N, Agarwal A, Gangwe A, Behera S, et al. Sympathetic ophthalmia: a comprehensive update. Indian J Ophthalmol. 2022;70(6):1931.
14. Cunningham ET, Kilmartin D, Agarwal M, Zierhut M. Sympathetic Ophthalmia. Ocul Immunol Inflamm. 2017;25(2):149-51.
15. Mahajan S, Invernizzi A, Agrawal R, Biswas J, Rao NA, Gupta V. Multimodal imaging in sympathetic ophthalmia. Ocul Immunol Inflamm. 2017;25(2):152–9.
16. Bousquet E, Duraffour P, Debillon L, Somisetty S, Monnet D, Brézin AP. Birdshot chorioretinopathy: a review. J Clin Med. 2022;11(16):4772.
17. Herbort CP, Probst K, Cimino L, Tran VT. Differential inflammatory involvement in retina and choroïd in birdshot chorioretinopathy. Klin Monatsbl Augenheilkd. 2004;221(5):351-6.
18. Verhoeff FH. An effective treatment for sympathetic uveitis. Trans Am Ophthalmol Soc. 1926;24:173-91.
19. Bazewicz M, Heissigerova J, Pavesio C, Willermain F, Skrzypecki J. Ocular sarcoidosis in adults and children: update on clinical manifestation and diagnosis. J Ophthal Inflamm Infect. 2023;13(1):41.
20. Pasadhika S, Rosenbaum JT. Ocular sarcoidosis. Clin Chest Med. 2015;36(4):669-83.
21. Mochizuki M, Smith JR, Takase H, Kaburaki T, Acharya NR, Rao NA. Revised criteria of International Workshop on Ocular Sarcoidosis (IWOS) for the diagnosis of ocular sarcoidosis. Br J Ophthalmol. 2019;103(10):1418-22.
22. Standardization of Uveitis Nomenclature (SUN) Working Group. Classification criteria for sarcoidosis-associated uveitis. Am J Ophthalmol. 2021;228:220-30.
23. Bodaghi B, Touitou V, Fardeau C, Chapelon C, LeHoang P. Ocular sarcoidosis. Presse Med. 2012;41(6):e349-54.
24. Leclercq M, Andrillon A, Maalouf G, Sève P, Bielefeld P, Gueudry J, et al. Anti-tumor necrosis factor α versus tocilizumab in the treatment of refractory uveitic macular edema. Ophthalmology. 2022;129(5):520-9.
25. Gnanaraj R, Shah AA, Palestine AG, Reddy AK. Uveitis in the setting of co-existing systemic sarcoidosis and multiple sclerosis. Ocul Immunol Inflamm. 2024;32(2):181-3.
26. Beccastrini E, Vannozzi L, Bacherini D, Squatrito D, Emmi L. Successful treatment of ocular sarcoidosis with rituximab. Ocul Immunol Inflamm. 2013;21(3):244-6.
27. Standardization of Uveitis Nomenclature (SUN) Working Group. Classification criteria for Vogt-Koyanagi-Harada disease. Am J Ophthalmol. 2021;228:205-11.

28. Abu El-Asrar AM, Al-Kharashi AS, Aldibhi H, Al-Fraykh H, Kangave D. Vogt-Koyanagi-Harada disease in children. Eye. 2008;22(9):1124-31.
29. Herbort CP, Tugal-Tutkun I, Khairallah M, Abu El Asrar AM, Pavésio CE, Soheilian M. Vogt–Koyanagi–Harada disease: recurrence rates after initial-onset disease differ according to treatment modality and geographic area. Int Ophthalmol. 2020;40(9):2423-33.
30. Deák GGy, Koreishi AF, Goldstein DA. Do not discount the diagnosis of VKH based on race: self-reported race and ethnicity of patients with Vogt-Koyanagi-Harada disease in a predominantly white population. J Ophthal Inflamm Infect. 2023;13(1):15.
31. Herbort CP, Mantovani A, Bouchenaki N. Indocyanine green angiography in Vogt–Koyanagi–Harada disease: angiographic signs and utility in patient follow-up. Int Ophthalmol. 2007;27(2–3):173-82.
32. Abu El-Asrar AM, Al Tamimi M, Hemachandran S, Al-Mezaine HS, Al-Muammar A, Kangave D. Prognostic factors for clinical outcomes in patients with Vogt-Koyanagi-Harada disease treated with high-dose corticosteroids. Acta Ophthalmologica. 2013;91(6):e486-93.
33. Pandey A, Balekudaru S, Venkatramani DV, George AE, Lingam V, Biswas J. Incidence and management of glaucoma in Vogt Koyanagi Harada disease. J Glaucoma. 2016;25(8):674-80.
34. Ahmad F, Deshmukh N, Webel A, Johnson S, Suleiman A, Mohan RR, et al. Viral infections and pathogenesis of glaucoma: a comprehensive review. Clin Microbiol Rev. 2023;36(4):e00057-23.
35. Mudie LI, Zick JD, Dacey MS, Palestine AG. Panuveitis following vaccination for COVID-19. Ocul Immunol Inflamm. 2021;29(4):741-2.

CHAPTER 5

Scleritis

Peter McCluskey, Alexander Newman, Sibel Kadayifcilar, Figen Bezci Aygun, Cristhian Urzúa, Marcelo Vega-Codd, Germán Mejía-Salgado, Meghan Berkenstock, Reema Bansal, Vishali Gupta, John H Kempen, Alejandra de-la-Torre

INTRODUCTION

Scleritis is a rare disease that occurs worldwide. It can be challenging to diagnose without a detailed, comprehensive history, examination, and review of systems. Watson's anatomically based classification, which also grades the severity of scleritis, is a straightforward, clinically useful framework for diagnosis and management.[1,2] Scleritis may be associated with significant, potentially life-threatening, systemic inflammatory diseases. Treatment involves systemic anti-inflammatory and immunomodulatory therapy (IMT). It may also be caused by local or systemic infection and require systemic antimicrobial and judicious anti-inflammatory therapy.

PRACTICAL TIPS IN THE MANAGEMENT OF SCLERITIS

Clinical Assessment

The diagnosis of scleritis is fundamentally based on a careful clinical assessment that includes a detailed history and careful clinical examination of both eyes. A thorough review of systems is vital to detect symptoms that might suggest an associated systemic disease. Watson's classification of scleritis is a useful framework **(Flowchart 1)**.[1,2]

The hallmark symptom of scleritis is pain. It is dull, aching, centered on the eye, and often radiates to the forehead, scalp, ear, and jaw. Scleritis pain develops over days to several weeks and may become severe and incapacitating, preventing the patient from performing their everyday activities. It is characteristically worse at night, often awakening the patient from sleep early in the morning. It is typically poorly responsive to analgesics. Patients also complain of redness, photophobia, and mild blurred vision. They may note that the eye is tender.

On examination, visual acuity may be variably reduced. Ocular redness often has a characteristic violaceous hue, especially when examined in natural daylight. Involved eyes are tender to palpation and can be exquisitely tender with reflex withdrawal to attempt palpation in severe disease. There may be apparent scleral nodules and, in some cases, scleral necrosis **(Figs. 1A to D)**.[4] The hallmark

Flowchart 1: Scleritis classification.

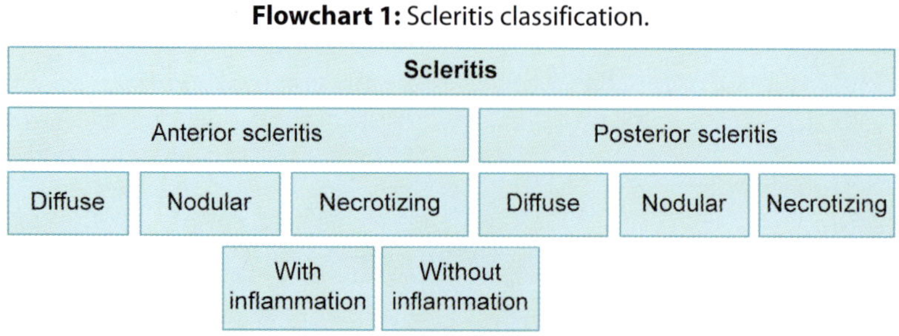

Source: Adapted from Watson and Hayreh;[1] Presented by Peter McCluskey in the International Uveitis Study Group (IUSG) grand rounds.[3]

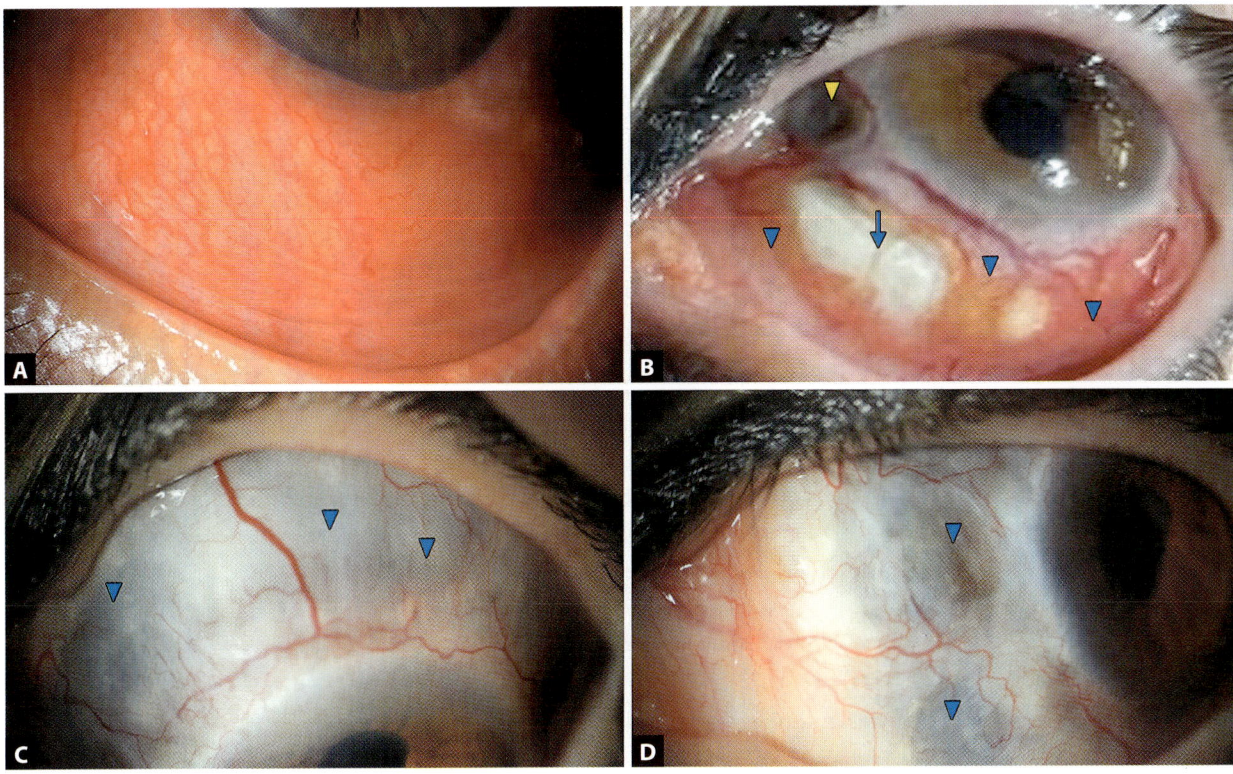

Figs. 1A to D: Slit-lamp findings in patients with scleritis. (A) Diffuse scleritis: characterized by generalized scleral edema and vascular injection involving both superficial and deep episcleral vessels. The eye is tender to palpation, with no evidence of nodular formation or necrosis; (B) Necrotizing scleritis with inflammation: a well-demarcated area of scleral necrosis is observed, appearing as a white, avascular zone due to loss of episcleral and scleral vasculature (blue arrow). Adjacent to the necrotic area, there is scleral thinning, through which the underlying uveal tissue becomes visible, imparting a dark bluish or grayish hue (yellow arrowhead). Surrounding these areas, intense congestion of deep episcleral and scleral vessels is noted (blue arrowheads); (C) Scleromalacia in the OD: noninflammatory scleral thinning. A zone of scleral transparency is observed, allowing visualization of the underlying uveal tissue, which gives a dark bluish appearance (blue arrowheads). No signs of active inflammation or necrosis are present; (D) Scleromalacia in the OS: noninflammatory scleral thinning with an area of scleral translucency, through which the underlying uveal tissue is visible, imparting a bluish hue (blue arrowheads). No evidence of active inflammation or necrosis.
Source: Courtesy of Alejandra de-la-Torre, member of the International Uveitis Study Group (IUSG).

clinical sign is scleral edema, detected clinically by outward displacement of the deep and superficial episcleral vascular plexus. The most superficial conjunctival plexus may need to be blanched with 2.5% phenylephrine to detect this sign. Using the red-free light beam during slit-lamp examination, often makes detection easier. Careful slit-lamp examination will also detect microvascular closure, the earliest sign of necrotizing scleritis (NS).[4]

Other clinical signs may exist, including stromal keratitis, peripheral ulcerative keratitis, uveitis, and elevated intraocular pressure **(Table 1)**. Approximately 80% of scleritis presentations exhibit other ophthalmic manifestations, least commonly for anterior nodular scleritis and ubiquitously for posterior scleritis.[2] There is a spectrum of clinical signs in patients with posterior scleritis largely dependent on which part of the sclera is the scleritis's focus **(Table 1)**.

Investigations

Investigations do not substitute clinical assessment, and patients do not need a "barrage" of investigations. Ancillary tests must be selective and targeted to rule in or rule out the disease that might be suspected from the clinical assessment or to confirm a likely syndromic diagnosis. The range of potential investigations is detailed in **Table 2**. Additional investigations may be required as part of the assessment needed to ensure that it is safe to use systemic IMT.

Pathology

There is limited understanding about the pathology of scleritis due to the scarcity of available histological specimens and the lack of a suitable animal model. Pathologically, scleritis is a chronic granulomatous

TABLE 1: Ophthalmic associations of scleritis.[2,4,5]

Ophthalmic association	*Rationale*
Scleromalacia	Following necrotizing disease
Peripheral corneal thinning/ peripheral ulcerative keratitis (PUK)	• Typically associated with granulomatosis with polyangiitis • Central perforation likely secondary to sicca from comorbid rheumatoid arthritis • High association with necrotizing scleritis • Associated PUK confers worse ocular prognosis and risk of vision loss • PUK is usually associated with potentially lethal systemic disease • Strong indication from commencing empiric immunomodulatory therapy
Stromal keratitis	Less likely to be associated with necrotizing scleritis and systemic disease compared with PUK
Open-angle glaucoma	• Trabeculitis • Elevated episcleral venous pressure • Steroid response
Closed-angle glaucoma	• Iris bombe with seclusion pupillae • Massive ciliochoroidal effusion or exudative retinal detachment from posterior scleritis
Hypotony	Following exudative or rhegmatogenous retinal detachment from posterior scleritis
Uveitis	Up to 40% incidence, variable severity, often seen with necrotizing/posterior scleritis
Cataract	• Steroid-induced • Associated with approximately 50% of presentations, typically severe
Anterior segment ischemia	Associated with circumferential anterior necrotizing scleritis
Phthisis	Associated with severe scleritis presentations
Posterior segment involvement	• Anterior scleritis in approximately 60% of presentations • Secondary angle closure • Optic neuropathy and optic perineuritis, either inflammatory or compressive • Microvascular occlusion • Retinal pigment epithelial rip • Circumscribed scleral elevation/mass lesion • Ciliochoroidal effusion syndrome • Exudative retinal detachment • Internal ophthalmoplegia

vasculitis characterized by a B-cell dominant inflammatory infiltrate with a range of features, including fibrinoid or zonal necrosis.[8] There may be prominent immune complex deposition. Immunohistochemistry reveals a proinflammatory cytokine profile, and that matrix metalloproteinases (MMPs) are the mechanism that affects scleral loss and necrosis, characterizing scleritis.[8,9]

Associated Systemic Disease

Scleritis may be undifferentiated or associated with a broad range of systemic diseases in up to 50% of patients. The associated diseases vary in different parts of the world. Rheumatoid arthritis remains the most common systemic disease, although its frequency in patients with scleritis appears to be decreasing. Scleritis typically develops in patients already diagnosed with rheumatoid arthritis.[4]

Scleritis may be a presentation of antineutrophil cytoplasmic antibody (ANCA)-associated vasculitis (AAV), most commonly granulomatosis with polyangiitis. Careful systems review will often uncover sinus, respiratory, or other symptoms that are clues to this diagnosis. Less commonly, other AAV, such as microscopic polyangiitis or eosinophilic polyangiitis, may develop scleritis. Other important systemic diseases associated with scleritis include relapsing polychondritis, human leukocyte antigen (HLA)-B27-related spondyloarthropathies, systemic vasculitis, spondylarthritis, immunoglobulin A (IgA) nephropathy, and inflammatory bowel disease. **Table 3** details the diseases associated with scleritis.

It has been recognized since the 1980s that NS is often associated with severe, potentially life-threatening disease and that without appropriate systemic IMT, there is up to a 50% mortality rate at 5 years.[13]

TABLE 2: Investigations utilized in the workup of scleritis when rationalized with the clinical phenotype.[2,4,6,7]

Laboratory investigations	***Comments***
Complete blood count	• Chronic inflammation leading to normocytic anemia/thrombocytosis/eosinophilia • Microcytic anemia due to chronic covert blood loss • Leukocytosis may indicate systemic response to infection
Renal function	Evaluation of creatinine and estimated glomerular filtration rate
Liver function tests	Albumin levels may indicate chronic inflammation or proteinuria
Erythrocyte sedimentation rate (ESR)	Nonspecific inflammatory marker
C-reactive protein (CRP)	Nonspecific inflammatory marker
Rheumatoid factor	Autoantibodies used in the diagnosis and prognosis on rheumatoid arthritis
Anticyclic citrullinated peptide	Diagnostic biomarker of rheumatoid arthritis
Antinuclear antibodies (ANAs)	• High sensitivity for the diagnosis of systemic lupus erythematosus (SLE) • Poor specificity, frequently positive in other rheumatic and nonautoimmune disorders • Interpreted in the clinical context and with the constellation of other autoantibodies
Extractable nuclear antigens (ENAs)	Used following positive ANA to diagnose connective tissue disorders
Antidouble-stranded DNA	Highly specific for the diagnosis of SLE
Antineutrophil cytoplasmic antibodies (ANCAs)	Specific for ANCA-associated vasculitis when indirect immunofluorescence interpreted with autoantibody testing
Angiotensin-converting enzyme (ACE)	Nonspecific test used in the evaluation of sarcoidosis
Treponemal/nontreponemal syphilis serology	Used to exclude syphilitic infectious etiology
Interferon gamma release assay/ Mantoux test	Used to exclude *Mycobacterium tuberculosis* infection
Polymerase chain reaction	Exclude Herpesviridae (HSV-1/HSV-2/VZV)
Microbiological sampling (swab/ scrape/tissue)	Speciate invasive bacterial infection
Urinalysis	Microhematuria or proteinuria may indicate associated glomerulonephritis
Imaging investigations	***Comments***
B-scan ultrasound	To diagnose posterior scleritis
Chest X-ray	• Exclude granulomatous lung/mediastinal disease • Exclude nodular/fibrotic/infiltrative lesions/alveolar hemorrhage/consolidation/tumor
Magnetic resonance imaging	Scleral enhancement, thickening, and periscleral cellulitis
Anterior segment angiography	Infrequently used to delineate ischemia
Ultrasound biomicroscopy	Evaluation of the iris–lens diaphragm in the context of posterior scleritis
Optical coherence tomography	*Posterior:* • Choroidal thickening/folds • Serous retinal detachments *Anterior:* • To distinguish from episcleritis • Detection of scleral abscess • Monitor scleral thickness

(HSV-1: herpes simplex virus type 1; VZV: varicella-zoster virus)

Infective Scleritis

Up to 10% of scleritis is infective in origin **(Table 4)**. It must always consider the potential for infection as a cause of scleritis, given that its management is typically the antithesis of noninfectious scleritis. Infectious scleritis may be exogenous and related to trauma or develop from contiguous spread from bacterial or fungal corneal infection such as herpes simplex virus or *Acanthamoeba*

TABLE 3: Common systemic associations of noninfectious scleritis.[2,4,10-12]

Systemic diseases	***Comments***
Connective tissue disease	*Rheumatoid arthritis:* • Associated with 10–33% of scleritis presentations • 0.2–6.3% of patients with rheumatoid arthritis develop scleritis • Symmetrical arthritis of small joints, particularly hands and feet, rheumatoid nodules, interstitial lung disease, and polyneuropathy
	Systemic lupus erythematosus: • Malar butterfly rash, polyarthritis, photosensitivity, pleuritis, adenopathy, glomerulonephritis, and myocarditis • Systemic investigations have low specificity in isolation
	Relapsing polychondritis: Recurrent inflammation of the auricular, nasal, and upper airway cartilaginous inflammation
	Others: HLA-B27 + Seronegative spondyloarthropathies
Systemic vasculitis	*Granulomatosis with polyangiitis*: • High rate of ocular involvement in limited and systemic cases, almost 50%, all ocular structures may be involved • Orbitopathy in approximately 50%, scleritis 16–38%, and peripheral ulcerative keratitis • Cytoplasmic pattern of indirect immunofluorescence and proteinase 3 antibody positivity highly specific • Classic systemic triad of upper/lower respiratory tract disease (sinusitis, crusting rhinitis, mastoiditis, saddle nose deformity, alveolar hemorrhage, pulmonary nodules), glomerulonephritis, and systemic vasculitis
	Eosinophilic granulomatosis with polyangiitis: • Obstructive airway disease, nasal polyps, and mononeuritis multiplex • Ocular manifestations in 6–20% of patients typically orbital inflammation or ischemic vasculitis
	Polyarteritis nodosa: Constitutional symptoms in 90%, necrotic cutaneous ulcers, livedo reticularis, peripheral neuropathy, hypertension, nephropathy, and mononeuritis multiplex
	Others: Microscopic polyangiitis, IgA vasculitis, sarcoidosis, giant cell arteritis, Behçet's disease, Cogan syndrome, Takayasu vasculitis, hypocomplementemic urticarial vasculitis, and cryoglobulinemia
Medication-induced	Bisphosphonates, cancer-related immunotherapy (nivolumab), topiramate, and etanercept
Miscellaneous	Foreign body, chemical injury, gout, and rosacea

TABLE 4: Classification and management of common causes of infectious scleritis.[2,10,12]

Organism	***Topical treatment***	***Systemic treatment***
Gram-positive bacteria	Fortified cephazolin, fluroquinolone, or fortified vancomycin	Ciprofloxacin, vancomycin
Gram-negative bacteria	Fortified aminoglycosides (gentamicin, tobramycin, amikacin), fluroquinolones	Ciprofloxacin, gatifloxacin, gentamicin
Spirochetes	–	Benzathine penicillin
Mycobacteria	Amikacin, fluoroquinolones	Ethambutol, isoniazid, rifampin, pyridoxine, ciprofloxacin
Nocardia	Amikacin, polymyxin, trimethoprim	Amikacin, ciprofloxacin
Fungi	Natamycin, voriconazole, amphotericin-B	Voriconazole, ketoconazole
Acanthamoeba	Polyhexamethylene biguanide, propamidine, chlorhexidine, voriconazole	Miltefosine, voriconazole
Virus (Herpesviridae)	–	Acyclovir, valacyclovir, famciclovir
Parasites	–	Albendazole, clindamycin, amoxycillin/ clavulanic acid

infection. In many parts of the world, infective scleritis develops following ocular surgery, most commonly after pterygium surgery, mainly when drugs such as mitomycin C have been applied intraoperatively. Severe recalcitrant scleritis can develop as part of herpes zoster ophthalmicus **(Fig. 2)**. Tuberculous scleritis is not uncommon in tuberculosis (TB)-endemic regions and is often a characteristic nodular "caseating" anterior scleritis **(Figs. 3A and B)**. Scleritis is an unusual but recognized ocular manifestation of syphilis.[14] Rarely, scleritis can occur superficially in the areas of florid intraocular inflammation in patients with toxoplasmic retinochoroiditis or eyes with severe acute retinal necrosis.[4]

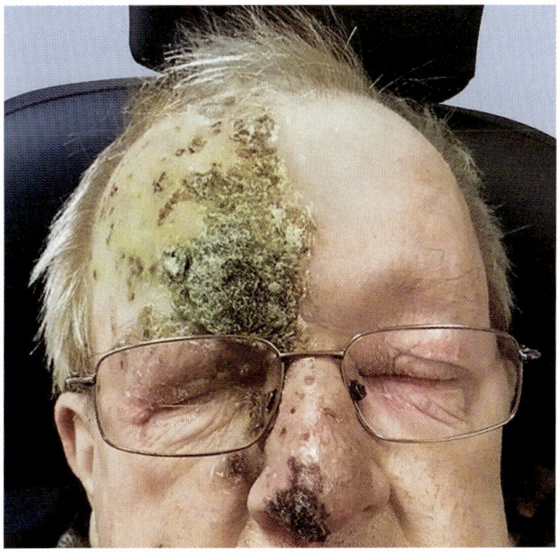

Fig. 2: Scleritis in a patient with herpes zoster ophthalmicus.
Source: Presented by Peter McCluskey in the International Uveitis Study Group (IUSG) grand rounds.[3]

Treatment

The mainstay of treatment for patients with scleritis is a stepped escalation algorithm of systemic anti-inflammatory and combination IMT. Topical and subconjunctival corticosteroids are beneficial adjunctive treatments in the selected patients. A representative algorithm is detailed in **Flowchart 2**. Treatment is proportional to the severity of the scleritis, its location, the threat to vision, and the threat to the integrity of the eye.

Patients with non-NS usually respond to a 6- to 10-week course of oral nonsteroidal anti-inflammatory drugs (NSAIDs) or oral corticosteroids. Treatment needs to be individualized and aligned with any comorbidities. A small number of patients develop relapsing scleritis that requires a steroid-sparing drug such as methotrexate or mycophenolate for 12–18 months to prevent further episodes.

Necrotizing and posterior scleritis represent significant threats to vision and the integrity of the globe. Such patients require high-dose oral corticosteroids and a steroid-sparing drug, as they will require immunosuppression for a minimum of 2–3 years. Patients with very severe or poorly responding scleritis will need treatment with a biological agent. Both B cell-depleting drugs and tumor necrosis factor (TNF) blockers are efficacious. Given the pathology of scleritis, B cell-depleting biologics, such as rituximab, are the preferred drug.

Patients who develop scleritis often have a previously diagnosed associated systemic disease that is on treatment; liaising closely with the patient's treating physician regarding the best therapy is critical.

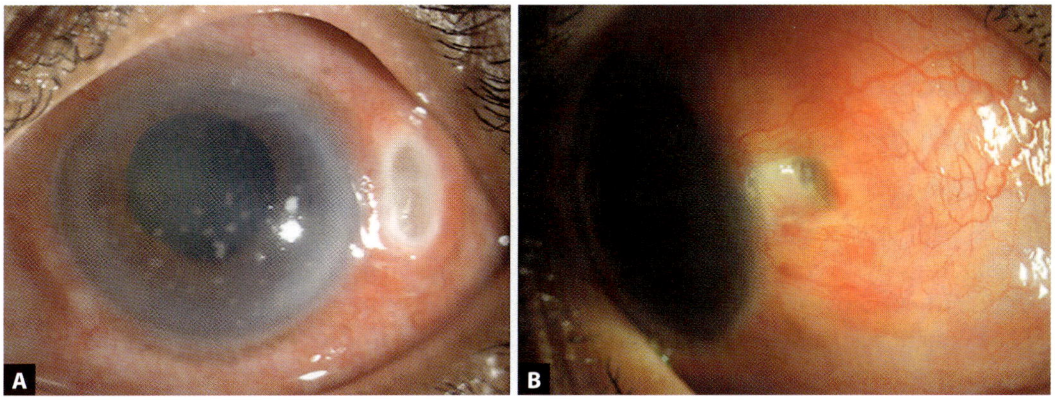

Figs. 3A and B: Scleritis secondary to *Mycobacterium tuberculosis* infection.
Source: Adapted from Murthy et al.;[10] Presented by Peter McCluskey in the International Uveitis Study Group (IUSG) grand rounds.[3]

Flowchart 2: Suggested treatment algorithm for noninfective scleritis.

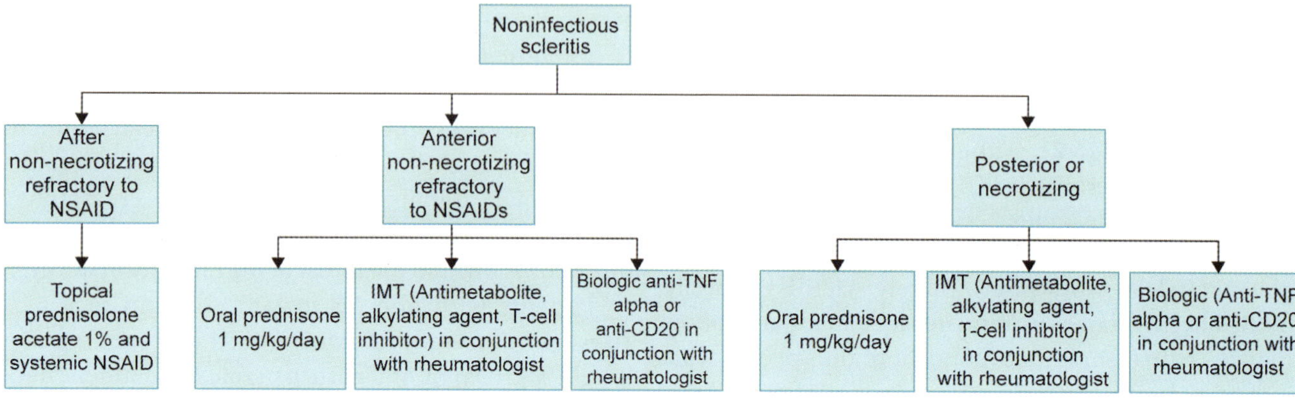

(NSAIDs: nonsteroidal anti-inflammatory drugs; IMT: immunomodulatory therapy; TNF: tumor necrosis factor)
Source: Modified from Stem et al.;[15] Presented by Peter McCluskey in the International Uveitis Study Group (IUSG) grand rounds.[3]

Infective scleritis requires prolonged systemic and local antimicrobial therapy, with drug selection guided by the antimicrobial susceptibility profile of the causative organism. Topical, subconjunctival, and local irrigation are all helpful and combined with systemic therapy. Surgical debridement is often required to obtain specimens for microbiology workup and debride the sclera. Judicious anti-inflammatory treatment may also be needed to control the associated inflammatory response.

INFECTIOUS SCLERITIS CASE

Case Presentation

Personal Data

- Male
- 64 years old
- *Past medical history:* Coronary artery disease, hypothyroidism, and hypertension
- *Previous ocular surgery:* Scleral buckling for macula-off rhegmatogenous retinal detachment due to a horseshoe tear

History of Present Illness

Redness in left eye (OS) and ocular pain 3 weeks after retinal detachment surgery; initial management with topical antibiotics and corticosteroids did not improve the symptoms. The patient also had upper eyelid swelling and tearing. At presentation, the patient was using ciprofloxacin 0.5% drops four times daily, dexamethasone 0.4% four times daily, tropicamide 0.5% one-time daily, and indomethacin 25 mg oral twice daily.

Physical Examination

The patient presented with visual acuity of 20/20 in OD and 20/200 in OS, associated with prominent redness and tenderness in OS, and extrusion of scleral buckling **(Fig. 4 and Table 5)**.

Differential Diagnosis

Infectious scleritis was the initial differential diagnosis. Subsequently, a conjunctival swab smear and culture were taken, which resulted in a positive result for gram-positive cocci; the patient was hospitalized for appropriate management.

Treatment

Intravenous (IV) sulbactam ampicillin 1,500 mg four times daily and topical moxifloxacin five times daily.

Two days later, the conjunctival swab culture results positive for methicillin-resistant *Staphylococcus aureus* (MRSA). Specifically, it was resistant to ampicillin, cefoxitin, gentamicin, and ciprofloxacin. Notably, it was sensitive to linezolid, teicoplanin, and vancomycin. Therefore, treatment was escalated to IV vancomycin 1 gram twice a day + fortified drops twice a day.

Follow-up

Ten days later, the patient showed significant improvement in the symptoms and ocular signs and was discharged with oral antibiotics. Two months later, the patient presented a prominent regression without further management. One year later, complete resolution of scleritis was evident with minimum subretinal fluid **(Figs. 5A to D)**.

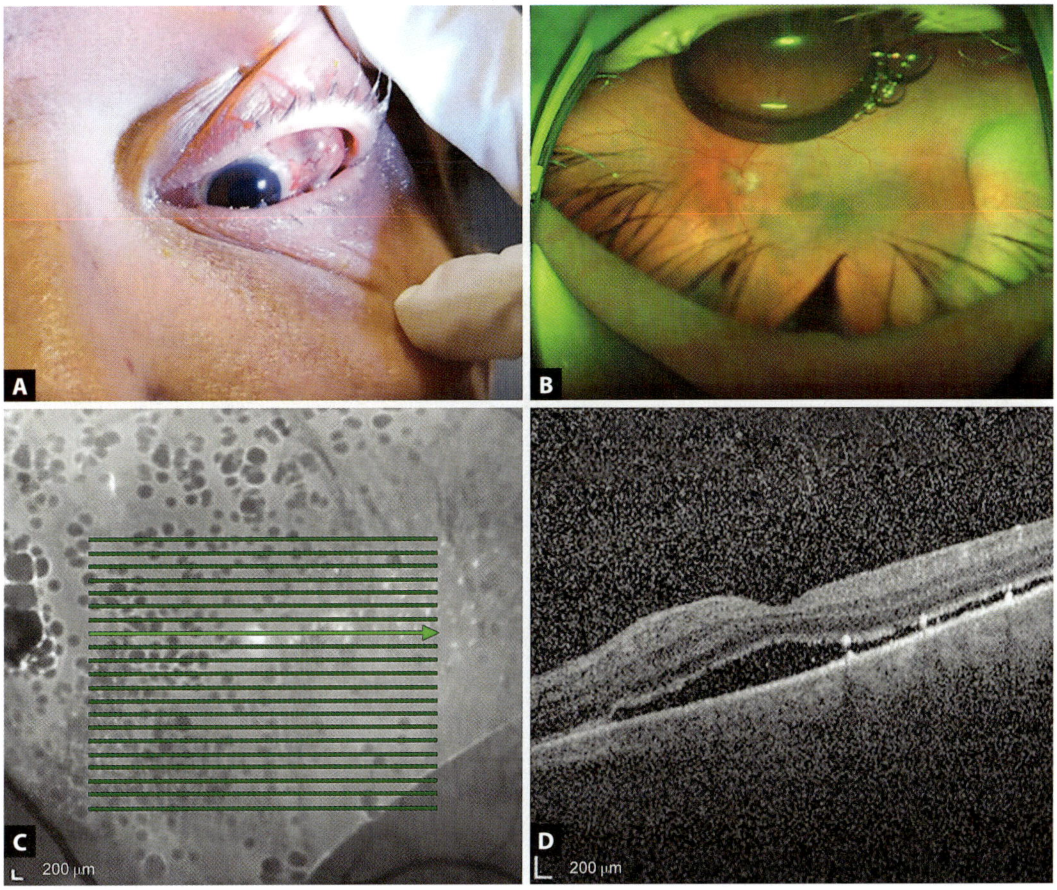

Figs. 4A to D: Initial clinical picture of infectious scleritis case. (A) Prominent redness and tenderness in the upper temporal region with visible radial scleral buckling on the surface of sclera underneath Tenon's capsule; (B) Gas bubble superiorly; (C) Attached retina with effective cryotherapy scar and temporally circumferential scleral buckling; (D) Residual retinal detachment.
Source: Presented by Figen Bezci Aygun in the International Uveitis Study Group (IUSG) grand rounds.[3]

TABLE 5: Physical examination of the patient having infectious scleritis case.

OD	*Parameters*	*OS*
20/20	BCVA	20/200
14 mm Hg	IOP	15 mm Hg
Normal	Conjunctiva	Temporal conjunctival injection
Quiet and normal	Sclera	Prominent redness and tenderness in the upper temporal region, visible radial and circumferential scleral buckling on the surface of sclera underneath Tenon's capsule
Clear	Cornea	Clear
ACC: 0+ cells	Anterior chamber	ACC: 0+ cells
Normal	Iris	Normal
Clear	Lens	Clear
Normal	Vitreous	Normal
Normal	Fundus	Attached retina with effective cryotherapy scar and temporally with circumferential scleral buckling, gas bubble superiorly

(ACC: anterior chamber cellularity; BCVA: best-corrected visual acuity; IOP: intraocular pressure)

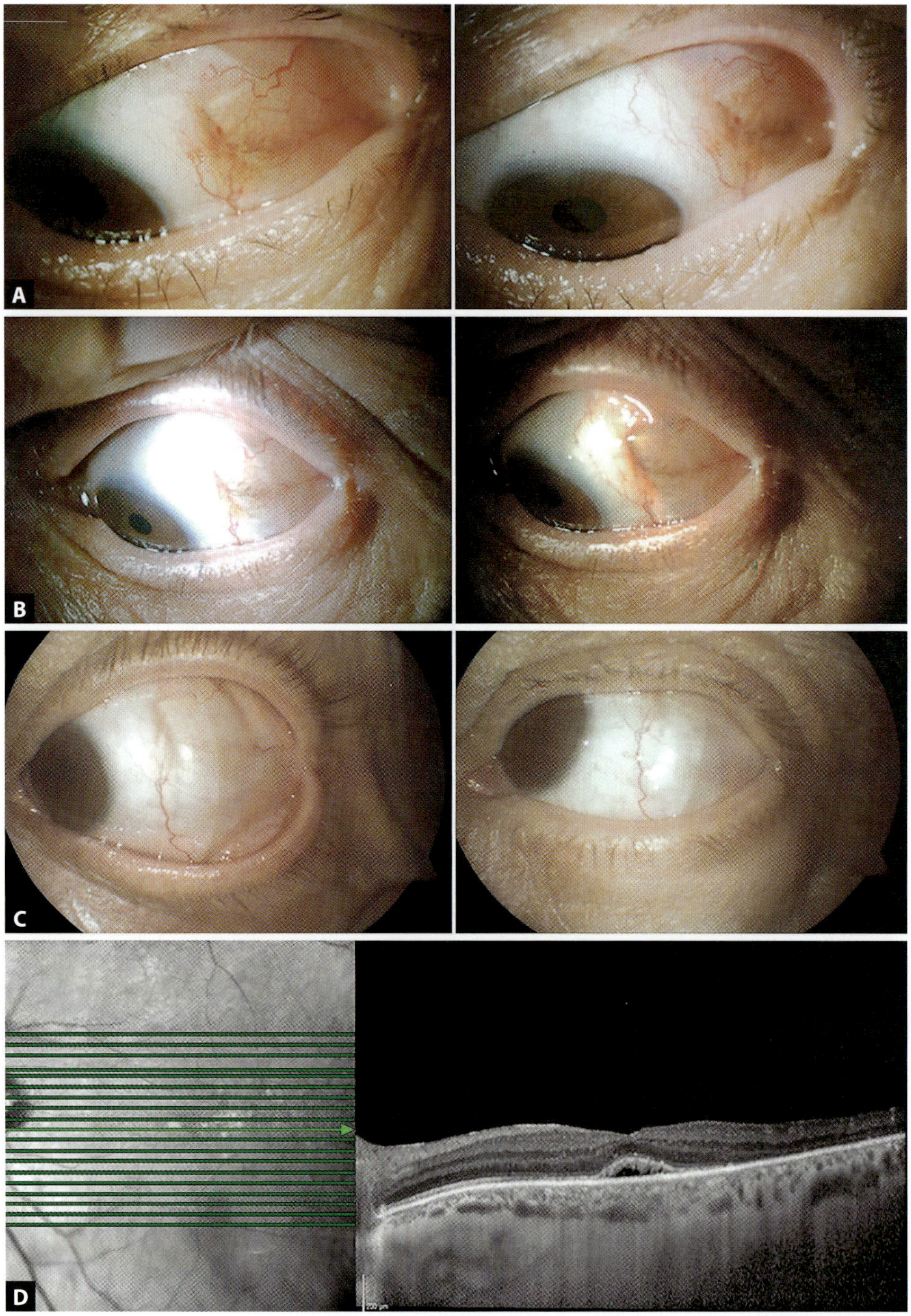

Figs. 5A to D: Follow-up of infectious scleritis case. (A) A 10-day follow-up photography showing improvement of redness and scleral tenderness; (B) A 2-month follow-up photography showing prominent regression of scleritis; (C) A 1-year follow-up photography shows complete scleritis resolution; (D) Minimum subretinal fluid in the optical coherence tomography (OCT).
Source: Presented by Figen Bezci Aygun in the International Uveitis Study Group (IUSG) grand rounds.[3]

Discussion

Infectious scleritis constitutes approximately 10% of scleritis cases in the Western world. The primary cause is exogenous in origin, often due to trauma or ocular surgeries. Less frequently, infectious scleritis can occur secondary to systemic endogenous infections, such as syphilis and TB. Predisposing factors include uses of antimetabolites such as mitomycin C, local radiotherapy, and the chronic use of topical corticosteroids.[10]

Patients typically experienced pain following initial postoperative healing. Persistent pain that is unresponsive to anti-inflammatory therapy may indicate infectious scleritis or surgically induced necrotizing scleritis (SINS). Accurate diagnosis relies on microbiological analysis and slit-lamp examination.[10]

A study by Hodson et al.[16] reported that the median onset of symptoms is approximately 2 months postinciting, with *Pseudomonas aeruginosa* being the most isolated pathogen. This aligns with other reports on scleritis secondary to scleral buckles, which corresponds to 6% of all SINS cases.[17] Notably, the onset of explant infection typically occurs 2–8 months postimplantation and is characterized by chronic irritation rather than severe pain, conjunctival erosion, and purulent discharge. Commonly implicated microorganisms include *Pseudomonas*, nontuberculous mycobacteria, and fungi, often associated with sponge-type implants.[18]

Solid silicone implants have increased recently due to their economic feasibility and biocompatibility. However, implantation may compromise local tissue integrity, fostering biofilm formation, particularly by mycobacteria, thus impeding antibiotic efficacy and the host immune response.[19] In India, gram-positive cocci, predominantly *Staphylococcus epidermidis,* known for its ability to form biofilm, has been reported as a common pathogen in scleral buckle infections.[20]

A recent study on scleritis following scleral buckling surgery reported an incidence of only two cases per 1,000 surgical procedures, suggesting a declining incidence compared to previous years. *S. epidermidis* emerged as the predominant pathogen, with the average onset of infection occurring approximately 30 days postimplantation. In approximately 80% of cases, there was evidence of scleral, buccal, or suture exposure. However, in 18% of cases, no signs of explant or conjunctival erosion were observed, akin to the current case, where the conjunctiva remained fully intact.[21]

There are only five reports concerning scleritis due to MRSA,[17,22-25] with one case documented as postdengue viral fever.[22] Although rare, SINS should always be considered in the differential diagnosis of patients with ocular pain and red eye occurring 1 month or more after ocular surgery. This clinical entity constitutes a complex diagnosis characterized by multifactorial components, including trauma, infection, ischemia, toxicity, and autoimmunity. Infectious scleritis may manifest independently or concurrently with SINS.[17,22-25]

Treatment necessitates empirical antibiotic therapy pending culture and sensitivity results. Resistance patterns, such as those encountered with *S. aureus*, require tailored management for optimal outcomes. Steroid use in the acute phase is contraindicated.[26] Decision-making regarding buckle removal hinges on individual case characteristics. Removal of the buckle within 3–6 months increases the risk of a new detachment in 70–82% of cases.[26] In this case, scleritis occurred during the third week postsurgery, coinciding with residual subretinal fluid. Consequently, the approach prioritized infection management before considering buckle removal. Encouragingly, favorable outcomes were achieved within 2 months, leading to the decision to retain the buckle.

NECROTIZING SCLERITIS CASE

Case Presentation

Personal Data

- Hispanic male, 55 years old
- Ambulance driver
- *Medical history:* Bronchial asthma (2011) and operated testicular cancer (2008)
- *Immunity:* COVID-19 (six doses) and influenza vaccine 2024
- *Family medical history:* Nonreported

History of Present Illness

4 years of recurrent deep red eye, bilateral progressive and asymmetric hearing loss, vertigo syndrome, tinnitus, headache, erythema of the auricle, polyarthralgia, and joint pain.

Physical Examination

The patient presented with a best-corrected visual acuity (BCVA) of 20/25 in OU, with bilateral redness. There was no evidence of inflammatory cells in the anterior chamber or vitreous **(Figs. 6, 7 and Table 6)**.

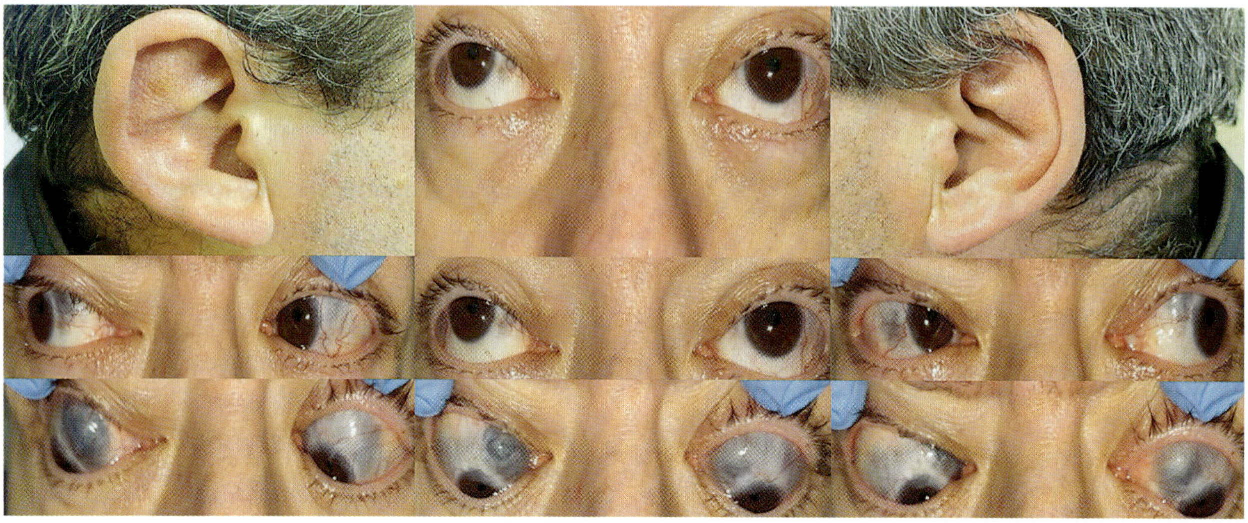

Fig. 6: External examination of necrotizing scleritis case. Sequelae of bilateral necrotizing scleritis with uveal protrusion are observed as dark, elevated lesions secondary to scleral thinning (scleromalacia). Moreover, the right ear has a floppy appearance because of previous active chondritis. In the left ear, active auricular chondritis was observed.
Source: Presented by Marcelo Vega in the International Uveitis Study Group (IUSG) grand rounds.[3]

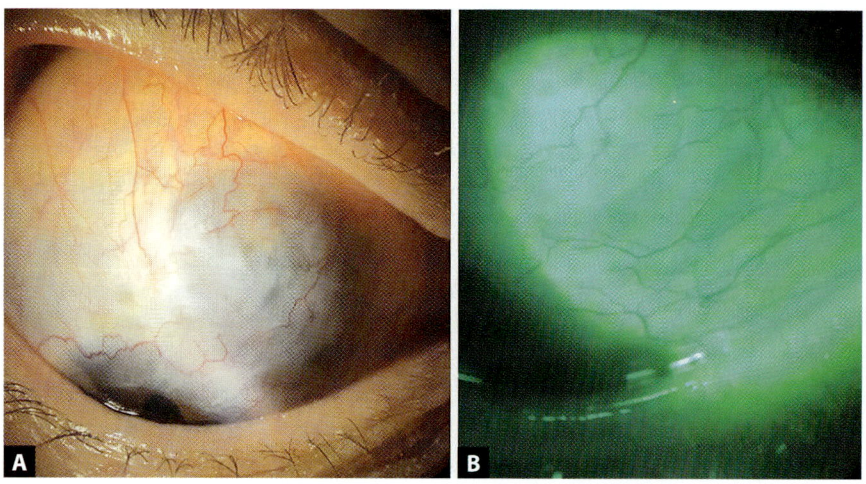

Figs. 7A and B: Slit-lamp examination of necrotizing scleritis case. Diffuse and red-free light photographs of the left eye. Red-free light photography facilitates visualization of the blood vessels and areas of capillary nonperfusion.
Source: Presented by Marcelo Vega in the International Uveitis Study Group (IUSG) grand rounds.[3]

Ancillary Test

- Complete blood count, renal function test, and liver function test were within normal limits.
- *Tests conducted to rule out noninfectious diseases* revealed negative antinuclear antibodies (ANAs), extractable nuclear antibodies (ENAs), and ANCA.
- *Tests conducted to rule out noninfectious diseases* also revealed negative Venereal Disease Research Laboratory (VDRL), microhemagglutination assay for *Treponema pallidum* (MHATP), and interferon gamma release assays (IGRAs).

Final Diagnosis

- Relapsing polychondritis
- Bilateral anterior NS

Treatment

- Oral prednisone 60 mg/day

TABLE 6: Physical examination of the patient having necrotizing scleritis (NS) case.

OD	***Parameters***	***OS***
20/25	BCVA	20/25
14 mm Hg	IOP	16 mm Hg
Moderate diffuse hyperemia	Conjunctiva	Moderate diffuse hyperemia
Clear	Cornea	Clear
No hypopyon ACC: 0+, flare 0+	AC	No hypopyon ACC: 0+, flare 0+
No posterior synechiae	Iris	No posterior synechiae
Retropupillary pigment and nuclear sclerosis	Lens	Retropupillary pigment and nuclear sclerosis
Anterior vitreous cells 0	Vitreous	Anterior vitreous cells 0
Optic disc and macula appear normal Retina without lesions	Fundus	Optic disc and macula appear normal Retina without lesions

(ACC: anterior chamber cellularity; BCVA: best-corrected visual acuity; IOP: intraocular pressure)

- Oral methotrexate 25 mg/weekly
- Folic acid 5 mg/week

Course

After treatment, the patient presented regression of scleral inflammation without other recurrences for >12 months.

Discussion

In cases with NS, some specific critical points regarding the clinical approach should be considered:

- *Ophthalmic examination*: In addition to the routine use of the slit lamp to evaluate this condition and potential ocular complications (such as peripheral ulcerative keratitis or anterior uveitis), red-free light and a macroscopic view with daylight may help the clinician assess the areas of necrosis or capillary nonperfusion and identify the typical violaceous color of the affected sclera in patients with active scleritis and identifying areas of scleromalacia.
- *Systemic conditions*: de la Maza et al. described an increased frequency of associated systemic disorders in NS in a large cohort of 500 patients with scleritis. Moreover, in around 60% of these patients, NS was the first manifestation of the systemic disease.[27] Indeed, an increased risk of systemic conditions in NS has been described, with an odds ratio of seven times in this subset of patients.[28] According to the published literature, rheumatoid arthritis and granulomatosis with polyangiitis are NS's most reported systemic associations.[12] Therefore, actions should be taken to rule out systemic disorders in NS based on a thorough systemic evaluation and review of systems **(Figs. 8A and B)**.
- *Ocular complications:* Scleral thinning is a potential source of complications in patients with scleritis. NS carries a risk of globe perforation, which requires complex surgical procedures **(Figs. 9A and B)**. In a Japanese case series, all subjects with NS had at least one ocular complication, including cataracts, ocular hypertension, and uveitis.[29] In addition, de la Maza et al. have described that ocular complications are more frequent in patients with NS, with a statistically significant difference in decreased vision, anterior uveitis, and peripheral ulcerative keratitis.[27] Similarly, reduced vision was found more frequent in NS in a multicentric and international cohort study from the Asia-Pacific region.[30]
- *Immunomodulatory therapy as first-line therapy*: Regarding the therapeutic approach, NS tends to be refractory to systemic corticosteroids; thus, IMT is needed.[29] In addition, de la Torre et al. described a higher frequency of a chronic course of the disease in cases of NS, which would also indicate the use of IMT.[28] Finally, some evidence has reported the positive impact of the indication of IMT on mortality. In two case series, authors found a decrease in mortality rate in patients with NS treated with IMT.[13]

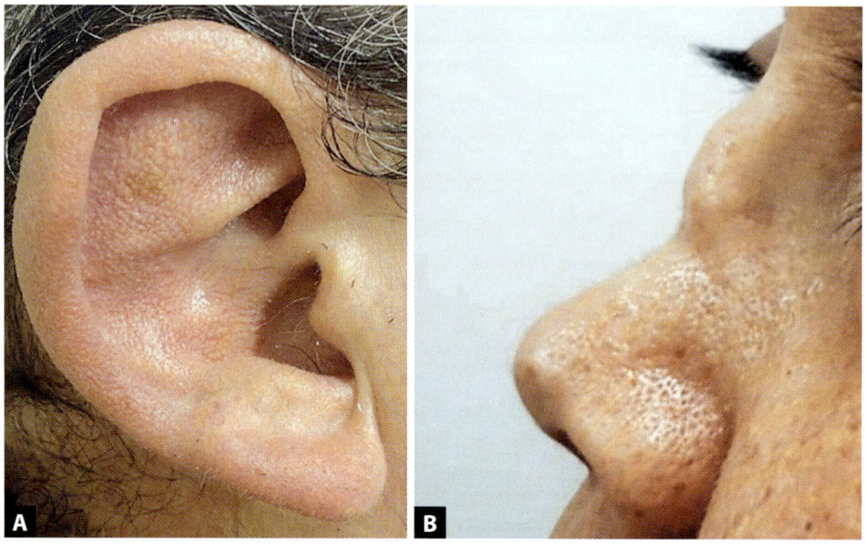

Figs. 8A and B: Extraocular findings in patients with systemic disease-associated scleritis. Typical findings of patients with relapsing polychondritis include (A) Deformity of auricular cartilage producing a floppy appearance secondary to previous chondritis and (B) Saddle nose deformity.
Source: Presented by Cristhian Urzúa in the International Uveitis Study Group (IUSG) grand rounds.[3]

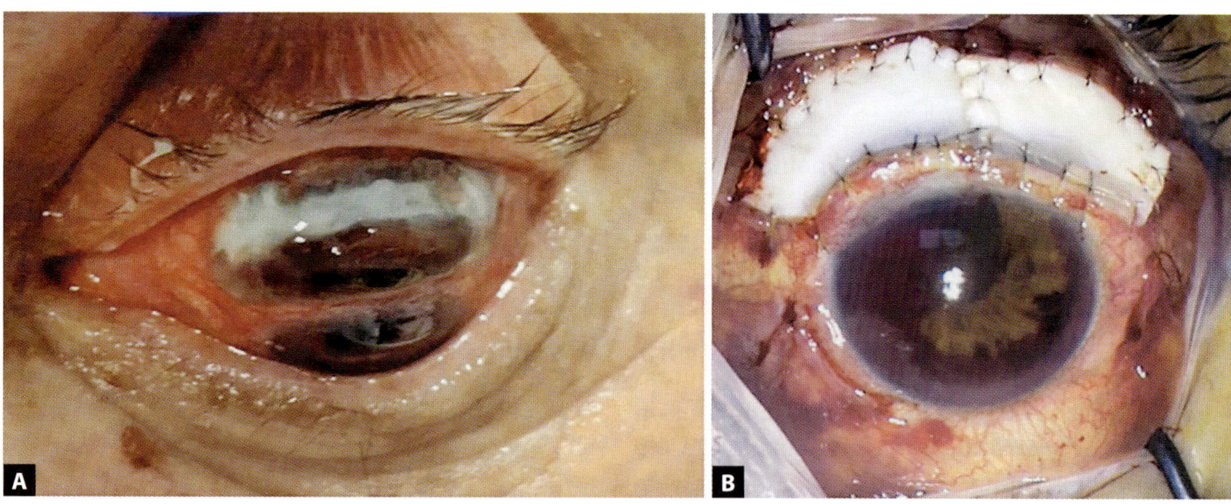

Figs. 9A and B: Complications of necrotizing scleritis. (A) Globe perforation in a patient with necrotizing scleritis; (B) Surgical repair of globe perforation using scleral patch.
Source: Presented by Cristhian Urzúa in the International Uveitis Study Group (IUSG) grand rounds.[3]

NONINFECTIOUS SCLERITIS CASE

Case Presentation

Personal Data

- Female
- 34 years old
- No previous eye diseases

History of Present Illness

The patient reported red eye and ocular pain in the OS 2 weeks after the second dose of the COVID-19 vaccine (September 2022). Initially, it was treated symptomatically with a short course of topical steroids with partial improvement. Three months later, after the persistent symptoms, anterior and posterior blepharitis were

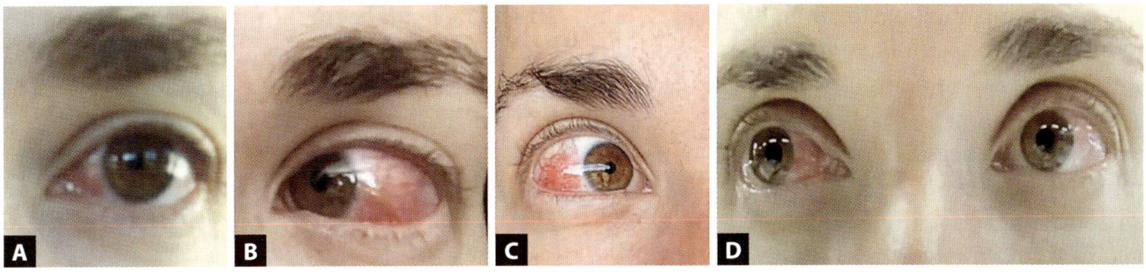

Figs. 10A to D: Clinical course of noninfectious scleritis case. (A) First episode of red eye in the OS; (B) Recurrence of red eye in the OS; (C) First episode of red eye in the OD; (D) Recurrence of red eye in both eyes.
Source: Presented by Alexander Newman in the International Uveitis Study Group (IUSG) grand rounds.[3]

considered the most probable diagnosis, prompting a trial of doxycycline and intermittent use of oral NSAIDs. The patient continues to experience a fluctuating course of red eye treated with artificial tears, topical antibiotics, and steroids for 3 years **(Figs. 10A to D)**. Subsequently, she presented with bilateral red eyes that progressively worsened over 4 months. She reported increasing pain that woke her at night, extreme sensitivity to light, ophthalmoplegia, lid edema, and severe functional impairment affecting her daily activities.

Physical Examination

The patient presented with a BCVA of 20/20 in OU, bilateral moderate ocular redness, normal IOP, absence of anterior chamber or vitreous cells, and normal fundus **(Table 7)**.

TABLE 7: Physical examination of the patient having noninfectious scleritis case.

OD	*Parameters*	*OS*
20/20	BCVA	20/20
14 mm Hg	IOP	14 mm Hg
Moderate ocular redness	Conjunctiva	Moderate ocular redness
Normal	Cornea	Normal
ACC: 0+	Anterior chamber	ACC: 0+
Normal	Iris	Normal
Clear	Lens	Clear
Normal	Vitreous	Normal
Normal	Fundus	Normal

(ACC: anterior chamber cellularity; BCVA: best-corrected visual acuity; IOP: intraocular pressure)

Ancillary Test

- *Negative/within normal limits*: Complete blood count, QuantiFERON gold, angiotensin-converting enzyme (ACE), ANAS, ENAS, HLA-B27, human immunodeficiency virus (HIV), renal and liver function tests, chest scan, colonoscopy, hepatitis B and C, erythrocyte sedimentation rate (ESR), and C-reactive protein (CRP).
- *Positive/out of normal limits:* ANCA was positive with indirect immunofluorescence, but the three myeloperoxidase and proteinase antibodies were negative.

Final Diagnosis

Bilateral noninfectious, no necrotizing anterior scleritis

Treatment

Prednisolone: 60 mg orally per day

Course

Within 3 days of initiating treatment and by the 2-week review, the patient exhibited completely white, uninflamed, and comfortable eyes. Due to her desire for pregnancy, she remained on a tapering monotherapy regimen with steroids. Additional investigations for steroid-sparing agents, such as azathioprine or TNF blockers, were not pursued. Remarkably, she achieved an excellent outcome, remaining disease-free and off treatment for approximately 6 months.

Discussion

The challenge of diagnosing scleritis is significant due to its implications, such as the necessity for systemic therapy, particularly in young patients, and a potential association with severe systemic diseases. Clinicians may initially try local therapies to mitigate symptoms without resorting to more aggressive treatments. However, as illustrated in this case, scleritis often requires robust therapy to control inflammation and prevent complications. This case also underscores the importance of a thorough clinical history in making an accurate diagnosis. Adequate follow-up and photographic records demonstrated scleral involvement, including nodular changes and vascular remodeling, indicating long-standing scleritis rather than episcleritis. The patient likely experienced a continuous low-grade scleritis attack for approximately 2 years, which was never adequately controlled. Upon initiation of systemic therapy, the condition improved rapidly.[31]

This case also highlights the importance of correctly interpreting positive ANCA serology. ANCA testing follows a two-step methodology: initial screening using indirect immunofluorescence to identify staining patterns (perinuclear, cytoplasmic, or atypical), followed by antigen-specific immunoassays for confirmation. These tests have high sensitivity and are critical for ruling out diseases.[32] Recent advancements have led laboratories to favor direct antigen-specific immunoassays over traditional screening immunofluorescence, for which positive ANA results can confound. This shift improves diagnostic accuracy and reduces the likelihood of misinterpretation.[32]

When considering systemic diseases associated with scleritis, it is essential to distinguish between rheumatic connective tissue disorders and vasculitides. There is significant overlap in the caliber of affected vessels, with ANCA-associated vasculitides typically involving small to medium vessels. In contrast, immune complex-mediated diseases primarily affect capillaries. This distinction is vital for understanding the underlying pathophysiology and guiding treatment.[32]

Small vessel vasculitides, such as those associated with ANCA, can involve larger vessels, leading to complications in organs such as the kidneys and lungs. The immune complex and granulomatous inflammation target capillaries and venules, fitting the scleral involvement in these diseases. The episcleral vasculature, characterized by areas of low flow or vasculostasis, is prone to antibody and immune complex deposition, contributing to the pathology of scleritis.[3]

In summary, accurate diagnosis of scleritis requires a comprehensive understanding of clinical history, proper interpretation of serological tests, and awareness of the systemic associations. Clinicians must use appropriate examination techniques, consider systemic conditions, anticipate ocular complications, and incorporate systemic therapy when necessary. The insights from this case emphasize the need for consistent, knowledgeable care to manage this complex condition effectively.

PEARLS FROM THE EXPERTS ON FREQUENTLY ASKED QUESTIONS[3]

Infectious Scleritis

1. When should explant removal be considered in scleritis secondary to a scleral buckle?

Answer: The decision to remove the explant should be based on the time elapsed since the surgery. During the first 6 months, removing the explant carries a significant risk of causing a new retinal detachment. Therefore, it is advisable to prioritize preserving the explant during this period. After 6 months, the risk of retinal detachment decreases, making explant removal a safer option if clinically indicated.

2. Are subconjunctival antibiotics, such as vancomycin, considered in cases of infectious scleritis?

Answer: Yes. In the case discussed, the patient showed improvement on the first day of vancomycin administration. The nodular appearance decreased, and frequent topical vancomycin drops were administered with a gradual dose reduction. Subconjunctival antibiotics remain a viable treatment option.

3. When encountering a patient with infectious scleritis, should noninfectious causes be investigated alongside the infection, or should the focus be solely on culture, smear, and polymerase chain reaction (PCR)?

Answer: Initial steps should include culturing and swabbing and starting IV antibiotic therapy. Additionally, underlying diseases, such as autoimmune conditions or immune suppression, should be investigated from the patient's medical history. Even in the absence of such a history, it is essential to consider autoimmune diseases and rheumatologic conditions, as they can often coexist with infectious scleritis.

4. For countries with limited laboratory diagnosis and antibiotic availability, is it advisable to inject if unsure about infection?

Answer: Local steroids should be avoided if there is doubt about infection. Oral steroids are preferred as they can be discontinued if the situation worsens. Local injections are risky if the infection status is unclear.

5. Should a swab and culture be taken for a patient with two purulent scleral nodules, or is a biopsy needed?
Answer: Initially, a swab and culture should be taken. If results are inconclusive, a scleral biopsy should be considered.

6. When infectious scleritis is suspected, in which cases would IV empiric antibiotics be preferred over oral antibiotics?
Answer: IV antibiotics are preferred in cases of severe disease. The sclera has a poor vascular supply, so high-dose drugs are needed to achieve optimal levels in the sclera; therefore, IV administration is necessary, at least initially.

7. Are gram-positive cocci considered normal conjunctival flora?
Answer: Yes, but the swab will show florid growth in infectious scleritis.

8. Was the patient a known carrier of MRSA, or was the bacterium acquired during retinal detachment surgery? Are patients screened for MRSA?
Answer: The patient was not a known MRSA carrier. The bacterium might have been acquired before the operation, especially since the patient was hospitalized for the procedure after traveling from another city. Patients are not regularly screened for MRSA.

9. Is it possible to have varicella-zoster virus (VZV) scleritis when the actual shingles are on the torso (not the facial area)? What is the dosage of valacyclovir for VZV scleritis?
Answer: While not commonly seen, VZV scleritis can occur with shingles on the torso. The dosage for VZV scleritis is 1 gram of valacyclovir three times a day for 7–10 days, followed by a maintenance dose of 1 gram daily for 3 months.

10. Are subconjunctival antibiotics routinely used at the end of surgery?
Answer: Yes. Subconjunctival antibiotics are routinely administered at the end of surgery, usually in a different quadrant from the explant.

11. How common is SINS in the present day scenario? Are there global data for SINS?
Answer: Global data are unknown and now scarce. Over the last 10 years, all cases encountered have been infectious rather than SINS.

Noninfectious Scleritis

1. In the era of biologics, if resources and availability are not an issue, should treatment begin with conventional disease-modifying antirheumatic drugs (DMARDs) and then move to rituximab or anti-TNF as second-line treatments or should rituximab be started directly?
Answer: Ideally, treatment would start directly with rituximab in severe cases due to its effectiveness in treating scleritis. However, conventional DMARDs are typically used initially due to resource limitations and with an escalated treatment approach. If side effects occur or the response is suboptimal, rituximab is introduced. In the future, it is anticipated that treatment may begin with steroids and rituximab directly.

2. Is cyclophosphamide still used in the treatment of scleritis?
Answer: IV cyclophosphamide has decreased over the past 9 years, particularly for ANCA-associated vasculitis. Rituximab has largely replaced cyclophosphamide as the preferred treatment option.

3. What are the special considerations for pediatric scleritis compared to adults?
Answer: Pediatric scleritis is rare. As with adults, therapy consists of escalated anti-inflammatory or antimicrobial treatment depending on the origin of scleritis. Dosages should be adjusted for age and weight, and communication with pediatricians is essential.

4. What are the tips on performing a scleral biopsy?
Answer: Scleral biopsy is challenging due to friable conjunctiva and bleeding. Sampling from the lesion's growing edge is preferred if possible. Even episcleral tissue can provide enough material for diagnosis. If uncertain, an excellent conjunctival smear or scraping may suffice. Samples should be transported in a cold box and inoculated promptly.

5. How is posterior scleritis combined with posterior uveitis?
Answer: Posterior scleritis often involves spillover inflammation into the choroid, retina, and optic disc and can present with changes such as choroidal folds and subretinal mass.

6. How prevalent is scleritis in general?
Answer: Scleritis is rare. At an eye hospital serving 7 million people, six to eight new patients are seen each year.

7. When should investigations be repeated if initial results are negative but the disease persists?

Answer: Retesting should be considered if new symptoms suggestive of a systemic disease develop. Symptoms are typically reviewed every 6–12 months.

8. What is the dose of the subtenon triamcinolone acetonide injection?

Answer: The dose is 0.05 mL of triamcinolone acetonide 40 mg/mL (i.e., 2 mg).

9. How frequently are subconjunctival triamcinolone acetonide injections administered in cases needing repeat injections?

Answer: The injections last for 6–10 weeks; if a second injection is needed, it is typically administered around 10–12 weeks later.

10. Can surgically induced non-NS?

Answer: Mild nonnecrotizing scleral inflammation can follow scleral buckling and other extraocular surgeries. It is usually mild and transient, resolving with topical steroid therapy.

11. Can subconjunctival triamcinolone acetonide be injected instead of subtenon? If so, what dosage?

Answer: A subconjunctival injection in the fornix is typically used for scleritis rather than a subtenon injection.

12. Is relapsing polychondritis a definitive diagnosis, or should the underlying disease be further investigated?

Answer: Relapsing polychondritis can occur alone or accompanied by various immunomodulated diseases (polyautoimmunity). Recent literature suggests that this disease may be related to VEXAS syndrome.

13. How common are masquerade syndromes or metastasis in the sclera?

Answer: Masquerade syndromes or metastasis in the sclera are scarce, but they occur. Lymphoma is probably the most common, with cases involving the lung, breast, and melanoma also seen.

FINAL WRAP-UP

In conclusion, scleritis is a rare but significant inflammatory eye disease. Accurate diagnosis relies on meticulous clinical assessment and selective, targeted investigations to confirm or exclude specific underlying disorders. Watson's classification system has proven to be a reliable and practical tool for assessing the location and severity of scleritis.

Up to 50% of patients with scleritis may have an associated systemic disease, with the risk increasing in correlation with the severity of the condition. NS serves as a marker for potentially life-threatening systemic vasculitis. An infectious etiology for scleritis should always be considered, especially in cases of NS. TB and fungal infections can also present as nodular anterior scleritis, with tuberculous nodular scleritis being relatively common in TB-endemic regions.

Inflammatory scleritis responds well to a stepped approach of systemic anti-inflammatory and IMT proportional to the severity of the condition. Biological therapies have shown effectiveness in cases of severe or poorly responsive scleritis. Conversely, treating infectious scleritis is complex, often requiring a combination of local and systemic antimicrobial therapy and surgical debridement.

REFERENCES

1. Watson PG, Hayreh SS. Scleritis and episcleritis. Br J Ophthalmol. 1976;60(3):163-91.
2. Okhravi N, Odufuwa B, McCluskey P, Lightman S. Scleritis. Surv Ophthalmol. 2005;50(4):351-63.
3. Webinars: IUSG Grand Round 05 (May 11, 2024). [online] Available from https://youtu.be/Pe8YOcLP6jk?si=Tl-BpfVbsrgP9c6h. [Last accessed March, 2025].
4. Majumder PD, Agrawal R, McCluskey P, Biswas J. Current approach for the diagnosis and management of noninfective scleritis. Asia Pac J Ophthalmol (Phila). 2020;10(2):212-23.
5. de la Maza MS, Foster CS, Jabbur NS, Baltatzis S. Ocular characteristics and disease associations in scleritis-associated peripheral keratopathy. Arch Ophthalmol. 2002;120(1):15-9.
6. Phan TG, Wong RCW, Adelstein S. Autoantibodies to extractable nuclear antigens: making detection and interpretation more meaningful. Clin Diagn Lab Immunol. 2002;9(1):1-7.
7. Diogo MC, Jager MJ, Ferreira TA. CT and MR imaging in the diagnosis of scleritis. AJNR Am J Neuroradiol. 2016;37(12):2334-9.
8. Wakefield D, Di Girolamo N, Thurau S, Wildner G, McCluskey P. Scleritis: immunopathogenesis and molecular basis for therapy. Prog Retin Eye Res. 2013;35:44-62.
9. Vergouwen DPC, Rothova A, Berge JCT, Verdijk RM, van Laar JAM, Vingerling JR, et al. Current insights in the pathogenesis of scleritis. Exp Eye Res. 2020;197:108078.
10. Murthy SI, Sabhapandit S, Balamurugan S, Subramaniam P, Sainz-de-la-Maza M, Agarwal M, et al. Scleritis: differentiating infectious from non-infectious entities. Indian J Ophthalmol. 2020;68(9):1818-28.

11. Sfiniadaki E, Tsiara I, Theodossiadis P, Chatziralli I. Ocular manifestations of granulomatosis with polyangiitis: a review of the literature. Ophthalmol Ther. 2019;8(2):227-34.
12. Majumder PD, Agarwal S, Shah M, Srinivasan B, K P, Iyer G, et al. Necrotizing scleritis: a review. Ocul Immunol Inflamm. 2024;32(7):1405-19.
13. Foster CS, Forstot SL, Wilson LA. Mortality rate in rheumatoid arthritis patients developing necrotizing scleritis or peripheral ulcerative keratitis. Ophthalmology. 1984;91(10):1253-63.
14. Samalia P, Sims J, Niederer R. Necrotizing syphilitic scleritis: the resurgence of syphilis in New Zealand. Asia Pac J Ophthalmol (Phila). 2021;10(4):417.
15. Stem MS, Todorich B, Faia LJ. Ocular pharmacology for scleritis: review of treatment and a practical perspective. J Ocul Pharmacol Ther. 2017;33(4):240-6.
16. Hodson KL, Galor A, Karp CL, Davis JL, Albini TA, Perez VL, et al. Epidemiology and visual outcomes in patients with infectious scleritis. Cornea. 2013;32(4):466-72.
17. Rich RM, Smiddy WE, Davis JL. Infectious scleritis after retinal surgery. Am J Ophthalmol. 2008;145(4):695-9.
18. Dev S, Mieler WF, Mittra RA, Prasad A. Acute macular edema associated with an infected scleral buckle. Arch Ophthalmol. 1998;116(8):1117-9.
19. Holland SP, Pulido JS, Miller D, Ellis B, Alfonso E, Scott M, et al. Biofilm and scleral buckle-associated infections. A mechanism for persistence. Ophthalmology. 1991;98(6):933-8.
20. Pathengay A, Karosekar S, Raju B, Sharma S, Das T. Microbiologic spectrum and susceptibility of isolates in scleral buckle infection in India. Am J Ophthalmol. 2004;138(4):663-4.
21. Chhablani J, Nayak S, Jindal A, Motukupally SR, Mathai A, Jalali S, et al. Scleral buckle infections: microbiological spectrum and antimicrobial susceptibility. J Ophthalmic Inflamm Infect. 2013;3(1):67.
22. Goyal M, Murthy SI. Infectious scleritis due to methicillin-resistant staphylococcus aureus after dengue viral fever. Ocul Immunol Inflamm. 2022;30(6):1544-6.
23. Wertheim MS, Cook SD, Knox-Cartwright NE, Le Van D, Tole DM. Electrolysis-needle cauterization of corneal vessels in patients with lipid keratopathy. Cornea. 2007;26(2):230-1.
24. Lee JE, Oum BS, Choi HY, Lee JS. Methicillin-resistant Staphylococcus aureus sclerokeratitis after pterygium excision. Cornea. 2007;26(6):744-6.
25. Maskin SL. Infectious scleritis after a diabetic foot ulcer. Am J Ophthalmol. 1993;115(2):254-5.
26. Lindsey PS, Pierce LH, Welch RB. Removal of scleral buckling elements: causes and complications. Arch Ophthalmol. 1983;101(4):570-3.
27. de la Maza MS, Molina N, Gonzalez-Gonzalez LA, Doctor PP, Tauber J, Foster CS. Clinical characteristics of a large cohort of patients with scleritis and episcleritis. Ophthalmology. 2012;119(1):43-50.
28. de-la-Torre A, Cabrera-Pérez M, Durán C, García S, Cuevas M, Carreño N, et al. Clinical patterns and risk factors in scleritis: a multicentric study in Colombia. Graefes Arch Clin Exp Ophthalmol. 2022;260(12):3957-67.
29. Keino H, Watanabe T, Taki W, Nakashima C, Okada AA. Clinical features and visual outcomes of Japanese patients with scleritis. Br J Ophthalmol. 2010;94(11):1459-63.
30. Lane J, Nyugen E, Morrison J, Lim L, Stawell R, Hodgson L, et al. Clinical features of scleritis across the Asia-Pacific region. Ocul Immunol Inflamm. 2019;27(6):920-6.
31. Ogra S, Sims JL, McGhee CNJ, Niederer RL. Ocular complications and mortality in peripheral ulcerative keratitis and necrotising scleritis: the role of systemic immunosuppression. Clin Exp Ophthalmol. 2020;48(4):434-41.
32. Jennette JC, Falk RJ. B cell-mediated pathogenesis of ANCA-mediated vasculitis. Semin Immunopathol. 2014;36(3):327-38.

CHAPTER

6 Ocular Toxoplasmosis

Alejandra de-la-Torre, Germán Mejía-Salgado, Justine R Smith, Lisia Barros Ferreira, Daniel Vitor Vasconcelos-Santos, Laura Camila Ramírez-Márquez, Rubens Belfort Jr, Guilherme Macedo Souza, Meghan Berkenstock, Reema Bansal, Vishali Gupta, John H Kempen

INTRODUCTION

Ocular toxoplasmosis (OT) has significant epidemiological and medical relevance. Approximately one-third of the global population has anti-*Toxoplasma gondii* immunoglobulin G (IgG) antibodies, indicating previous exposure to the parasite. Among those infected, 2–18% experience ocular involvement, making OT the leading cause of posterior uveitis.[1-3] In several countries, it is the primary cause of uveitis in adults and children.[4,5]

This recurrent infection can result in visual impairment and blindness. Currently, there is no ideal treatment, and the efficacy of available therapies remains controversial.[6,7] Therefore, understanding and addressing OT is paramount due to its significant impact on patients suffering from this disease.

Human infection can occur through various routes: direct exposure to oocysts in the environment, contaminated food, or water; ingestion of tissue cysts in undercooked meat from chicken, beef, or pork (which has shown a stronger association with toxoplasmosis transmission than contact with cats); or, less commonly, organ transplantation from a donor with tissue cysts.[6,8] While cats are the definitive parasite hosts and excrete oocysts into the environment, domestic cats' infection risk is minimal, provided they are vaccinated and proper precautions are taken when cleaning their litter.[1,9]

Although any consumption of contaminated meat from warm-blooded animals can theoretically transmit toxoplasmosis, the risk depends on the type of animal and preparation of the meat. Cysts can survive in raw or undercooked meat but not adequately cooked meat.[7] For instance, lamb meat has been documented as a potential source of *T. gondii* infection in an Australian population, with parasite DNA detected in 43% of tested samples.[10] In Colombia, pork was the most contaminated, followed by beef and chicken.[11]

One of this parasite's primary transmission methods is consuming water contaminated with oocysts. Even treated water from cities can be contaminated, as oocysts can survive detergents, disinfectants such as sodium hypochlorite, and even chlorination.[12] While most waterborne toxoplasmosis outbreaks have been described in developing countries,[13] cases have also been reported in high-income countries, underscoring the importance of educating the population about not drinking tap water and improving methods to eliminate the parasite.[14]

PRACTICAL TIPS IN THE MANAGEMENT OF OCULAR TOXOPLASMOSIS

Practical Tips in Diagnosis of Ocular Toxoplasmosis

The most important clue for diagnosing OT is its clinical presentation. The immune response to the infection typically results in a scar characterized by hyperpigmented edges and an atrophic center. While the immune system can control the parasites, it cannot eliminate them entirely; they remain encysted within retinal cells. These persistent cysts explain the frequent reactivations at the periphery of old lesions. These reactivations present as active, yellowish-white satellite lesions adjacent to the old scars. These satellite lesions result from the proliferation and invasion of tachyzoites into cells neighboring the previous retinal lesion **(Figs. 1A to C)**.

A survey among uveitis experts revealed that 56.8% of cases were diagnosed using a combination of clinical examination and *T. gondii* serology. In comparison, 35.9%

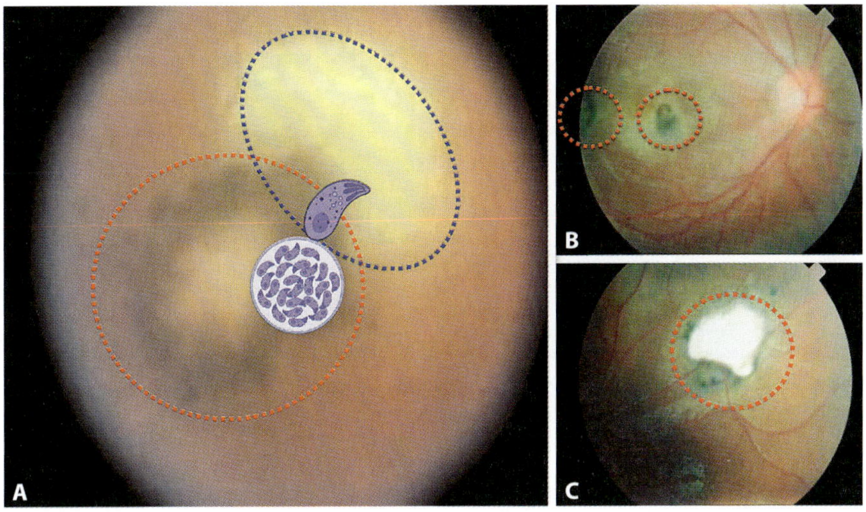

Figs. 1A to C: Clinical picture of ocular toxoplasmosis. (A) Old chorioretinal scar with hyperpigmented borders and an atrophic center (red circle), where tissue cysts containing bradyzoites remain encysted. These are illustrated as a rounded structure from which bradyzoites transform into tachyzoites and exit the infected cell to invade neighboring cells. The lesion is accompanied by a yellowish-white creamy satellite active focus (purple circle), where we can observe inflammation triggered by tachyzoites invading adjacent retinal cells; (B) Inactive hyperpigmented chorioretinal scars; (C) Inactive atrophic scar with complete destruction of the retina and choroid, exposing the underlying sclera.
Source: Presented by Alejandra de-la-Torre at the International Uveitis Study Group (IUSG) Grand Rounds.

of cases were diagnosed based on clinical examination alone. Additionally, 5.2% of cases used a combination of clinical assessment, *T. gondii* serology, and ocular fluid testing, while 2.1% of cases relied on clinical examination and ocular fluid testing.[15]

The symptoms of OT vary depending on the patient's age. In children, the condition often presents with decreased visual acuity and strabismus secondary to amblyopia, nystagmus, leukocoria, microphthalmos, and microcornea. In adults, the symptoms include a decrease in visual acuity, floaters, photophobia, pain, and hyperemia.[2,16]

The location of the lesions also significantly influences the symptomatology. When the posterior segment is affected, including retinochoroiditis and vitritis, patients may experience floaters, decreased visual acuity, blurred vision, and visual field compromise. When both the posterior and anterior segments are involved, additional symptoms such as pain, hyperemia, photophobia, and a further decrease in visual acuity are common.[16,17]

Posterior uveitis, specifically unifocal retinochoroiditis **(Figs. 2A to C)**, is the most common finding and is often associated with vitritis. However, it can also be associated with vasculitis or papillitis. In some cases, anterior involvement is present, manifesting as granulomatous or nongranulomatous inflammation.[18,19] Additional anterior segment findings may include posterior synechiae, fibrin, and iris nodules. These manifestations are secondary to potential reactivations and inflammation in the posterior segment, which can also lead to elevated intraocular pressure (IOP).[18]

Ocular toxoplasmosis can be classified into congenital and acquired forms, each with distinct clinical presentations and characteristics. Congenital OT typically affects both eyes and often presents with more severe manifestations due to more frequent macular compromise. In contrast, acquired OT usually affects only one eye, and lesions are typically focal and can occur anywhere in the fundus.

Serological tests (IgG, IgM) detect antibodies against *T. gondii* for diagnostic purposes. Additionally, a low IgG avidity test, defined as occurring within the past 3 months, supports the diagnosis of a recent primary infection if the avidity is <30 IU/mL.[2]

Recurrences

Recurrences of OT usually develop as satellite lesions. These active retinochoroidal lesions form at the edge of an old, pigmented scar. The transition of bradyzoites to tachyzoites plays a crucial role in this process. Recurrences often exhibit a clustering pattern following an acute episode. This means that the risk of presenting another recurrence in a shorter time notably increases after the first recurrence occurs.[20,21]

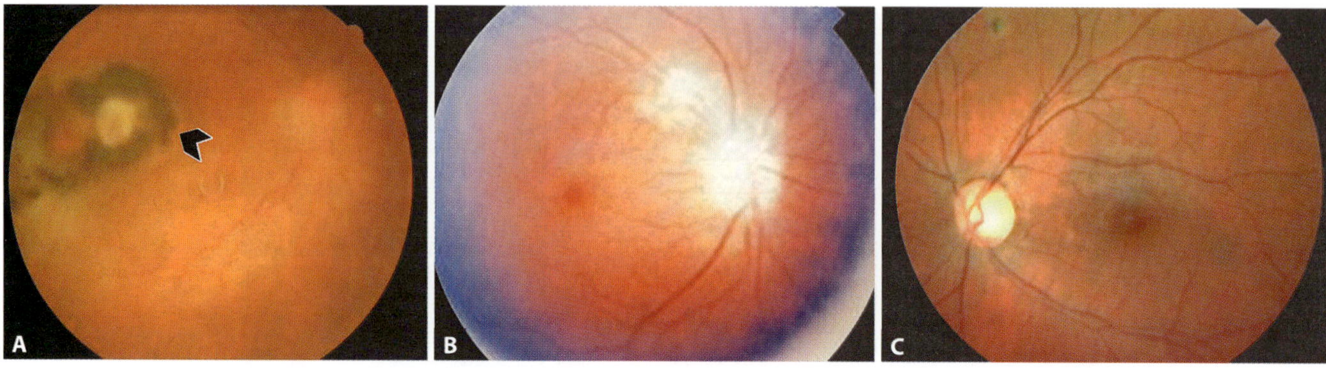

Figs. 2A to C: Location of ocular toxoplasmosis retinochoroidal lesions. (A) Macular; (B) Optic disc; (C) Mid-periphery.
Source: Presented by Alejandra de-la-Torre in the International Uveitis Study Group (IUSG) grand rounds.[1]

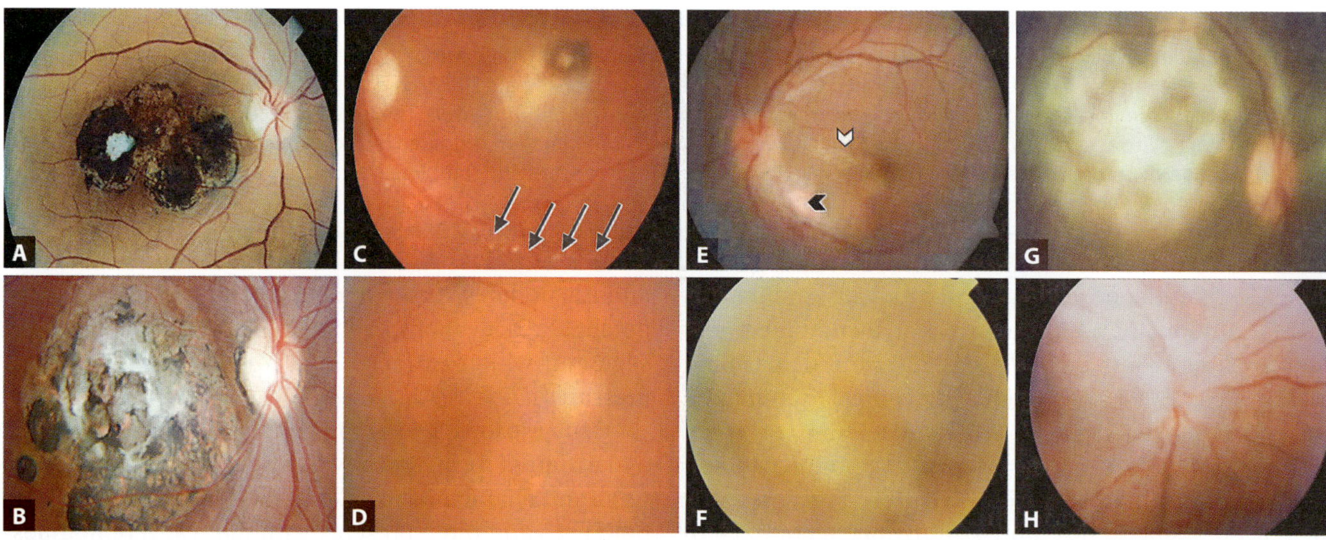

Figs. 3A to H: Forms of presentation of ocular toxoplasmosis. (A) Extensive coalescent hyperpigmented macular retinochoroidal scars; (B) Large macular retinochoroidal scar with atrophic and hyperpigmented areas; (C) Kyrieleis phenomenon; (D) Vitritis; (E) Neuroretinitis; (F) Headlight in the fog sign suggestive of active lesions; (G) Multifocal extensive chorioretinitis; and (H) Papillitis.
Source: Presented by Alejandra de-la-Torre in the International Uveitis Study Group (IUSG) grand rounds.[1]

The previous use of systemic steroids without concomitant antibiotics or the application of subconjunctival steroid injections has been associated with a high recurrence rate.[21] This underscores the importance of appropriate and combined treatment strategies to manage OT effectively.

In addition to the typical retinochoroidal scars, OT can also present with the Kyrieleis phenomenon, neuroretinitis, multifocal and extensive retinochoroiditis, vitritis, the "headlight in the fog" sign, and papillitis, among other manifestations **(Figs. 3A to H)**.

Significant clinical differences exist in OT between South America and Europe/North America, focusing on the inflammatory response, parasite characteristics, and immune response deviations. In South American patients, a severe inflammatory response is associated with decreased intraocular levels of interferon-gamma (IFN-γ) and interleukin (IL)-17 and increased levels of IL-6 and IL-13. This cytokine profile indicates a shift toward a Th2 response, correlating with more severe ocular involvement. In contrast, European patients exhibit a typical Th1 inflammatory response.[22] Additionally, IL-5 and vascular endothelial growth factor (VEGF) have been associated with a higher recurrence rate of OT **(Figs. 4A and B)**. Genetic polymorphisms in cytokines, including tumor necrosis factor-α (TNF-α), interferon gamma (IFN-γ), IL-1α, IL-1β, and IL-10, have been identified in patients with OT. These polymorphisms require further

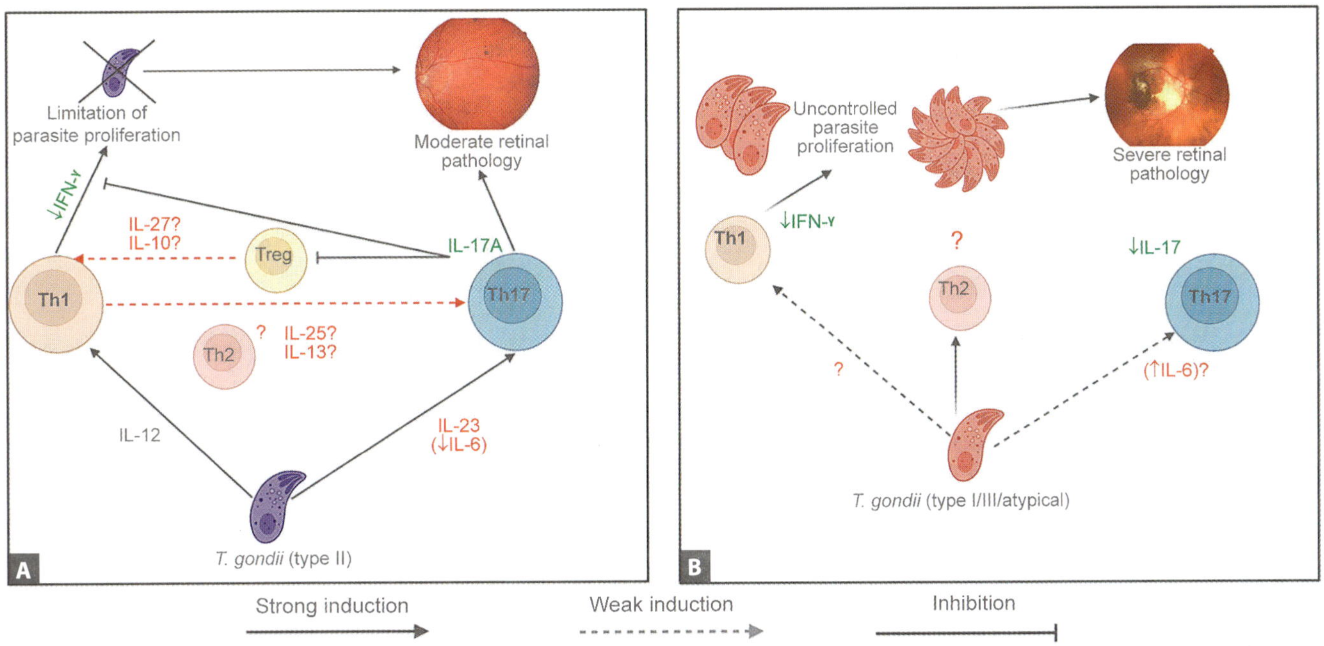

Figs. 4A and B: Intraocular immune response differences and clinical consequences regarding *Toxoplasma gondii* strains. (A) Type II *Toxoplasma gondii* strains (predominant in Europe and North America). This strain triggers Th1 and Th17 immune responses. Research suggests that IL-17A is crucial in retinal pathology and inhibits the protective IFN-γ driven response. Neutralizing IL-17A appears to reverse these effects, at least partially. This pathological process typically self-limits over time, resulting in moderate retinal damage and relatively small lesions. IL-17A suppresses regulatory T (Treg) cells and possibly Th2 cells, although many aspects (highlighted in red) remain unclear. Specifically, induction and regulation of IL-17A production (involving IL-6 and IL-23), potential roles of other IL-17 family members, and precise functions of Th2 and Treg cells in the interaction between IL-17A and IFN-γ require further elucidation; (B) Atypical and highly variable strains (observed in South America). These strains induce minimal production of both IFN-γ and IL-17A. Interestingly, IL-6 levels are elevated in these patients. The relative lack of IFN-γ permits uncontrolled parasite replication, leading to severe pathology with numerous and larger lesions. The immunological regulation of this process is much less understood than type II infection. (IFN-γ: interferon gamma; IL: interleukin)
Source: Modified from Pfaff et al.;[22] Presented by Alejandra de-la-Torre in the International Uveitis Study Group (IUSG) grand rounds.[1]

investigation to understand their correlation with disease severity.[22]

According to the diagnostic algorithm for OT, patients with suspected infectious uveitis undergo an enzyme-linked immunosorbent assay (ELISA) in serum for anti-*Toxoplasma* IgG and IgM antibodies. If the results are positive, further testing of the aqueous humor sample for *Toxoplasma* and other pathogens is conducted using polymerase chain reaction (PCR) to detect *T. gondii* DNA in ocular fluids or the Goldmann–Witmer coefficient (GWC) to determine if antibodies against *T. gondii* are being produced within the eye. It is important to note that a negative GWC or PCR result, although informative, does not completely rule out OT. Therefore, clinical diagnosis remains paramount and should be the primary consideration in evaluating suspected cases.[23]

Workup: Optical Coherence Tomography Findings

Optical coherence tomography (OCT) can reveal several key features in acute OT cases. Ocular lesions typically begin in the most superficial layers of the retina and may extend until they reach the choroid. The most common clinical presentation includes the development of lesions around preexisting scars. Common OCT findings in these cases include a thickened (65%) and hyperreflective (61%) retina, choroidal thickening (55%) and hyperreflectivity (61%), hyperreflective vitreous dots (80%), and deposits (36%).[24] These changes may also involve the sclera in severe cases in immunocompromised patients.[25]

Differential Diagnoses

The differential diagnosis for *T. gondii* retinochoroiditis varies based on the timing of presentation, either early

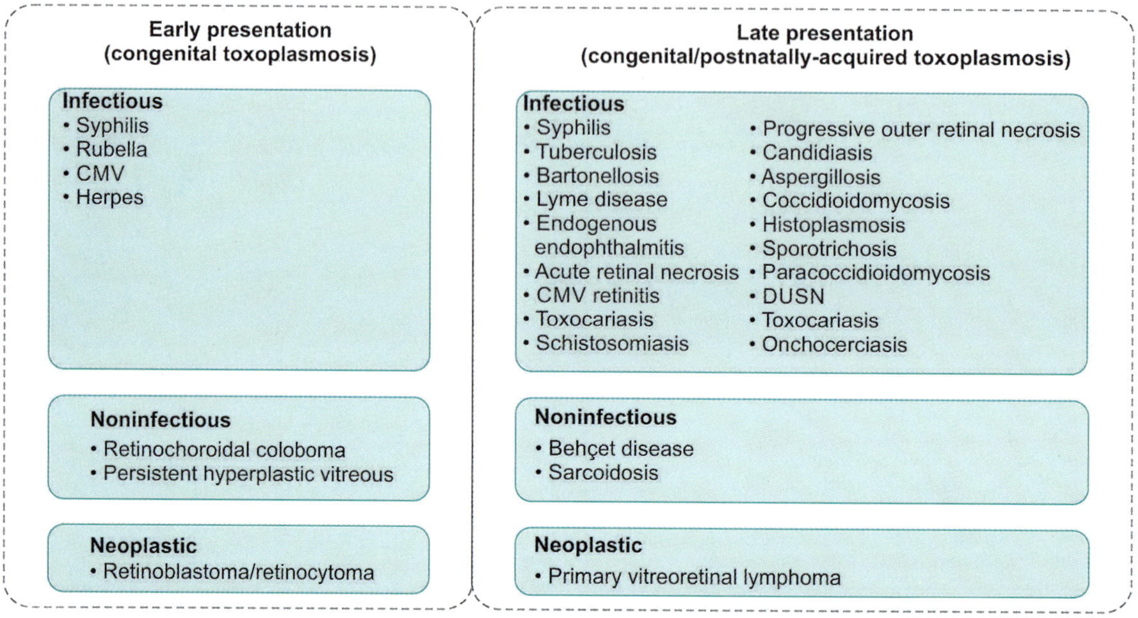

Fig. 5: Differential diagnoses of ocular toxoplasmosis. (CMV: cytomegalovirus; DUSN: diffuse unilateral subacute neuroretinitis)
Source: Modified from Gomez-Marín and de-la-Torre;[26] Presented by Alejandra de-la-Torre in the International Uveitis Study Group (IUSG) grand rounds.[1]

(congenital toxoplasmosis) or late (congenital/postnatally acquired toxoplasmosis), and includes both infectious and noninfectious causes **(Fig. 5)**.[26]

Clinical Pearls in Ocular Toxoplasmosis Diagnosis

Although the clinical presentation in OT is frequently typical, serology is useful:

- To confirm the diagnosis in typical cases
- To provide information about the time of acquisition/onset of infection
  - *IgG:* Memory antibodies, which mean old chronic infection
  - *IgM:* Recent infection

Given the high prevalence of positive anti-*Toxoplasma* IgG in the general population, a positive serology does not confirm a diagnosis. PCR in intraocular fluids is useful for confirming diagnosis, detecting coinfections, or ruling out differential diagnoses, especially in atypical cases. However, a negative PCR result could not rule out 100% of the diagnosis (sensitivity ranging from 72 to 83% PCR alone[27,28] and 53–93% combining PCR and GWC).[23,29] Images are useful for determining disease activity, monitoring it, and detecting complications.[30]

Practical Tips in the Treatment of Ocular Toxoplasmosis

There is currently no standardized therapy for treating OT. Ophthalmologists often use various therapies alone or in combination. A systematic review of the literature that analyzes the effectiveness of different treatments and a survey of practices conducted by uveitis experts identified 24 different regimens used to treat OT.[31] The most common therapies used to treat OT are listed in **Table 1**.

Trimethoprim-sulfamethoxazole (TMP-SMX) is the most frequently prescribed drug, followed by clindamycin (26.6%). Medications such as azithromycin, sulfadiazine, spiramycin, acetyl spiramycin, and atovaquone are less commonly used. Intravitreal clindamycin is used in 8.85% of cases, typically up to three times. Corticosteroids can be used either orally or topically. However, their administration should be approached with caution and always after antiparasitic treatment to ensure safety and efficacy.[15]

In typical OT, achieving a favorable visual outcome is often challenging. In a study conducted in São Paulo among 311 eyes with inactive disease, normal vision (≥20/40) was observed in 156 eyes (50.1%), while mild visual impairment (20/50–20/60) was seen in 29 eyes (9.3%). Moderate visual

TABLE 1: Recommended doses of classical therapy for ocular toxoplasmosis.

	First-line therapy for ocular toxoplasmosis	
	Adult dose	***Pediatric dose***
Oral pyrimethamine[33,34]	100 mg oral dose on the first 2 days (for a total load dose of 200 mg), followed by 25–75 mg daily for a minimum of 4–6 weeks in active acquired or recurrent infections (ideally until the active lesion completely resolves)	The first dose is 2 mg/kg, followed by 1 mg/kg daily for 1 year in congenital forms and for a minimum of 4–6 weeks in active acquired or recurrent infections (ideally until the active lesion completely resolves)
Oral sulfadiazine[33,34]	4 g daily (500 mg every 6 hours) for a minimum of 4–6 weeks in active acquired or recurrent infections (ideally until the active lesion completely resolves)	50 mg/kg two times daily, equivalent to 100 mg/kg per day for 1 year for congenital infection and for a minimum of 4–6 weeks in active acquired or recurrent infections (ideally until the active lesion completely resolves)
Oral folinic acid[33,34]	15 mg daily	7.5 mg daily
	Other therapies	
	Adult dose	***Pediatric dose***
Oral trimethoprim (TMP) and sulfamethoxazole (SMX)[34-36]	TMP (160 mg)/SMX (800 mg) every 12 hours or two pills of TMP (80 mg)/SMX (400 mg) for a minimum of 4–6 weeks in active acquired or recurrent infections (ideally until the active lesion completely resolves)	No pediatric dosing guidelines have been reported for the use of TMP-SMX in children with congenital forms of the infection. However, the following dosages are commonly used. Notably, it should always be prescribed as part of a multidisciplinary approach involving a pediatric infectious disease specialist: • For children younger than 2 months of age, use is not recommended. • For children 2 months of age and older, the dose is based on body weight. The usual dose is 40 mg/kg of body weight of SMX and 8 mg/kg of body weight of TMP, given in two divided doses every 12 hours for a minimum of 4–6 weeks, ideally until the active lesion completely resolves – Weighing 40 kg: Four teaspoonfuls (20 mL) of oral liquid or two tablets (or one double-strength tablet) two times a day for a minimum of 4–6 weeks, ideally until the active lesion completely resolves – Weighing 30 kg: Three teaspoonfuls (15 mL) of oral liquid or 1.5 tablet two times a day for a minimum of 4–6 weeks, ideally until the active lesion completely resolves – Weighing 20 kg: Two teaspoonfuls (10 mL) of oral liquid or one tablet two times a day for a minimum of 4–6 weeks, ideally until the active lesion completely resolves – Weighing 10 kg: One teaspoonful (5 mL) of oral liquid two times a day for a minimum of 4–6 weeks, ideally until the active lesion completely resolves • Children weighing 40 kg (88 pounds) or more should have the adult dosages
Oral azithromycin[34]	500 mg daily for a minimum of 4–6 weeks in active acquired or recurrent infections (ideally until the active lesion completely resolves)	10–30 mg/kg daily for a minimum of 4–6 weeks in active acquired or recurrent infections (ideally until the active lesion completely resolves)

Contd...

Contd...

	Other therapies	
	Adult dose	***Pediatric dose***
Oral corticosteroids[34]	• 0.5–1 mg/kg daily, not exceeding a total of 60 mg/day • This dosage should be used in cases of severe vitritis or lesions localized in zone I with a high risk of blindness, beginning 48 hours after initiating antimicrobial therapy • The dosage should be gradually reduced and finished before the end of the antimicrobial treatment • It should be used in combination with classic therapy or with any other antimicrobial therapy	
Intravitreal clindamycin plus dexamethasone[33,37,38]	1–1.5 mg/0.1 mL (clindamycin) and 400 µg/0.1 mL (dexamethasone) every 2 weeks; generally, two injections are enough. However, three to four injections can be administered according to treatment response until the lesion is inactive	Pediatric doses have not been standardized. However, similar doses have been reported effectively in a 12-year-old child
	Intravitreal therapy reduces the risk of systemic drug adverse effects. It should be given as an adjunct therapy, not as monotherapy, except in cases where systemic therapy is contraindicated, such as early pregnancy (before 18 weeks) and severe drug adverse effects	
	Prophylaxis	
	Adult dose	***Pediatric dose***
TMP and SMX[39]	TMP (160 mg)/SMX (800 mg) 3 days a week for a minimum of 1 year for lesions at zone I with a high risk of blindness	Pediatric doses have not been standardized
	During treatment, it should be monitored complete blood count, liver, and renal function tests at baseline, in the second week, and then every 4–6 weeks	

impairment (20/70–20/200) affected 25 eyes (8.0%), and severe visual impairment (>20/200–20/400) was present in 23 eyes (7.4%). Notably, blindness (>20/400) occurred in 78 eyes (25.0%).[32]

Blindness was found to be associated with several factors, including macular lesions, with an odds ratio (OR) of 9.95 [95% confidence interval (CI): 2.45–47.15], any complication, with an OR of 10.26 (95% CI: 3.82–30.67), and atypical OT, with an OR of 4.99 (95% CI: 1.14–22.85).[32]

Clinical Pearls in Ocular Toxoplasmosis Treatment

- Preventing recurrence is possible through prophylactic therapy.
- There is no ideal treatment because there are no available therapies to eradicate the tissue cysts.
- Not treating is not an option. Peripheral lesions should also be treated.
- Treatment is usually given for at least 4–6 weeks. However, it should be given until the retinochoroiditis is entirely resolved.
- Steroids should be given only in combination with antibiotic/antiparasitic therapy.

TYPICAL OCULAR TOXOPLASMOSIS CASE

Case Presentation

Personal Data

- Boy
- 15 years old
- Caucasian
- Past ocular history: OT in the right eye (OD) 2.5 years ago treated with sulfamethoxazole 800 mg + trimethoprim 160 mg every 12 hours for 6 weeks, azithromycin 250 mg/day for 6 weeks, and deflazacort 30 mg with progressive tapering.
- There is no history of recurrences.
- Visual acuity (VA) after first episode 20/70 OD and 20/20 OS
- No other past/current medical condition
- Previous laboratory testing:
  - *T. gondii* serology: IgM negative and IgG positive
  - *Complete blood count (CBC):* Hematocrit 45.3%, Hb 15.4 g/dL, platelets 161,000/µL, white blood count 5,300/µL, and neutrophils 2,400/µL

History of Present Illness

Blurry vision, myodesopsia, and a central black spot in OD for 5 days; patient denied photophobia, pain, or hyperemia.

Physical Examination

The patient presented with visual acuity of 20/400 OD and 20/20 OS. A slit-lamp examination revealed a slightly hyperemic conjunctiva with no cells in the anterior chamber OU. IOP was within normal limits OU. The fundoscopy of the OD showed a hyperemic optic disc with a whitish area of retinitis with intraretinal hemorrhages adjacent to pigmented retinochoroidal scars and vascular sheathing **(Table 2 and Fig. 6)**.

Diagnosis

Recurrence of OT.

Workup

Fundus fluorescein angiography (FFA) and optical coherence tomography were performed to characterize the lesions **(Figs. 7 and 8)**.

Treatment

The patient restarted treatment with sulfamethoxazole 800 mg and trimethoprim 160 mg, administered every 12 hours until the lesion appeared inactive (7 weeks), combined with oral corticosteroids 30 mg 2 days after starting antibiotic therapy, administered for 2 weeks with gradual tapering (12 mg for 1 week, then 6 mg for 1 week).

During the 7-week follow-up, fundus examination revealed an increase in the total area of scarring. OCT showed loss of retinal architecture and atrophy. Due to macular involvement, the patient's visual acuity remained at 20/400 OD **(Figs. 9A and B)**. Prophylactic therapy was suggested, but the patient refused to take it.

Discussion

This case represents a typical presentation of recurrent toxoplasmic retinochoroiditis in a young patient with characteristic central lesion symptoms, including decreased visual acuity, floaters, and visual field defects without associated redness, hyperemia, or photophobia. Consequently, it is crucial to perform a comprehensive ophthalmological examination, including pupillary dilation, to visualize the fundus in patients with these symptoms. Clinically, the case reveals a satellite lesion adjacent to a previous macular scar, consistent with conversion of bradyzoites into tachyzoites that invade adjacent cells, causing inflammation and tissue destruction, further compromising the patient's central visual field.

In this case, IgG was positive, and IgM was negative, leaving uncertainty about whether the prior scar resulted from an acquired or congenital infection, especially in this 15-year-old patient with a previous episode treated at age 13. The suspicion leans toward congenital toxoplasmosis;

TABLE 2: Physical examination of the patient having typical ocular toxoplasmosis case.

OD	***Parameter***	***OS***
20/400	BCVA	20/20
14 mm Hg	IOP	14 mm Hg
Slightly hyperemic conjunctiva	Conjunctiva	Slightly hyperemic conjunctiva
Clear	Cornea	Clear
ACC: 0+ cells	Anterior chamber	ACC: 0+
Normal	Iris	Normal
Clear	Lens	Clear
0.5+ cells	Vitreous	Normal
• Mildly hyperemic optic disc with blurred margins • Whitish area of retinitis with intraretinal hemorrhages, adjacent to pigmented retinochoroidal scars • Vascular sheathing	Fundus	Normal

(ACC: anterior chamber cellularity; BCVA: best-corrected visual acuity; IOP: intraocular pressure)

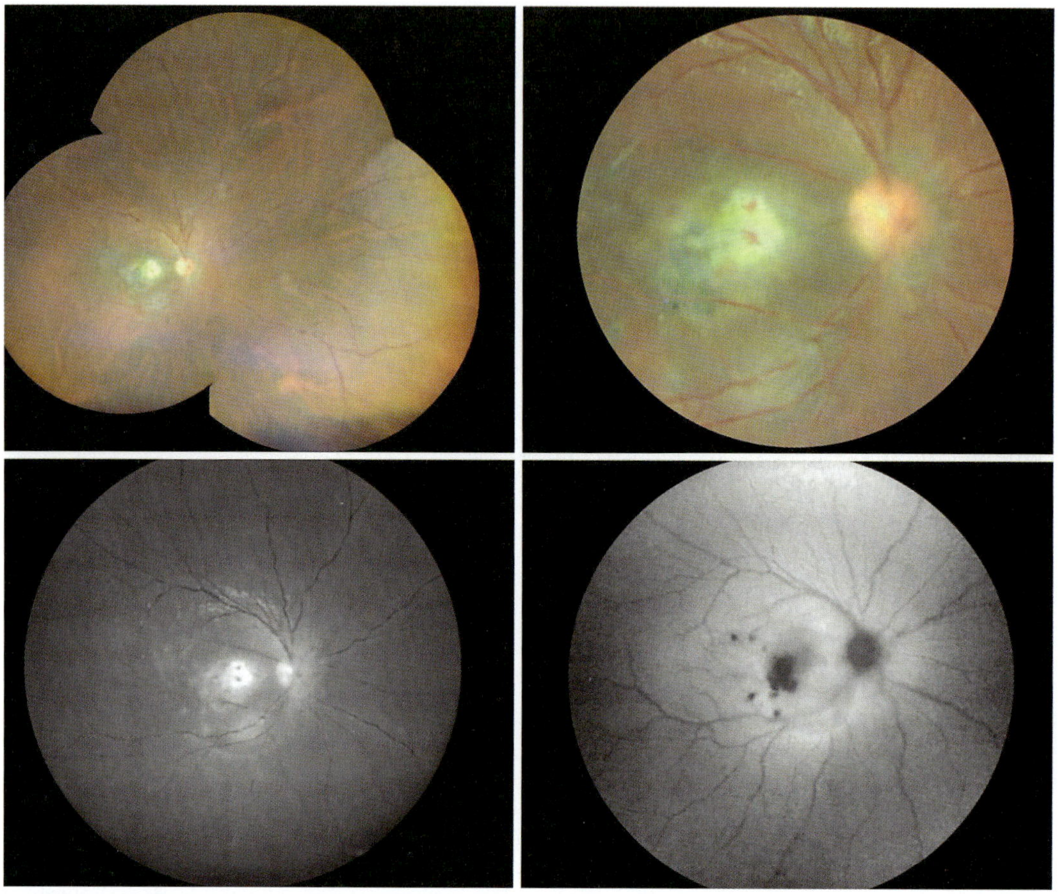

Fig. 6: Initial clinical picture. Whitish area of retinitis with intraretinal hemorrhages adjacent to pigmented retinochoroidal scars.
Source: Presented by Lisia Barros Ferreira in the International Uveitis Study Group (IUSG) grand rounds.[1]
Courtesy: Alejandra de-la-Torre.

however, it is noted that a significant percentage of infections in patients under 18 years old are acquired.[40] Thus, while clinical diagnosis is essential, serological testing is necessary. In cases of acquired toxoplasmosis, prophylactic treatment following acute-phase therapy is crucial to prevent recurrences, particularly in patients with a high risk of severe visual impairment, such as in this case where the prior lesion also involved the macula.

Regarding therapy, the patient received the most used treatment for active OT, although not the classic regimen of pyrimethamine, sulfadiazine, and corticosteroids. TMP-SMX was used, typically resulting in the resolution of inflammation. In this case, steroids were added due to the central lesion, although vitritis was minimal.

The recurrence occurred 2.5 years after the initial episode, highlighting that while the risk of recurrence is higher within the first 2 years following an active lesion, recurrences can occur at any point in life. This patient would benefit from prophylactic therapy due to the lesion's location and heightened risk of visual compromise. However, the patient declined prophylaxis.

ATYPICAL OCULAR TOXOPLASMOSIS CASE

Case Presentation

Personal Data

- Female
- 52-year-old
- No previous diseases

History of Present Illness

Ocular pain and decreased vision in OS for 1 week, otherwise healthy; she denied other systemic symptoms,

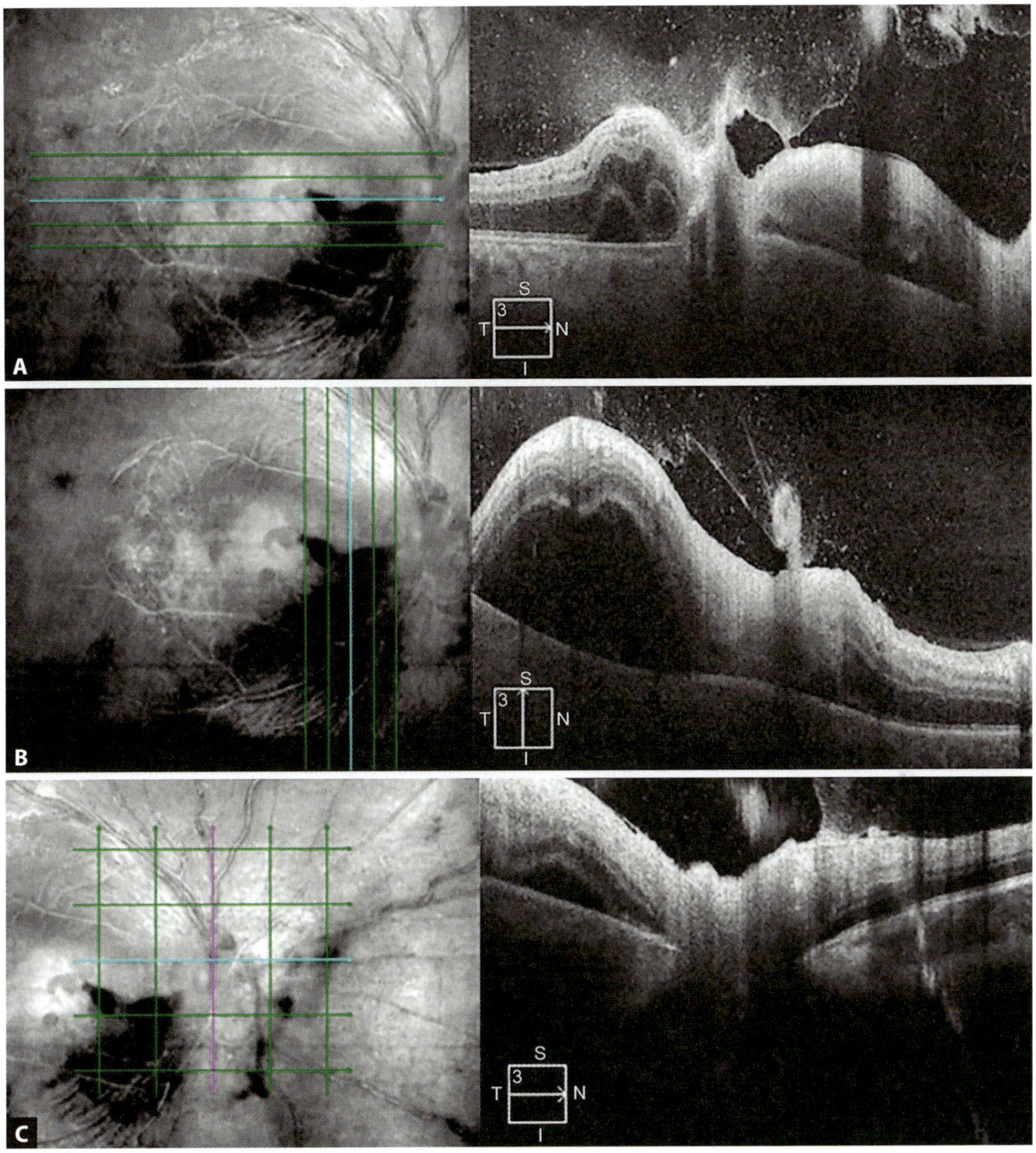

Figs. 7A to C: Optical coherence tomography (OCT) findings at the initial examination. (A) Horizontal and (B) Vertical cut centered on the macula featuring vitritis, posterior vitreous detachment, and a prominent neurosensory retinal detachment, creating multiple subretinal spaces with complete disorganization of retinal layers. The underlying choroid architecture shows alterations with areas of hyporeflectivity likely indicating inflammation; (C) Vertical cut centered on the optic disc showing swelling and hyperreflective changes.
Source: Presented by Lisia Barros Ferreira in the International Uveitis Study Group (IUSG) grand rounds.[1]
Courtesy: Alejandra de-la-Torre.

trauma, allergies, travels, or contact with TB and the use of corticosteroids.

Physical Examination

She presented with a visual acuity of 20/20 in OD and 20/70 in OS. IOP was high (36 mm Hg) in OS; anterior chamber inflammation was evident in OS, with severe vitritis and necrotizing retinochoroidal lesion up to the optic disc **(Table 3 and Fig. 10)**.

Multimodal imaging was performed to characterize the lesion. A hyperautofluorescent lesion was observed in the fundus autofluorescence photo **(Fig. 10B)** corresponding to the necrotizing lesion observed in the fundus photograph **(Fig. 10A)**. FFA revealed a hypofluorescent

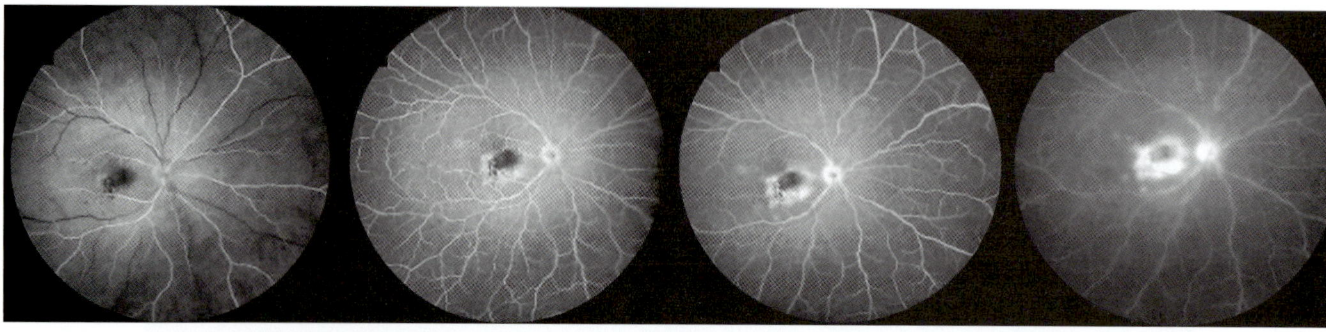

Fig. 8: Fundus fluorescein angiography (FFA) findings at the initial examination. The FFA sequence shows early hypofluorescence at the center of the active lesion, with later phases revealing hyperfluorescence at the borders with fuzzy margins, indicating leakage. Additionally, hyperfluorescence of the optic disc with late leakage is observed, along with venular late leakage, primarily in the temporal arcades.
Source: Presented by Lisia Barros Ferreira in the International Uveitis Study Group (IUSG) grand rounds.[1]
Courtesy: Alejandra de-la-Torre

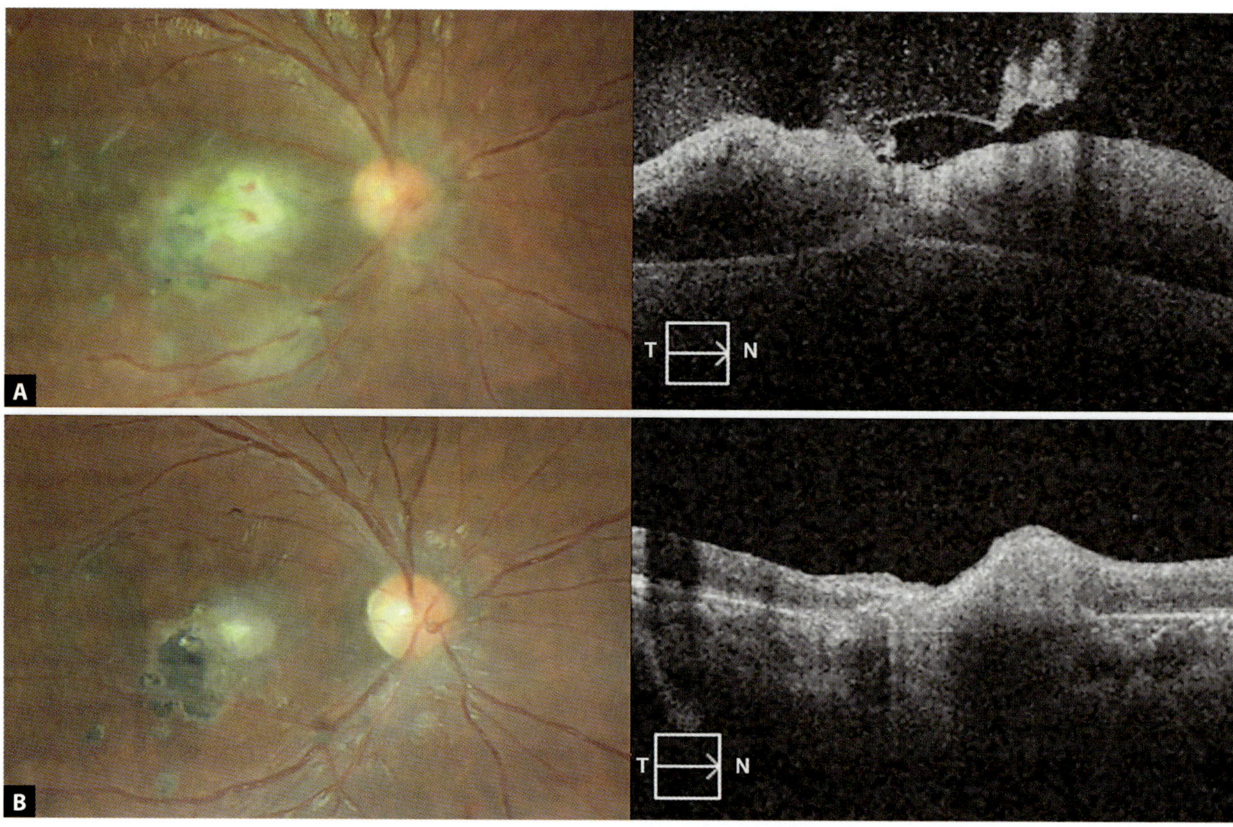

Figs. 9A and B: Comparison of fundus and optical coherence tomography (OCT) images between initial clinical presentation and 7-week post-treatment. (A) Initial clinical picture; (B) Follow-up at week 7.
Source: Presented by Lisia Barros Ferreira in the International Uveitis Study Group (IUSG) grand rounds.[1]
Courtesy: Alejandra de-la-Torre

region around the lesion, with hyperfluorescent edges and late-stage leakage **(Figs. 10C and D)**. OCT centered on the macula showed intense vitritis **(Fig. 10E)**. In the lesion area, there was evidence of full-thickness retinal thickening, hyperreflectivity of the internal layers, interruptions of the retinal pigment epithelium (RPE), and choroidal thickening **(Fig. 10F)**.

TABLE 3: Physical examination of the patient having atypical ocular toxoplasmosis case.

OD	*Parameter*	*OS*
20/20	BCVA	20/70
12 mm Hg	IOP	36 mm Hg
Normal	Conjunctiva	Mild ciliary injection
Clear	Cornea	Mild corneal edema, numerous granulomatous KP
0+ cells, 0+ flare	Anterior chamber	3+ cells, 2+ flare
Normal	Iris	Normal
Clear	Lens	Clear
0+ cells	Vitreous	3+ cells
Normal	Fundus	Impossible to see due to intense vitritis. However, a necrotizing with region was evident up to the optic disc

(BCVA: best-corrected visual acuity; IOP: intraocular pressure; KP: keratic precipitate)

Differential Diagnosis

Two possibilities were considered: (1) atypical toxoplasmosis due to the larger lesion or (2) necrotizing herpetic retinitis. A serological test and an anterior chamber tap were ordered.

Treatment

It was decided to initiate treatment for both conditions with pyrimethamine, sulfadiazine, folinic acid, and valacyclovir 2 grams three times daily.

Course

During the 7-day follow-up, there was a partial reduction in vitritis. The serology results were negative for human immunodeficiency virus (HIV) and positive for IgG *Toxoplasma*, *herpes simplex virus* (HSV), and *varicella-zoster virus* (VZV). PCR results were negative for *Toxoplasma*, *HSV*, and *VZV*. Based on these findings, prednisolone treatment was initiated. In subsequent follow-ups, there was further reduction in vitritis and lesion size, resulting in visual acuity of 20/25 by day 45 **(Fig. 11)**.

At the final follow-up, the FFA revealed a window defect at the lesion site. The OCT showed thinning and disorganization of the neurosensory retina **(Fig. 12A)** and a thin and hyperreflective choroid **(Fig. 12B)**.

Whether it was atypical toxoplasmosis or necrotizing viral retinitis remained unresolved. However, it was answered 6 years later when the patient experienced an episode of emotional distress and reactivation of the lesion, resulting in a decrease in vision to 20/60. The new lesion appeared as a satellite lesion, more typical of toxoplasmosis than herpetic retinitis. An alternative treatment regimen was initiated, including pyrimethamine, azithromycin, folinic acid, and prednisolone (starting 2 days later). This treatment improved vision to 20/30 at week 3 and 20/20 at week 7 **(Figs. 13A to C)**.

Six weeks later, the patient presented with a new recurrence, and treatment was restarted. Following this second recurrence, prophylactic therapy was initiated with TMP-SMX (160/800 mg) three times a week.

Discussion

Ocular toxoplasmosis can present in various atypical forms **(Figs. 14 and 15)**, which include:

- *Toxoplasmic neuroretinitis*: Inflammation affecting both the retina and the optic nerve.
- *Punctate outer retinal toxoplasmosis*: Characterized by multifocal gray-white lesions at the deep retina and RPE level, which are associated with little or no overlying vitreous reaction.
- *Multifocal retinochoroiditis*: Can be necrotizing (associated with elderly patients/immunosuppressed or recently acquired toxoplasmosis) or punctate (associated with early congenital toxoplasmosis and recently acquired toxoplasmosis).
- *Extensive retinochoroiditis*: This form simulates acute retinal necrosis or necrotizing herpetic retinopathy and is associated with recently acquired toxoplasmosis.
- *Frosted branch angiitis*: A condition marked by widespread retinal vasculitis.

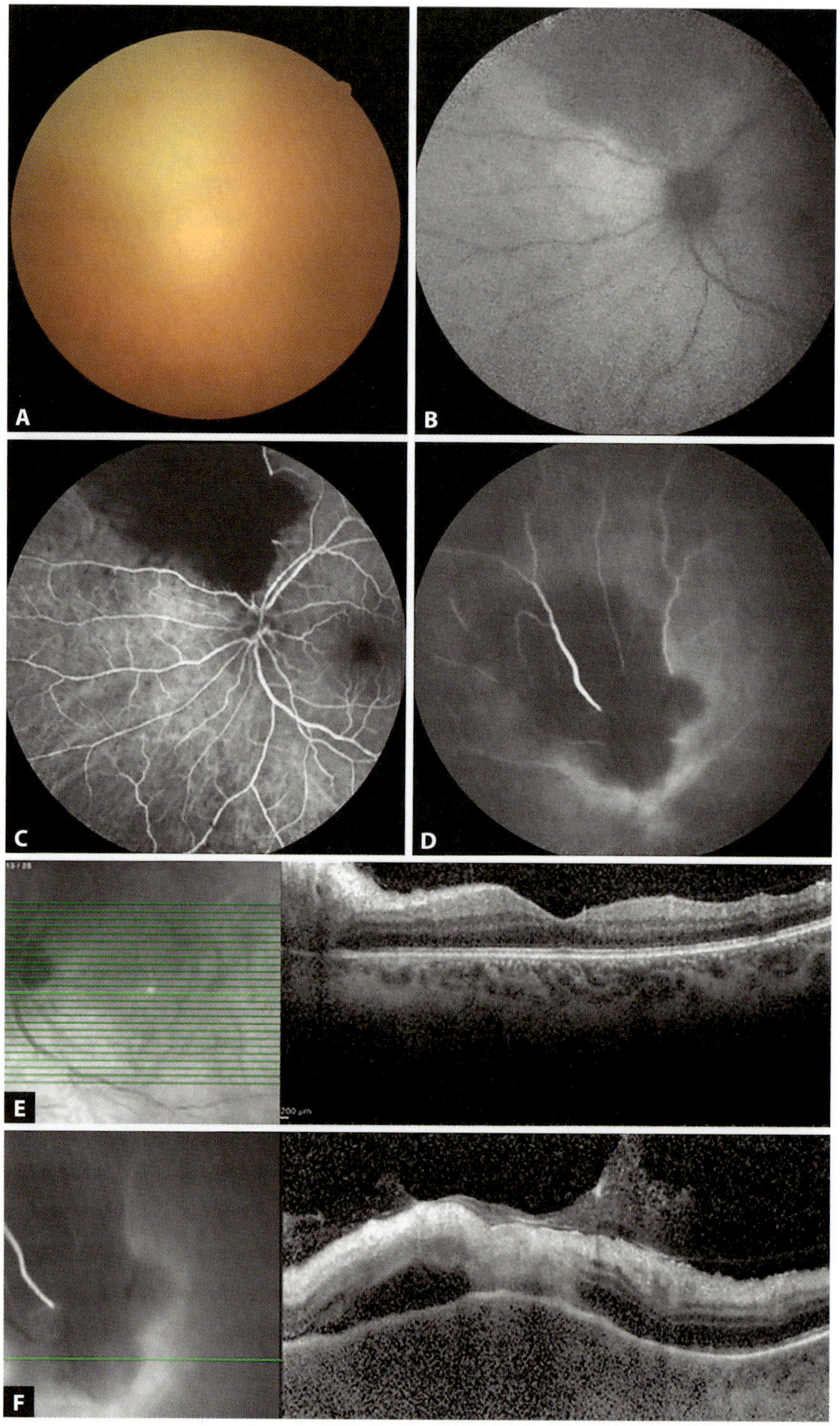

Figs. 10A to F: Multimodal imaging. (A) Fundus photograph with severe vitritis and headlight in the fog suggesting active retinochoroidal lesion up to the optic disc; (B) An autofluorescence image that highlights a hypoautofluorescent area in the place of a retinochoroidal lesion observed in the fundus photo; (C and D) A fluorescein angiography image shows a hypofluorescent lesion due to poor retinal perfusion secondary to retinochoroidal necrosis; (E) Horizontal optical coherence tomography (OCT) cut centered on the macula showing some small areas of vitreous macular traction with the normal distribution of retinal layers; (F) Horizontal OCT cut centered on the lesion evidencing vitreous opacities, disruption of inner and outer retinal layers, areas of subretinal fluid, diffuse macular edema, and choroidal thickening.
Source: Presented by Laura Camila Ramirez-Marquez in the International Uveitis Study Group (IUSG) grand rounds.[1]

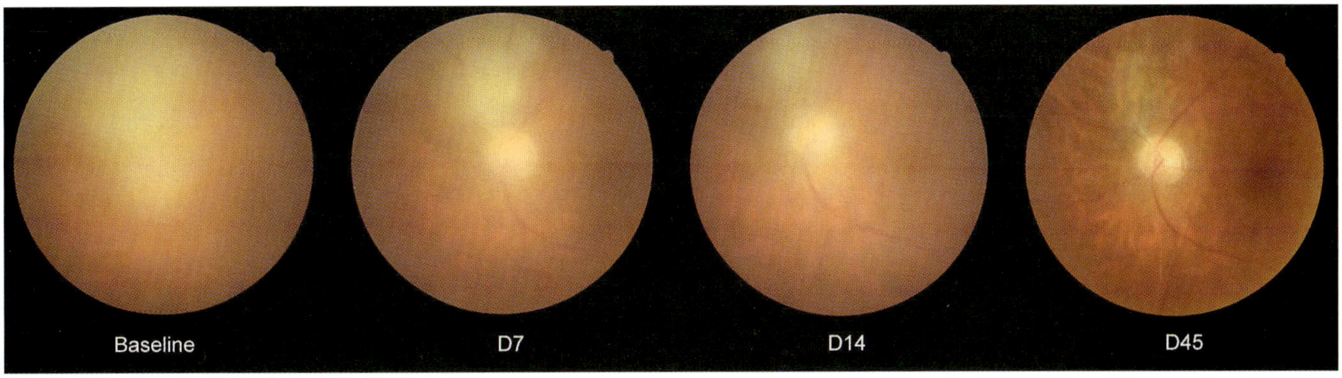

Fig. 11: Follow-up fundus photographs. Reduction of vitritis and resolution of the activity of the retinochoroidal lesion with the absence of hyperpigmented edges during follow-up.
Source: Presented by Laura Camila Ramirez-Marquez in the International Uveitis Study Group (IUSG) grand rounds.[1]

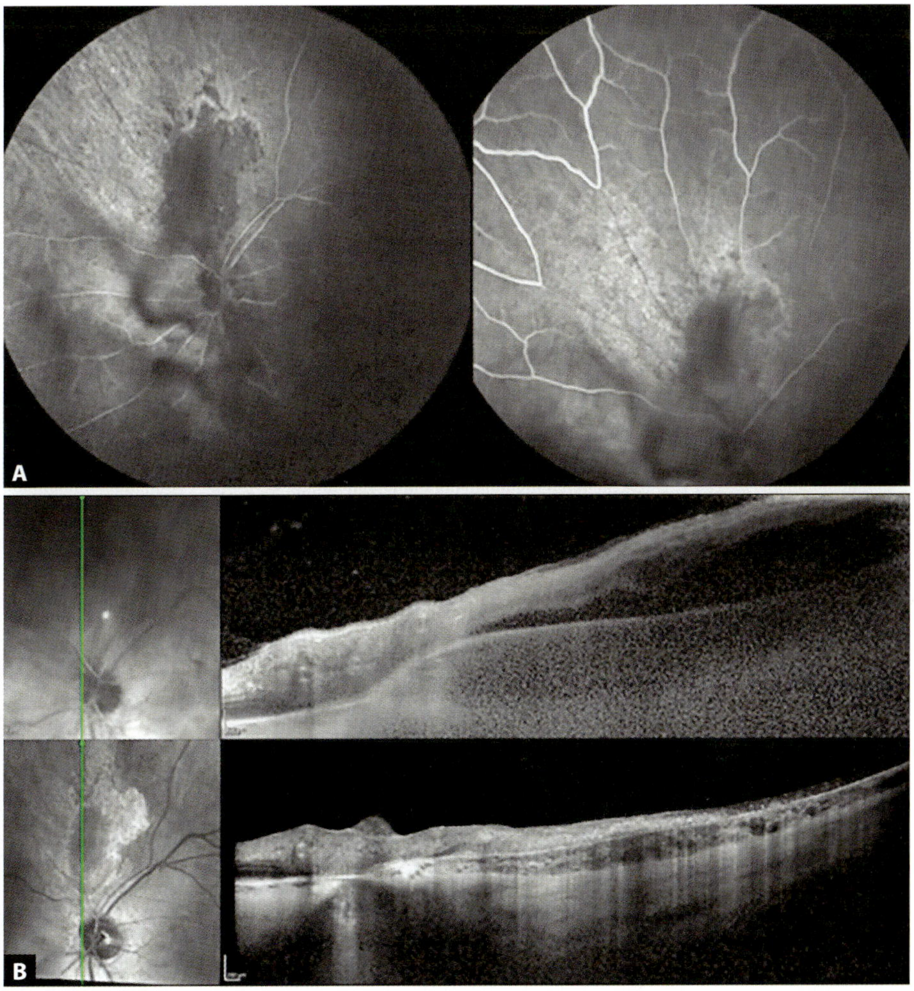

Figs. 12A and B: Multimodal imaging at day 45 of follow-up. (A) Fluorescein angiography with reduced hyperfluorescence of the edges with (B) residual disorganization of the retinal layers and subretinal fluid at the level of the retinochoroidal lesion.
Source: Presented by Laura Camila Ramirez-Marquez in the International Uveitis Study Group (IUSG) grand rounds.[1]

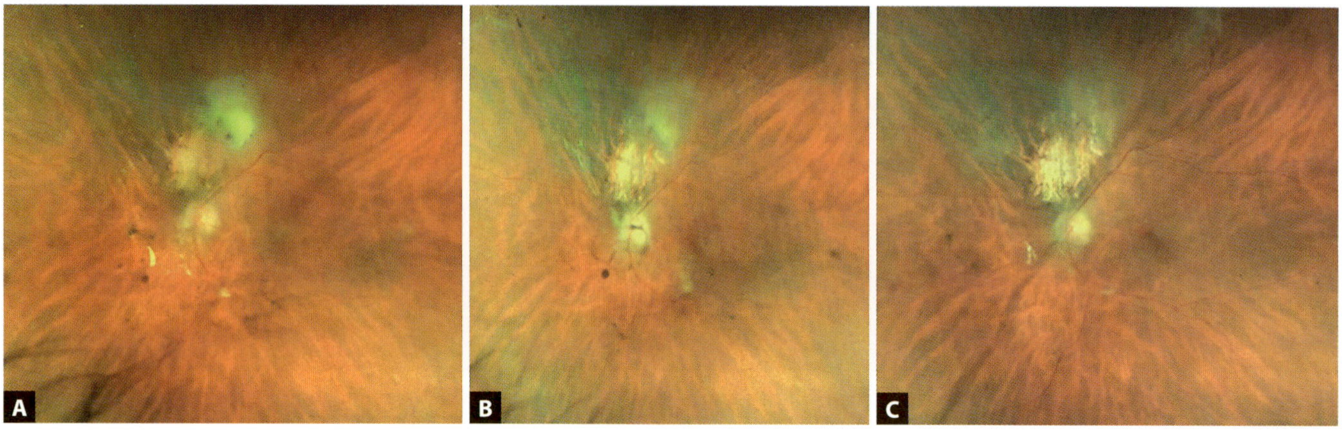

Figs. 13A to C: First recurrence. (A) 6 years after the first episode; (B) 3 weeks after the start of pyrimethamine, azithromycin, folinic acid, and prednisolone, achieving 20/30 in visual acuity and a reduction of the inflammatory activity of the lesion; (C) 7-week follow-up with treatment achieving 20/20 and a complete resolution.
Source: Presented by Laura Camila Ramirez-Marquez in the International Uveitis Study Group (IUSG) grand rounds.[1]

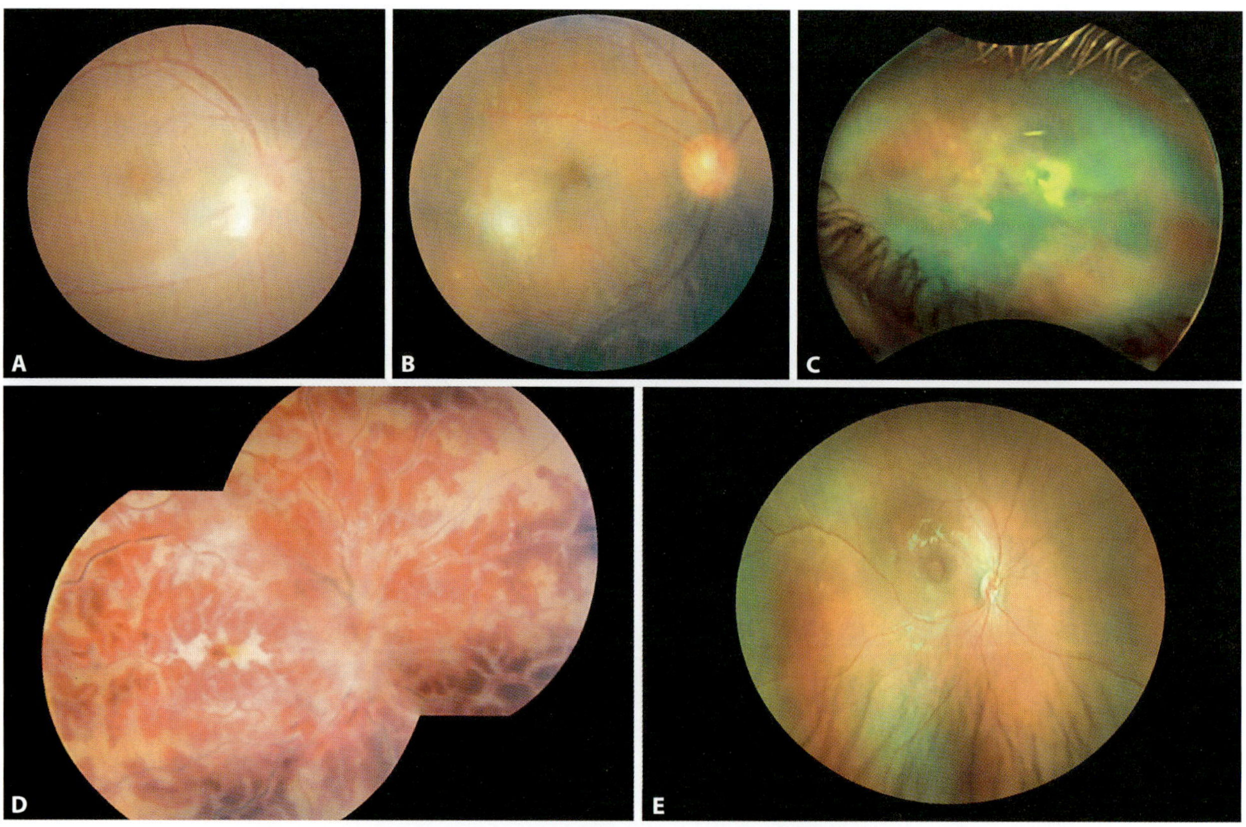

Figs. 14A to E: Atypical forms of ocular toxoplasmosis. (A) Toxoplasmic neuroretinitis; (B) Punctate "outer" retinal toxoplasmosis; (C) Multifocal extensive necrotizing retinochoroiditis; (D) Frosted branch angiitis; (E) Multifocal punctate.
Source: Presented by Daniel Vítor Vasconcelos-Santos in the International Uveitis Study Group (IUSG) grand rounds.[1]

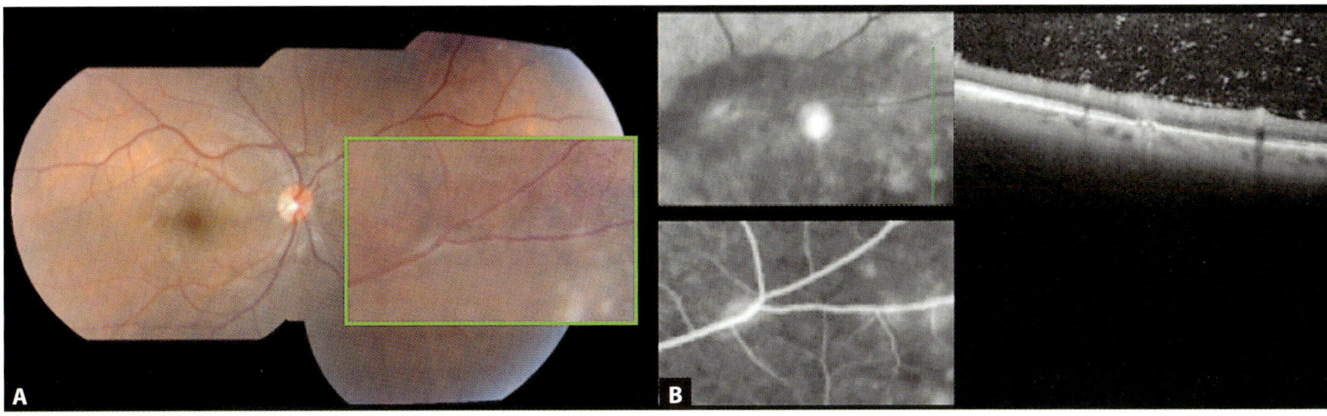

Figs. 15A and B: Multimodal imaging of multifocal punctate retinitis. Multifocal punctate retinitis is characterized by (A) Small white infiltrates in the fundus typically observed in early congenital toxoplasmosis but can also occur in recent postnatally acquired toxoplasmosis; (B) These lesions can be observed more clearly in the optical coherence tomography (OCT) as hyperreflective dots.
Source: Presented by Daniel Vítor Vasconcelos-Santos in the International Uveitis Study Group (IUSG) grand rounds.[1]

- *Intraocular inflammation (anterior uveitis, retinal vasculitis, vitritis) without retinochoroiditis*: These cases are extremely rare and may be attributed to periphery lesions that cannot be easily observed.

It is important to be aware of these atypical forms, especially in patients with predisposing conditions such as immunosuppressive states (HIV, chemotherapy, cancer), careless use of steroids (oral, intravenous, intramuscular, intravitreal), or recent seroconversion for toxoplasmosis.

Multimodal imaging and molecular testing are beneficial in these atypical cases. Classical therapy should be administered in more severe cases. Additionally, secondary prophylaxis should be considered more frequently in atypical cases.

OCULAR TOXOPLASMOSIS CASE WITH TREATMENT CHALLENGES

Case Presentation

Personal Data

- Male
- 59 years old
- No systemic diseases are known
- Smoker

History of Present Illness

Progressive vision loss, redness, and pain in both eyes for a week, worse in the left eye.

Physical Examination

The patient presented with a visual acuity of 20/50 in the OD and 20/200 in the OS, with high IOP, ciliary injection, anterior chamber cells, and vitreous cells in OU. In fundoscopy, intense vasculitis and focal exudative necrotizing retinitis are present in the OD, while in the OS, severe vitreous haze limits the visibility of the fundus **(Table 4, Figs. 16 and 17)**.

Workup

Fundus fluorescein angiography (FFA) **(Fig. 18)** and ocular ultrasound **(Fig. 19)** were performed to characterize the lesions.

Differential Diagnosis

In the case of bilateral acute hypertensive posterior uveitis, the following diagnoses were considered:

- *Infectious*: Viral retinitis/acute retinal necrosis, syphilis, tuberculosis, and toxoplasmosis
- *Noninfectious*: Sarcoidosis, Behçet's disease, antineutrophil cytoplasmic antibodies (ANCAs)-associated vasculitis
- *Masquerade syndrome*

Management

The IOP was successfully controlled with topical antiglaucomatous medications. During the etiological investigation, intravenous acyclovir was started empirically to treat presumed viral retinitis or acute retinal necrosis. Laboratory workup ruled out HIV, syphilis, and

TABLE 4: Physical examination of the patient having ocular toxoplasmosis case with treatment challenges.

OD	***Parameter***	***OS***
20/50	BCVA	20/200
25 mm Hg	IOP	36 mm Hg
Mild ciliary injection	Conjunctiva	Severe ciliary injection
Clear	Cornea	Corneal edema 2+
2+ anterior chamber cells and flare	Anterior chamber	3+ anterior chamber cells and flare
Trophic No posterior synechiae	Iris	Trophic No posterior synechiae
Vossius ring	Lens	Clear
Anterior vitreous cells 2+ and haze	Vitreous	Anterior vitreous cells 2+ and haze
Intense vasculitis (evident in fluorescein angiography) and focal exudative necrotizing retinitis in inferior quadrants	Fundus	Impossible–ocular ultrasound was performed

(BCVA: best-corrected visual acuity; IOP: intraocular pressure)

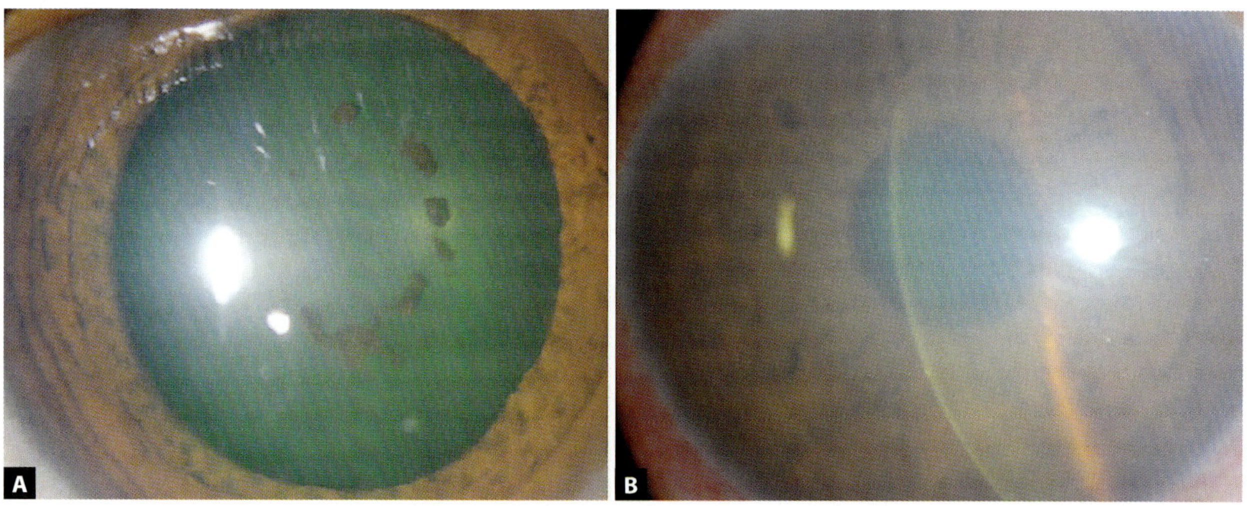

Figs. 16A and B: Slit-lamp examination. (A) Right eye with Vossius ring; (B) Left eye with 2+ corneal edema.
Source: Presented by Guilherme Macedo in the International Uveitis Study Group (IUSG) grand rounds.[1]

tuberculosis. Chest CT and rheumatological panel results were normal. The patient tested positive for IgG serology for toxoplasmosis and negative for IgM. Nevertheless, due to bilateral infection and partial improvement with antiviral therapy, oral prednisone at a dose of 1 mg/kg/day achieved a best-corrected visual acuity (BCVA) of 20/40 in the OD and 20/60 in the OS. After hospital discharge, the patient continued taking oral acyclovir at a maintenance dosage.

Evolution

After 1 month, the patient experienced a recurrence of symptoms in both eyes. Physical examination revealed granulomatous keratic precipitates in both eyes, increased exudation of the previous retinal lesion in the OD, adjacent hemorrhages, and two new retinochoroidal lesions. A large exudative necrotizing retinitis focus and vasculitis were observed in the OS **(Figs. 20 to 22)**. With these new findings, OT was considered the primary diagnosis; empirical anti-*T. gondii* therapy was initiated with SMX-TMP (800 mg + 160 mg) twice daily.

Over the subsequent month, the patient experienced significant weight loss and developed cervical lymphadenopathy. A comprehensive diagnostic workup revealed metastases in the cervical lymph nodes, bones, and liver, originating from an undifferentiated squamous

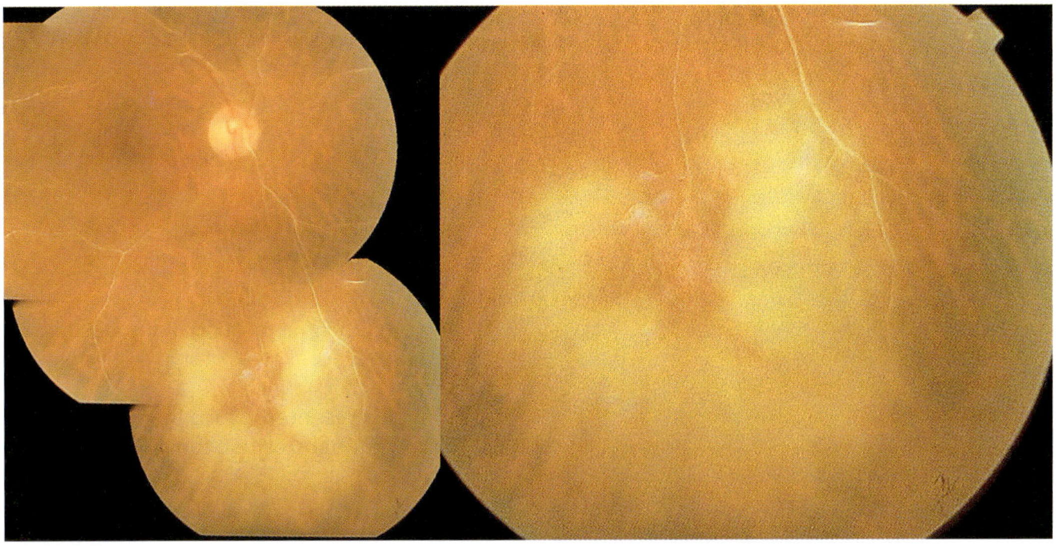

Fig. 17: Fundoscopy of the right eye. Focal exudative necrotizing retinitis in inferior quadrants with vascular sheathing in the four quadrants.
Source: Presented by Guilherme Macedo in the International Uveitis Study Group (IUSG) grand rounds.[1]

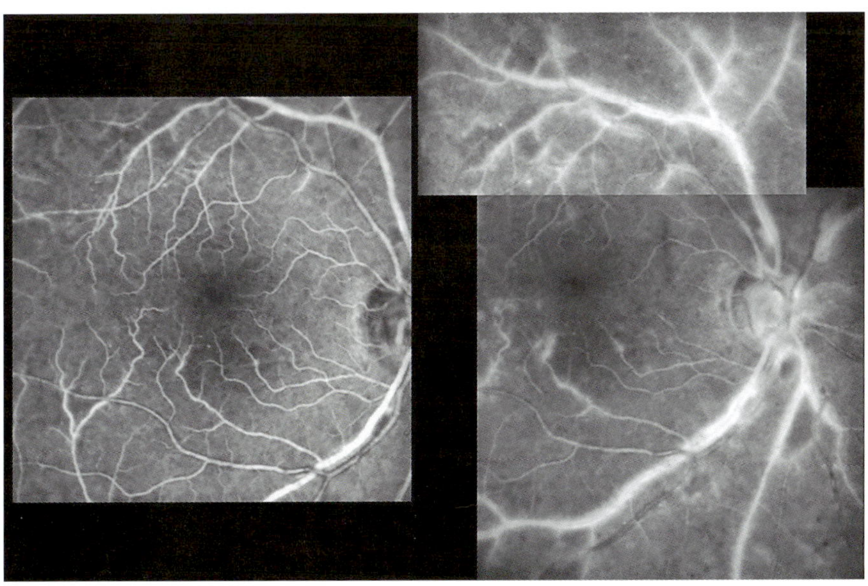

Fig. 18: Fundus fluorescein angiography of OD. Intense vasculitis is evident in fundus fluorescein angiography in the right eye.
Source: Presented by Guilherme Macedo in the International Uveitis Study Group (IUSG) grand rounds.[1]

cell carcinoma of unknown primary origin. He died 3 weeks later and donated his eyes for research purposes **(Figs. 23 and 24)**.

Discussion

The treatment of OT presents numerous challenges, including:

- *Diagnostic difficulties*: Establishing an accurate diagnosis can be challenging due to atypical presentations or difficulty in visualizing retinal details with significant media opacity. Additionally, the limited availability of molecular diagnostic techniques in many parts of the world remains a significant barrier. Relying on serological tests is not always ideal, as many of the population may be IgG positive without pathological significance.[41-44] PCR in intraocular fluids is helpful to confirm the diagnosis, coinfections, or differential diagnoses, mostly in atypical cases. However, a negative result could not rule out the diagnosis with 100% certainty.[23,29]

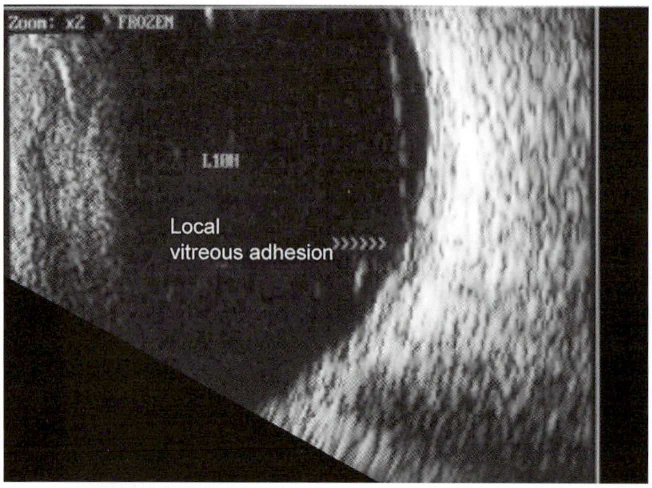

Fig.19: Ocular ultrasound of the OS. Inflammatory vitreous process, areas of atypical hyaloid adhesion, and attached retina.
Source: Presented by Guilherme Macedo in the International Uveitis Study Group (IUSG) grand rounds.[1]

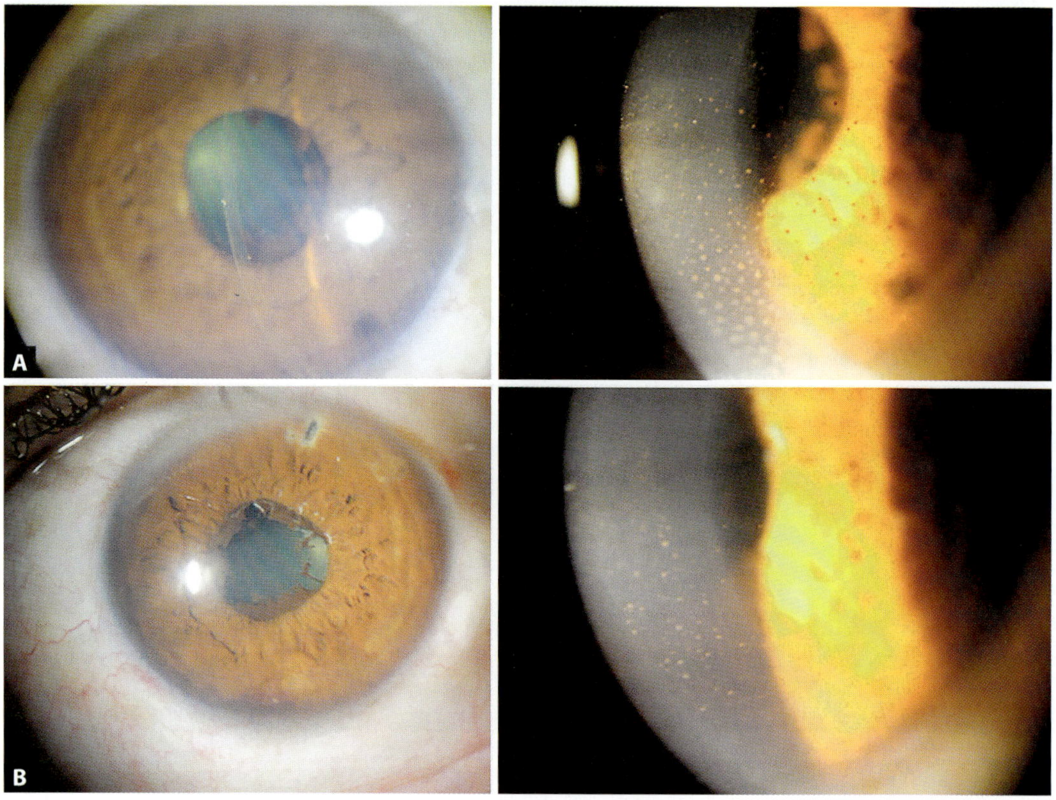

Figs. 20A and B: Slit-lamp examination during recurrence. (A) On slit-lamp examination, granulomatous keratic precipitates (KPs) were evident in the Arlt triangle, posterior synechiae, and pigment on the anterior capsule of the lens in the right eye; (B) Similar findings were observed in the left eye.
Source: Presented by Guilherme Macedo in the International Uveitis Study Group (IUSG) grand rounds.[1]

- *Medication-related obstacles*: The use of specific medications for OT treatment can be hindered by several factors, including drug allergies (common with sulfa drugs), serious side effects (such as bone marrow suppression caused by pyrimethamine), and teratogenic risks (associated with pyrimethamine and trimethoprim) in pregnant women during the first trimester.[45-48] Moreover, no treatment is available to target bradyzoites encysted in the retina.

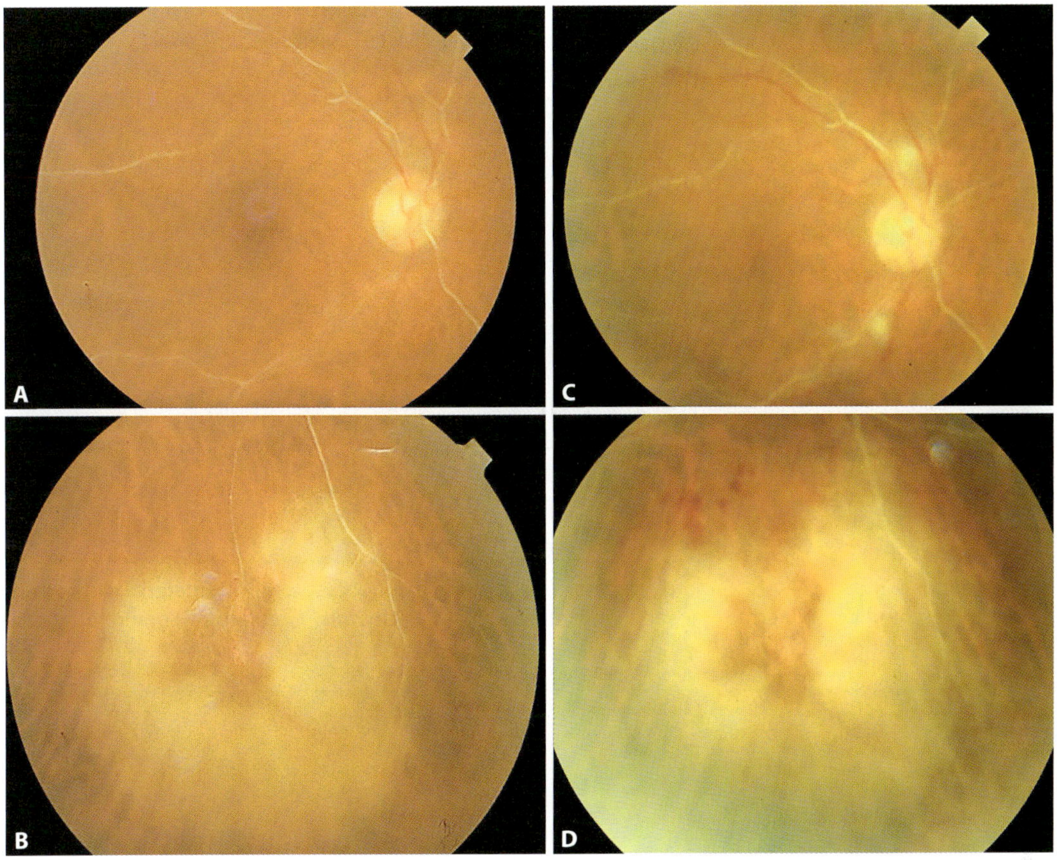

Figs. 21A to D: Comparison of fundus photos of the right eye at baseline and recurrence (1 month follow-up). (A and B) Baseline with one active retinochoroidal lesion at the inferior quadrant; (C and D) 1-month follow-up evidencing increased exudation of the previous retinal lesion, adjacent hemorrhages, and two new retinitis lesions. One is located near the optic disc and the other is in the inferotemporal arcade.
Source: Presented by Guilherme Macedo in the International Uveitis Study Group (IUSG) grand rounds.[1]

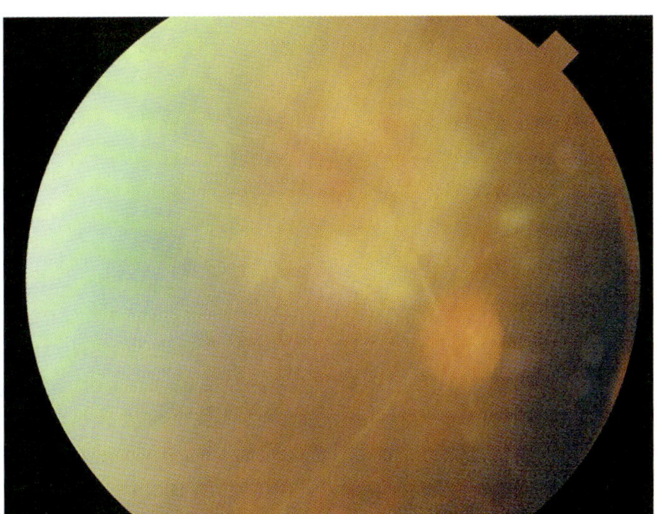

Fig. 22: Fundus exam of the OS at recurrence. Vitreous haze 2+ with an extensive yellowish-white lesion in the nasal superior arcade.
Source: Presented by Guilherme Macedo in the International Uveitis Study Group (IUSG) grand rounds.[1]

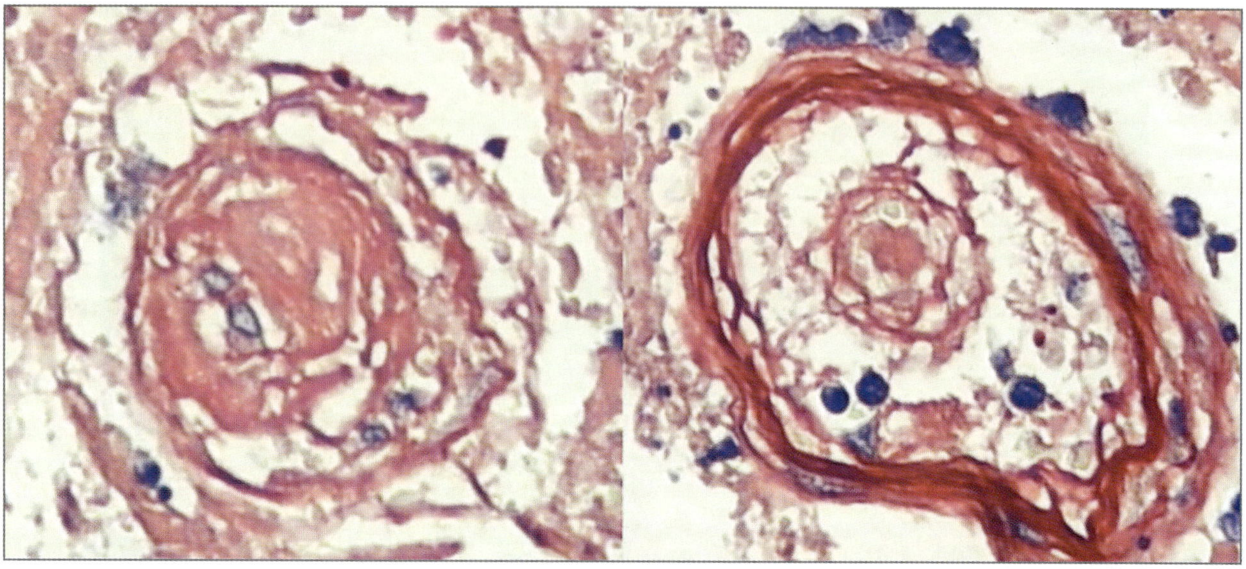

Fig. 23: Pathological findings of retinal vessels. Hematoxylin and eosin staining highlights thrombotic material within the vascular lumen.
Source: Presented by Guilherme Macedo in the International Uveitis Study Group (IUSG) grand rounds.[1]

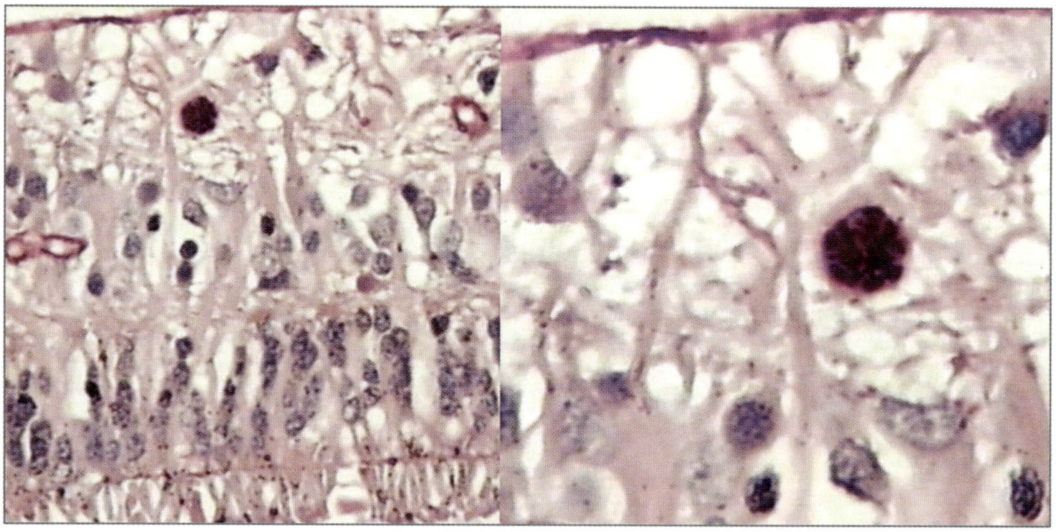

Fig. 24: Pathological findings or retinal tissue. Hematoxylin and eosin staining highlights the bradyzoite cysts of *Toxoplasma gondii* within the retinal layers.
Source: Presented by Guilherme Macedo in the International Uveitis Study Group (IUSG) grand rounds.[1]

- *Clinical and surgical complications*: Patients may develop a range of complications, such as choroidal neovascularization, retinal detachment, and macular holes, which can complicate treatment and recovery.[49,50] For proper management, obtaining an early diagnosis and initiating specific treatment promptly are important. No PCR analysis was available in the presented case, making the diagnostic conclusion more difficult.[51]

Herein, a case of initial misdiagnosis due to an atypical presentation (such as viral acute retinal necrosis) led to inappropriate treatment. Furthermore, another challenge in treating this patient was the comorbidities that led to a negative outcome—death of the patient. It is important to note the anatomopathological changes observed, which are consistent with what is found in the literature.[52-54]

PEARLS FROM THE EXPERTS ON FREQUENTLY ASKED QUESTIONS

Questions related to diagnosis

1. Should we conduct ocular PCR testing in pregnant patients before starting treatment?
Answer: PCR in intraocular fluids should be utilized only when there is uncertainty in the diagnosis of OT. In clinically typical cases, sending for IgG and IgM serology and an avidity test is sufficient.

2. Can IgM be positive more than once?
Answer: It is very unusual. However, this may be attributable to reinfection with another strain.

3. Is *Toxoplasma* serology recommended for all patients with uveitis and retinitis, or should it be limited to cases morphologically resembling toxoplasmosis?
Answer: Toxoplasma serology is warranted in cases of focal necrotizing retinochoroiditis. Serology is also ordered for atypical presentations, primarily for its negative predictive value.

4. What percentage of patients with acquired ocular toxoplasmosis also develop cerebral toxoplasmosis? Are there newer tests available for the rapid diagnosis of toxoplasmosis?
Answer: Cerebral involvement generally occurs in immunocompromised patients rather than in immunocompetent individuals. An immunochromatographic test for *Toxoplasma gondii*, developed by LDBIO Diagnostics, is a rapid diagnostic method used to detect anti-*Toxoplasma gondii* antibodies (IgG and/or IgM) in serum or plasma within a few hours.[55]

5. Can serology be a reliable diagnostic tool in cases of congenital toxoplasmosis or severely immunocompromised patients?
Answer: Yes; however, it can sometimes yield false-negative results.

6. When is it appropriate to conduct an IgG avidity test?
Answer: The avidity test should be requested when there is uncertainty about the time of infection acquisition to determine if prophylactic therapy is necessary.

7. Does transmission of toxoplasmosis through ingestion of oocysts result in more aggressive cases due to the parasite load?
Answer: Evidence suggests that oocysts are more likely to cause infection than bradyzoites. However, individuals are more commonly exposed to bradyzoites.

8. When should a GWC test be performed?
Answer: GWC is not routinely available in clinical practice. However, it has been reported that when performed combined with the PCR, its diagnostic performance increases more than that of the PCR alone. Notably, previous research indicates that disruption of the blood–aqueous barrier in severe cases may affect GWC results.

Questions related to treatment

1. When should corticosteroids be combined with anti-*Toxoplasma* treatment, and what is the protocol for their use, especially in cases involving the macula or optic disc?
Answer: Corticosteroids should be combined with anti-*Toxoplasma* therapy 48–72 hours after the start of antibiotic–antiparasitic therapy. It is recommended, especially when the macula or optic disc is involved.

2. What are the indications for initiating prophylactic anti-*Toxoplasma* therapy, and is there a specific population that meets the criteria for this treatment?
Answer: Prophylactic therapy is recommended to prevent recurrences in patients with vision-threatening lesions involving the macula or optic nerve, those with frequent recurrences (more than once every 2 years), first active acquired lesions, elderly patients with recent reactivation, or immunocompromised individuals.

3. How long is prophylactic treatment typically administered?
Answer: There is no definitive answer, but it is generally recommended to administer prophylactic treatment for 1 year and then re-evaluate the patient.

4. Should patients with typical chorioretinal scars for toxoplasmosis, negative IgM, and positive IgG serology be treated?
Answer: Inactive scars are generally not treated. However, secondary prophylaxis may be considered for frequently recurring lesions. IgG levels are not indicative of active infection. If the lesion is typical and active, treatment should be initiated regardless of IgG serology indicating a chronic infection.

5. What is the drug of choice for prophylaxis in individuals allergic to sulfa drugs?
Answer: For patients allergic to sulfa drugs, pyrimethamine (administered three times a week) with folinic acid supplementation or azithromycin (administered twice weekly) can be used. Although there are no published data on clindamycin, it could also be used as prophylactic

therapy (300 mg every 12 hours, three times weekly); nevertheless, further studies are necessary to confirm this.

6. What should be done if a patient does not respond to treatment after 6–8 weeks?

Answer: If there is no response to classical therapy, switching to an alternative therapy or adjusting the doses may be necessary. Supplementation with intravitreal therapy might also be warranted.

7. In atypical cases of OT, should both antiviral and anti-*Toxoplasma* treatments be initiated?

Answer: Combining antiviral therapy with anti-*Toxoplasma* treatment is recommended in cases with large or multiple lesions suggestive of herpes viral disease. The duration of symptoms can also provide a clue; rapid progression typically indicates herpes virus, whereas prolonged symptoms suggest toxoplasmosis.

8. Would you initiate treatment in a recurrent ocular toxoplasmosis case with underlying poor vision due to an old macular scar (counting finger vision)?

a. *Answer:* Yes, treatment would be initiated to prevent additional complications.

9. Is there any information on microbiome changes related to long-term antibiotic prophylaxis?

a. *Answer:* There is no conclusive information on microbiome changes related to long-term antibiotic prophylaxis. This remains an important area for future research.

10. What would you recommend for patients undergoing immunosuppressive therapy for systemic lymphoma intolerant to standard toxoplasmosis treatments such as pyrimethamine or clindamycin?

a. *Answer:* In such cases, azithromycin could be used. Intravitreal therapy may be considered as an alternative, although it is less effective than systemic therapy.

FINAL WRAP-UP

In conclusion, OT is a common cause of infectious posterior uveitis. The most important risk factors include consuming undercooked meat, poorly washed vegetables, or contaminated water. Its typical presentation consists of retinochoroidal scars (in an inactive state) with satellite lesions during recurrences. However, other atypical presentations should be considered to avoid being overlooked. The typical therapy includes pyrimethamine + sulfadiazine + folinic acid or TMP-SMX, accompanied by corticosteroids (in cases with severe vitritis or lesions with vision-threatening locations). Alternative therapies, such as oral azithromycin or clindamycin, can be used. clindamycin + dexamethasone injection is also helpful as an adjuvant therapy. Classical therapy is preferred for more severe cases. Moreover, prophylactic therapy with TMP-SMX helps prevent future recurrences.

REFERENCES

1. International Uveitis Study Group (IUSG). Uveitis grand rounds 06: ocular toxoplasmosis. 2024. [online] Available from https://youtu.be/5N4ABEjyEhY?si=7jZPywoEuCEF-24l. [Last accessed March, 2025]
2. Holland GN. Ocular toxoplasmosis: a global reassessment. Am J Ophthal. 2003;136(6):973-88.
3. Petersen E, Kijlstra A, Stanford M. Epidemiology of ocular toxoplasmosis. Ocul Immunol Inflamm. 2012;20(2):68-75.
4. de-la-Torre A, Mejía-Salgado G, Cifuentes-González C, Rojas-Carabali W, Cuevas M, García S, et al. Epidemiology, clinical features, and classification of 3,404 patients with uveitis: Colombian uveitis multicenter study (COL-UVEA). Graefes Arch Clin Exp Ophthalmol. 2024;262(8):2601-5.
5. Cifuentes-González C, Rojas-Carabali W, Mejia-Salgado G, Pineda-Sierra JS, Muñoz-Vargas PT, Boada-Robayo L, et al. Colombian ocular inflammatory diseases epidemiology study (COIDES): prevalence, incidence and sociodemographic characterisation of scleritis in Colombia, 2015–2020. BMJ Open Ophthalmol. 2022;7(1):e001096.
6. Kijlstra A, Petersen E. Epidemiology, pathophysiology, and the future of ocular toxoplasmosis. Ocul Immunol Inflamm. 2014;22(2):138-47.
7. Furtado JM, Winthrop KL, Butler NJ, Smith JR. Ocular toxoplasmosis I: parasitology, epidemiology and public health. Clin Exper Ophthalmol. 2013;41(1):82-94.
8. Flatt A, Shetty N. Seroprevalence and risk factors for toxoplasmosis among antenatal women in London: a re-examination of risk in an ethnically diverse population. Eur J Public Health. 2013;23(4):648-52.
9. Zamora-Vélez A, Triviño J, Cuadrado-Ríos S, Lora-Suarez F, Enrique Gómez-Marín J. Detection and genotypes of *Toxoplasma gondii* DNA in feces of domestic cats in Colombia. Parasite. 2020;27:25.
10. Dawson AC, Ashander LM, Appukuttan B, Woodman RJ, Dubey JP, Whiley H, et al. Lamb as a potential source of *Toxoplasma gondii* infection for Australians. Aust N Z J Public Health. 2020;44(1):49-52.
11. Medina Hernández JD, Osorio Delgado LA, Zabala Gonzalez D, De Almeida Vitor RW, Gómez JE, Carranza JC, et al. Molecular detection of *Toxoplasma gondii* in meat for human consumption in Ibague, Colombia. Biomedica. 2022;42(1):136-46.
12. Shapiro K, Bahia-Oliveira L, Dixon B, Dumètre A, De Wit LA, VanWormer E, et al. Environmental transmission of

Toxoplasma gondii: oocysts in water, soil, and food. Food Waterborne Parasitol. 2019;15:e00049.
13. Rosado-García FM, Guerrero-Flórez M, Karanis G, Hinojosa MDC, Karanis P. Water-borne protozoa parasites: the Latin American perspective. Int JHygEnviron Health. 2017;220(5):783-98.
14. Krueger WS, Hilborn ED, Converse RR, Wade TJ. Drinking water source and human *Toxoplasma gondii* infection in the United States: a cross-sectional analysis of NHANES data. BMC Public Health. 2014;14(1):711.
15. Yogeswaran K, Furtado JM, Bodaghi B, Matthews JM, International Ocular Toxoplasmosis Study Group, Smith JR. Current practice in the management of ocular toxoplasmosis. Br J Ophthalmol. 2023;107(7):973-9.
16. Vedula SS, Nguyen QD. Corticosteroids for ocular toxoplasmosis. In: The Cochrane Collaboration (Ed). Cochrane Database of Systematic Reviews. Chichester, UK: John Wiley & Sons Ltd; 2008.
17. Holland GN. Ocular toxoplasmosis: a global reassessment. Part II: disease manifestations and management. Am J Ophthalmol. 2004;137(1):1-17.
18. Goh EJH, Putera I, La Distia Nora R, Mahendradas P, Biswas J, Chee SP, et al. Ocular toxoplasmosis. Ocul Immunol Inflamm. 2023;31(7):1342-61.
19. de-la-Torre A, López-Castillo CA, Gómez-Marín JE. Incidence and clinical characteristics in a Colombian cohort of ocular toxoplasmosis. Eye. 2009;23(5):1090-3.
20. Holland GN, Crespi CM, Ten Dam-van Loon N, Charonis AC, Yu F, Bosch-Driessen LH, et al. Analysis of recurrence patterns associated with toxoplasmic retinochoroiditis. Am J Ophthalmol. 2008;145(6):1007-13.
21. de-la-Torre A, Rios-Cadavid AC, Cardozo-Garcia CM, Gomez-Marin JE. Frequency and factors associated with recurrences of ocular toxoplasmosis in a referral centre in Colombia. Br J Ophthalmol. 2009;93(8):1001-4.
22. Pfaff AW, de-la-Torre A, Rochet E, Brunet J, Sabou M, Sauer A, et al. New clinical and experimental insights into Old World and neotropical ocular toxoplasmosis. Int J Parasitol. 2014;44(2):99-107.
23. de-la-Torre A, Valdés-Camacho J, De Mesa CL, Uauy-Nazal A, Zuluaga JD, Ramírez-Páez LM, et al. Coinfections and differential diagnosis in immunocompetent patients with uveitis of infectious origin. BMC Infect Dis. 2019;19(1):91.
24. Oliver GF, Ferreira LB, Vieira BR, Arruda S, Araújo M, Carr JM, et al. Posterior segment findings by spectral-domain optical coherence tomography and clinical associations in active toxoplasmic retinochoroiditis. Sci Rep. 2022;12(1):1156.
25. Pichi F, Curi ALL, Vasconcelos-Santos DV, Marchese A, Cicinelli MV, Miserocchi E, et al. Optical coherence tomography findings in infectious posterior uveitis. Ocul Immunol Inflamm. 2022;30(3):652-63.
26. Gomez-Marin JE, de-la-Torre A. (2020). Chapter 5—Ocular disease due to Toxoplasma gondii. [online] Available from https://linkinghub.elsevier.com/retrieve/pii/B9780128150412000050. [Last accessed February, 2025].
27. Talabani H, Asseraf M, Yera H, Delair E, Ancelle T, Thulliez P, et al. Contributions of immunoblotting, real-time PCR, and the Goldmann–Witmer coefficient to diagnosis of atypical toxoplasmic retinochoroiditis. J Clin Microbiol. 2009;47(7):2131-5.
28. Sugita S, Ogawa M, Inoue S, Shimizu N, Mochizuki M. Diagnosis of ocular toxoplasmosis by two polymerase chain reaction (PCR) examinations: qualitative multiplex and quantitative real-time. Jpn J Ophthalmol. 2011;55(5):495-501.
29. Taravati P, Lam D, van Gelder RN. Role of molecular diagnostics in ocular microbiology. Curr Ophthalmol Rep. 2013;1(4):181-9.
30. Cunningham ET, Smit DP, Zierhut M. Imaging ocular toxoplasmosis. Ocul Immunol Inflamm. 2022;30(3):525-6.
31. Feliciano-Alfonso JE, Muñoz-Ortiz J, Marín-Noriega MA, Vargas-Villanueva A, Triviño-Blanco L, Carvajal-Saiz N, et al. Safety and efficacy of different antibiotic regimens in patients with ocular toxoplasmosis: systematic review and meta-analysis. Syst Rev. 2021;10(1):206.
32. Arruda S, Vieira BR, Garcia DM, Araújo M, Simões M, Moreto R, et al. Clinical manifestations and visual outcomes associated with ocular toxoplasmosis in a Brazilian population. Sci Rep. 2021;11(1):3137.
33. Soheilian M, Ramezani A, Azimzadeh A, Sadoughi MM, Dehghan MH, Shahghadami R, et al. Randomized trial of intravitreal clindamycin and dexamethasone versus pyrimethamine, sulfadiazine, and prednisolone in treatment of ocular toxoplasmosis. Ophthalmology. 2011;118(1):134-41.
34. de-la-Torre A, Stanford M, Curi A, Jaffe GJ, Gomez-Marin JE. Therapy for ocular toxoplasmosis. Ocul Immunol Inflamm. 2011;19(5):314-20.
35. Soheilian M, Sadoughi MM, Ghajarnia M, Dehghan MH, Yazdani S, Behboudi H, et al. Prospective randomized trial of trimethoprim/sulfamethoxazole versus pyrimethamine and sulfadiazine in the treatment of ocular toxoplasmosis. Ophthalmology. 2005;112(11):1876-82.
36. Mayo Clinic. (2025). Sulfamethoxazole and trimethoprim (oral route). [online] Available from https://www.mayoclinic.org/drugs-supplements/sulfamethoxazole-and-trimethoprim-oral-route/description/drg-20071899. [Last accessed February, 2025].
37. Lasave AF, Díaz-Llopis M, Muccioli C, Belfort R, Arevalo JF. Intravitreal clindamycin and dexamethasone for zone 1 toxoplasmic retinochoroiditis at twenty-four months. Ophthalmology. 2010;117(9):1831-8.
38. Verma L, Thulasidas M, Gupta A. Intravitreal clindamycin as first-line therapy for toxoplasmic retinochoroiditis: a case series. Clin Ophthalmol. 2020;14:4279-85.
39. Silveira C, Belfort R, Muccioli C, Holland GN, Victora CG, Horta BL, et al. The effect of long-term intermittent

trimethoprim/sulfamethoxazole treatment on recurrences of toxoplasmic retinochoroiditis. Am J Ophthalmol. 2002;134(1):41-6.

40. Glasner PD, Silveira C, Kruszon-Moran D, Martins MC, Burnier M, Silveira S, et al. An unusually high prevalence of ocular toxoplasmosis in Southern Brazil. Am J Ophthalmol. 1992;114(2):136-44.
41. Crosson JN, Kuthyar S, Shantha JG, Debiec MR, Laird PW, Hwang CS, et al. Toxoplasmosis chorioretinitis mimicking acute retinal necrosis associated with local corticosteroid. Int J Retin Vitr. 2020;6(1):21.
42. Fine HF, Burke SP, Albini TA. Toxoplasmosis retinitis masquerading as acute retinal necrosis. Ophthalmic Surg Lasers Imaging Retina. 2016;47(10):895-9.
43. Moshfeghi D, Dodds EM, Couto CA, Santos CI, Nicholson DH, Lowder CY, et al. Diagnostic approaches to severe, atypical toxoplasmosis mimicking acute retinal necrosis. Ophthalmology. 2004;111(4):716-25.
44. Balansard B. Necrotising retinopathies simulating acute retinal necrosis syndrome. Br J Ophthalmol. 2005;89(1):96-101.
45. Khan DA, Knowles SR, Shear NH. Sulfonamide hypersensitivity: fact and fiction. J Allergy Clin Immunol Pract. 2019;7(7):2116-23.
46. Dibbern DA, Montanaro A. Allergies to sulfonamide antibiotics and sulfur-containing drugs. Ann Allergy Asthma Immunol. 2008;100(2):91-101.
47. Daniel D, Bacchi S, Casson R, Chan W. Sulfonamides in ophthalmology: adverse reactions: Evidence-based use of sulfa drugs in ophthalmology. Int Ophthalmol. 2024;44(1):214.
48. Ben-Harari RR, Goodwin E, Casoy J. Adverse event profile of pyrimethamine-based therapy in toxoplasmosis: a systematic review. Drugs R D. 2017;17(4):523-44.
49. Goh EJ, Putera I, La Distia Nora R, Mahendradas P, Biswas J, Chee SP, et al. Ocular toxoplasmosis. Ocul Immunol Inflamm. 2023;31(7):1342-61.
50. Amaral DC, Lane M, Aguiar EH, Marques GN, Cavassani LV, Rodrigues MP, et al. Surgical management of retinal detachment and macular holes secondary to ocular toxoplasmosis: a systematic review and meta-analysis. Int J Retina Vitreous. 2024;10(1):23.
51. Kalogeropoulos D, Sakkas H, Mohammed B, Vartholomatos G, Malamos K, Sreekantam S, et al. Ocular toxoplasmosis: a review of the current diagnostic and therapeutic approaches. Int Ophthalmol. 2022;42(1):295-321.
52. Shima AL, Johnson LK, Skerratt LF, Zeiss C. Ocular anatomy and pathology in lumholtz's tree-kangaroo (dendrolagus lumholtzi). J Zoo Wildl Med. 2021;51(4):868-78.
53. Roberts F, Mets MB, Ferguson DJ, O'Grady R, O'Grady C, Thulliez P, et al. Histopathological features of ocular toxoplasmosis in the fetus and infant. Arch Ophthalmol. 2001;119(1):51-8.
54. Butler NJ, Furtado JM, Winthrop KL, Smith JR. Ocular toxoplasmosis II: clinical features, pathology and management. Clin Exp Ophthalmol. 2013;41(1):95-108.
55. Zhou Y, Leahy K, Grose A, Lykins J, Siddiqui M, Leong N, et al. Novel paradigm enables accurate monthly gestational screening to prevent congenital toxoplasmosis and more. PLoS Negl Trop Dis. 2024;18(5):e0011335.

CHAPTER 7

Ocular Tuberculosis

Vishali Gupta, Atul Arora, Ahana Sen, Sudharshan S, Luca Cimino, Pietro Gentile, Talluri Ronnie Abhishek, Soumyava Basu, Germán Mejía-Salgado, Meghan Berkenstock, Reema Bansal, John H Kempen, Alejandra de-la-Torre

INTRODUCTION

Ocular tuberculosis (OTB) is estimated to account for approximately 4.0% of all uveitis cases, making it one of the leading causes of infectious uveitis.[1] In endemic countries such as India and Indonesia, 22.9–48.0% of all infectious uveitis cases may be due to tuberculosis (TB).[1-3] OTB has protean manifestations and can affect nearly every part of the eye, with varied manifestations representing both infective and immune-mediated phenotypes.[1-3] This chapter aims to provide a few practical, day-to-day tips for managing OTB.

PRACTICAL TIPS FOR MANAGING A PATIENT WITH OCULAR TUBERCULOSIS

Pathogenesis

Ocular TB is a form of extrapulmonary disease where the eye gets affected due to the hematogenous spread of *Mycobacterium tuberculosis* (MTB) from the lungs. Following inhalation, the MTB forms a primary infectious focus in the lungs; this may be contained by host immunity, and, thus, the patient does not develop pulmonary TB. The MTB-laden macrophages enter the eye through a hematogenous route, and highly vascularized choroid may be the first available entry spot where they reside.[4,5] Retinal pigment epithelium (RPE) cells have toll-like receptors that recognize pathogen-associated molecular patterns. Recognition of pathogens by these receptors elicits an immune response, including cytokine release.[6] The resultant disease is, thus, believed to be an immunological response to MTB antigens, and the typical example of this is serpiginous-like choroiditis (SLC).[7] While the MTB is lodged in the choroid and/or RPE, the body tries to contain the infection by monocytic infiltration, resulting in granuloma formation.[7] Even a single organism in the RPE layer can incite granuloma formation. Understanding this aspect is important as it highlights the interplay of treatment comprising systemic steroids, antituberculosis therapy (ATT), and sometimes immunosuppression.

In some cases, the granulomas become very large and form a tuberculoma. It has been shown that vitreous humor from eyes with these granulomas has an elevated level of vascular endothelial growth factor (VEGF), which is required for the growth of the granulomas.[7] Thus, anti-VEGF therapy has an important role to play as an adjunct host-directed therapy in these eyes.

While this understanding about the pathogenesis explains posterior segment inflammation, the development of granulomatous anterior uveitis without posterior segment involvement cannot be described yet.

Clinical Features[8,9]

Anterior Uveitis

Tuberculosis can cause granulomatous uveitis, which may be characterized by the presence of anterior segment inflammation with broad-based synechiae, mutton-fat keratic precipitates, pupillary border iris nodules (Koeppe nodules), or iris stromal nodules (Busacca nodules) **(Figs. 1A to C)**.

Intermediate Uveitis

Tuberculosis may cause intermediate uveitis characterized by vitritis, large snowballs in the vitreous cavity, and diffuse vascular leak on fluorescein angiography **(Fig. 2)**. Pars plana snowbanking, a classic feature of pars planitis, is not usually seen in patients with TB-induced intermediate uveitis.

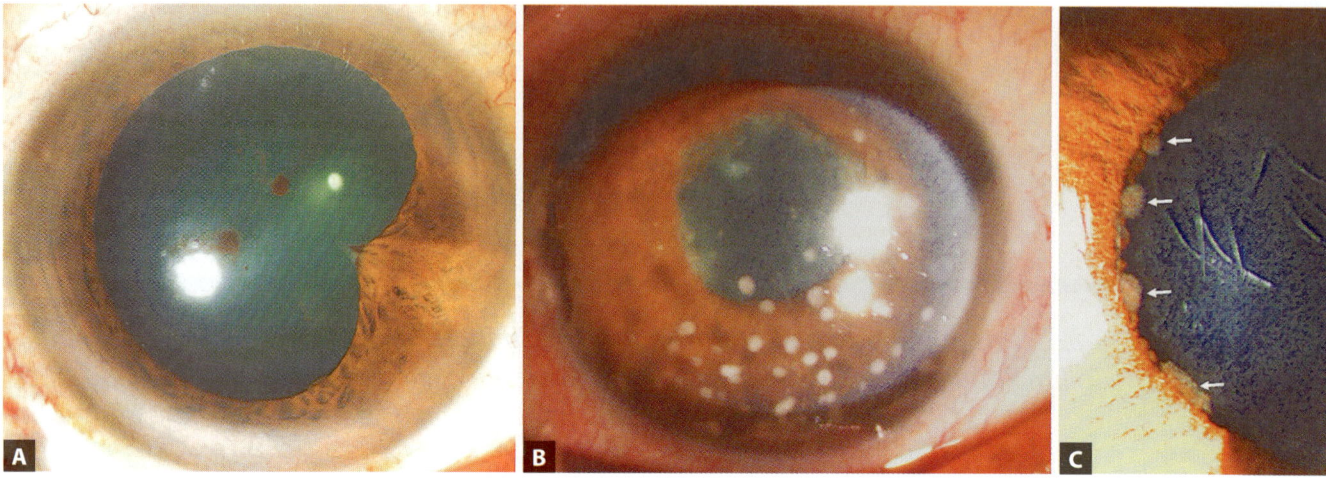

Figs. 1A to C: Clinical features of tubercular anterior uveitis. Anterior segment photograph of a patient with tubercular anterior uveitis showing (A) broad-based posterior synechiae, (B) mutton-fat keratic precipitates, and (C) Koeppe nodules (white arrows).
Courtesy (Fig. 1B): Reema Bansal, PGIMER, Chandigarh, India.
Source: Presented by Vishali Gupta in the International Uveitis Study Group (IUSG) grand rounds.[10]

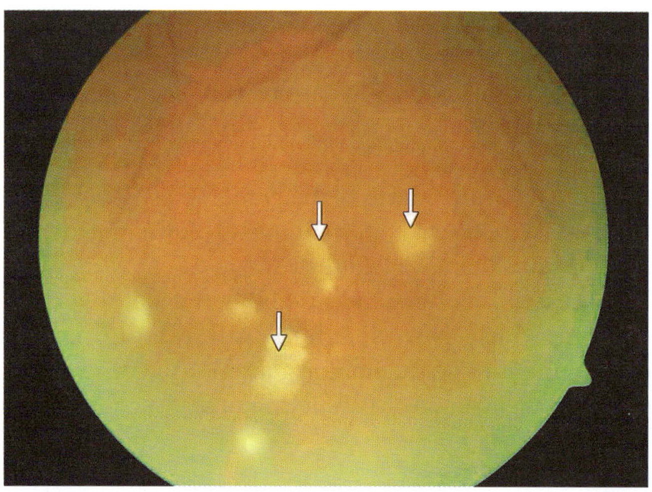

Fig. 2: Clinical features of tubercular anterior uveitis. Fundus photography evidencing moderate vitritis and large snowballs (white arrows).
Source: Presented by Vishali Gupta in the International Uveitis Study Group (IUSG) grand rounds.[10]

Posterior Uveitis

Posterior uveitis is the most common presentation of OTB, possibly because MTB first reaches the choroid through a hematogenous route. The common posterior segment manifestations include choroidal tubercle/tuberculoma **(Figs. 3A to D)**, SLC, or multifocal choroiditis. Outer retinal involvement is commonly seen on optical coherence tomography (OCT). However, TB usually does not present as isolated retinitis, and there are only few isolated reports of TB retinitis.

Retinal vasculitis is a common presentation of TB, and it is characterized by occlusive periphlebitis that may be associated with paravenous choroiditis (mostly healed) patches. Many of these cases may develop neovascularization (mainly at the junction between the perfused and nonperfused retina) **(Figs. 4A and B)**, which results in recurrent vitreous hemorrhages. In the past, these patients were erroneously termed "Eales' disease." However, Eales', by definition, is an idiopathic disease; thus, these patients should be labeled as TB vasculitis.

Serpiginous-like choroiditis: the first report of TB as an etiology for SLC appeared in 2003, in which the authors showed a significant reduction in the number of recurrences following the addition of ATT.[11] This publication highlighted the fact that choroidal TB may present as multifocal progressive or diffuse choroiditis resembling serpiginous choroiditis (SC). Recognition of this phenotype is important to investigate and add ATT in a timely manner, as these eyes show a good response to systemic ATT. SLC may begin as multifocal lesions resembling acute posterior multifocal placoid pigment epitheliopathy (APMPPE) that may progress and coalesce to look like SC with an active edge. The presence of the anterior segment or vitreous inflammation (primarily mild), snowballs, vasculitis, unilaterality, and multifocality indicate the disease as TB-SLC rather than SC. TB choroiditis can initially present as multifocal choroiditis or focal choroiditis that

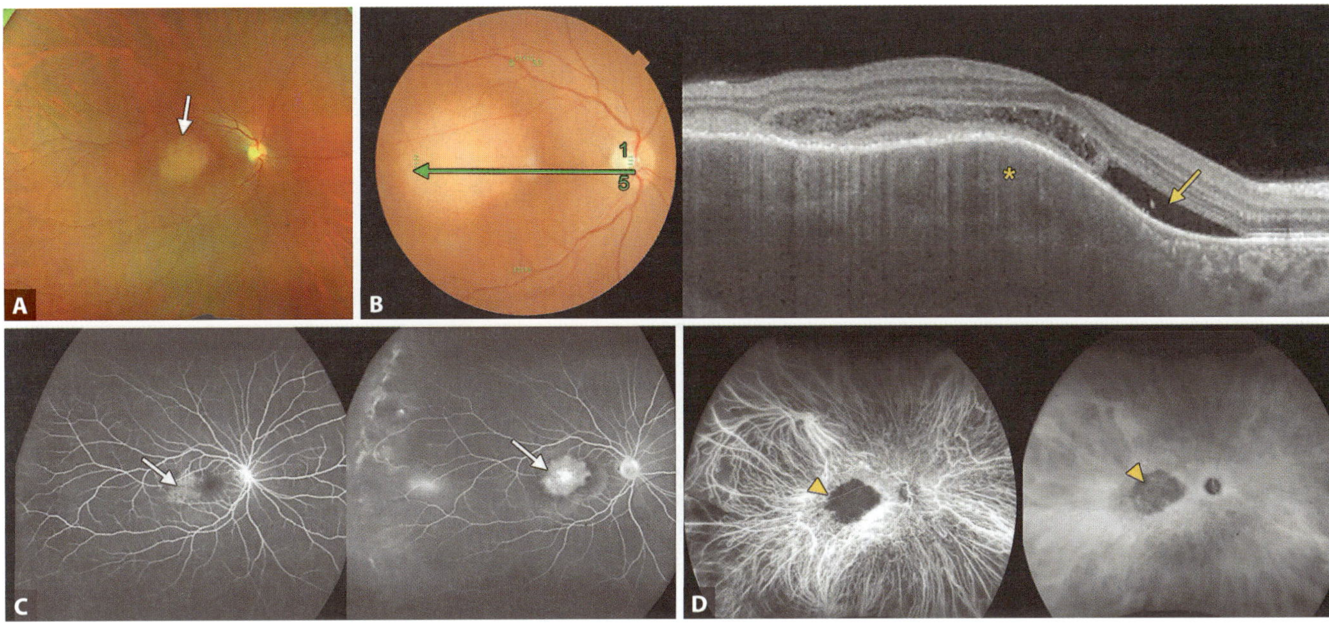

Figs. 3A to D: Choroidal tuberculoma. (A) Ultrawide-field fundus photograph (Optos California ultrawide-field imaging 200 DTx icg, Scotland, United Kingdom) of a patient with tubercular choroidal granuloma (white arrow); (B) Swept-source optical coherence tomography (SS-OCT) line scan passing through the lesion shows choroidal granuloma (asterisk) with overlying subretinal fluid (yellow arrow); (C) Ultrawide-field fundus fluorescein angiography (Optos California ultrawide-field imaging 200 DTx icg, Scotland, United Kingdom) shows a hypofluorescent lesion in the early phase (left), with the surface becoming progressively hyperfluorescent in later phases of angiogram (right); (D) The lesion appeared hypofluorescent in both early and late phases of indocyanine green angiography.
Source: Presented by Vishali Gupta in the International Uveitis Study Group (IUSG) grand rounds.[10]

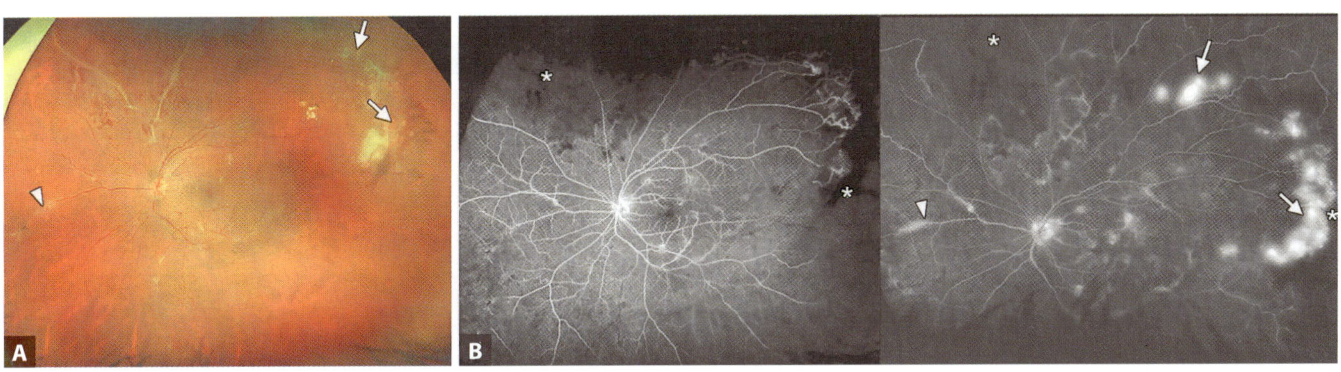

Figs. 4A and B: Tuberculosis-associated retinal vasculitis. (A) Ultrawide-field fundus photograph (Optos California ultrawide-field imaging 200 DTx icg, Scotland, United Kingdom) of a patient with ocular tuberculosis shows perivascular retinal infiltrates (periphlebitis) (white arrowhead) and neovascularization at the junction of the perfused and nonperfused retina (white arrows); (B) Corresponding fluorescein angiography shows (left) occlusive vasculitis resulting in peripheral capillary nonperfusion areas (asterisk) and (right) active leakage in later phases of the angiogram (white arrows).
Source: Presented by Vishali Gupta in the International Uveitis Study Group (IUSG) grand rounds.[10]

may resemble APMPPE and progress to develop into SLC **(Figs. 5A to D)**. Sometimes, TB SLC may present as placoid lesion, mostly seen in the posterior pole. These placoid lesions are yellowish white, plaque-like that progress along the edge in a serpentine fashion. The edge of these lesions may be more yellow and even appear to have a volume **(Figs. 6A and B)**.

Panuveitis

Tuberculosis may present as panuveitis that may be difficult to treat and has a poor prognosis. Patients with panuveitis who have received immunosuppressive therapy and corticosteroids over a long duration without any ATT have the worst prognosis.

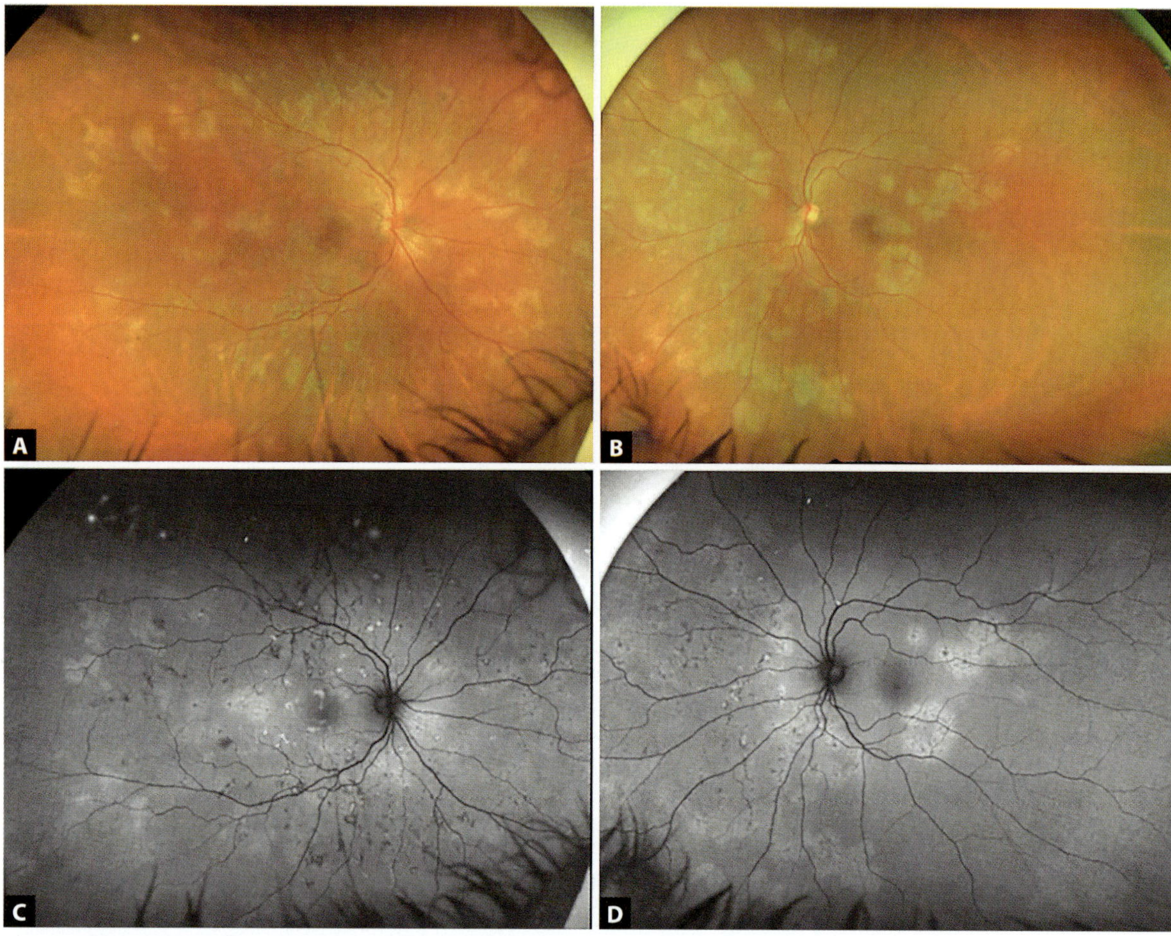

Figs. 5A to D: Serpiginous-like choroiditis (SLC). (A and B) Ultrawide-field fundus photograph (Optos California ultrawide-field imaging 200 DTx icg, Scotland, United Kingdom) showing active multifocal SLC lesions; (C and D) Corresponding fundus autofluorescence (FAF) shows stippled hyperautofluorescent corresponding to the active lesions.
Source: Presented by Vishali Gupta in the International Uveitis Study Group (IUSG) grand rounds.[11]

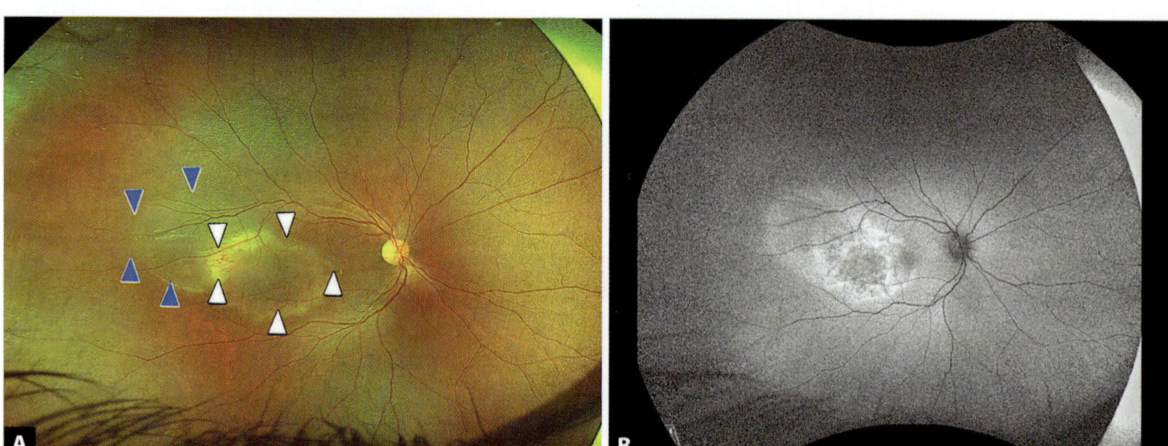

Figs. 6A and B: (A) Fundus photograph R/E of a 39-year-man with placoid lesion of TB SLC. White arrowheads demarcate the lesion that has a intense yellow temporal border associated with ring of exudative fluid (blue arrowheads); (B) Hyper-autofluorescence of active edges.
Source: Presented by Vishali Gupta in the International Uveitis Study Group (IUSG) grand rounds.[10]

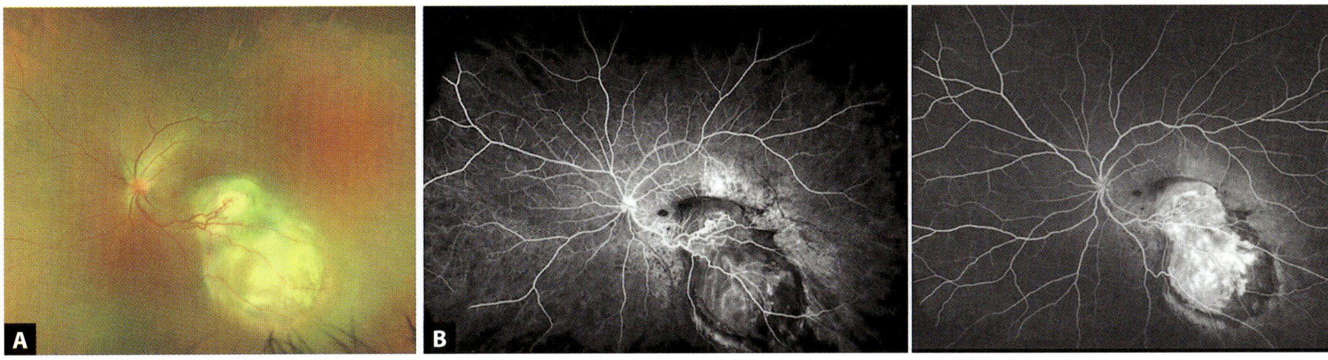

Figs. 7A and B: Retinal angiomatous proliferation. (A) Ultrawide-field fundus photograph (Optos California ultrawide-field imaging 200 DTx icg, Scotland, United Kingdom) showing a large choroidal granuloma with overlying RAP lesion; (B) Corresponding fluorescein angiography shows the lesion to be hypofluorescent in early phases with late hyperfluorescence (left). Leakage from the RAP lesion can also be appreciated in later phases of the angiogram (right).
Source: Presented by Vishali Gupta in the International Uveitis Study Group (IUSG) grand rounds.[10]

Ancillary Investigations

Fundus Photography

It allows documentation of fundus lesions and monitoring of response/non-response to therapy. Conventional color photographs using true-color imaging are preferred over confocal scanning laser ophthalmoscope (cSLO)-based pseudocolor images.[12] If the predominant pathology is peripheral, ultrawide-field (UWF) imaging with a 200° field of view in one single frame offers a distinct advantage regarding disease characterization and monitoring. UWF imaging is useful (i) to detect peripheral pathology, including snowballs, choroiditis patches, vasculitis, neovascularization, etc., and (ii) to document paradoxical worsening as the worsening may be characterized by the development of new lesions in the periphery that can be better identified on UWF photography.[13] Fundus photography of TB granuloma reveals a single, large, yellowish lesion with overlying retinal hemorrhages or retinal angiomatous proliferation (RAP) **(Figs. 7A and B)**. Most of these manifestations are not associated with active pulmonary disease.

Rarely, may one see typical miliary tubercles that are multiple, one-fourth to one-third of disc diameter (DD) in size, and choroidal lesions scattered throughout the fundus in a patient with miliary TB. The diagnosis here is not a challenge, as the patient has obvious systemic miliary TB **(Fig. 8)**.

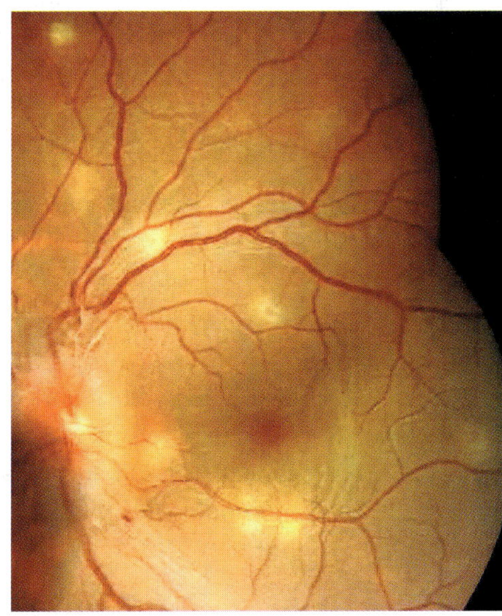

Fig. 8: Choroidal tubercles in a patient with miliary tuberculosis (TB). Fundus photograph of the left eye showing multiple choroidal tubercles in a patient with miliary TB.
Source: Presented by Vishali Gupta in the International Uveitis Study Group (IUSG) grand rounds.[10]

Fundus Fluorescein Angiography

Fundus fluorescein angiography (FFA) is conventionally used to (i) identify active lesions of choroiditis, e.g., an active edge of SLC will show initial hypo- with late hyperfluorescence of the edge and diffusion of dye into the adjacent healthy retina **(Fig. 9)** and (ii) in cases with TB retinal vasculitis, it is used to identify areas of capillary nonperfusion as TB vasculitis is occlusive in nature **(Figs. 4A and B)**. Many times, new vessels may be seen at the border of perfused and nonperfused retinas. UWF angiography, if available, is preferred as the nonperfusion, and neovascularization may be limited to the extreme periphery.[14]

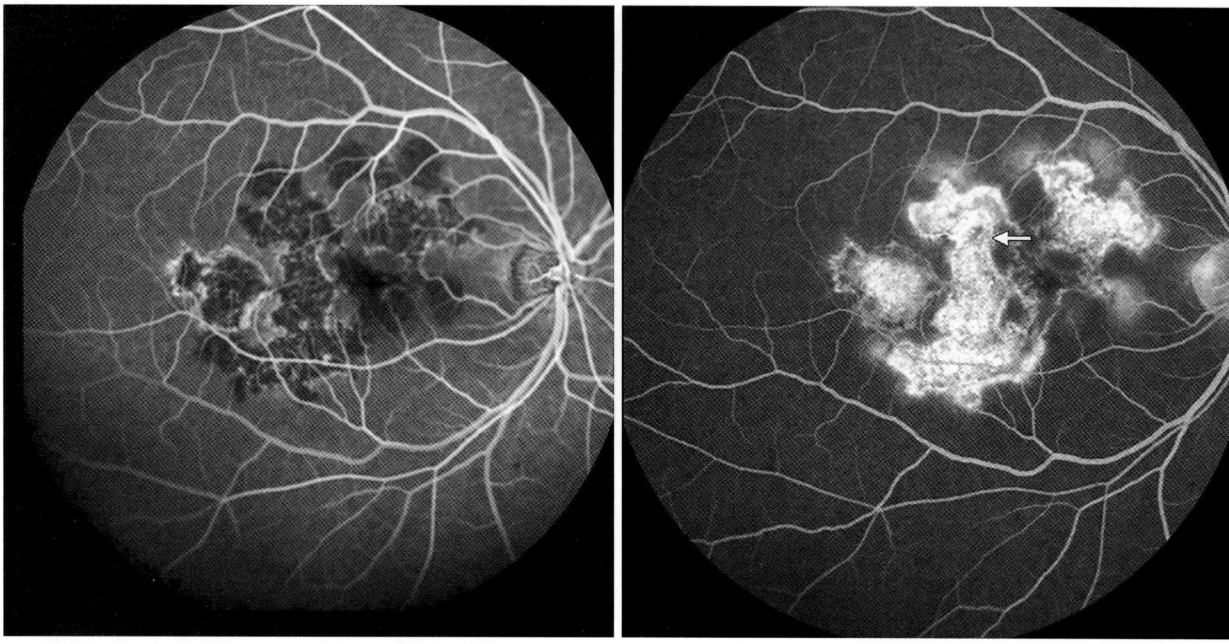

Fig. 9: Typical fundus fluorescein angiography (FFA) findings in ocular tuberculosis (TB). FFA in a patient with TB serpiginous-like choroiditis (SLC) shows early hypofluorescence of the edges (right), with late hyperfluorescence associated with dye leakage into the adjacent healthy retina.
Source: Presented by Vishali Gupta in the International Uveitis Study Group (IUSG) grand rounds.[10]

Fundus Autofluorescence

Fundus autofluorescence is a noninvasive imaging modality often used to detect disease activity in posterior uveitis. FAF stages have been described to represent various stages of SLC with active lesions appearing hyperautofluorescent and becoming gradually hypoautofluorescent as they heal[14] **(Fig. 10)**. Thus, this modality may be used to identify active lesions, demonstrate a response to therapy, and look for paradoxical worsening. Again, UWF imaging is preferred.

Optical Coherence Tomography

In TB SLC, active lesions that are hyperautofluorescent on FAF show hyperreflective areas the outer retina on OCT **(Fig. 11)**. The inner retinal layers are mainly either not involved or show minimal distortion. During healing, the outer retinal layers undergo atrophy corresponding to hypoautofluorescent lesions on FAF.[15]

Enhanced depth imaging OCT or swept-source OCT (SS-OCT) is useful in detecting choroidal granulomas characterized by large hypo- or isoreflective areas of increased homogeneity within the choroid with increased transmission the OCT signal. TB granulomas are seen as large, solitary lesions with overlying hyperreflectivity in the outer retina. In contrast, sarcoid granulomas are multiple and stromal and do not have associated hyperreflective changes in the outer retina.[16]

Indocyanine Green Angiography

Ocular TB affects the choriocapillaris—outer retina complex in SLC, appearing as multifocal areas of choriocapillaris ischemia. These lesions may show as hypofluorescent in the early phase and remain hypofluorescent in the late phase, indicating capillary ischemia or full-thickness granulomas **(Fig. 12)**. Large granulomas/tuberculomas will be seen as hypofluorescent lesions that remain hypofluorescent in the late phase. Since granulomas in TB are VEGF driven, they may present with RAP that can be delineated very well on indocyanine green angiography (ICGA).[16]

Optical Coherence Tomography Angiography

Optical coherence tomography angiography (OCTA) is used to delineate areas of choriocapillaris flow void and can be used to monitor the disease course and response to therapy **(Fig. 13)**. However, the most practical use of OCTA

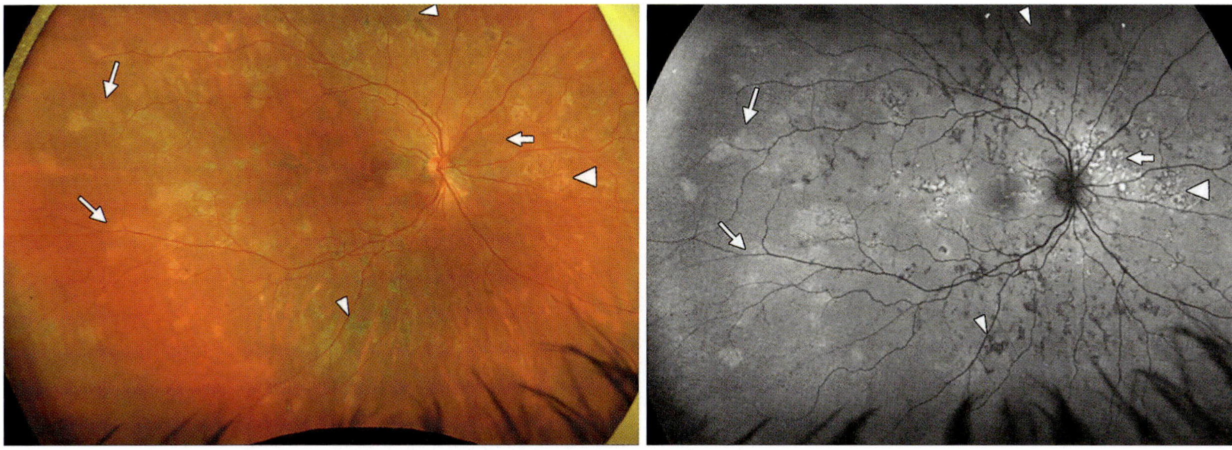

Fig. 10: Ultrawide-field imaging in a patient with ocular tuberculosis. Ultrawide-field fundus photograph (right) (Optos California ultrawide-field imaging 200 DTx icg, Scotland, United Kingdom) and fundus autofluorescence (FAF) (left) showing the different stages of serpiginous-like choroiditis lesions. Fresh lesions (stage I) temporal to the macula have fuzzy margins and appear hyperautofluorescent on FAF (white arrows). As the lesions start healing, a thin rim of hypoautofluorescence emerges at the lesion's periphery, indicating the onset of healing (stage II), while the central area of hyperautofluorescence becomes more pronounced (white double arrows). In stage III, there is a reduction in central hyperautofluorescence coupled with an increase in peripheral hypoautofluorescence, resulting in a stippled appearance of the lesion (white double arrowheads). Finally, upon healing, the lesions have well-demarcated margins and are hypoautofluorescent (white arrowheads).
Source: Presented by Vishali Gupta in the International Uveitis Study Group (IUSG) grand rounds.[10]

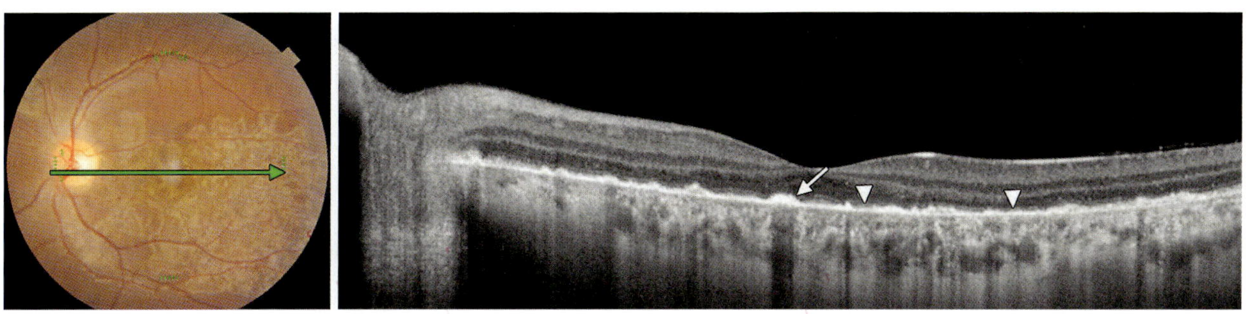

Fig. 11: Optical coherence tomography findings in active ocular tuberculosis. Swept-source optical coherence tomography line scan passing through the serpiginous-like choroiditis lesions shows hyperreflective areas involving the outer retina (white arrow). Additionally, outer retinal atrophy and retinal pigment epithelium (RPE) disruption can also be noted (white arrowheads).
Source: Presented by Vishali Gupta in the International Uveitis Study Group (IUSG) grand rounds.[10]

is to detect vascular abnormalities, including neovascular tufts, tangled vessels, and neovascular membranes underneath the choroiditis.[17]

Laboratory Diagnosis

The most important point to remember before ordering tests for TB is that the clinician should suspect OTB based on the phenotypic presentation, and it is important to rule out other possible etiologies in the differential diagnosis. For example, in a patient with placoid chorioretinitis, a positive test for TB has no meaning if syphilis has not been tested and ruled out. Global uveitis experts from the Collaborative Ocular Tuberculosis Study (COTS) group agreed that there is no single gold standard test for diagnosing OTB due to protean clinical manifestations, variable endemicity, and disease prevalence in the general population.

Diagnosing pulmonary TB relies on histopathological evidence from smear or culture positivity in sputum samples. However, such confirmation is not feasible for OTB due to the paucity of samples and paucibacillary disease. The next best alternative is to detect the MTB

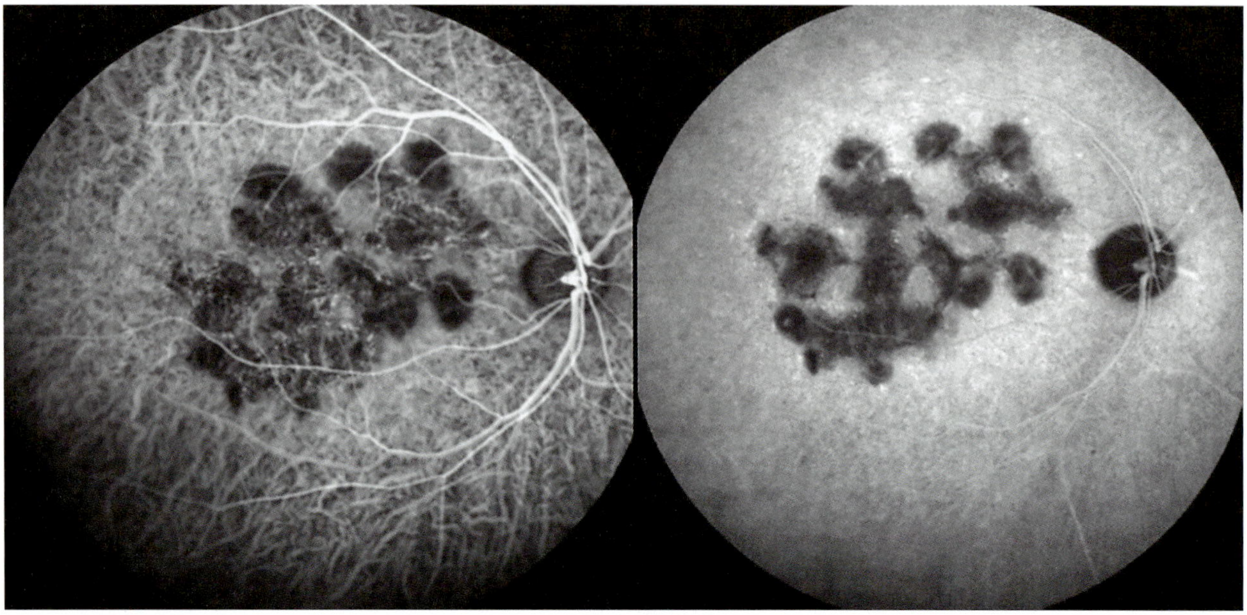

Fig. 12: ICGA findings in ocular tuberculosis (TB). ICGA in a patient with TB SLC shows (left) lesions that are hypo in the early phase and (right) remain hypo in the late phase. (ICGA: indocyanine green angiography; SLC: serpiginous-like choroiditis)
Source: Presented by Vishali Gupta in the International Uveitis Study Group (IUSG) grand rounds.[10]

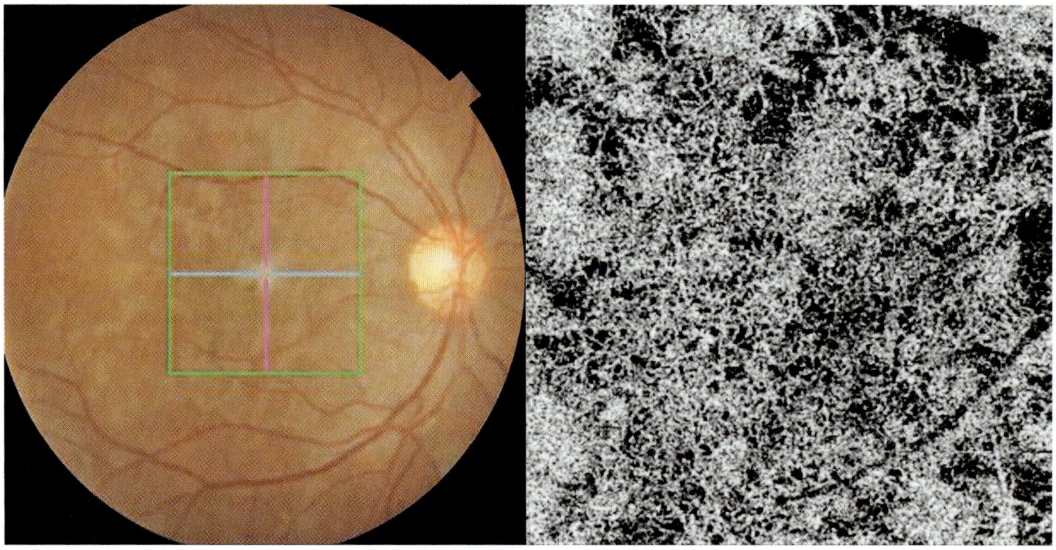

Fig. 13: Optical coherence tomography angiography (OCTA) findings in ocular tuberculosis. Swept-source OCTA scan of a patient with serpiginous-like choroiditis shows flow voids in the choriocapillaris layer.
Source: Presented by Vishali Gupta in the International Uveitis Study Group (IUSG) grand rounds.[10]

genome using polymerase chain reaction (PCR), but this method is nonstandardized and has limited specificity. As a result, PCR for MTB detection in intraocular fluids is not commonly used, and a negative result does not rule out TB.[18] This leaves us with a choice of looking at the indirect evidence, including the tuberculin skin test (TST)/ Mantoux skin test, interferon gamma release assay (IGRA), and chest imaging.

The tuberculin skin test is a century-old test based on the principle of detecting immunological memory against MTB antigens. TST is readily available, low cost, and easy to perform, with a reported sensitivity of 70.9–95.8% in diagnosing OTB. However, variations in the administration and interpretation can affect the TST objective reliability of the test. The test may become negative in patients with energy like miliary TB or severe immunosuppression. Attention should be paid while measuring TST as it is the area of induration, not erythema, that should be carefully measured. Normally, an induration of >10 × 10 mm after 72 hours of injecting 10 tuberculin units (TUs) of purified protein derivative (PPD) is considered positive for OTB.[19,20] Bacillus Calmette-Guérin (BCG) vaccination could produce false-positive results in the first years after immunization, and TST will also be positive in nontuberculous mycobacterial (NTM) infections. The IGRAs assess interferon gamma (INF-γ) production by T lymphocytes in response to MTB antigens [early secretion antigenic target-6 (ESAT-6) and culture filtrate protein-10 (CFP-10)]. Since these antigens are absent in BCG and NTM, thus false positivity due to NTM infections or BCG is unlikely. Overall, the reported sensitivity of IGRA is less than TST.[20,21] In practice, limited resources in many TB-endemic regions hinder the use of IGRAs due to their high cost, technical difficulties, and inability to differentiate between active and latent TB.

Radiological evidence is generally obtained from the chest X-rays or contrast-enhanced computed tomography (CECT) chest. The chest radiography mainly reveals hilar lymphadenopathy with calcified nodes, parenchymal scarring, or fibrosis that is indicative of old exposure to the disease, and one should not look for active pulmonary disease in these patients. Results from COTS showed that in their patient cohort, 26.9% had radiologic features suggestive of inactive TB on chest X-ray, while 68.6% had positive findings on chest computed tomography (CT), indicating that CT chest is better than chest X-ray in detecting past exposure to TB.[22] A whole-body positron emission tomography (PET) scan may be done to detect metabolically active lymphadenopathy, but it is not performed routinely.[23]

Treatment

When to Treat?

There has been considerable uncertainty among uveitis experts about when to treat OTB. This confusion arose for several reasons: (i) The diagnosis of OTB is based on collaborative evidence, including Mantoux, QuantiFERON-TB Gold (QFT-G), and chest imaging. Thus, the treatment is based solely on indirect evidence. (ii) COTS-1 has shown that >90% of patients will not have evidence of active pulmonary disease at the time of diagnosis of OTB. In several countries, ATT is administered by infectious disease (ID) experts who look for evidence of active pulmonary TB to initiate treatment. Thus, it is very important to work in close coordination with ID experts and inform them about the need to administer ATT for ocular disease and not for concomitant pulmonary TB. (iii) A very common concern among uvea specialists is that tests for TB may be positive in many patients, including those who have uveitis due to causes other than TB. Thus, it will lead to many patients receiving ATT unnecessarily. The answer to this concern lies in knowing the pretest probability of the test and performing TB tests only when the phenotype is suggestive of TB. It is also very important to rule out all other possible etiologies in the differential diagnosis and ensure that the ocular inflammation is consistent with TB.

To address these concerns, the COTS group, in association with the International Uveitis Study Group (IUSG), International Ocular Inflammation Society (IOIS), and Foster Ocular Immunology Society (FOIS), has developed consensus guidelines for initiating ATT for specific clinical phenotypes.[24,25] Two major factors that influenced the therapeutic decision to initiate ATT included the patient's specific phenotypic expression and geographic origin. Different permutations and combinations of endemicity, first versus recurrent episode, active versus inactive disease, and immunological/radiological tests created 486 questions for Delphi and distributed among five phenotypes. The summary of recommendations is given as follows:

- *Serpiginous-like choroiditis:* There was a strong consensus on treating this phenotype, which is likely associated with TB. Most of the experts recommended treating SLC in the following cases:
  - Serpiginous-like choroiditis with positive immunological tests (PPD skin test and IGRA) and one radiological test (CT chest or X-ray) positive.
  - Both immunological tests are positive (PPD skin test or IGRA), and radiological tests are negative or not done/not available.
  - One immunological test is positive (either PPD skin test or IGRA), and the second test is either negative or not done/not available. One radiological test is also positive.
  - One immunological test is positive (PPD skin test or IGRA), the second test is not done/not available, and the radiological test is negative or not done/not available.

- *Tuberculoma:*
  - Antituberculosis therapy is recommended for patients with positive immunological tests (PPD and IGRA) and a positive radiological test.
  - Antituberculosis therapy is also recommended in patients with both immunological tests positive but absent radiological evidence.
- *Tubercular multifocal or unifocal choroiditis:*
  - Antituberculosis therapy is recommended when immunological (PPD and IGRA) and radiological tests are positive.
  - There is moderate consensus that ATT should be initiated when only one immunological test is positive, in the presence of a positive radiological test.
- *Anterior uveitis:*
  - Recurrent granulomatous anterior uveitis in case both immunological tests (PPD skin test and IGRA) are positive, and one radiological test (CT chest or X-ray) is positive.
  - Recurrent granulomatous anterior uveitis in case one immunological test (PPD skin test and IGRA) is positive, and one radiological test (CT chest or X-ray) is positive.
- *Intermediate uveitis:*
  - For intermediate uveitis, there is moderate consensus to start ATT if both immunological tests and radiological evidence of TB are positive, irrespective of the endemicity.
  - ATT may be considered in endemic regions if one immunological test is positive alongside radiological evidence.
- *Panuveitis:*
  - Antituberculosis therapy is recommended for all patients with panuveitis if both immunological and radiological tests are positive, regardless of endemicity.
  - Antituberculosis therapy may be initiated in a nonendemic region even if only one immunological test is positive, along with radiological findings.
- *Retinal vasculitis:*
  - Antituberculosis therapy is advised for active retinal vasculitis in endemic regions when both immunological tests (PPD skin test and IGRA) and radiological tests are positive.
  - Antituberculosis therapy is also recommended for active retinal vasculitis in endemic regions when either of the two immunological tests (PPD skin test or IGRA) is positive along with a positive radiological test.

Collaborative Ocular Tuberculosis Study Calculator[26]

The COTS calculator is an online tool designed to initiate ATT for patients with OTB. It was developed using consensus data from 81 global experts who evaluated 486 clinical scenarios using the Delphi method. It was specifically created to provide an accessible and straightforward decision-making tool for clinicians, especially in real-world settings where resources may be limited, and clinical uncertainty often complicates the management of OTB. By integrating multiple clinical parameters—such as clinical phenotypes, endemicity, immunological tests (TST, IGRA), and radiological evidence—the tool offers a practical approach to guide treatment decisions. The calculator assigns a score from 1 to 5, indicating the probability of initiating ATT based on expert consensus, where a score of 5 reflects a strong recommendation to start therapy. The COTS calculator aims to provide a low-cost, evidence-based clinical decision tool, enhancing the clinician's ability to make informed decisions in diverse healthcare settings. However, further validation studies are needed to confirm its utility and reliability in clinical practice.

Drugs and Duration of Therapy

Since ATT regimens are different for different countries, the COTS group did not comment on the types of drugs to be used and the duration of therapy. In practice, clinicians must be careful about either not giving ethambutol or giving it for a short duration for the first 2 months. In clinical practice, four drugs (isoniazid, rifampicin, pyrazinamide, and ethambutol) are given for 2 months, followed by isoniazid and rifampicin for seven more months. Monitoring liver functions every 6–8 weeks, while the patient is on ATT, is important. The regimen may be revised if liver enzymes are elevated, in consultation with a hepatologist.

Concomitant Use of Corticosteroids

In phenotypes that represent an immune-mediated response to TB (e.g., SLC, multifocal choroiditis, vasculitis), systemic corticosteroids can be initiated along with ATT. In case SLC approaches fovea-threatening vision, systemic corticosteroids can be initiated at presentation, while awaiting reports, and ATT may be added later if indicated. When the inflammation recurs during tapering, corticosteroid-sparing immunosuppressants may be started in these patients. However, if the ocular phenotype is suggestive of actively multiplying bacteria, as in a subretinal abscess, or the patient is suspected of having concomitant active systemic disease, oral corticosteroids may be avoided without the cover of ATT.

Adjunct Local Therapy

Local therapy may be added in two situations, given as follows:

1. In the case of large, vascularized granulomas, local injections of anti-VEGF therapy may be useful in reducing vascularity. Moreover, TB granulomas depend on VEGF for growth, and blocking VEGF reduces granuloma size.[27] A recent study indicated the beneficial role of adding intravitreal moxifloxacin to anti-VEGF therapy as these act as host-directed therapies and help in earlier resolution.[28]
2. Local therapy is also indicated to supplement systemic therapy in patients who show paradoxical worsening on the initiation of ATT. The paradoxical worsening typically occurs 2–3 weeks after the initiation of ATT and is more commonly seen in patients receiving low-dose concomitant corticosteroids. This may be characterized by the enlargement of previous lesions or the development of new lesions, and is mainly due to an increase in inflammatory cytokines.[29] Many of these lesions may appear in the periphery; thus, UWF imaging may be useful in the early detection of paradoxical worsening. The treatment includes increasing the dose of systemic corticosteroids to 1–1.5 mg/kg body weight along with local injections of dexamethasone implant[30] or intravitreal methotrexate.[31] COTS consensus advocated using these therapies at the discretion of treating physicians as the number of studies is limited, and no uniform consensus could be made. However, it is important to continue and not to stop ATT.

Nonresponse to Therapy

If the patient is not responding to ATT or has a recurrence after the ATT treatment, there could be several reasons, and you may have to apply these reasons depending upon the knowledge and context. The following points may be considered:

- *Diagnosis might be inaccurate:* TB can often mimic other conditions. For instance, fibrinous central serous chorioretinopathy, vitreoretinal lymphoma, or metastasis may present similarly to TB. If there is any uncertainty, it is crucial to reassess the patient as if they were a new case, as a correct diagnosis might have been overlooked.
- *Paradoxical worsening:* Sometimes, paradoxical worsening may be mistaken for a nonresponse to ATT. As described in the previous section, paradoxical worsening has a specific time of onset and responds to the addition of corticosteroids.
- *Atypical Mycobacterium:* Rarely, the infection may be due to atypical mycobacteria and not MTB. In such cases, the patient will need diagnostic sampling and testing with molecular diagnostics and next-generation sequencing.
- *Recurrent inflammation after completing ATT:* This is a complicated situation as there are several possibilities given as follows (**Flowchart 1**):
    - *Poor compliance:* Poor compliance can occur if the patient has not taken the full course of ATT or stopped treatment independently. Therefore, following up with the patient is essential to ensure they understand the importance of adhering to the treatment plan. If the ophthalmologist observes poor compliance at the time of recurrence, it is important to refer the patient back to the physician to reinitiate ATT.
    - *Non-TB etiology:* It could be a TB masquerade that responded initially to concomitant steroids and has recurred. This is especially important if the phenotype was not typical for TB, and the patient was still diagnosed and treated as ocular TB. In such a scenario, all investigations must be repeated to rule out other possible etiologies.

  If the above two possibilities have been ruled out, and one attributes the recurrence to TB, one should look at the phenotype at the time of recurrence. TB recurrence often presents as nongranulomatous anterior uveitis without posterior segment involvement. One may perform FFA/ICGA to rule out posterior segment involvement in cases of doubt. For pure anterior segment recurrence, topical steroids with mydriatics are often sufficient, and one may not need to add systemic therapy. Such patients may be followed up for the development of any fundus lesions. However, if the recurrence is in the form of posterior or panuveitis, one would need to look for any history of contact with a multidrug-resistant TB patient leading to reinfection. These cases could represent reactivation of an endogenous infection or re-exposure and would require more detailed investigation, including gene sequencing for resistance genes and coordination with physicians to select an appropriate regimen for reinitiating ATT.
- *Recurrence of autoimmune inflammation following completion of ATT:* Sometimes, TB can induce an

Flowchart 1: Diagrammatic representation of a plan for managing nonresponsive patients.

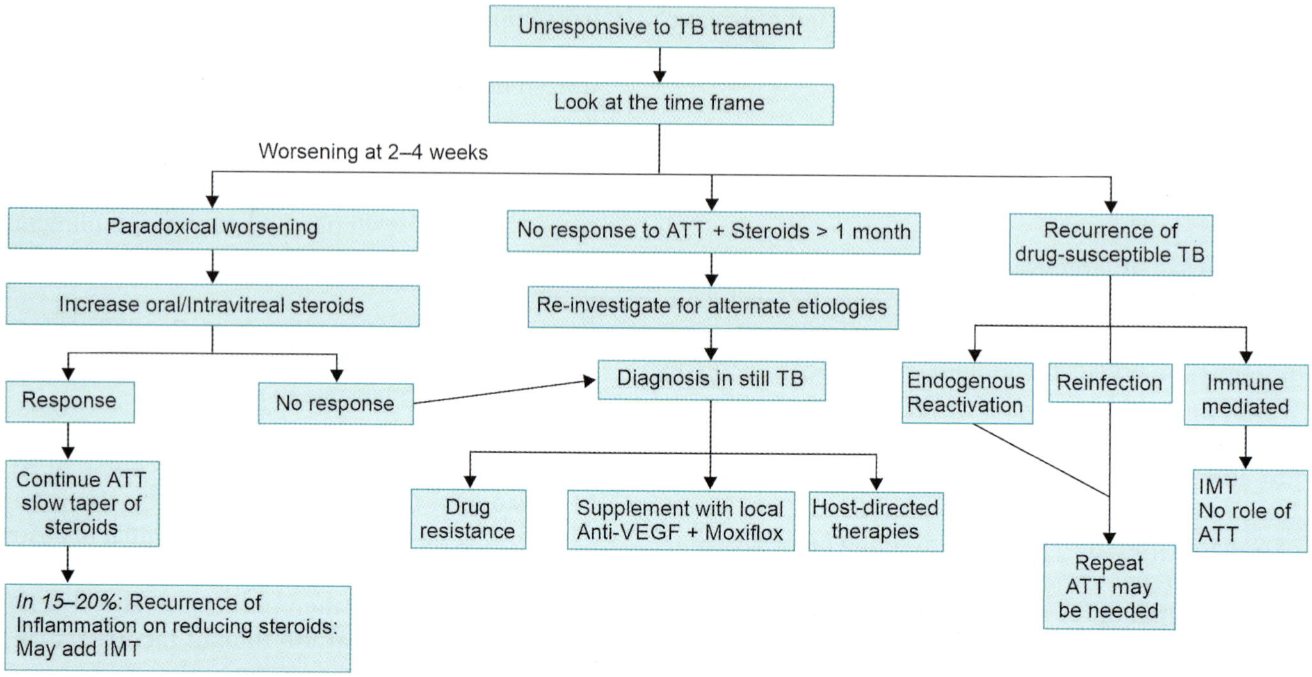

(ATT: antituberculosis therapy; IMT: immunomodulatory therapy; TB: tuberculosis; VEGF: vascular endothelial growth factor)

autoimmune response that may manifest as recurrence once ATT and steroids are over. In such a scenario, the phenotype is generally distinct, typically manifesting as vitritis with or without retinal vasculitis. Such relapses are likely to respond to immunosuppressive therapy.

SERPIGINOUS-LIKE CHOROIDITIS

Case Series Presentation

Case 1

Personal data at presentation:

- Female, 17 years old
- No known systemic disease
- She was on oral prednisolone 30 mg/day.
- There was no history of TB or TB contact.

History of present illness: Progressive worsening of vision in the right eye (OD) over the previous 2 weeks, with similar symptoms in the left eye (OS) beginning 4 days ago.

Ocular examination: The patient presented with a best-corrected visual acuity (BCVA) of 1/60 (equivalent to 20/1200 Snellen) in the OD and 6/12 (equivalent to 20/40) in the OS. Anterior chamber examination was unremarkable in both eyes. Fundoscopy revealed active choroidal lesions at the posterior pole in both eyes **(Fig. 14A)**.

Uveitis workup:

- Mantoux positive
- QuantiFERON-TB gold positive

Considering the typical phenotype, active bilateral presentation with both QFT-G and Mantoux tests being positive, initial treatment included initiating a full course of antitubercular regimen. Since the posterior pole was involved, the patient received three doses of intravenous methylprednisolone, followed by a tapering course of oral prednisolone.

At 1-month follow-up, there was no further inflammatory activities, which held true even after 5 years of follow-up **(Fig. 14B)**.

Case 2

Personal data:

- Female, 22 years old
- No history of TB or known TB contact

History of present illness: Previously treated for SLC in both eyes with oral prednisone at 60 mg/day with a tapering schedule. The lesions had fully resolved following treatment.

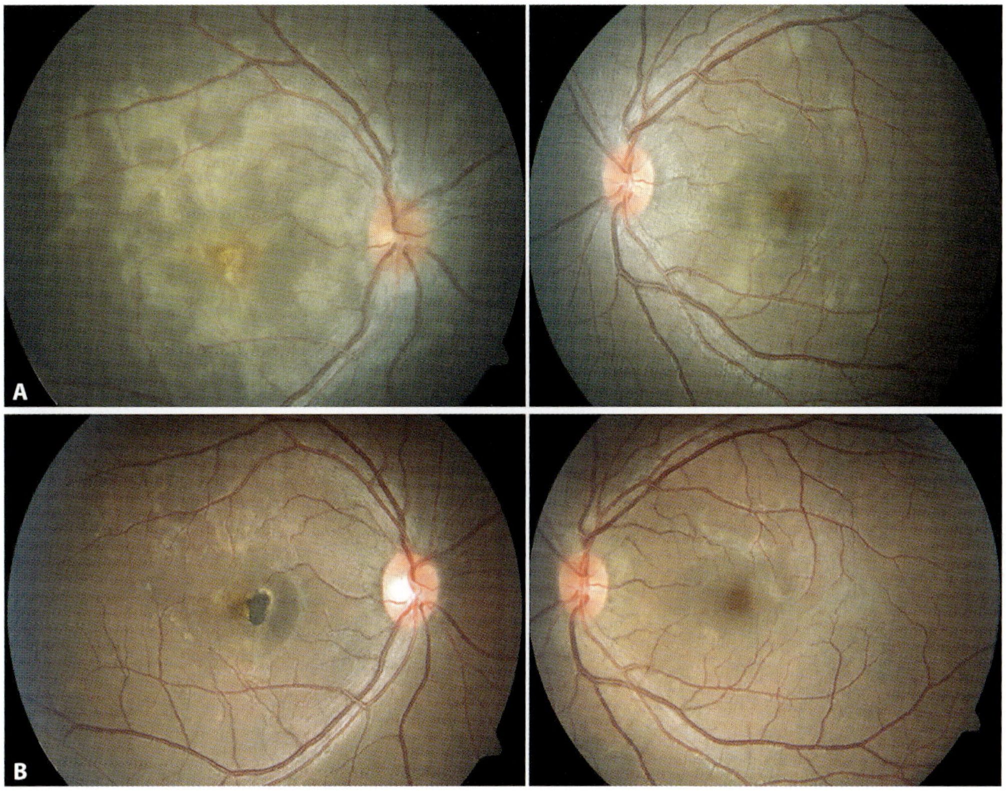

Figs. 14A and B: Fundoscopy at baseline and during follow-up. Fundus photograph showing (A) active choroidal lesions at the posterior pole in both eyes and (B) no new lesions or further inflammatory activities at 5-year follow-up.
Source: Presented by Ahana Sen in the International Uveitis Study Group (IUSG) grand rounds.[10]

Uveitis workup:

- *Mantoux test:* Negative
- *Quantiferon-TB Gold:* Positive
- *High-resolution computed tomography (HRCT):* Normal
- *Venereal Disease Research Laboratory (VDRL) and Treponema pallidum hemagglutination assay (TPHA):* Negative

Ocular examination: Fundus examination revealed inactive choroidal lesions in both eyes **(Fig. 15A)**.

Treatment: After 8 months, the patient experienced a recurrence of inflammation in the form of new active choroidal lesions in both eyes **(Fig. 15B)**. This time, ATT was initiated alongside oral corticosteroids.

Follow-up: After 9 months, there was no further inflammatory activity, and the anti-TB treatment had been completed. One month following this, she had a blurring of vision in her OD. Fundus examination revealed healed choroidal lesions with cystoid macular edema (CME) in both eyes, confirmed by OCT **(Fig. 16)**.

At this point, mycophenolate mofetil 1 gram twice daily, along with oral prednisolone at 40 mg/day was started with a slow weekly taper. At 1-month follow-up, the CME had resolved, and no further inflammatory activity was observed.

Final Follow-up: After 1 year, the BCVA was 20/20 in OU. At her last visit, 6 months later, there was no recurrence of inflammatory activity.

Case 3

Personal data:

- Male, 36 years old.
- No history of TB or known TB contact

History of present illness: The patient reported reduced vision in the OS over the past week.

Physical examination: BCVA was 20/20 in the OD and 20/40 in the OS; examination of the anterior segment was normal in OU. Fundus examination revealed active choroidal lesions at the posterior pole in the OS.

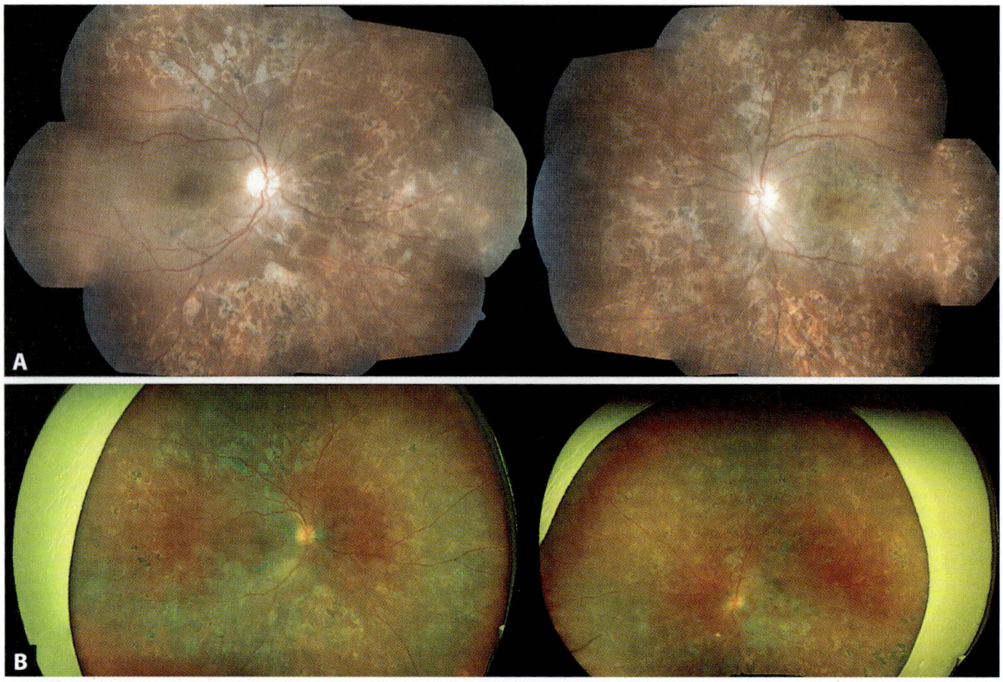

Figs. 15A and B: Fundoscopy at baseline and during follow-up. (A) Inactive choroidal lesions in the periphery at baseline; (B) Fresh choroidal lesions at 8 months follow-up in both eyes.
Source: Presented by Ahana Sen in the International Uveitis Study Group (IUSG) grand rounds.[10]

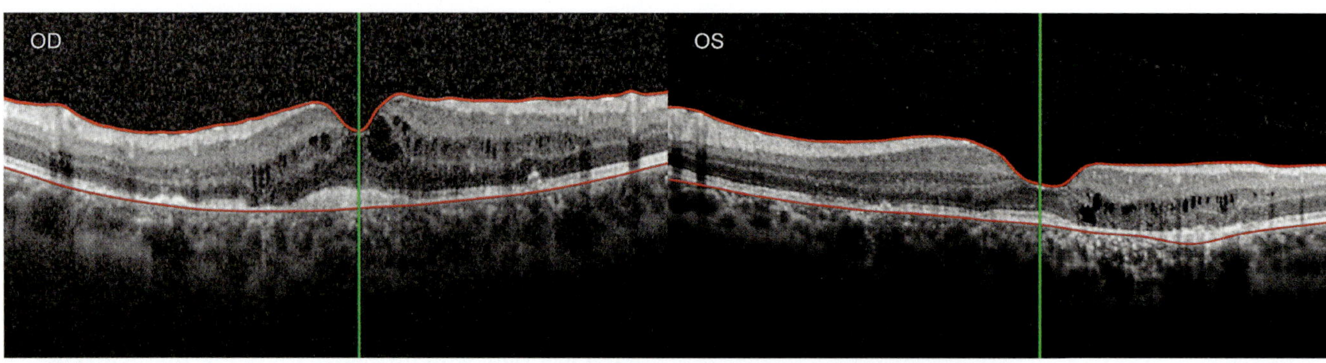

Fig. 16: Optical coherence tomography (OCT) findings at 10-month follow-up. OCT shows cystoid macular edema in both eyes.
Source: Presented by Ahana Sen in the International Uveitis Study Group (IUSG) grand rounds.[10]

Fluorescein angiography showed hyperfluorescence of the optic disc and hypofluorescence corresponding to the choroidal lesions in the early phase, margins of which showed staining in later phases of the angiogram, giving rise to the "ring of fire" appearance **(Figs. 17A and B)**.

Uveitis workup:

- *Mantoux test:* Negative
- *Quantiferon-TB Gold:* Negative
- *Rapid Plasma Reagin (RPR) and TPHA:* Negative
- *Toxoplasma antibodies:* Negative
- High-resolution computed tomography of the chest suggestive of old granulomatous disease sequelae

Initial treatment: Oral corticosteroids were prescribed at 60 mg/day with weekly tapering, calcium supplements, and antacids.

Follow-up: One month later, BCVA was 20/20 in OU. Previous lesions had healed, but fresh choroidal lesions were seen along the superior arcade **(Fig. 18A)**. ATT was initiated, and the oral corticosteroid dose was hiked up again to the initial dose of 60 mg/day. There were early

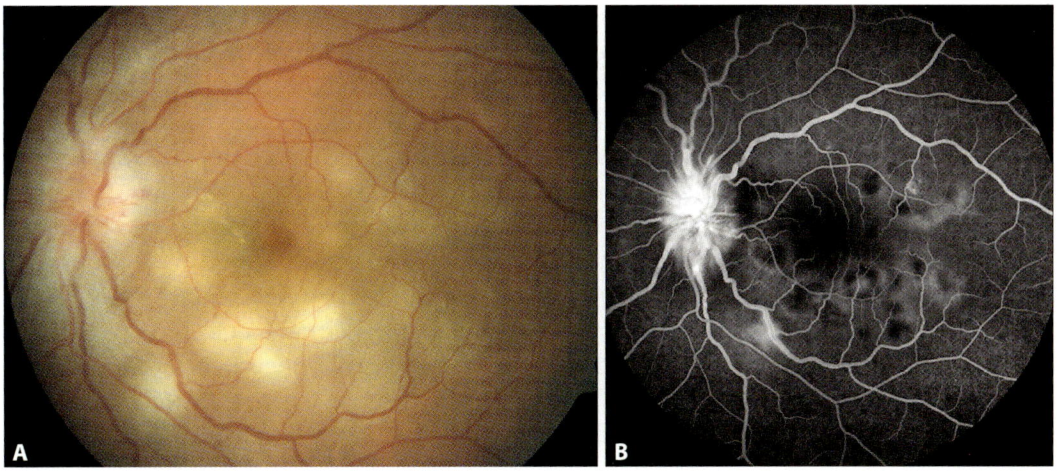

Figs. 17A and B: Fundus fluorescein angiography. (A) Fundus examination of the OD showing choroidal lesions at the posterior pole and optic disc edema; (B) Fluorescein angiography revealing hyperfluorescence of the disc and hypofluorescence corresponding to the choroidal lesions, margins showing staining in the later phases of angiogram giving rise to the "ring of fire" appearance.
Source: Presented by Ahana Sen in the International Uveitis Study Group (IUSG) grand rounds.[10]

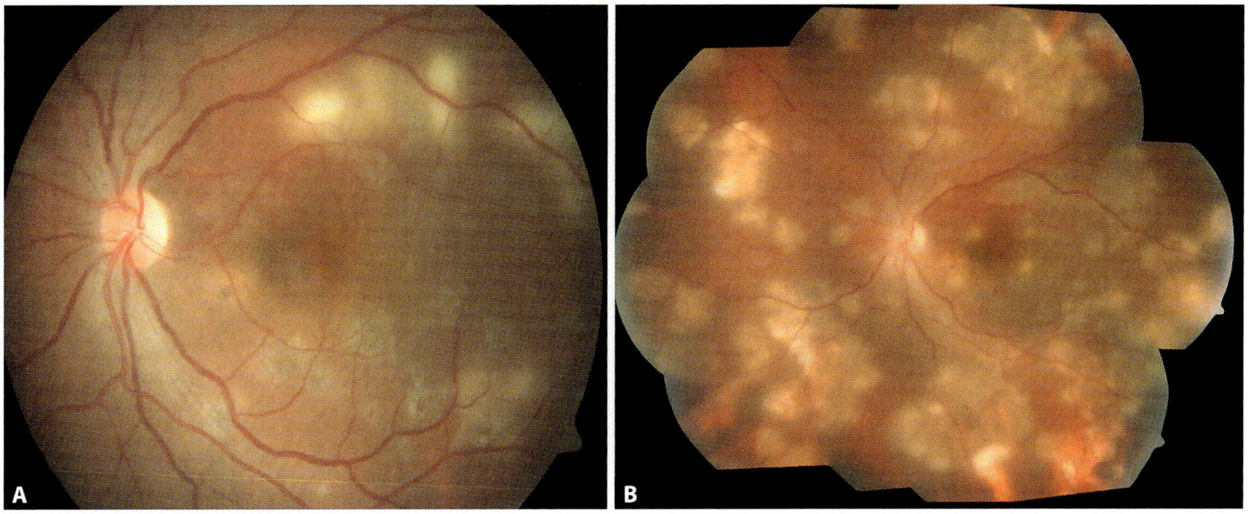

Figs. 18A and B: Paradoxical reaction after antituberculosis treatment. Fundus photograph of left eye. (A) At 1-month follow-up, it shows healed lesions along the inferior arcade and new lesions along the superior region; (B) One month after initiating ATT, the resolution of previous lesions, but new and partially resolving lesions at the posterior pole and mid-periphery, was observed.
Source: Presented by Ahana Sen in the International Uveitis Study Group (IUSG) grand rounds.[10]

signs of choroiditis resolution. But in the following month, vision deteriorated to 20/60. Multiple choroidal lesions in active and resolving stages were seen at the posterior pole and mid-periphery. The patient was diagnosed with a paradoxical reaction to ATT **(Fig. 18B)**.

Treatment: Intravenous methylprednisolone was administered in three doses, along with mycophenolate mofetil (1 gram twice daily) and oral corticosteroids (60 mg/day with slow weekly tapering). ATT was continued. One month later, no new lesions were observed, and the inflammation was under control.

Discussion

Serpiginous-like choroiditis, as a phenotype, is more often associated with a tuberculous etiology, especially in endemic regions, and is supported by ancillary laboratory tests or radiology. ATT and steroids can lead to complete resolution of inflammation, as noted in Case 1.

The course of SLC is varied; they can have an aggressive course, develop reactivations, or even have paradoxical worsening. It is hypothesized that Mycobacterium may persist in the RPE cells, leading to reactivation.

Kawali et al. classified SLC into placoid, advanced dendritic, and dendritic morphologies based on the appearance of the lesion.[32] Placoid SLC is associated with a poor visual prognosis, while advanced dendritic and dendritic forms tend to have a better outcome; inflammatory serum cytokine profiling has demonstrated elevated levels of proinflammatory cytokines in patients experiencing paradoxical worsening, correlating with higher bacillary loads.[29] Imaging studies have indicated that the opacity and size of lesions at baseline can predict poor therapeutic response and disease progression.

High Recurrence Risk with Corticosteroid Monotherapy

Studies have demonstrated that the use of ATT, compared with corticosteroids alone, reduces recurrences by approximately two-thirds.[11] Corticosteroid monotherapy is associated with a higher risk of disease progression and the development of new lesions, as illustrated in the second case.[33]

Notably, SLC does not always recur in the form of choroiditis. As noted in Case 2, the recurrence of inflammation was in the form of CME. Immunosuppressive therapy following ATT can reduce the chances of recurrence of inflammation. Following ATT, anti-inflammatory therapies such as local corticosteroid injections (e.g., Ozurdex) and biological agents such as adalimumab are also viable treatment options.[34,35]

Negative Immunoreactive Tests

Patients with OTB can present with negative immunoreactive tests, as seen in Case 2, in which both the Mantoux test and QFT-G were negative. HRCT of the chest, however, showed old granulomatous disease sequelae, and ATT was started on this basis. A study reports that up to 10% of patients with OTB exhibit negative results on immunoreactivity tests, despite fitting the typical clinical profile and experiencing recurrences.[36] In such cases, HRCT findings or recurrences of a typical phenotype can guide treatment decisions with ATT.[37]

Worsening Despite Treatment

If ocular inflammation worsens despite treatment, it is crucial to reassess the diagnosis. Paradoxical worsening is a relatively more common occurrence. In some cases, worsening of inflammation may result from rapid tapering of anti-inflammatory therapy or drug resistance.[38]

Case 3 was diagnosed as SLC with paradoxical worsening after initiation of ATT. A UWF imaging study found that approximately 36% of patients exhibited paradoxical worsening, with 18% showing lesions in the peripheral fundus.[13]

To summarize, the initial treatment of SLC without ancillary tests or radiological positivity can be with a trial course of adequate corticosteroids. However, in typical phenotypes and positive ancillary tests, ATT is advisable as there is a high chance of relapse with corticosteroid monotherapy. Reactivation while on/after ATT can be presented as choroiditis, vitritis, or even CME alone, which may need additional immunomodulatory therapies (IMTs). Aggressive spread of choroiditis can occur while on ATT and systemic steroids. The treatment of this paradoxical worsening needs high-dose systemic steroids, usually with IMTs. Drug resistance is the other differential that must be considered in such situations.

TUBERCULOSIS RETINAL VASCULITIS

Case Presentation

Personal Data

- Male, 56 years old
- Tunisian
- History of syphilis infection in 2010
- Diagnosed with colon cancer in 2021

History of Present Illness

The patient reported decreased vision and floaters in the OD over the past 3 weeks. He denied any previous ocular surgery or trauma and had no systemic symptoms.

Physical Examination

The patient presented with a visual acuity of 20/25 in the OD and 20/20 in the OS, with normal intraocular pressure (IOP) in OU and no anterior chamber cells. Fundoscopy of the OD revealed diffuse retinal hemorrhages, venous perivascular sheathing, moderate vitritis, and retinal neovascularization inferior to the optic disc. In the OS, neovascularization was observed in the nasal midperipheral retina **(Figs. 19A and B)**. Multimodal imaging was requested, evidencing active leakage in OU **(Figs. 20A and B)** and serous retinal detachment in the OD **(Figs. 21A and B)** **(Table 1)**.

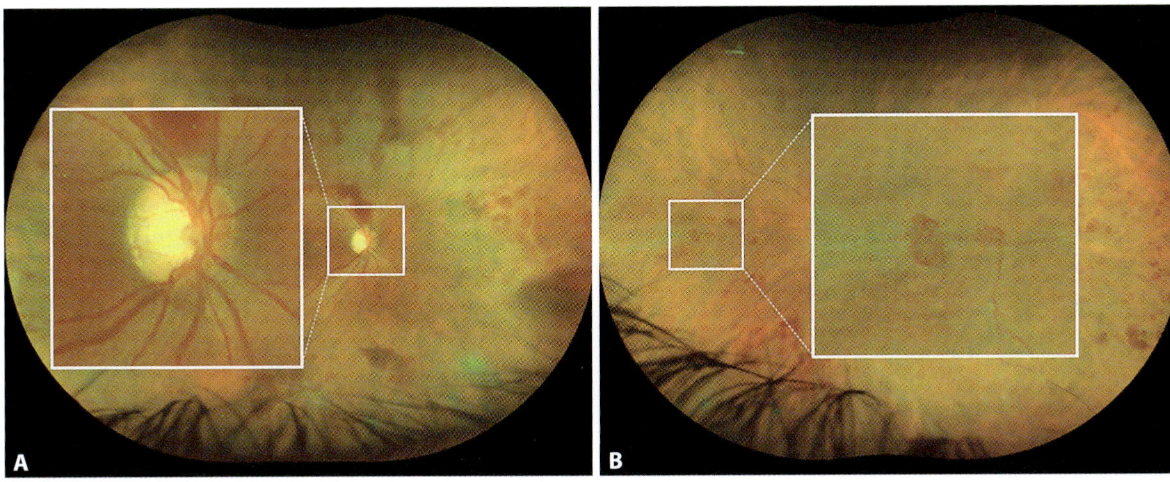

Figs. 19A and B: Fundoscopy findings. (A) OD with diffuse retinal hemorrhages, veins, perivascular sheathing, moderate vitritis, and retinal neovascularization inferiorly to the optic disc; (B) OS with neovascularization inferiorly in the nasal mid-peripheral retina.
Source: Presented by Pietro Gentile in the International Uveitis Study Group (IUSG) grand rounds.[10]

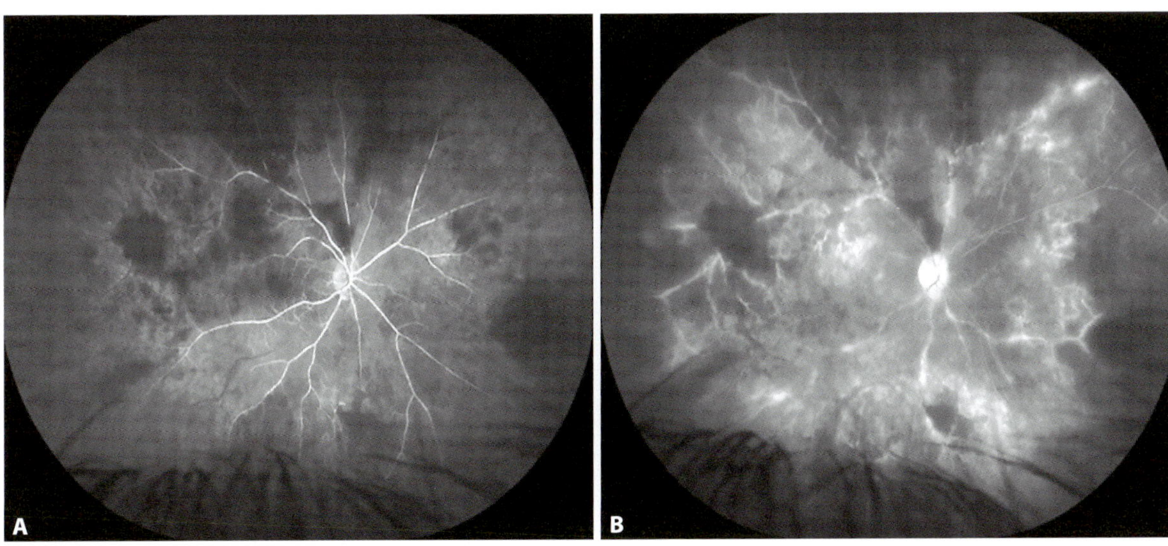

Figs. 20A and B: Fundus fluorescein angiography findings. (A) OD with active vasculitis, lead leakage confirming retinal neovascularization, and diffuse retinal ischemia in the periphery in all quadrants; (B) OS with active vasculitis, lead leakage confirming retinal neovascularization more prominent than OD.
Source: Presented by Pietro Gentile in the International Uveitis Study Group (IUSG) grand rounds.[10]

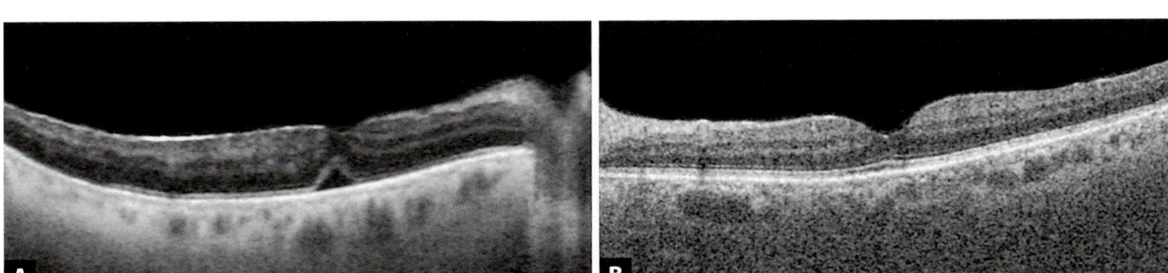

Figs. 21A and B: Optical coherence tomography findings. (A) OD presence of serous retinal detachment; (B) OS: No abnormalities were found.
Source: Presented by Pietro Gentile in the International Uveitis Study Group (IUSG) grand rounds.[10]

TABLE 1: Physical examination of the patient having TB retinal vasculitis.

OD	Parameters	OS
20/25	BCVA	20/20
15 mm Hg	IOP	18 mm Hg
Quiet	Conjunctiva	Quiet
Normal, clear	Cornea	Normal, clear
No cells ACC: 0+	Anterior chamber	No cells ACC: 0+
No synechiae	Iris	No synechiae
Clear	Lens	Clear
Unremarkable	Vitreous	Unremarkable
Diffuse retinal hemorrhages, veins, perivascular sheathing, and moderate vitritis; retinal neovascularization inferiorly to the optic disc	Fundus	Neovascularization inferiorly in the nasal mid-peripheral retina

(ACC: anterior chamber cellularity; BCVA: best-corrected visual acuity; IOP: intraocular pressure; TB: tuberculosis)

Uveitis Workup

The patient presented with occlusive venous vasculitis and moderate vitritis in the OD, characterized by perivascular sheathing, retinal hemorrhages, retinal ischemia, and neovascularization.

- Routine laboratory examinations were within normal limits. Syphilis serology did not indicate active infection. The patient tested negative for human immunodeficiency virus (HIV) and had an indeterminate QuantiFERON result. Consequently, a Mantoux test was performed, which returned positive (18 × 18 mm).
- A chest CT scan revealed apical nodules consistent with healed TB. Sputum analysis for Mycobacterium was negative.
- An ID specialist evaluated the patient and ruled out active systemic signs of TB.

Diagnosis

Based on the COTS classification, the patient was diagnosed with presumed OTB, specifically tubercular retinal vasculitis.

Treatment

The patient was started on a 12-month regimen of ATT, including rifampin, isoniazid, pyrazinamide, and ethambutol, combined with oral prednisone at 0.7 mg/kg, with a tapering schedule.

Follow-up

Shortly before the initiation of systemic treatment, the patient experienced a vitreous hemorrhage in the OD, which was managed 1 month later with vitrectomy, phacoemulsification, and laser photocoagulation. Despite this, a recurrence of vitreous hemorrhage occurred, though it resolved spontaneously, allowing completion of laser photocoagulation. The OS remained free of vitreous hemorrhage but was treated with laser photocoagulation 2 months later, alongside a course of three intravitreal ranibizumab injections due to retinal neovascularization; mild visual loss in his left eye from 20/20 to 20/25 was noted with increasing floaters 24 weeks after the start of treatment. At the time, the patient was under rifampin, isoniazid, and 5 mg/day of oral prednisone **(Figs. 22A to D)**.

The patient developed diabetes, which contraindicated the use of high-dose oral steroids. Additionally, immunosuppressive drugs were not recommended due to the recent history of malignancy. A local approach (24 weeks) was taken, and a 0.7-mg dexamethasone intravitreal implant was administered in the OS **(Figs. 23A to D)**. Six months later, a repeat injection of the dexamethasone intravitreal implant was required in the left eye.

Discussion

Lessons Learned from the Case

- Collaborative Ocular Tuberculosis Study Group: Since 2015, COTS has played a critical role in standardizing nomenclature, allowing for precise communication among physicians and improving patient care in cases of OTB.
- Key points for diagnosis:
    - Retinal vasculitis more commonly involves veins rather than arteries.
    - Occlusive vasculitis is a typical feature of tubercular retinal involvement.
    - UWF imaging is recommended for monitoring retinal vasculitis.
    - Collaboration with other specialists is essential for better interpretation and correlation between clinical phenotypes and diagnostic tests.
- *Management considerations:* The diagnostic approach differs significantly between endemic and nonendemic

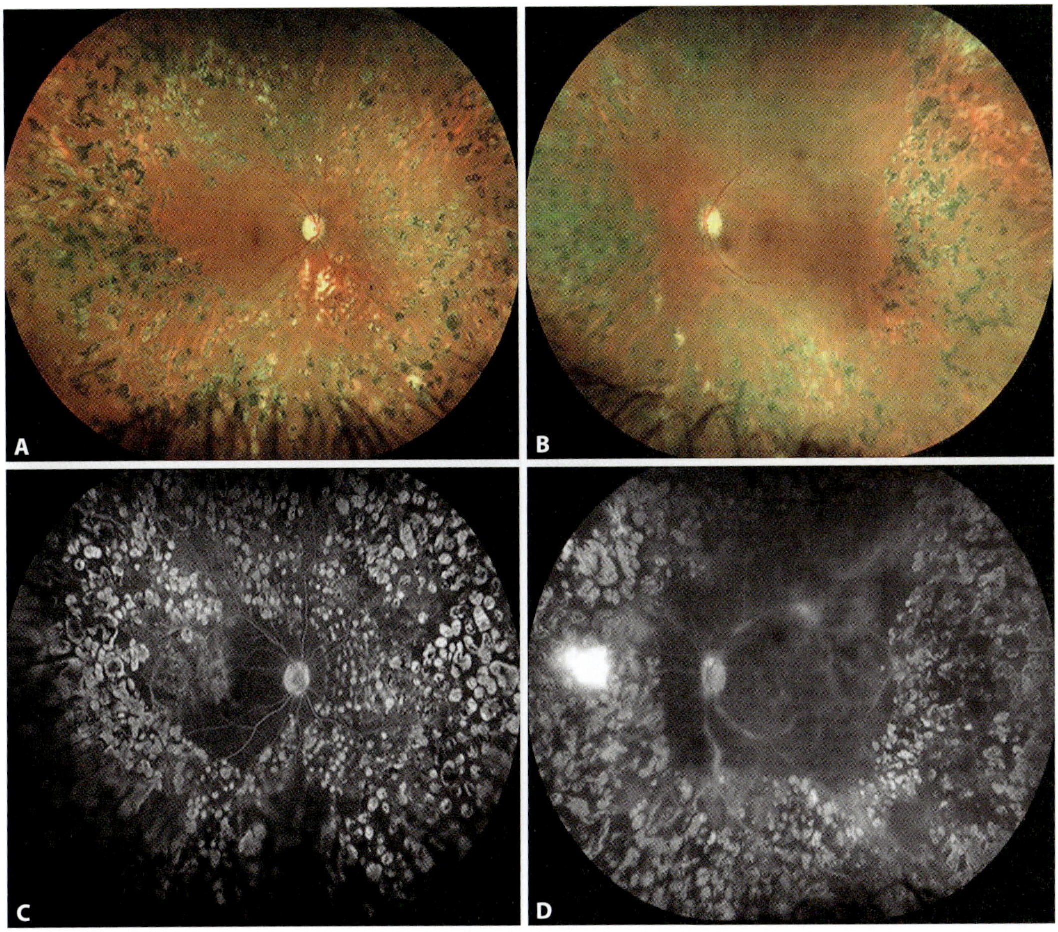

Figs. 22A to D: Fundoscopy and fundus fluorescein angiography at 24-week follow-up. (A and B) Fundoscopy images at 24 weeks of follow-up showing moderate vitritis in the OS; (C and D) Fundus fluorescein angiography revealed no signs of active inflammation or vasculitis in the OD; however, active vasculitis and recurrent retinal neovascularization were noted in the OS.
Source: Presented by Pietro Gentile in the International Uveitis Study Group (IUSG) grand rounds.[10]

regions, emphasizing the importance of understanding the pretest likelihood of OTB. The disease phenotype is crucial in guiding this diagnostic process.[39]

Treatment Strategies

Systemic steroids play a vital role in managing sight-threatening conditions involving vasculitis of the posterior pole, hemorrhages, vitritis, choroidal lesions, or in cases of paradoxical worsening.[40]

Intravitreal dexamethasone implants are particularly useful when systemic steroids are contraindicated, such as in cases of diabetes or recent malignancy.[30]

To manage retinal vasculitis associated with TB, a combination of systemic steroids and ATT is essential to prevent reactivation. Photocoagulation is necessary for neovascularization linked to ischemic areas.

It is crucial to consider the timing of vitrectomy, particularly in recurrent hemorrhages, often associated with active fibrovascular proliferation.[41]

TUBERCULOSIS CHOROIDAL GRANULOMA

Case Series Presentation

Case 1

Personal data:

- Female, 29 years old
- No history of systemic diseases

History of present illness: The patient presented with a sudden decrease in vision in the OS, accompanied by constant pain for the past 10 days.

Physical examination: The patient presented with a BCVA of 20/20 in the OD and 20/40 in the OS. No cells

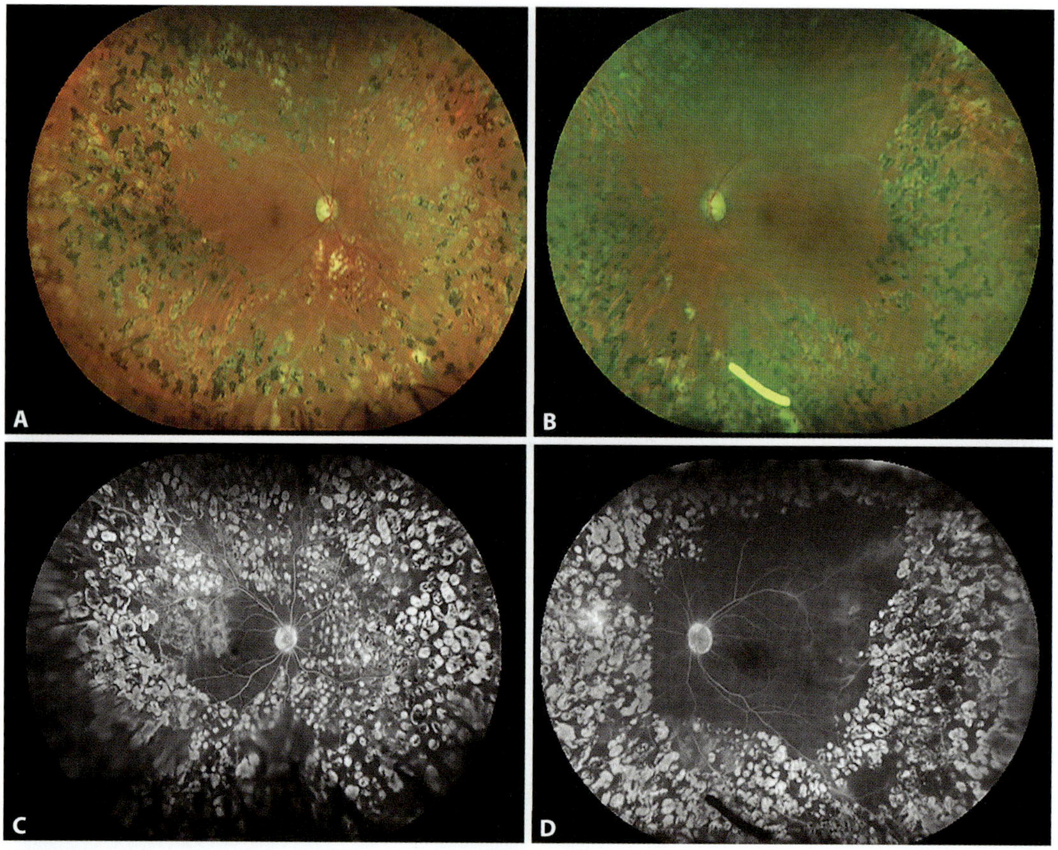

Figs. 23A to D: Funduscopy and fundus fluorescein angiography at 28-week follow-up. (A and B) Funduscopy images at 28 weeks of follow-up (1 month after 0.7 dexamethasone intravitreal implant in OS showing a resolution of vitritis in the OS; (C and D) Fundus fluorescein angiography revealed no signs of active inflammation or vasculitis in the OD; however, an acceptable control of both vasculitis and retinal neovessels was achieved in the OS.
Source: Presented by Pietro Gentile in the International Uveitis Study Group (IUSG) grand rounds.[10]

were observed in the anterior chamber of either eye. Fundoscopy of the OD was unremarkable, but the OS revealed subretinal nodular lesions superior to the optic disc, along with optic disc edema and an exudative retinal detachment **(Fig. 24A and Table 2)**.

Multimodal imaging was ordered, evidencing pinpoint leaks in the early phases of FFA and a hypofluorescent spot around the optic disc, which became hyperfluorescent in the late phases, confirming choroidal involvement **(Figs. 24B and C)**. The OCT revealed the "contact sign" with neurosensory retinal detachment and full-thickness choroidal elevation **(Figs. 25A and B)**.

Uveitis workup:

- Mantoux test showed 20 mm induration at 48 hours.
- Elevated erythrocyte sedimentation rate (28 mm in the first hour).
- Chest X-ray revealed bilateral hilar prominence.
- VDRL and HIV tests were negative.

Anatomical diagnosis: Posterior uveitis with scleritis in the OS.

Morphological diagnosis: Nodular scleritis with choroiditis in the OS.

Etiological diagnosis: Presumed OTB.

Treatment: The patient was started on a four-drug antitubercular regimen along with oral prednisolone 40 mg/day with weekly tapering. After 15 days of treatment, the lesion in the OS had completely resolved, with a BCVA of 20/40.

Follow-up: Four months later, the patient, still on ATT, presented with diminished vision (20/40) in the OS.

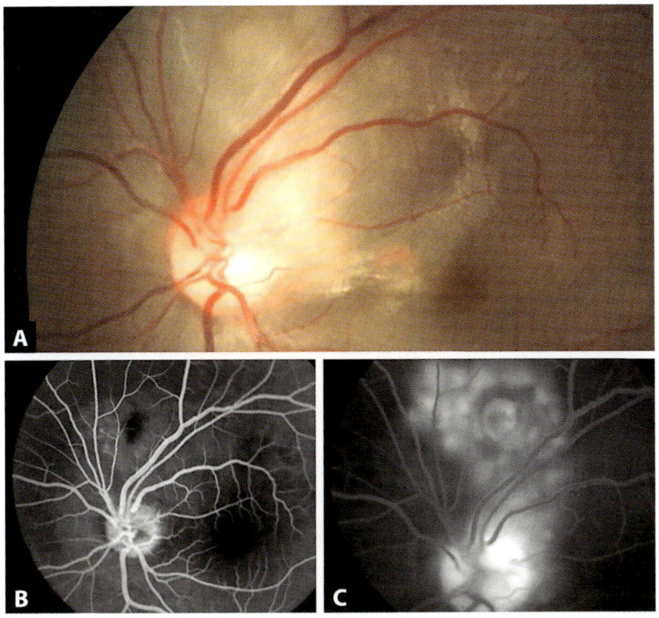

Figs. 24A to C: Color fundus photograph and fluorescein angiography at baseline. (A) Color fundus photograph [FF450plus camera (Carl Zeiss Meditec AG, Jena, Germany)] of the left eye (OS) of a patient showing multiple bright yellow-orangish subretinal nodular lesions half to one disc diameter (DD) in size, superior and superotemporal to the optic disc, accompanied by optic disc edema and an exudative retinal detachment; (B) Fundus fluorescein angiography [FF450plus camera (Carl Zeiss Meditec AG, Jena, Germany)] of the OS showed pinpoint leaks in the early phases with (C) hypofluorescent spots that exhibit intralesional hyperfluorescence in the late phases, suggestive of choroidal involvement.

Source: Presented by Ronnie Abhishek in the International Uveitis Study Group (IUSG) grand rounds.[10]

Fundus examination showed disc edema and multiple choroidal granulomas at different locations. The OD also showed a choroidal lesion in the inferior temporal region. The OCT showed full-thickness choroidal involvement and subretinal hyperreflective material through these lesions **(Figs. 26A to D)**. Moreover, the FFA showed intralesional hyperfluorescence in the later phases, suggesting choroidal involvement with subvascular lesions from the earlier episode **(Figs. 27A and B)**.

TABLE 2: Physical examination of the patient having TB choroidal granuloma.

OD	***Parameters***	***OS***
20/20	BCVA	20/40
11 mm Hg	IOP	11 mm Hg
Quiet	Conjunctiva	Quiet
Normal, clear	Cornea	Normal, clear
No cells ACC: 0+	Anterior chamber	No cells ACC: 0+
No synechiae	Iris	No synechiae
Clear	Lens	Clear
Unremarkable	Vitreous	Unremarkable
Unremarkable	Fundus	Subretinal nodular lesions, which are superior to the disc with optic disc edema and exudative retinal detachment

(ACC: anterior chamber cellularity; BCVA: best-corrected visual acuity; IOP: intraocular pressure; TB: tuberculosis)

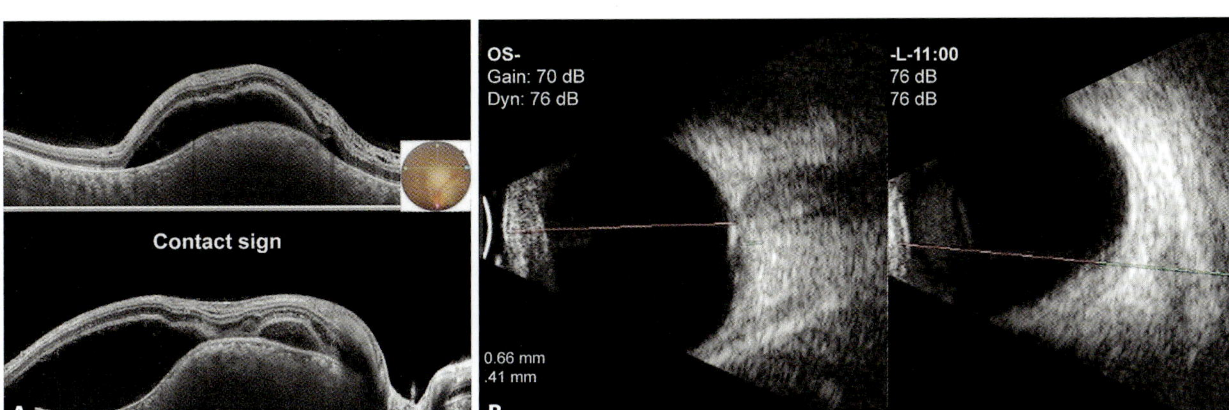

Figs. 25A and B: Optical coherence tomography (OCT) and B-scan ultrasound. (A) Swept-source OCT (Topcon DRI OCT Triton® plus, Japan) 12 mm horizontal and vertical line scan passing through the lesion demonstrating a contact sign with neurosensory detachment and full-thickness choroidal elevation; (B) B-scan ultrasound (Marvel B Scan, Appasamy Associates, Chennai, India) axial and longitudinal scans showing choroidal thickening with subtenon fluid, suggestive of scleritis.

Source: Presented by Ronnie Abhishek in the International Uveitis Study Group (IUSG) grand rounds.[10]

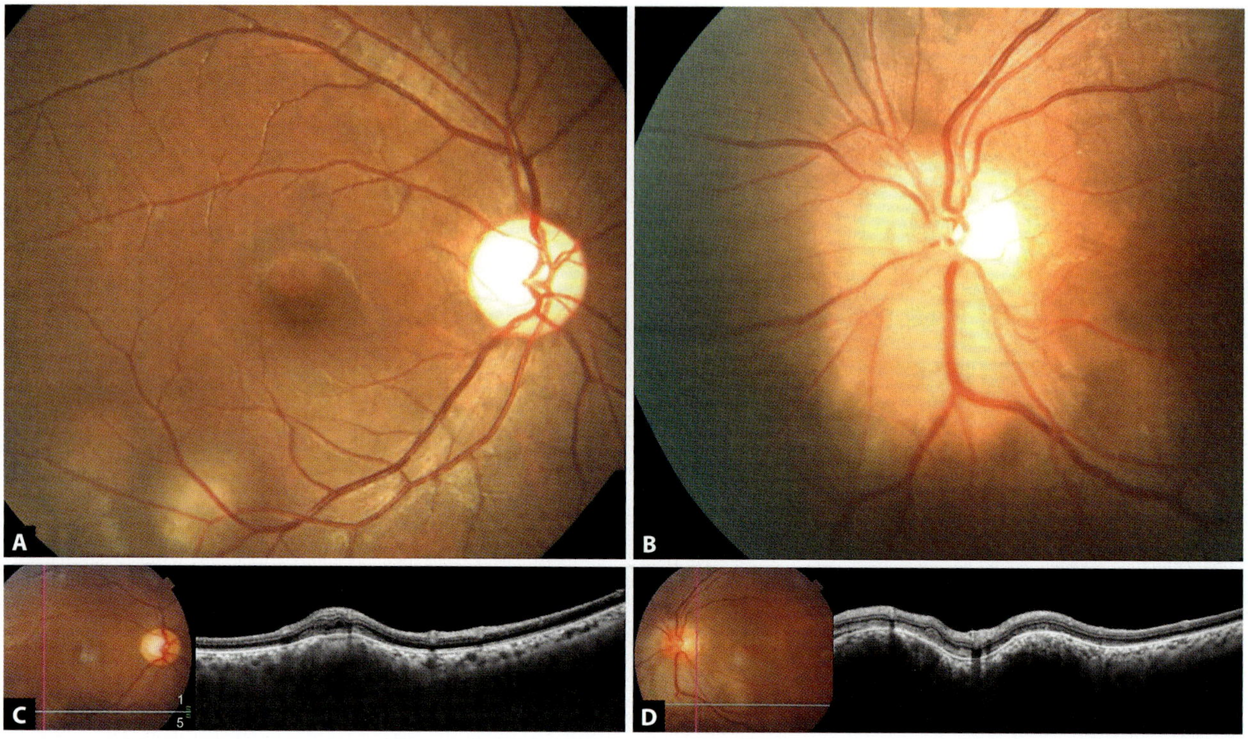

Figs. 26A to D: Color fundus photographs and optical coherence tomography (OCT) at 4-month follow-up. (A and B) Color fundus photographs [FF450plus camera (Carl Zeiss Meditec AG, Jena, Germany)] showing in the OD a dull yellowish choroidal lesion along the inferior temporal arcade 0.5 DD in size and in the OS with disc edema and multiple bright yellow-orangish choroidal granulomas inferior to the disc; (C and D) Swept-source OCT (Topcon DRI OCT Triton® plus, Japan) images documenting a full-thickness choroidal involvement of the lesions.

Source: Presented by Ronnie Abhishek in the International Uveitis Study Group (IUSG) grand rounds.[10]

The patient was started on azathioprine 100 mg while continuing ATT and tapering prednisolone. After 1 month, the lesions had completely resolved, and the BCVA in the OS improved to 20/25 **(Figs. 28A to D)**.

Five years and 8 months later, the patient returned with complaints of decreased vision, redness, and pain in the OD. Visual acuity was 20/60 in OD and 20/40 in the OS. The examination of the left eye (OS) was unremarkable. However, in the OD, there was conjunctival redness, 2+ anterior chamber cells, iris nodules, and posterior synechiae. Fundus examination revealed a subretinal lesion suggestive of a choroidal granuloma **(Figs. 29A to C)**.

Uveitis workup:
- Quantiferon-TB Gold: Negative
- HRCT of the thorax: Normal
- TPHA: Negative

Treatment: The patient was restarted on ATT along with tapering doses of oral prednisolone. Within 1 month, the lesions had completely resolved, and the CME subsided with no further inflammatory activity.

Final follow-up: After 1 year (6 years and 8 months after the initial assessment), the BCVA was 20/20 both eyes, with no further recurrence.

Case 2

Personal data: Male, 37 years old.

History of present illness: The patient reported a decrease in vision in the OD over the past week.

Physical examination: Visual acuity in the OD was limited to counting fingers. The conjunctiva was quiet, cornea was clear, and there was no evidence of anterior chamber inflammation or synechiae. Fundoscopy of the OD revealed a nodular subretinal lesion temporal to the optic disc, retinal whitening, optic disc edema, and an exudative retinal detachment. The OS examination was unremarkable **(Fig. 30)**.

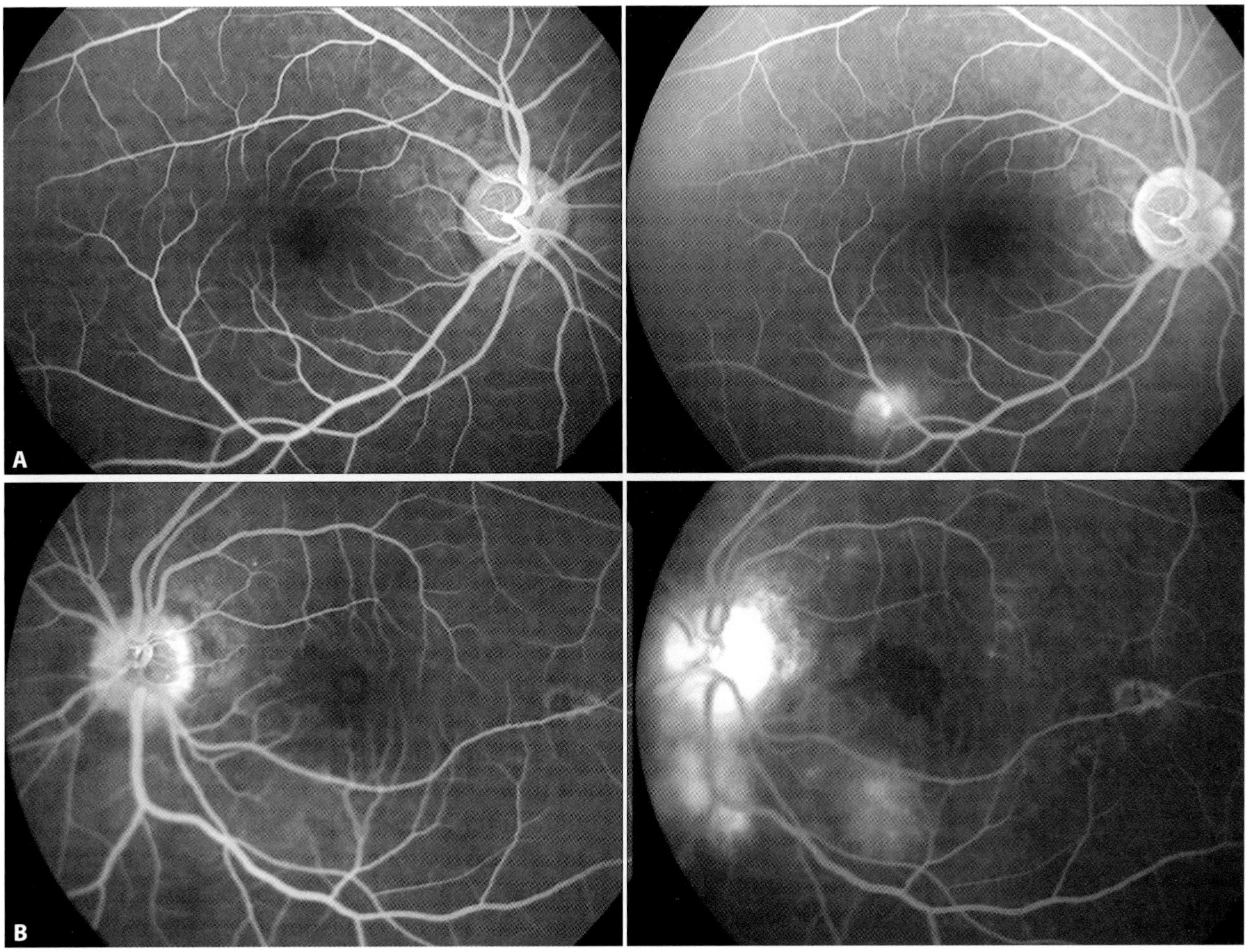

Figs. 27A and B: Fundus fluorescein angiography at 4-month follow-up. (A) Fundus fluorescein angiography [FF450plus camera (Carl Zeiss Meditec AG, Jena, Germany)] OD with hypofluorescent spots in the inferior arcade in the early phase (left) turn to intralesional hyperfluorescence, suggestive of choroidal involvement (right). (B) OS with subvascular lesion, which was from the earlier episode.
Source: Presented by Ronnie Abhishek in the International Uveitis Study Group (IUSG) grand rounds.[10]

B-scan ultrasound of the right eye demonstrated nodular thickening of the sclerochoroidal complex, characterized by moderate-to-high outer reflectivity and lower inner reflectivity. Additionally, a T-sign was noted, indicating fluid suggestive of scleral involvement **(Fig. 31)**.

Treatment: The patient was started on intravenous methylprednisolone 500 mg for 3 days, followed by tapering doses of oral prednisolone.

Follow-up: After 10 days of treatment, the patient's vision improved to counting fingers at 2 m, with almost complete lesion resolution. However, 4 months later, he returned with complaints of pain and hazy vision in the OD, with a BCVA of 20/320. Fundus examination revealed findings like the initial presentation **(Figs. 32A and B)**.

A further uveitis workup revealed a normal erythrocyte sedimentation rate (7 mm in the first hour) and no systemic abnormalities. The Mantoux test was negative. The patient also reported a history of TB contact from an eyebrow lesion 2–3 years earlier. Based on these findings, the patient was started on a four-drug ATT regimen without corticosteroids.

Two weeks after initiating ATT, the collateral lesion had completely resolved with ATT alone. Five months post-treatment, the patient remained stable. Three years later, the patient presented again with diminished vision in the right eye, with a BCVA of 20/125. He was once more started on ATT monotherapy without immunosuppression. After 2 weeks, the lesion resolved completely, and the patient remained recurrence free for 1.5 years **(Fig. 33)**.

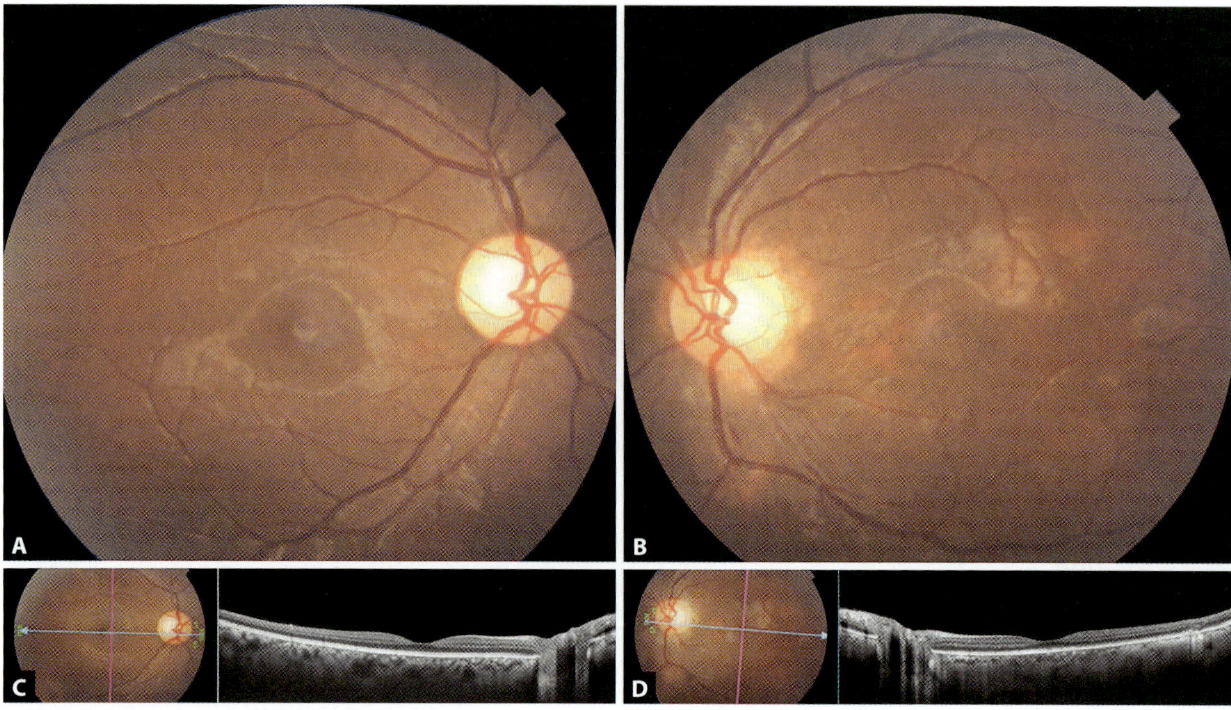

Figs. 28A to D: Color fundus photographs and optical coherence tomography (OCT) following 1 month of antituberculosis therapy (ATT), prednisolone, and azathioprine. (A and B) Color fundus photograph [FF450plus camera (Carl Zeiss Meditec AG, Jena, Germany)] images showing completely resolved lesions in both eyes with (C and D) organization of retinal layers and resolution of choroidal lesions in the swept-source OCT (Topcon DRI OCT Triton® plus, Japan).
Source: Presented by Ronnie Abhishek in the International Uveitis Study Group (IUSG) grand rounds.[10]

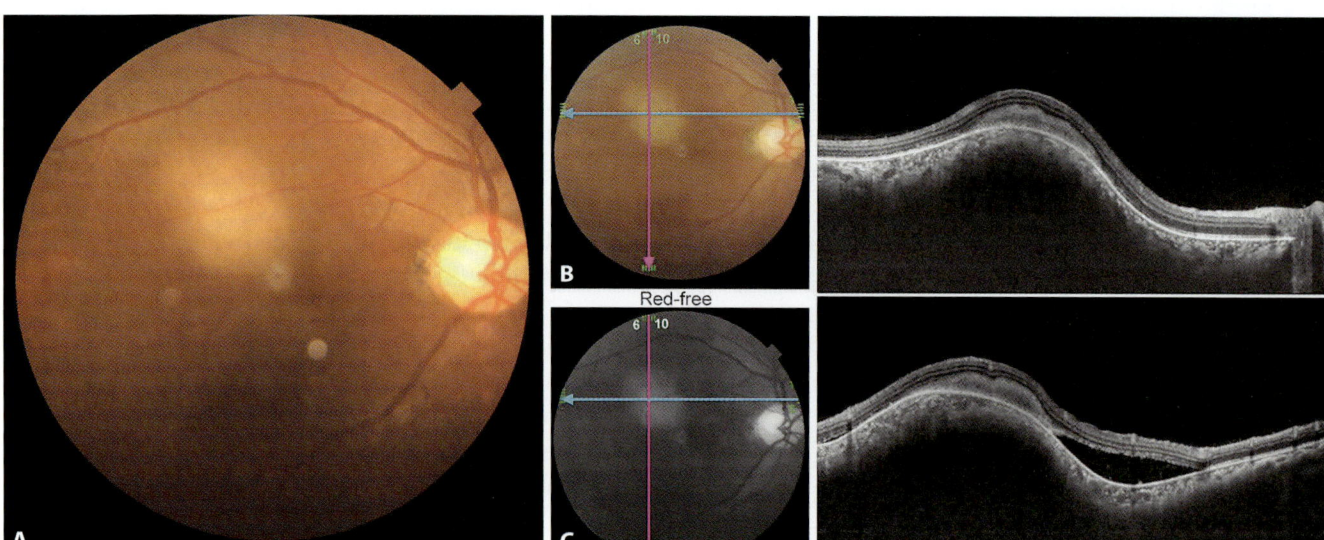

Figs. 29A to C: Color fundus photograph of the OS 5 years and 8 months after the first assessment. (A) Color fundus photograph [FF450plus camera (Carl Zeiss Meditec AG, Jena, Germany)] showing in the OD a dull yellowish choroidal lesion superotemporal to fovea 1 DD in size; (B and C) Swept-source optical coherence tomography (OCT) (Topcon DRI OCT Triton® plus, Japan) 12 mm horizontal and vertical line scan passing through the lesion demonstrating a contact sign with neurosensory detachment and full-thickness choroidal elevation.
Source: Presented by Ronnie Abhishek in the International Uveitis Study Group (IUSG) grand rounds.[10]

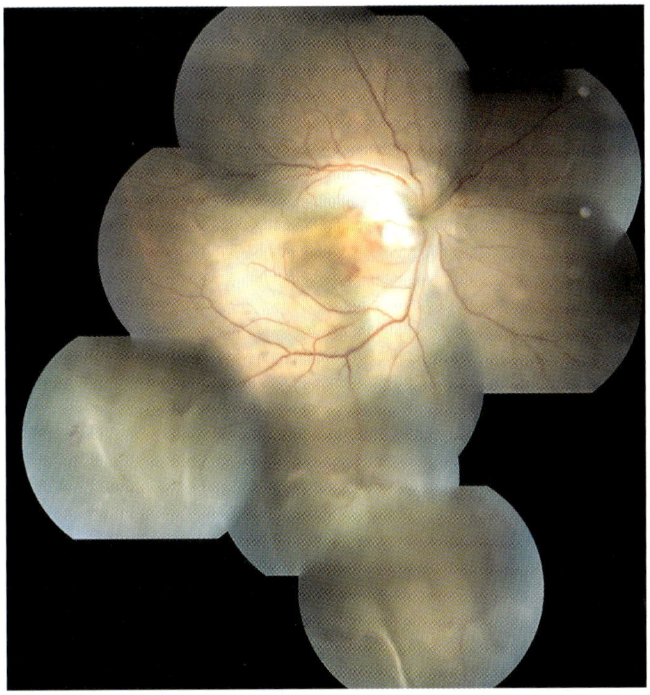

Fig. 30: Fundoscopy examination. Montage color fundus photograph [FF450plus camera (Carl Zeiss Meditec AG, Jena, Germany)] of the OD showing a bright yellow-orange nodular subretinal lesion 4 DD in size temporal to the optic disc, accompanied by retinal whitening, optic disc edema, and an exudative retinal detachment.

Source: Presented by Ronnie Abhishek in the International Uveitis Study Group (IUSG) grand rounds.[10]

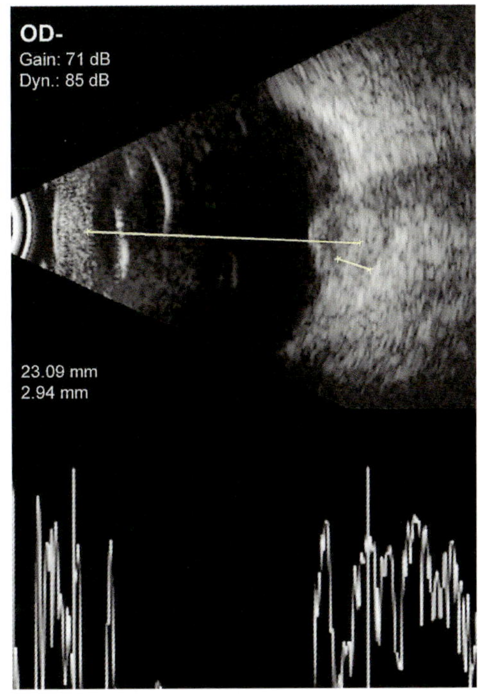

Fig. 31: B-scan ultrasound at baseline. B-scan ultrasound (Marvel B Scan, Appasamy Associates, Chennai, India) axial scan showing nodular thickening of the sclerochoroidal complex, characterized by moderate-to-high outer reflectivity and lower inner reflectivity, along with the presence of a T-sign, indicating fluid suggestive of scleral involvement.

Source: Presented by Ronnie Abhishek in the International Uveitis Study Group (IUSG) grand rounds.[10]

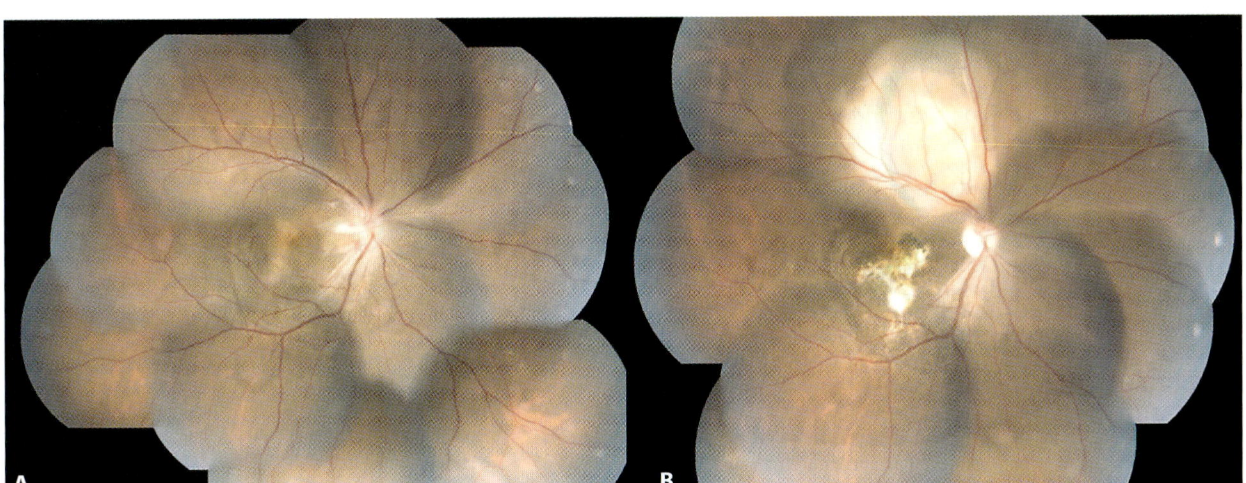

Figs. 32A and B: Color fundus photograph 10 days after corticosteroid pulses and 4-month follow-up. (A) Montage color fundus photograph [FF450plus camera (Carl Zeiss Meditec AG, Jena, Germany)] of the OD showing almost complete lesion resolution; (B) Montage color fundus photograph [FF450plus camera (Carl Zeiss Meditec AG, Jena, Germany)] of the OD at 4-month follow-up, revealing a bright yellowish subretinal lesion (at a different location) superior to the disc 7 DD in size.

Source: Presented by Ronnie Abhishek in the International Uveitis Study Group (IUSG) grand rounds.[10]

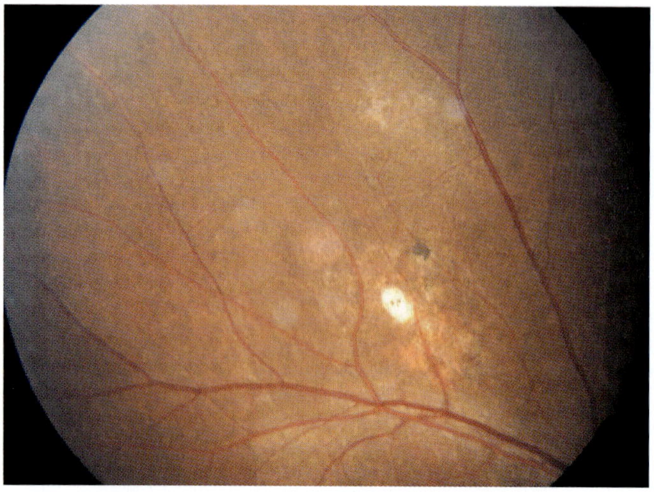

Fig. 33: Follow-up fundoscopy. Color fundus photograph [FF450plus camera (Carl Zeiss Meditec AG, Jena, Germany)]. The new lesion resolved completely within 2 weeks of initiating antituberculosis therapy (ATT).

Source: Presented by Ronnie Abhishek in the International Uveitis Study Group (IUSG) grand rounds.[10]

Discussion

One of the major issues highlighted by these cases is the post-ATT recurrence of inflammation. In such instances, several critical factors must be considered, including drug compliance, the possibility of a nontuberculous etiology, and drug resistance. When dealing with recurrent drug-susceptible TB, it could either be due to reactivation or reinfection. Typically, reactivation occurs early in the disease course, while reinfection manifests much later. Relapse is essentially a combination of both reactivation and reinfection.

Another essential concept is endogenous reactivation at an extrapulmonary site. In a study from Mexico, autopsy findings in individuals with no known history of TB showed mycobacterial DNA in the reticuloendothelial cells of various organs, including the liver, spleen, kidneys, and brain.[41,42] Although the eye was not studied, this raises the possibility that ocular tissues, specifically the RPE, might serve as a similar reservoir for mycobacteria. Professor Narsing Rao's histopathological study in 2006 provided evidence of mycobacteria residing within the RPE, suggesting that the RPE may serve as an anatomical niche for TB in the eye.[7]

The RPE, with its excellent phagocytic ability, functions similarly to macrophages, and thus may serve as a potential harbor for mycobacteria. However, unlike macrophages, mycobacteria seem to survive longer within the RPE cells, likely due to the RPE's high tolerance to oxidative stress and its resistance to antibiotics.[42,43] Beyond the RPE, other ocular cells may also harbor mycobacteria, particularly choroidal macrophages, and perivascular macrophages, which are abundant around retinal blood vessels. These cells could also serve as reservoirs, contributing to recurrent inflammation even after ATT.

When dealing with late persistent or recurrent inflammation, it is critical to first confirm whether TB is truly the underlying cause. This often requires a careful review of the clinical pattern and additional or repeat laboratory testing. If inflammation persists, drug resistance should also be considered. Testing for resistance can be performed molecularly, which is common in ocular samples or through conventional bacteriological techniques.[44]

Once non-TB etiology and drug resistance have been ruled out, we need to decide whether persistent/recurrent inflammation is related to mycobacterial infection. The likelihood of mycobacterial infection increases if the recurrence has a granulomatous appearance such as a choroidal granuloma or nodular scleritis or granulomatous anterior uveitis. This is based on the hypothesis that mycobacteria may persist in an anatomical niche, possibly within the RPE or other tissues such as choroid, and could be responsible for reactivation and recurrent inflammation after the completion of ATT. Such patients require a repeat course of anti-TB therapy. In other scenarios, such as nongranulomatous anterior uveitis, vitritis, or episcleritis, we tend to treat with anti-inflammatory therapy alone, local, and/or systemic and may also include IMT.

PEARLS FROM THE EXPERTS ON FREQUENTLY ASKED QUESTIONS

1. Intermediate uveitis associated with TB is known for its high recurrence rate. Is there an endogenous recurrence model specifically for TB-related intermediate uveitis?

Answer: The intermediate uveitis in question is likely not caused by TB; other etiologies must be excluded.

2. Are cases of tubercular neuroretinitis with severe optic disc edema common?

Answer: No, such cases are not common but have been reported in the literature.

3. Ethambutol toxicity is often underdiagnosed. What is your opinion on this?

Answer: We agree. Ethambutol toxicity is indeed highly underdiagnosed and requires greater awareness and vigilance.

4. In cases requiring both ATT and oral steroids, do you initiate both treatments concurrently or do you start ATT first and follow-up with oral steroids a week later?
Answer: If the phenotype is typically immune, such as in SLC, I start steroids at the same time or sometimes even before ATT, especially if the lesions are very close to the fovea and threaten vision. ATT can be added later, as it prevents recurrences rather than treating an active ID. The immune mechanism often requires steroids for proper management.

5. In cases of tubercular occlusive retinal vasculitis, should one wait 1 or 2 weeks for oral steroids to take effect before performing laser treatment, given the risk of inflammation worsening?
Answer: Yes, you can administer anti-VEGF if new vessels are present, but laser treatment should only be performed once the inflammation is under control.

6. In the case of TB retinal vasculitis, would subconjunctival triamcinolone be as effective or inferior in comparison to intravitreal dexamethasone?
Answer: Intravitreal dexamethasone is more effective and is less likely to increase IOP. Sometimes, TB retinal vasculitis may be associated with the formation of new vessels, and anti-VEGF treatment would be preferred.

7. How common are complications of tuberculous uveitis? Specifically, how common are cataracts and glaucoma in tuberculous uveitis cases?
Answer: These complications are not very common. They tend to occur in cases with panuveitis that have not received ATT.

8. How can one differentiate between ED and TB-related retinal vasculitis?
Answer: In most cases of TB, occlusive retinal vasculitis is present. Thanks to the COTS, the current terminology for occlusive TB vasculitis is TB retinal vasculitis. Historically, ED also referred to cases of nonocclusive vasculitis, a key distinction.

9. Can a vitreous biopsy be performed for presumed OTB for cytology and microbiology?
Answer: We generally do not perform a vitrectomy in such cases due to the low sensitivity of microbiological tests for TB, at least in nonendemic countries.

10. Can SLC affect only the perimacular zone (posterior pole)?
Answer: TB-associated SLC is mostly seen in the posterior pole and not in the peripapillary region, as with SC.

11. For Dr. Sudarshan's case 3, since both Mantoux and QuantiFERON tests were negative, why was ATT initiated? Could the improvement be due to IMT?
Answer: Phenotypically, the case resembled TB. In some patients, QuantiFERON tests can be negative. The inflammation was recurring aggressively despite the use of steroids. IMT was started only after paradoxical worsening.

12. In cases of late recurrence, should we start another ATT course?
Answer: Topical treatments are sufficient if there is only an anterior segment recurrence. Immunosuppression and steroids should be considered if there is vitritis and some vascular leakage. In cases of SLC recurrence or granuloma recurrence, reinfection should be considered. It is essential to test for TB; if reinfection is suspected, a second course of ATT should be added. It is also crucial to verify that the patient has complied with the initial treatment and completed the first course of ATT.

13. What is your opinion on intravitreal injections of steroids or methotrexate for macular edema?
Answer: Intravitreal Ozurdex can be administered for both paradoxical worsening and macular edema, but adequate coverage with ATT is necessary. Local injections should be avoided in cases involving large granulomas, as they may indicate multibacillary disease, in which local steroids are contraindicated. Methotrexate has a very short half-life and requires close monitoring when used.

14. How long would you continue IMT in cases of paradoxical reactivation?
Answer: IMT is typically continued for about a year, with regular monitoring using FFA and ICGA to ensure the disease is inactive before stopping treatment.

15. In non-HIV patients, do CD4 cell counts, CD3/CD4 ratios, or any other immune markers correlate with the treatment response to ATT in TB or the prognosis of OTB?
Answer: We are unsure if these markers play a role, as we do not routinely test them in non-HIV patients. They are considered only in cases where the patient has multiple infections or if the condition worsens despite proven treatment.

16. Is there any indication for restarting ATT in a patient with OTB, or do we always augment immunosuppression in patients previously treated with ATT?
Answer: Topical treatments may suffice if there is only recurrence in the anterior segment. However, IMT and

corticosteroids should be considered in cases of vitritis with some vascular leakage. If there is a recurrence of SLC or granuloma, this could indicate reinfection, and it is recommended to repeat TB testing. If reinfection is suspected, a second course of ATT should be added. It is also essential to verify that the patient was compliant with the initial course of treatment and completed the full course.

17. In a patient with active intermediate tubercular uveitis, treated with anti-TB medication, steroids, and immunosuppressants, who completed a 6-month course of ATT but still has persistent low-grade inflammation, should we restart another cycle of ATT or increase the immunosuppressant dosage?

Answer: No, I would increase immunosuppression. In some cases, pars plana vitrectomy helps to clear the media and reduce the need for immunosuppression.

18. In a severe case of presumed OTB with bilateral panuveitis, complicated by total cataract, macular edema, and hypotony (6 mm Hg), with partial response to ATT and azathioprine, is there a role for biological treatment to prepare for cataract surgery? Or is biological treatment contraindicated in OTB?

Answer: You can administer Ozurdex during cataract surgery. However, biological treatments carry a risk of reactivating systemic TB and, therefore, should be avoided.

19. Do you routinely perform a chest CT scan on all your ocular TB patients, given its higher sensitivity (90%)? Is it advisable to perform routine chest CT scans?

Answer: Yes, this is to look for evidence of old infection, including calcified hilar nodes or Ghon's focus.

20. When a chest scan is needed, is it better to request a contrast-enhanced computed tomography (CECT) or an HRCT? Is there any basic rule to determine which one to send in each case?

Answer: CECT is generally preferred in most cases.

21. Does occlusive vasculitis in OTB often affect the central (posterior pole) as well?

Answer: Rarely, mainly, it affects the periphery.

FINAL WRAP-UP

In conclusion, this chapter highlights the complexity of diagnosing and managing OTB due to its varied clinical manifestations. It can affect multiple parts of the eye, with presentations ranging from anterior uveitis to posterior segment inflammation, including SLC, choroidal tubercles, and retinal vasculitis. ATT and corticosteroids are crucial for controlling inflammation and preventing recurrence. However, challenges such as paradoxical worsening, recurrence after ATT, and the need for careful diagnostic workup are also significant considerations.

Moreover, the chapter underscores the importance of utilizing multimodal imaging techniques such as fundus photography, fluorescein angiography, and OCT to monitor disease progression and treatment response. Collaboration with ID specialists is critical, ensuring appropriate use of ATT based on indirect evidence such as immunological tests and radiological findings. Ultimately, the chapter highlighted the need for a tailored approach to treatment, recognizing the diverse presentations and the possibility of reactivation or autoimmune inflammation post-treatment.

REFERENCES

1. Alli HD, Ally N, Mayet I, Dangor Z, Madhi SA. Global prevalence and clinical outcomes of tubercular uveitis: a systematic review and meta-analysis. Surv Ophthalmol. 2022;67(3):770-92.
2. Putera I, La Distia Nora R, Utami N, Karuniawati A, Yasmon A, Wulandari D, et al. The impact of aqueous humor polymerase chain reaction and serological test results for establishing infectious uveitis diagnosis: an Indonesian experience. Heliyon. 2022;8(10):e10988.
3. Dogra M, Singh R, Agarwal A, Sharma A, Singh SR, Gautam N, et al. Epidemiology of uveitis in a tertiary-care referral institute in North India. Ocul Immunol Inflamm. 2017;25(sup1):S46-53.
4. Moule MG, Cirillo JD. *Mycobacterium tuberculosis* dissemination plays a critical role in pathogenesis. Front Cell Infect Microbiol. 2020;10:65.
5. Heiden D, Saranchuk P, Keenan JD, Ford N, Lowinger A, Yen M, et al. Eye examination for early diagnosis of disseminated tuberculosis in patients with AIDS. Lancet Infect Dis. 2016;16(4):493-9.
6. Detrick B, Hooks JJ. The RPE Cell and the Immune System. In: Klettner AK, Dithmar S (Eds). Retinal Pigment Epithelium in Health and Disease. Cham: Springer International Publishing; 2020. pp. 101-14.
7. Rao NA, Saraswathy S, Smith RE. Tuberculous uveitis: distribution of *Mycobacterium tuberculosis* in the retinal pigment epithelium. Arch Ophthalmol. 2006;124(12):1777-9.
8. Gupta V, Gupta A, Rao NA. Intraocular tuberculosis—an update. Surv Ophthalmol. 2007;52(6):561-87.
9. Gupta V, Shoughy SS, Mahajan S, Khairallah M, Rosenbaum JT, Curi A, et al. Clinics of ocular tuberculosis. Ocul Immunol Inflamm. 2015;23(1):14-24.

10. International Uveitis Study Group (IUSG). (2024). Uveitis Webinar—Grand Round 7. WEBINAR 37: Ocular Tuberculosis: Case-Based Approach. [online] Available from https://iusg.net/past-iusg-grand-rounds/. (www.youtube.com/watch?v=Pe8YOcLP6jk). [Last accessed February, 2025].
11. Gupta V, Gupta A, Arora S, Bambery P, Dogra MR, Agarwal A. Presumed tubercular serpiginouslike choroiditis: clinical presentations and management. Ophthalmology. 2003;110(9):1744-9.
12. Gupta K, Agarwal A, Arora A, Aggarwal K, Bansal R, Katoch D, et al. Multicolor confocal scanning laser ophthalmoscope imaging in posterior uveitis. Retina. 2022;42(7):1356-63.
13. Aggarwal K, Agarwal A, Deokar A, Singh R, Bansal R, Sharma A, et al. Ultra-wide field imaging in paradoxical worsening of tubercular multifocal serpiginoid choroiditis after the initiation of anti-tubercular therapy. Ocul Immunol Inflamm. 2019;27(3):365-70.
14. Gupta A, Bansal R, Gupta V, Sharma A. Fundus autofluorescence in serpiginouslike choroiditis. Retina. 2012;32(4):814-25.
15. Bansal R, Kulkarni P, Gupta A, Gupta V, Dogra MR. High-resolution spectral domain optical coherence tomography and fundus autofluorescence correlation in tubercular serpiginouslike choroiditis. J Ophthal Inflamm Infect. 2011;1(4):157-63.
16. Agarwal A, Aggarwal K, Pichi F, Meng T, Munk MR, Bazgain K, et al. Clinical and multimodal imaging clues in differentiating between tuberculomas and sarcoid choroidal granulomas. Am J Ophthalmol. 2021;226:42-55.
17. Agarwal A, Mahajan S, Khairallah M, Mahendradas P, Gupta A, Gupta V. Multimodal imaging in ocular tuberculosis. Ocul Immunol Inflamm. 2017;25(1):134-45.
18. Agarwal A, Agrawal R, Gunasekaran DV, Raje D, Gupta B, Aggarwal K, et al. The collaborative ocular tuberculosis study (COTS)-1 report 3: polymerase chain reaction in the diagnosis and management of tubercular uveitis: global trends. Ocul Immunol Inflamm. 2019;27(3):465-73.
19. Lalvani A, Pareek M. A 100 year update on diagnosis of tuberculosis infection. Br Med Bull. 2010;93:69-84.
20. World Health Assembly. (2014). Report on the financial and administrative implications for the Secretariat of resolutions proposed for adoption by the Executive Board or the Health Assembly. [online] Available from https://iris.who.int/handle/10665/162911. [Last accessed February, 2025].
21. Fernández-Zamora Y, Finamor LP, Silva LMP, Rodrigues DS, Casaroli-Marano RP, Muccioli C. Role of interferon-gamma release assay for the diagnosis and clinical follow up in ocular tuberculosis. Ocul Immunol Inflamm. 2023;31(2):304-11.
22. Testi I, Agrawal R, Mahajan S, Agarwal A, Gunasekeran DV, Raje D, et al. Tubercular uveitis: Nuggets from Collaborative Ocular Tuberculosis Study (COTS)-1. Ocul Immunol Inflamm. 2020;28(sup1):8-16.
23. Mehta S. Patterns of systemic uptake of 18-FDG with positron emission tomography/computed tomography (PET/CT) studies in patients with presumed ocular tuberculosis. Ocul Immunol Inflamm. 2012;20(6):434-7.
24. Agrawal R, Testi I, Mahajan S, Yuen YS, Agarwal A, Kon OM, et al. Collaborative ocular tuberculosis study consensus guidelines on the management of tubercular uveitis–report 1: guidelines for initiating antitubercular therapy in tubercular choroiditis. Ophthalmology. 2021;128(2):266-76.
25. Agrawal R, Testi I, Bodaghi B, Barisani-Asenbauer T, McCluskey P, Agarwal A, et al. Collaborative ocular tuberculosis study consensus guidelines on the management of tubercular uveitis–report 2: guidelines for initiating antitubercular therapy in anterior uveitis, intermediate uveitis, panuveitis, and retinal vasculitis. Ophthalmology. 2021;128(2):277-87.
26. Agrawal R, Ludi Z, Betzler BK, Testi I, Mahajan S, Rousellot A, et al. The collaborative ocular tuberculosis study (COTS) calculator–a consensus-based decision tool for initiating antitubercular therapy in ocular tuberculosis. Eye (Lond). 2023;37(7):1416-23.
27. Oehlers SH, Cronan MR, Scott NR, Thomas MI, Okuda KS, Walton EM, et al. Interception of host angiogenic signalling limits mycobacterial growth. Nature. 2015;517(7536):612-5.
28. Agarwal M, Gupta C, Mohan KV, Upadhyay PK, Dhawan A, Jha V. Adjunctive intravitreal anti-vascular endothelial growth factor and moxifloxacin therapy in management of intraocular tubercular granulomas. Ocul Immunol Inflamm. 2023;31(1):158-67.
29. Agarwal A, Deokar A, Sharma R, Singh N, Aggarwal K, Sharma S, et al. Longitudinal analysis of serum cytokine profile among patients with tubercular multifocal serpiginoid choroiditis: a pilot study. Eye (Lond). 2019;33(1):129-35.
30. Agarwal A, Handa S, Aggarwal K, Sharma M, Singh R, Sharma A, et al. The role of dexamethasone implant in the management of tubercular uveitis. Ocul Immunol Inflamm. 2018;26(6):884-92.
31. Julian K, Langner-Wegscheider BJ, Haas A, De Smet MD. Intravitreal methotrexate in the management of presumed tuberculous serpiginous-like choroiditis. Retina. 2013;33(9):1943-8.
32. Kawali A, Bavaharan B, Sanjay S, Mohan A, Mahendradas P, Shetty R. Serpiginous-like choroiditis (SLC)—morphology and treatment outcomes. Ocul Immunol Inflamm. 2020;28(4):667-75.
33. Bansal R, Gupta A, Gupta V, Dogra MR, Bambery P, Arora SK. Role of anti-tubercular therapy in uveitis with latent/manifest tuberculosis. Am J Ophthalmol. 2008;146(5):772-9.
34. Forrester JV, Kuffova L, Dick AD. Autoimmunity, autoinflammation, and infection in uveitis. Am J Ophthalmol. 2018;189:77-85.
35. Tagirasa R, Parmar S, Barik MR, Devadas S, Basu S. Autoreactive T cells in immunopathogenesis of

TB-associated uveitis. Invest Ophthalmol Vis Sci. 2017;58(13):5682-91.

36. Ireni S, Mooss VS, Kelgaonkar A, Babu K, Basu S. Tubercular serpiginous-like choroiditis in patients with negative TB-immunoreactivity tests. Ocul Immunol Inflamm. 2024;32(8):1549-55.
37. Mehta S. Utility of computed chest tomography (CT scan) in recurrent uveitis. Indian J Ophthalmol. 2004;52(4):321-2.
38. Ganesh SK, Abraham S, Sudharshan S. Paradoxical reactions in ocular tuberculosis. J Ophthal Inflamm Infect. 2019;9(1):19.
39. Hoyt C. BJO at a glance. Br J Ophthalmol. 2002;86(12):1323.
40. Martínez-Rubio C, López-Corell PM, Pascual-Camps I, Gallego-Pinazo R, Dolz-Marco R, Díaz-Llopis M. The best of the year in uveitis 2017. Pan Am J Ophthalmol. 2018;17(4):98-104.
41. El-Asrar AMA, Al-Kharashi SA. Full panretinal photocoagulation and early vitrectomy improve prognosis of retinal vasculitis associated with tuberculoprotein hypersensitivity (Eales' disease). Br J Ophthalmol. 2002; 86(11):1248-51.
42. Barrios-Payán J, Saqui-Salces M, Jeyanathan M, Alcántara-Vazquez A, Castañon-Arreola M, Rook G, et al. Extrapulmonary locations of mycobacterium tuberculosis DNA during latent infection. J Infect Dis. 2012; 206(8):1194-205.
43. Nazari H, Karakousis PC, Rao NA. Replication of Mycobacterium tuberculosis in retinal pigment epithelium. JAMA Ophthalmol. 2014;132(6):724-9.
44. Liu R, Dang JN, Lee R, Lee JJ, Kesavamoorthy N, Ameri H, et al. Mycobacterium dormancy and antibiotic tolerance within the retinal pigment epithelium of ocular tuberculosis. Microbiol Spectr. 2024;12(8):e0078824.

CHAPTER

8 Ocular Syphilis

Mark Westcott, Ahmed Sallam, Francesco Pichi, Mudit Tyagi, Ahmed Shakarchi, Yanny Pérez Jimenez, Shravya Choudhary Bala, Germán Mejía-Salgado, Meghan Berkenstock, Reema Bansal, John H Kempen, Alejandra de-la-Torre, Vishali Gupta

INTRODUCTION

Syphilis is a sexually transmitted infection caused by the spirochete *Treponema pallidum*. Historically, it has been a significant public health concern, with periodic fluctuations in incidence. Over the past decade, there has been a resurgence of syphilis cases worldwide, particularly linked to unsafe sexual practices. This resurgence has been notably observed among men who have sex with men (MSM), a population at higher risk for sexually transmitted infections due to behavioral and epidemiological factors.[1] The countries most affected by this resurgence include the United Kingdom, several European countries, the United States, South Asia, and China.[1]

This chapter aims to provide a few practical, day-to-day tips for diagnosing and managing ocular syphilis.

PRACTICAL TIPS FOR MANAGING A PATIENT WITH OCULAR SYPHILIS

Classic Classification[2]

Syphilis can be classified into two broad categories: (1) Acquired and (2) Congenital. The acquired form of the disease follows a well-known progression through several stages given as follows:

- *Primary syphilis*: This is the initial stage, characterized by the appearance of a chancre at the site of infection.
- *Secondary syphilis*: It occurs after the primary stage and is marked by systemic symptoms, including skin rashes and mucocutaneous lesions.
- *Latent syphilis*: This stage is divided into early and late latency. Early latent syphilis occurs within 2 years of infection, while late latent syphilis occurs beyond this period. During latency, there are no clinical symptoms, but the infection remains active.
- *Tertiary syphilis*: If left untreated, syphilis may progress to the tertiary stage, characterized by the development of gummas—granulomatous lesions that can affect multiple organ systems.
- *Quaternary syphilis*: This advanced stage involves severe damage to the cardiovascular system (CVS) and central nervous system (CNS), leading to life-threatening complications.

In contrast, *congenital syphilis* is transmitted from an infected mother to the fetus. It can manifest as follows:

- *Early congenital syphilis*: Symptoms appear within the first few weeks or months of life.
- *Latent congenital syphilis*: The disease may remain asymptomatic for years before manifesting.
- *Late congenital syphilis*: This stage is characterized by significant physical and neurological stigmata, resulting from prolonged infection during fetal development.

The modern understanding of syphilis acknowledges significant overlap between its stages, particularly concerning CNS involvement. Ocular and otic involvement are now recognized as specific forms of neurosyphilis. These complications frequently occur concomitantly with secondary syphilis, although they can also present in other stages of the disease. In early or secondary phases, ocular involvement is associated with active inflammatory signs (such as anterior chamber cells, vitreous haze, and placoid lesions). Conversely, in late stages, such as tertiary syphilis, patients typically exhibit no signs of active inflammation but instead show sequelae such as optic nerve pallor or a pseudoretinitis pigmentosa pattern. Although tertiary syphilis can have ocular consequences, the focus remains on the active inflammatory manifestations seen in earlier stages, such as syphilitic uveitis, which requires prompt diagnosis and treatment to prevent severe visual loss.

Systemic Evaluation

Before utilizing the slit lamp for ocular examination, several systemic signs can serve as important clues for diagnosing syphilis. One notable indicator is the presence of a maculopapular rash, mainly when observed on the palms. This clinical finding highlights the importance of maintaining a broad diagnostic perspective, as ophthalmologists should focus on ocular manifestations and consider systemic signs that may guide diagnosis.

It is not uncommon for patients with syphilis to report hearing loss, often presenting as acute sensorineural hearing loss. When a patient presents with both uveitis and hearing loss, syphilis should always be considered as a potential diagnosis. This combination of symptoms warrants a thorough differential diagnosis, as several conditions can present similar findings. These include, but are not limited to, the following:

- Vogt–Koyanagi–Harada (VKH) syndrome
- Lyme disease
- Sarcoidosis
- Susac syndrome
- Granulomatosis with polyangiitis
- Cogan syndrome

Epidemiology

Syphilis remains an overwhelmingly male-dominated disease, mainly affecting men in regions such as the United Kingdom, Europe, the United States, and Asia. However, recent data show a gradual increase in the number of syphilis cases in both men and women. UK data, which closely reflect trends in Europe, reveal a steady rise in diagnoses over the past decade, with most cases occurring in men, while women are approximately eight times less common than in men. However, both sexes are seeing an overall increase in incidence.[3] When considering the epidemiology of syphilitic uveitis, the pattern closely mirrors that of syphilis in general.

Men who have sex with men represent the demographic most at risk, at 69% of all cases in the United Kingdom.[3] While the incidence of syphilis in men who have sex with women is lower, there has also been a slight increase in this population, though still significantly less than in MSM.

The epidemiology of ocular syphilis is far less understood. There is a notable lack of comprehensive data on this topic, with most information derived from single-center case series.

The British Ocular Syphilis Study (BOSS) was the first national prospective study conducted in the United Kingdom to investigate the manifestations of ocular syphilis.[4] This epidemiological survey, spanning 3 years from 2009 to 2011, aimed to characterize the disease's incidence, clinical presentation patterns, and treatment outcomes. The inclusion criteria required patients to present with active intraocular inflammation and positive treponemal serology, with the exclusion of late syphilis and other disorders.

A total of 41 cases were included, involving 63 eyes, with an annual UK incidence of 0.3 cases per million people. The disease was overwhelmingly more common in men, with a male-to-female ratio of 9:1. One of the key findings was the broad age distribution, with patients presenting syphilitic uveitis at ages ranging from 21 to 75 years, with a mean age of 49 years. This highlighted the importance of testing all adult patients with intraocular inflammation, as ocular syphilis is not confined to younger populations.[4]

Regarding treatment outcomes, the response to antimicrobial therapy was remarkably good, with 92% of patients achieving a final visual acuity of at least logarithm of the minimum angle of resolution (logMAR) 0.3. Approximately one-third of the patients were human immunodeficiency virus (HIV) positive, many of whom were newly diagnosed during their ophthalmologic evaluation. Notably, neither the presenting visual acuity nor the duration of symptoms significantly influenced the visual prognosis, underscoring the treatable nature of this disease.[4]

Anatomically, most patients presented with panuveitis, while others showed optic neuritis. Isolated anterior uveitis caused by treponemal disease was rare, indicating that syphilis typically involves the middle or posterior segments of the eye.

Clinical Phenotypes

Syphilitic uveitis presents with a wide spectrum of phenotypes, many of which can mimic other retinal or inflammatory diseases. The key phenotypes include:

- *Anterior and intermediate uveitis*

- *Posterior placoid chorioretinitis* **(*Figs. 1A to C*)**:
    - Characterized by large, well-circumscribed plaques at the posterior pole
    - Involves the choriocapillaris and retinal pigment epithelium (RPE), with distinctive dusky discoloration
    - Often associated with minimal anterior chamber activity and a relatively quiet eye
    - Optical coherence tomography (OCT) typically shows sub-RPE deposits and significant ellipsoid zone disruption, leading to poor visual acuity
    - The condition responds well to penicillin therapy, improving retinal structure and vision
- *Retinitis with vasculitis* **(*Fig. 2*)**:
    - It can closely mimic viral causes, such as acute retinal necrosis (ARN).
    - Typically presents with peripheral retinitis and vasculitis, often leading to diagnostic challenges.
    - Aqueous viral polymerase chain reaction (PCR) testing would be expected to be negative, but positive treponemal serology confirms syphilitic etiology.
- *Inner punctate retinitis (Funny white dots)* **(*Figs. 3A to C*)**:
    - A rare phenotype characterized by small, nummular foci at the junction between the vitreous and inner retina.
    - It likely represents collections of inflammatory cells or possibly treponemal organisms.
    - This unique presentation is uncommon and has few mimics.
- *Optic neuritis* **(*Figs. 4A and B*)**:
    - Syphilis can cause optic nerve swelling as a manifestation of optic neuritis, often associated with sensory neural hearing loss.

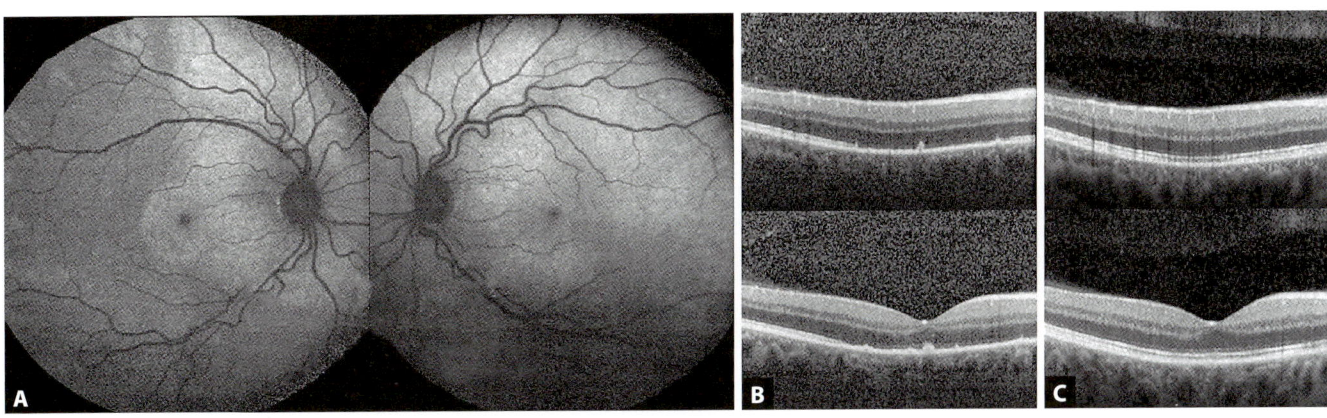

Figs. 1A to C: Posterior placoid chorioretinitis phenotype. (A) Autofluorescence imaging showing large, confluent hyperautofluorescent patches extending across the macula and involving the optic disc indicative of retinal pigment epithelium (RPE) involvement; (B) Optical coherence tomography (OCT) scans at presentation through the macula showing prominent sub-RPE deposits, which appeared as hyperreflective areas beneath the RPE. The ellipsoid zone was also disrupted, correlating with poor visual acuity (20/200 Snellen chart); (C) Repeat OCT scans following treatment with penicillin showed substantial restoration of the ellipsoid zone and resolution of the sub-RPE deposits. This recovery of retinal structure was accompanied by improved visual function.
Source: Presented by Mark Westcott in the International Uveitis Study Group (IUSG) grand rounds.[5]

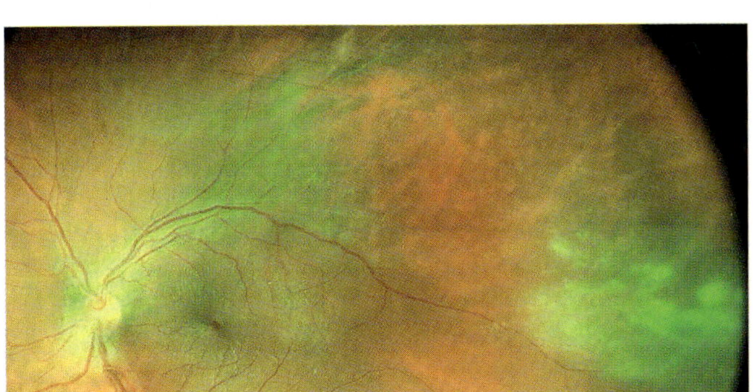

Fig. 2: Treponemal mimicking acute retinal necrosis. Color fundus photograph shows multiple white retinal lesions in the temporal periphery, accompanied by subtle vasculitis.
Source: Presented by Mark Westcott in the International Uveitis Study Group (IUSG) grand rounds.[5]

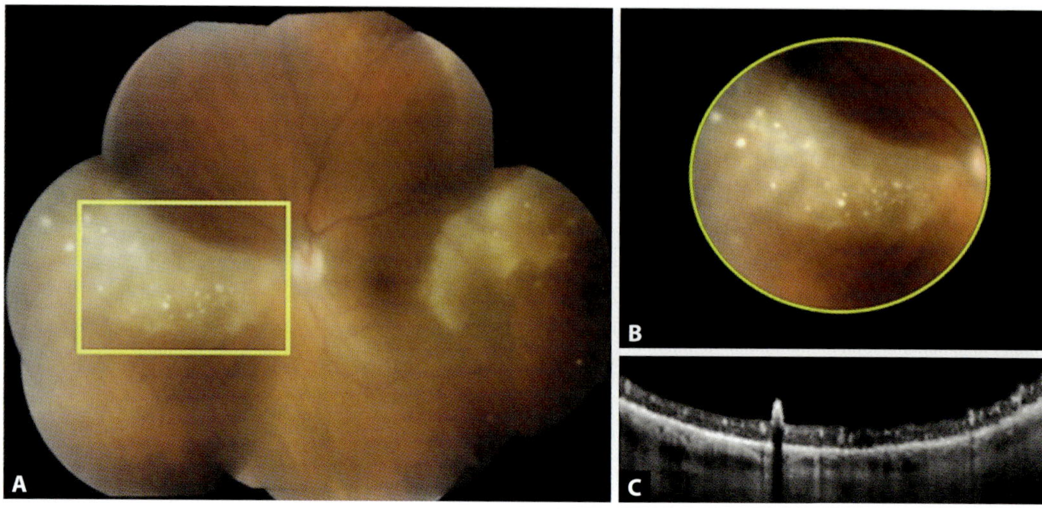

Figs. 3A to C: Inner punctate retinitis secondary to ocular syphilis. (A and B) Small, nummular white lesions scattered across the inner retina; (C) Primarily at the interface between the vitreous and the retina.
Source: Presented by Mark Westcott in the International Uveitis Study Group (IUSG) grand rounds.[5]

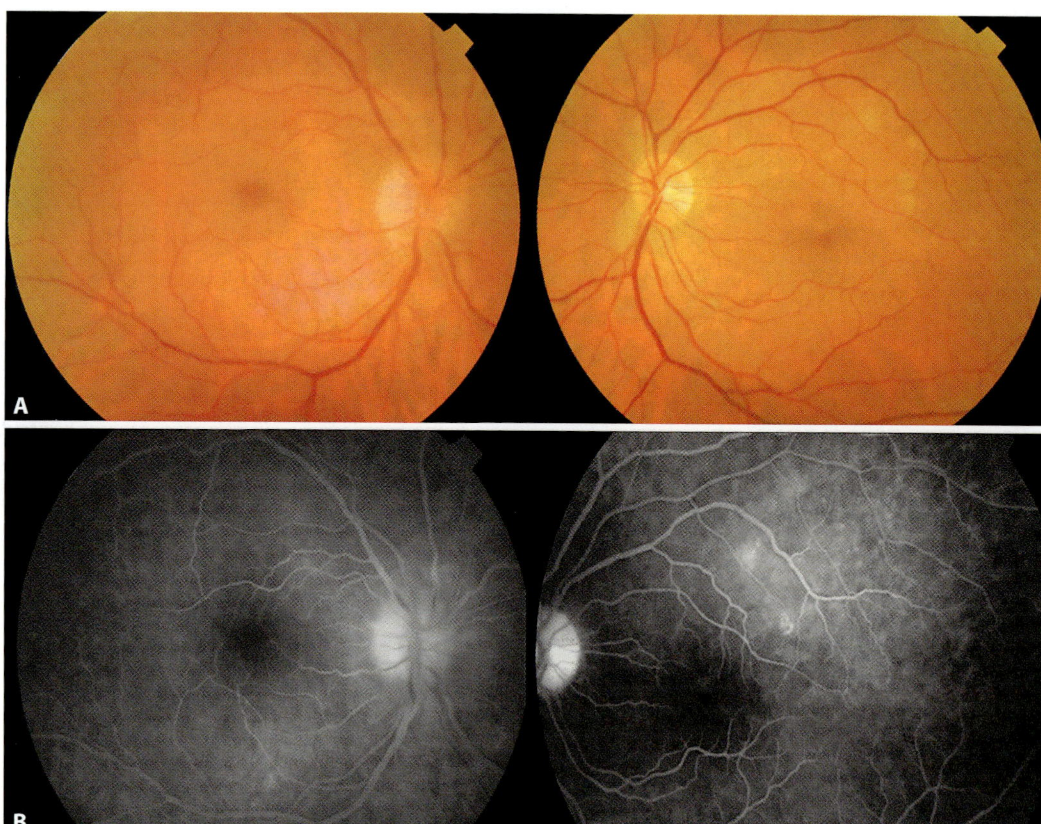

Figs. 4A and B: Ocular syphilis with optic neuritis. (A) Color fundus images reveal swelling around the optic nerve head in the right eye and in the left with mild disc hyperemia, with some subtle signs of inflammation. Additionally, there were hints of changes in the left eye's retina, indicating that the involvement extended beyond the optic nerve; (B) Fundus fluorescein angiography evidencing in the right eye subtle leakage around the optic disc in the left eye, confirming active inflammation of the optic nerve. In the left eye, there was evidence of diffuse retinal pigment epithelium (RPE) leakage, which was less pronounced but still indicative of ocular involvement.
Source: Presented by Mark Westcott in the International Uveitis Study Group (IUSG) grand rounds.[5]

- Fluorescein angiography may reveal subtle disc leakage, sometimes accompanied by diffuse RPE leakage in the fellow eye.
- It is not unusual for syphilitic disease to present with asymmetric findings between the eyes, such as optic neuritis in one eye and retinitis or placoid chorioretinitis in the other.

Each of these phenotypes emphasizes the importance of thorough systemic assessment and serological testing, as syphilis can manifest in various ways within the same patient. Prompt recognition and treatment are critical for favorable visual outcomes.

Serological Testing (Fig. 5)

The serological testing for syphilis relies heavily on both treponemal-specific and nontreponemal tests. Treponemal-specific tests, such as the fluorescent treponemal antibody absorption (FTA-ABS) test and the *Treponema pallidum* particle agglutination (TPPA) assay, are highly sensitive and specific for *T. pallidum*. These tests typically become positive 4–6 weeks after infection and remain positive for life, regardless of whether the patient is treated. This persistence means that even in cases where infection is successfully treated, these tests will not revert to negative.

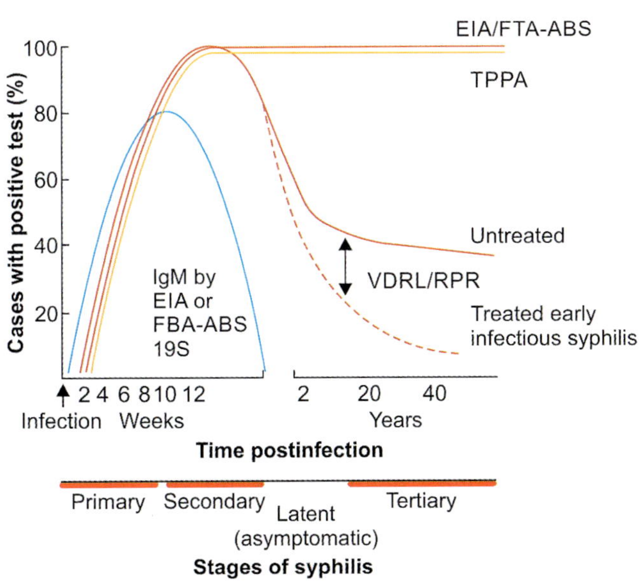

Fig. 5: Serology in untreated syphilis. (EIA: enzyme immunoassay; FTA-ABS: fluorescent treponemal antibody absorption; RPR: rapid plasma reagin; TPPA: *Treponema pallidum* particle agglutination; VDRL: Venereal Disease Research Laboratory)

Source: Presented by Mark Westcott in the International Uveitis Study Group (IUSG) grand rounds.[5]

Nontreponemal tests, such as the rapid plasma reagin (RPR) and the Venereal Disease Research Laboratory (VDRL) test, are used as markers of active infection. These tests detect antibodies that indicate the presence of an ongoing infection, and their titers tend to decline following successful treatment. However, these are not specific to syphilis and must not be relied upon for diagnosis but serve as valuable indicators of disease activity and response to therapy.

In untreated cases, the disease progresses from the primary to the secondary stage, where patients with syphilitic uveitis are often seen. If left untreated, the infection can move into the latent and eventually tertiary stages. In these advanced stages, treponemal-specific tests remain positive, while nontreponemal tests typically show low or negative titers, reflecting the diminished infectious activity. These patients may present years later with neuro-ophthalmic sequelae, such as optic nerve pallor or retinitis pigmentosa-like patterns, characteristic of the late effects of syphilis.

Thus, the combination of treponemal-specific tests for diagnosis and nontreponemal tests for monitoring active infection is crucial for the effective management of syphilis, particularly in cases involving ocular manifestations.

Treatment Regimen for Syphilitic Uveitis[6]

The management of ocular syphilis follows the same principles as the treatment for neurosyphilis, as both involve the CNS and require high-dose penicillin. The standard regimen consists of intravenous benzylpenicillin at 12–24 million units (MU) per day, administered in divided doses every 4 hours for 14 days.

In cases where intravenous administration is impractical due to limited healthcare resources or patient factors, intramuscular procaine penicillin can be used as an alternative. The recommended dose is 1.8–2.4 MU daily, combined with oral probenecid 500 mg every 6 hours. Probenecid increases the antimicrobial effect by reducing penicillin's renal excretion, thereby enhancing its effectiveness.

For patients who cannot tolerate or refuse penicillin injections, ceftriaxone can be administered either intramuscularly or intravenously at a dose of 2 grams daily for 14 days. In rare cases where patients refuse both intravenous and intramuscular treatment, an oral regimen consisting of amoxicillin 2 grams three times daily, along with probenecid 500 mg every 6 hours for 4 weeks, may be considered as a last resort.

Despite these alternative options, high-dose penicillin remains the gold standard for treating syphilitic uveitis and is generally the most effective therapy.

In Allergic Patients[6]

In cases where patients with syphilitic uveitis report a penicillin allergy, alternative treatments must be considered. The Centers for Disease Control and Prevention (CDC) recommends ceftriaxone, given its very low risk of cross-reactivity in patients with a history of penicillin allergy. It can be administered intramuscularly or intravenously at 1–2 grams daily for 14 days. Skin testing for penicillin allergies may be performed before therapy to assess the risk, though cross-reactivity with ceftriaxone remains minimal.

Some guidelines recommend penicillin desensitization. However, due to the associated costs, time required, and complexity of the process, it is not a practical solution in many cases. Consequently, desensitization is often avoided in favor of other alternatives.

Limited data also support the use of doxycycline (200 mg twice daily for 4 weeks) as an alternative in penicillin-allergic patients, although its use is less well documented compared to ceftriaxone. Given the evidence available, ceftriaxone remains the preferred option for treating syphilitic uveitis in patients with penicillin allergies.

Role of Lumbar Puncture in Ocular Syphilis[7]

A common point of debate in the management of ocular syphilis is whether a lumbar puncture (LP) for cerebrospinal fluid (CSF) analysis is necessary. Current guidelines from the United Kingdom, Europe, and the CDC suggest that LP is generally not required for ocular or otic syphilis. In most instances, the results of CSF analysis do not alter clinical management, and the procedure is rarely deemed useful.

However, there are specific clinical scenarios where an LP might be considered. One such situation is when a patient presents with both uveitis and acute cranial nerve palsies, suggesting more extensive neurological involvement. In these cases, CSF analysis may provide valuable diagnostic information. Another indication for LP would be in patients whose infection markers, such as the RPR titers, fail to normalize after completing systemic treatment. Persistently elevated titers may indicate ongoing infection or treatment failure.

In very rare cases, an LP may be warranted in patients with ocular syphilis who exhibit worsening or persistent inflammation despite receiving the full course of treatment. This could raise concern for reinfection or treatment-resistant syphilis. In such instances, CSF analysis could help determine if *T. pallidum* is still present and contributing to the ongoing disease process.

Use of Steroids[6]

In managing syphilitic uveitis, the use of corticosteroids plays a nuanced role. The primary concern is avoiding the Jarisch–Herxheimer reaction, an inflammatory response triggered by rapid lysis of treponemal bacteria during antibiotic treatment, which can worsen symptoms due to a sudden release of cytokines. Oral prednisolone is often initiated, typically at a dose of 30–60 mg daily for 3 days, with antibiotics, such as penicillin, commenced 24 hours after starting antibiotics to minimize the risk of this reaction. While this protocol makes sense for preventing complications such as optic neuritis and severe uveitis, there is little direct evidence supporting its necessity.

In clinical practice, the approach to steroids depends on the severity of ocular involvement. For patients with confirmed syphilitic uveitis, particularly those beginning antimicrobial therapy, Professor Westcott recommends the use of steroids based on the phenotype.

- *Anterior uveitis ± vitritis*: Intensive topical corticosteroids are often used, but systemic steroids are rarely necessary.
- *Posterior placoid chorioretinitis*: These cases often exhibit minimal inflammation, so steroids are used sparingly, primarily to prevent the Herxheimer reaction rather than to treat inflammation directly.
- *Retinitis*: Corticosteroids are generally not required as retinitis tends to resolve swiftly with antimicrobial therapy.
- *Optic neuritis*: Historically, steroids have been given, although there is no strong evidence that they are needed beyond mitigating the Herxheimer reaction.

This steroid regimen is applied case by case, ensuring that each patient's ocular condition and response to antimicrobial therapy are closely monitored.

PLACOID CHORIORETINITIS PRESENTATION

Case Series Presentation

In this section, different cases of placoid chorioretinitis will be present.

Case 1

A 30-year-old male presented with a vision of 20/200 in the right eye (OD) and 20/40 in the left eye (OS). The patient had a previous history of gastric ulcer and brain bleeding.

On examination, the patient showed signs of retinitis **(Fig. 6A)**. The imaging revealed a placoid area of hyperautofluorescence in the posterior pole **(Fig. 6B)**, suggestive of syphilitic involvement. OCT findings highlighted a blurring of the retinal layers, consistent with retinal disruption. Cells were also noted in the overlying vitreous **(Fig. 6C)**. Despite the vitreous findings not being particularly diagnostic, the key feature was the posterior placoid hyperautofluorescence. The patient subsequently tested positive for syphilis and responded favorably to treatment, with significant clinical improvement.

Case 2

A 42-year-old female, initially referred for evaluation of papilledema, presented with cells in the anterior chamber. Notably, it is important to test routinely for syphilis in all patients with disc swelling due to its prevalence, particularly in cases with additional signs such as anterior chamber cells. Imaging revealed disc swelling with evidence of mild vitreous haze **(Fig. 7A)**. Autofluorescence **(Fig. 7B)** and OCT **(Fig. 7C)** confirmed disc edema, extending into the subretinal space in the macular region. The patient was positive for *T. pallidum*. Treatment was initiated, and the patient's vision and macular edema improved.

Case 3

A 38-year-old male with a history of latent neurosyphilis and HIV (last CD4 count of 409) presented with a vision

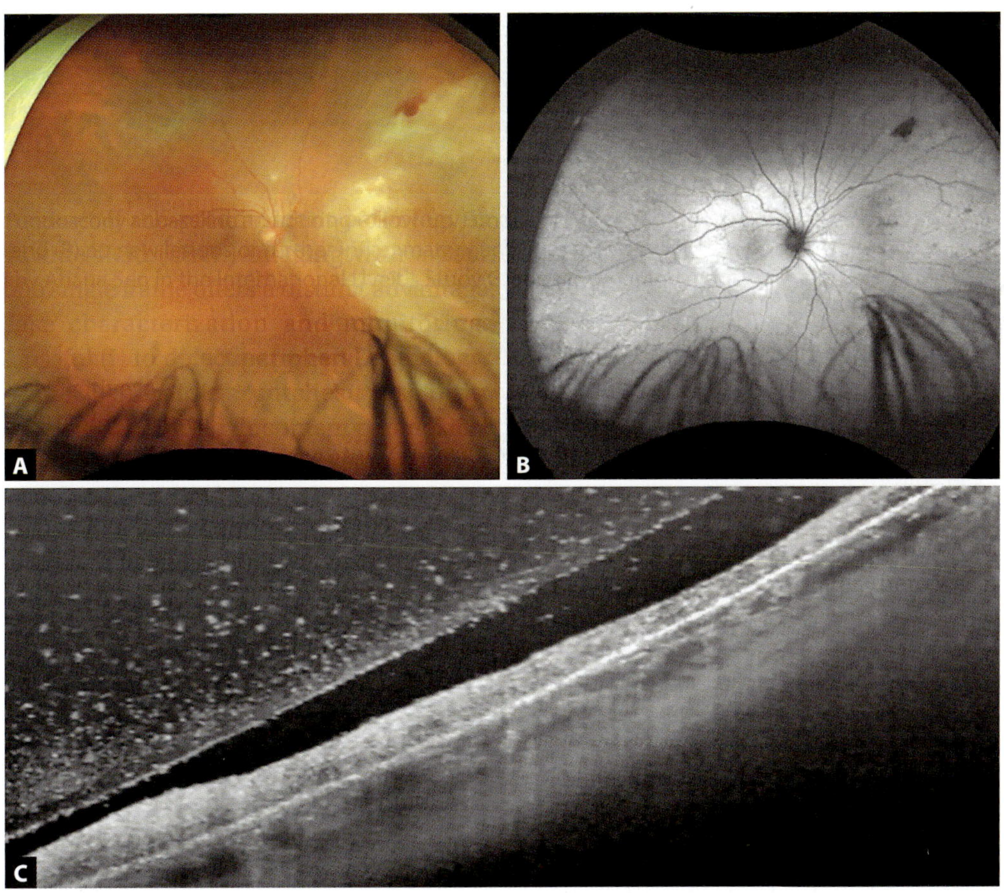

Figs. 6A to C: Case 1 of placoid chorioretinitis. (A) Color fundus photograph of the right eye showing areas of retinal whitening in the nasal periphery indicative of retinitis with vitreous hemorrhages; (B) Fundus autofluorescence image demonstrating a well-defined hyperautofluorescent placoid lesion at the posterior pole, characteristic of syphilitic chorioretinitis; (C) Optical coherence tomography scan showing retinal layer disorganization and blurred demarcation of the inner retinal layers, with notable vitreous opacities suggestive of inflammatory cells.

Source: Presented by Ahmed Shakarchy in the International Uveitis Study Group (IUSG) grand rounds.[5]

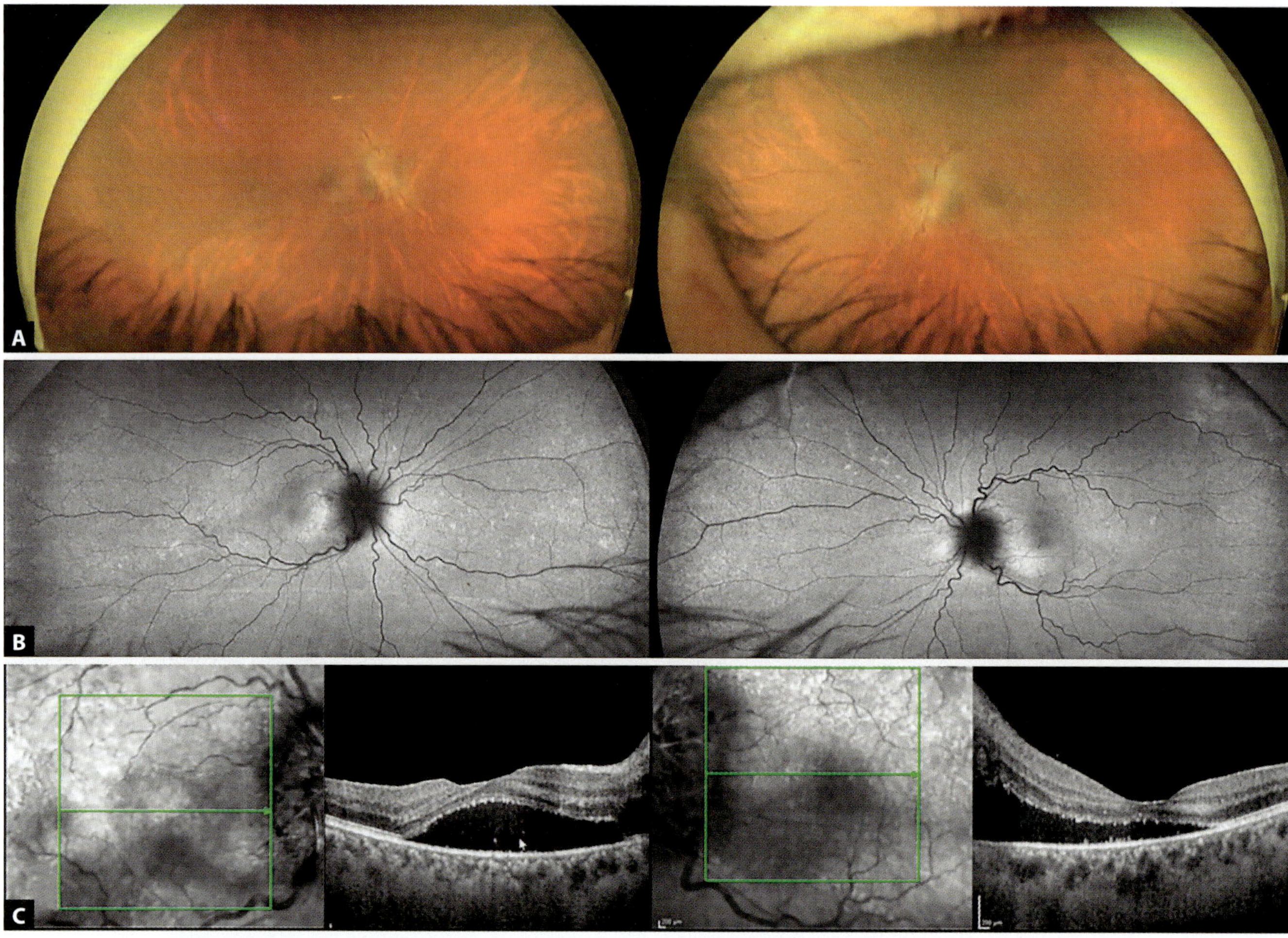

Figs. 7A to C: Case 2 of placoid chorioretinitis. (A) Color fundus photographs of both eyes showing optic disc swelling, with mild vitreous haze; (B) Fundus autofluorescence imaging highlighting hyperautofluorescence around the optic discs with an apparent elevated lesion on the macular region; (C) Optical coherence tomography scans showing the presence of subretinal fluid and disc edema, extending into the subretinal space in both eyes.
Source: Presented by Ahmed Shakarchy in the International Uveitis Study Group (IUSG) grand rounds.[5]

of counting fingers in the OD and 20/400 in the OS. The fundus examination showed severe vitritis (3+) in the OD and moderate (2+) in the OS **(Fig. 8A)**. In the autofluorescence, a placoid hyperautofluorescent pattern involving the optic disc and speckled autofluorescence in the retinal periphery were noted in both eyes (OU), which were more evident in the OS due to the significant vitreous haze in the OD **(Fig. 8B)**. Optical coherence tomography (OCT) and OCT angiography revealed attenuation of the choriocapillaris **(Fig. 8C and 8D)**. After treatment, the patient's vision improved to 20/200 in OD and 20/50 in OS, with vitritis and attenuation of choriocapillaris.

Case 4

A 33-year-old male with a history of treated syphilis and cytomegalovirus (CMV) retinitis dating back to 2016 **(Fig. 9A)** presented with vision deterioration after initially improving to 20/40 post-CMV treatment. Imaging before this episode resolved CMV retinitis and associated macular edema **(Fig. 9B)**. However, the outer retina was attenuated upon re-evaluation, raising suspicion of a syphilitic recurrence **(Fig. 9C)**. This prompted retesting for syphilis, which returned positive. The recurrence of outer retinal involvement was a critical factor in confirming the reactivation of syphilitic disease, and the patient was retreated accordingly.

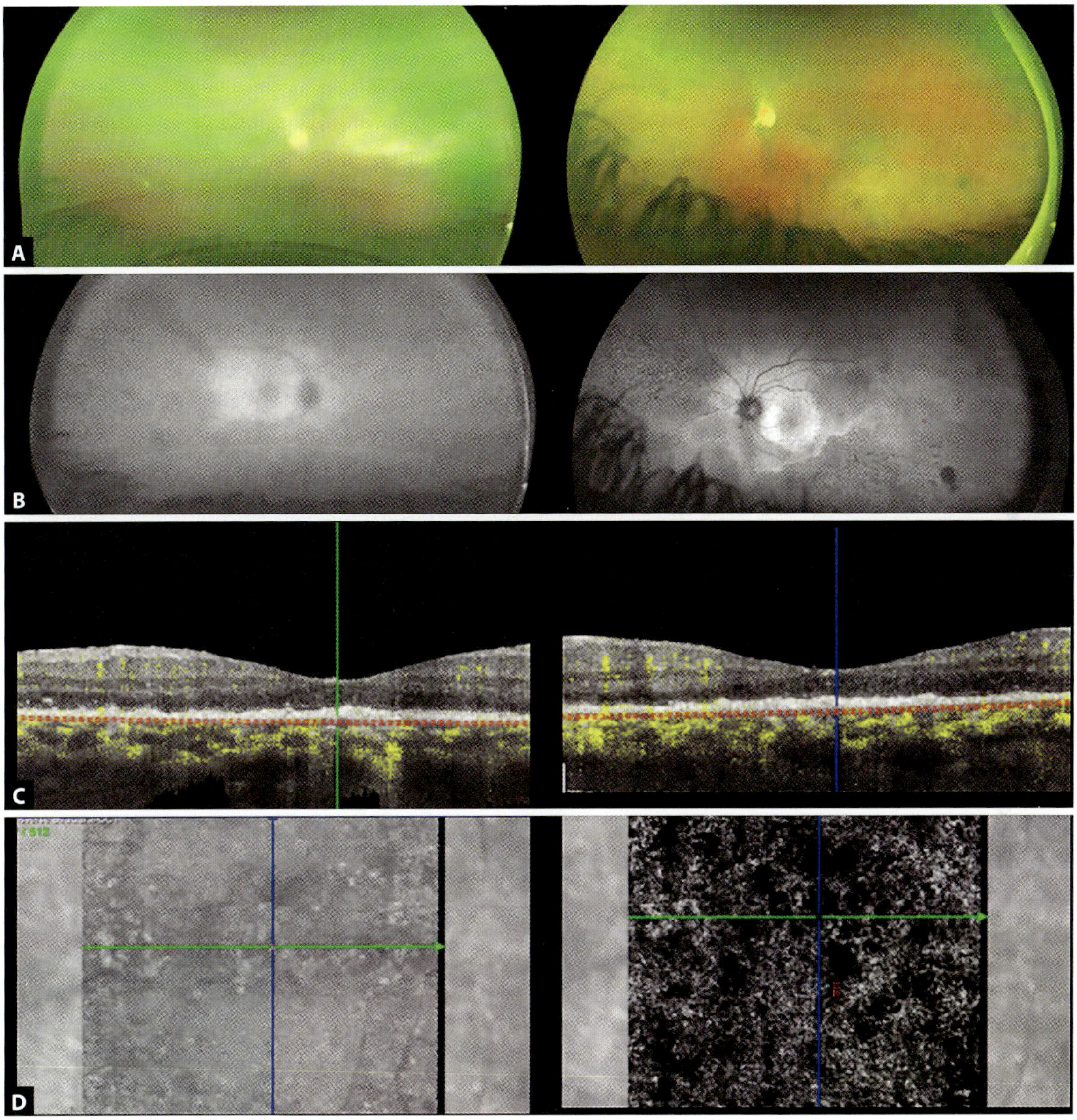

Figs. 8A to D: Case 3 of placoid chorioretinitis. (A) Color fundus photographs show significant vitreous haze in the OD and moderate haze in the OS; (B) Fundus autofluorescence reveals a placoid hyperautofluorescent pattern in the macula and speckled autofluorescence in the retinal periphery of both eyes, more prominent in the OS; (C and D) Optical coherence tomography (OCT) and OCT angiography showing attenuation of the choriocapillaris.
Source: Presented by Ahmed Shakarchy in the International Uveitis Study Group (IUSG) grand rounds.[5]

Discussion

In the United States, the approach to syphilis testing has shifted, with treponemal antibody tests now used as the first line of screening, followed by RPR or VDRL as confirmatory tests. If clinical suspicion remains high and a treponemal test is positive while the RPR is negative, a retest using another treponemal antibody test is typically performed. A therapeutic trial is usually initiated, following the CDC recommendations,[8] if this is also positive.

Intravenous penicillin is the standard treatment for syphilitic uveitis. Most patients are admitted to receive intravenous treatment or are sent home with a peripherally inserted central catheter (PICC) line for continued administration. Regarding the use of steroids, topical steroids are generally used for patients with

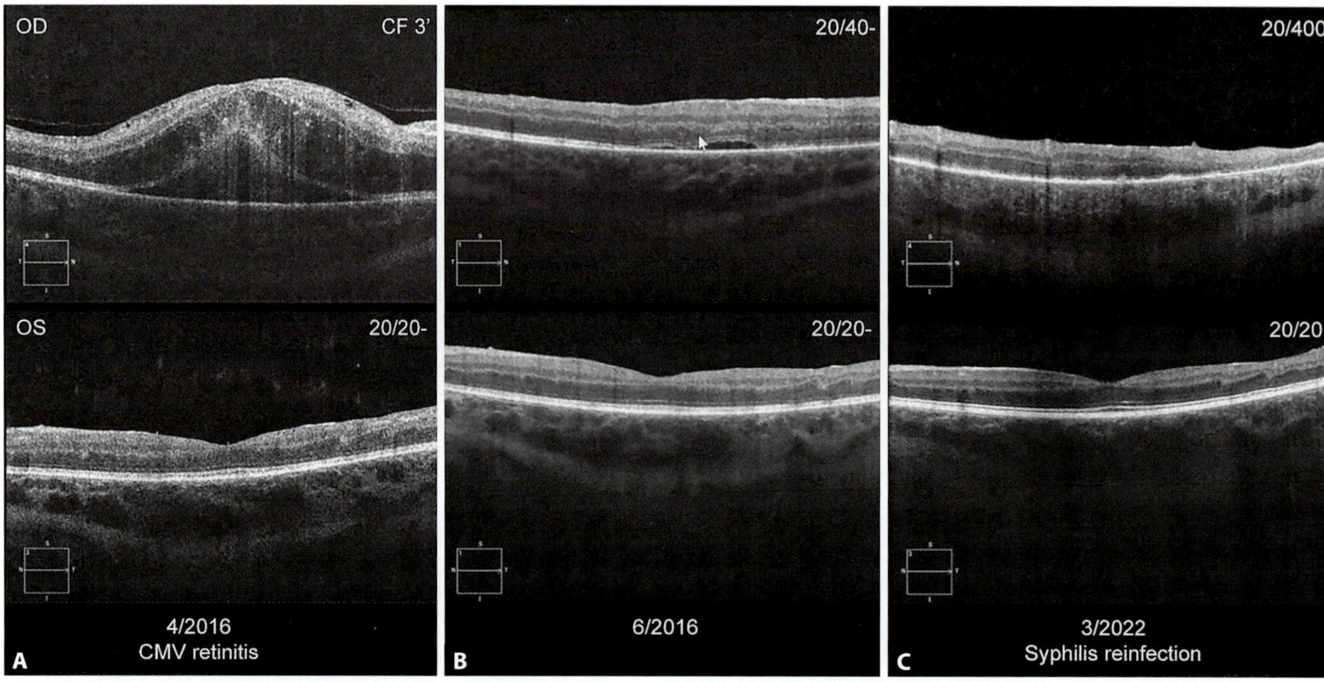

Figs. 9A to C: Case 4 of placoid chorioretinitis. (A) Initial OCT scan from April 2016 showing cystoid macular edema in the OD and resolved retinitis in the OS following CMV treatment; (B) Follow-up OCT from June 2016 indicates resolution of the macular edema in OD and stable retinal structure in OS, with visual acuity improving to 20/40 in OD and 20/20 in OS; (C) OCT from March 2022 reveals outer retinal attenuation in both eyes, particularly in OD, coinciding with vision loss to 20/400 in OD. The recurrence of outer retinal involvement led to retesting and confirmation of syphilis reactivation, prompting retreatment. (CMV: cytomegalovirus; OCT: optical coherence tomography)
Source: Presented by Ahmed Shakarchy in the International Uveitis Study Group (IUSG) grand rounds.[5]

significant anterior chamber reactions. In most cases, a 2-week course of 40 mg oral prednisone is administered, starting 2 days after initiating antimicrobial therapy, unless contraindications exist, which is stopped abruptly after this period. This approach avoids suppressing the pituitary–adrenal axis, making it a practical and widely adopted regimen.[9]

Syphilis remains a rising concern in urbanized areas worldwide, and clinicians are urged to maintain a high suspicion for the disease. Key indicators include placoid lesions in the retina and acute retinal necrosis, as syphilis can mimic various infectious and noninfectious ocular pathologies.[10] In cases of suspected acute retinal necrosis, clinicians should perform an anterior chamber tap, test for viral and toxoplasmic PCR, and initiate treatment with intravitreal antiviral therapy while awaiting blood test results of syphilis.[11]

Additionally, optic nerve involvement in uveitis should prompt consideration of syphilis, especially in patients with joint issues, rashes, or a history of multiple sexual partners, particularly MSM, as this group remains at high risk for syphilis. There are also differences between UK and US testing practices; in the United Kingdom, treponemal serology such as TPPA or FTA-ABS tests are used for diagnosis, while RPR or VDRL is reserved solely for monitoring disease activity, not for initial screening.

TYPICAL CASE OF SYPHILIS

Case Presentation

Personal Data

- Male
- 52 years old
- Originally from Pakistan
- Nonsmoker, no history of drug use
- *Allergies:* None reported

History of Present Illness

- The patient complained of decreased OS vision for 1 month, which was associated with pain and redness.
- The patient had been previously seen by an outside ophthalmologist and treated with cyclopentolate, prednisolone (three times a day), and tobramycin with dexamethasone drops in the OS, but there was no improvement.

- During the systems review, the patient denied any other symptoms.
- There was no history of ocular disease or trauma.
- *Past medical history:* It includes chronic kidney disease, essential hypertension, and hepatitis B; patient receiving amlodipine 5 mg and perindopril 5 mg.

Physical Examination

The patient presented with a visual acuity of 20/25 in the OD and 20/150 in the OS, with normal intraocular pressure (IOP) in OU and anterior chamber cells in the OS. Examination of the OD was unremarkable. Conversely, in the OS, 3+ vitreous cells and a faint area of retinitis were observed in the superonasal retina, surrounded by some ground-glass appearance **(Table 1 and Fig. 10)**.

Differential Diagnoses

At this stage, a differential diagnosis was considered for unilateral retinitis in the OS. The potential causes included viral retinitis, tuberculosis (TB), syphilis, CMV retinitis, progressive outer retinal necrosis (PORN), and ARN. Given that the patient was not immunocompromised, CMV retinitis and PORN were excluded. Multimodal imaging was then utilized for further evaluation.

Optical coherence tomography, fundus fluorescein angiography (FFA), and indocyanine green angiography (ICGA) of the OD were unremarkable. In the OS, hyperreflective dots were observed, correlating with vitritis, though no macular fluid was noted. Additionally, hyperreflective dots and RPE changes overlying the lesion suggest syphilitic involvement **(Fig. 11A)**. FFA of the OS showed focal areas of leakage, particularly in the superonasal region, associated with vasculitis and retinitis. The leakage intensified as the angiogram progressed **(Fig. 11B)**, while the ICG findings remained normal.

Workup

Following traditional diagnostic algorithms, serological testing was conducted, including RPR, FTA-ABS,

TABLE 1: Physical examination of the patient having a typical case of syphilis.

OD	*Parameters*	*OS*
20/25	BCVA	20/150
13 mm Hg	IOP	9 mm Hg
White and quiet	Conjunctiva/sclera	White and quiet
Normal and clear	Cornea	Pigment deposits
No cells	Anterior chamber	3+ cells
No synechiae	Iris	Irregular appearance
Clear	Lens	Pigment observed on the lens capsule
Unremarkable	Vitreous	BIO score 3+
Normal	Fundus	A faint area of retinitis was observed in the superonasal retina

(BCVA: best-corrected visual acuity; IOP: intraocular pressure)

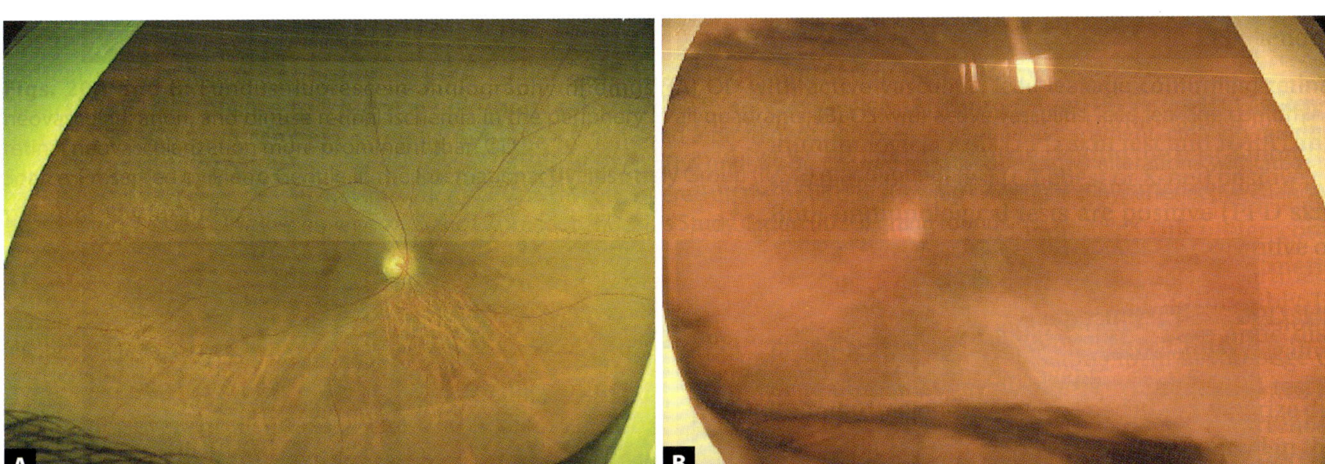

Figs. 10A and B: Fundus examination at baseline. Ultrawide-field fundus photographs showing (A) no significant abnormalities in the right eye and (B) severe vitritis and a faint area of retinitis in the superior nasal quadrant.
Source: Presented by Yanny Pérez Jimenez in the International Uveitis Study Group (IUSG) grand rounds.[5]

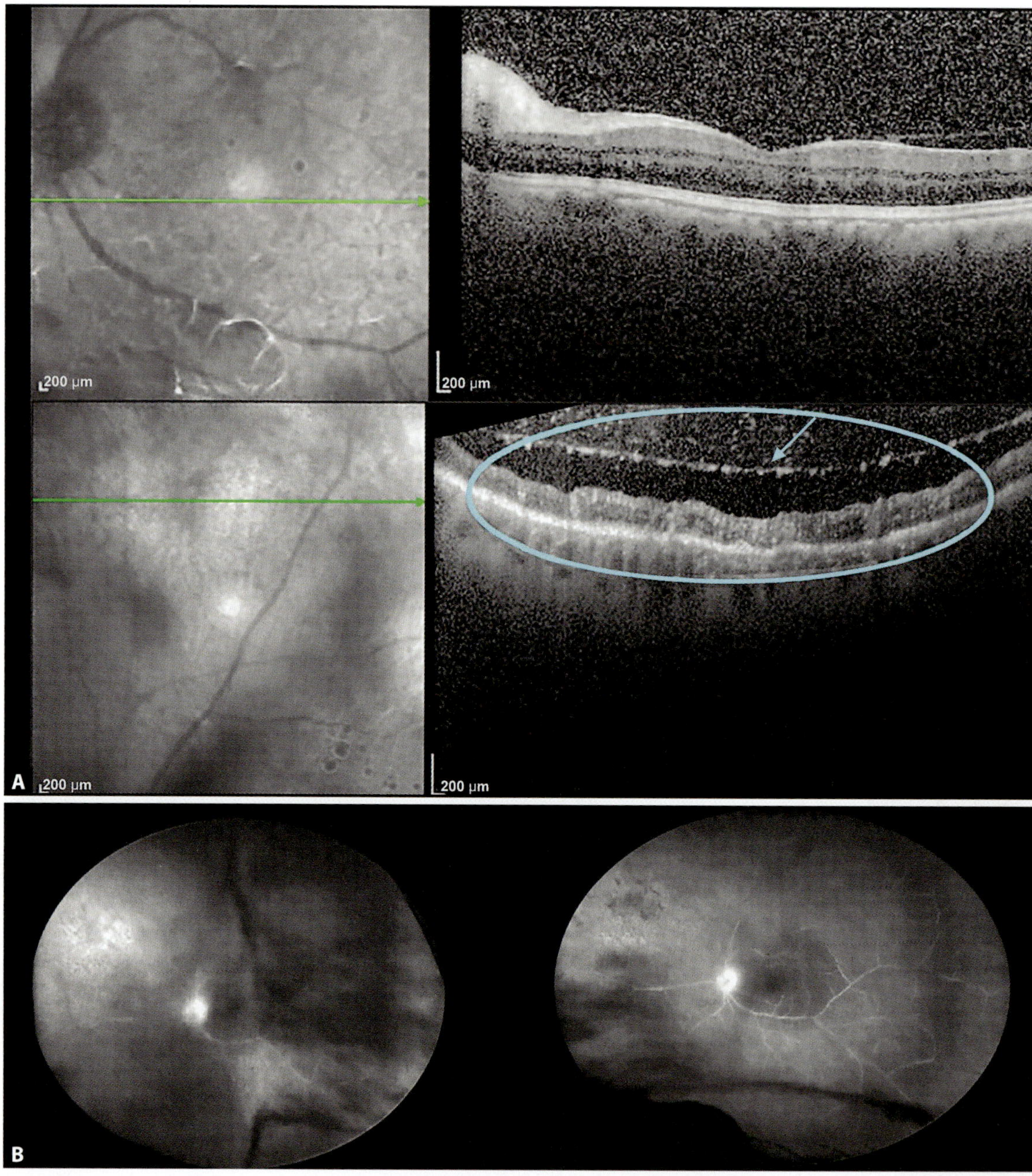

Figs. 11A and B: Multimodal imaging at baseline. (A) OCT in the OS shows hyperreflective dots overlying the posterior hyaloid in the macula (blue arrow), correlating with vitritis and RPE changes, without macular fluid; (B) Fluorescein fundus angiography of the OS reveals areas of focal leakage, particularly in the superonasal region, associated with vasculitis and retinitis. The leakage intensified in the later phases of the angiogram. (OCT: optical coherence tomography; RPE: retinal pigment epithelium)
Source: Presented by Yanny Pérez Jimenez in the International Uveitis Study Group (IUSG) grand rounds.[5]

QuantiFERON-TB Gold, *Toxoplasma* IgG/IgM, and HIV. Based on the differential, empirical treatment was initiated with sulfadiazine and pyrimethamine, to target toxoplasmosis, alongside valacyclovir for potential viral retinitis. Shortly after, the RPR test returned positive, confirmed by FTA-ABS. The tests for TB and toxoplasmosis were negative, as was the HIV test.

The patient was admitted, **(Fig. 12A)** and treatment was started with intravenous penicillin G at a dose of 3 MU every 4 hours for 10–14 days in consultation with infectious disease specialists. Prednisolone drops were also prescribed for the OS every 6 hours. At the 48-hour follow-up, elevated creatinine levels were noted, and the antibiotic dosage was adjusted. Oral prednisolone (40 mg once daily) was introduced, as the patient was already covered with antibiotics. Visual acuity had improved to 20/100, and anterior chamber cells were reduced to 2+. The fundus remained hazy, but the area of retinitis showed increased pigmentation, and OCT demonstrated fewer hyperreflective dots at the lesion site, with improving but persistent RPE changes **(Fig. 12B)**.

Three days after visual acuity had improved to 20/60, with reduced vitritis and anterior chamber cells (1+). Fluorescein angiography showed reduced leakage and increased pigmentation in the area of retinitis. After one week, best-corrected visual acuity (BCVA) had further improved to 20/50, reducing anterior chamber cells to 0.5+. The fluorescein angiogram revealed complete resolution of leakage, with only minimal late-phase staining. After five days, BCVA remained stable at 20/50, with no anterior chamber cells. Although RPR remained positive (1/64), the fluorescein angiography showed no further leakage, and the retinitis had fully healed **(Fig. 12C)**. The slightly hazy view observed in the ultrawide-field imaging was attributed to cataract development, but the lesion itself had completely resolved.

Discussion

In this case discussion, two key aspects were highlighted as follows:

- *Role of multimodal imaging*:[12,13] Multimodal imaging has provided the ability to classify syphilis-related

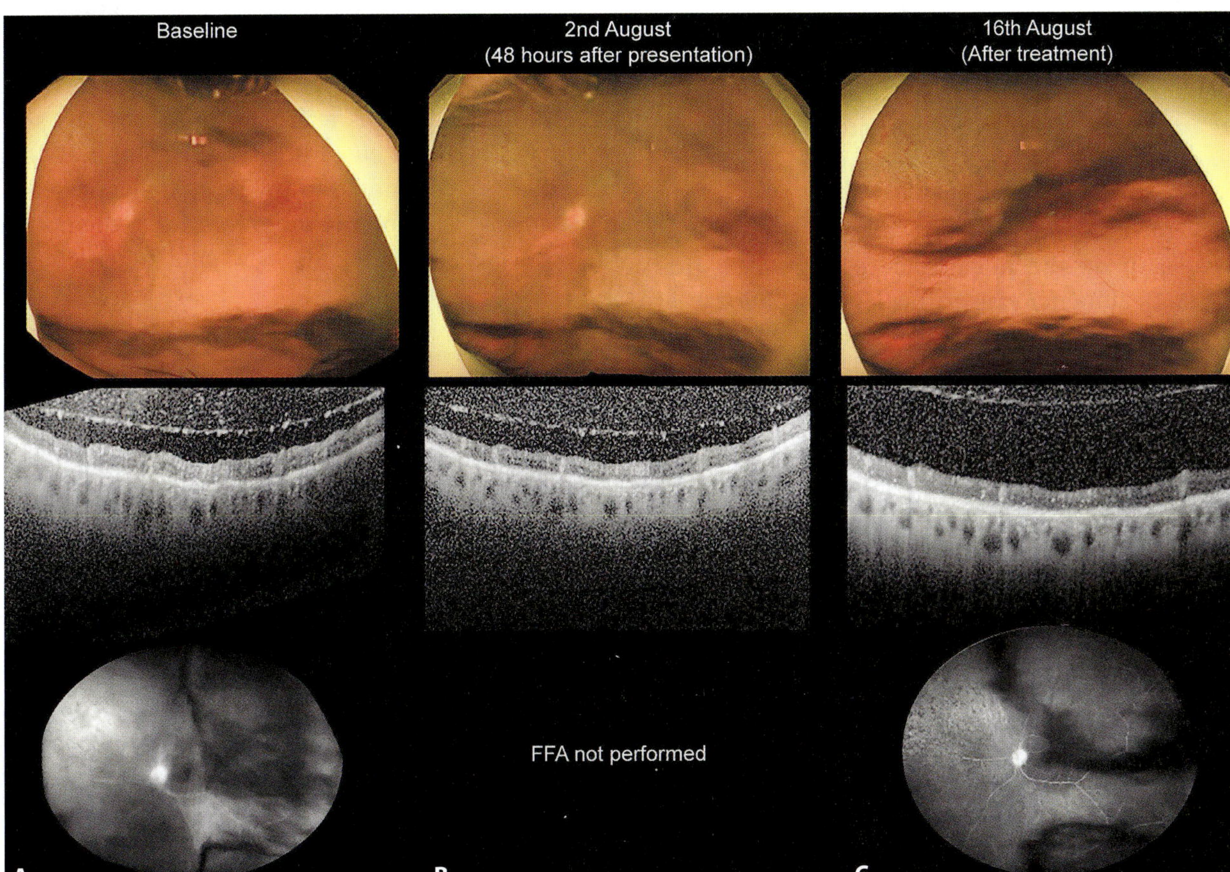

Figs. 12A to C: Multimodal imaging follow-up. A comparison of the baseline OCT with the scan from two weeks after baseline revealed significant improvement, with reduced vitritis and near-complete resolution of RPE changes. (OCT: optical coherence tomography; RPE: retinal pigment epithelium)

Source: Presented by Yanny Pérez Jimenez in the International Uveitis Study Group (IUSG) grand rounds.[5]

ocular manifestations into distinct categories. As syphilis is known for mimicking various conditions, such imaging techniques are crucial for distinguishing it from other diseases. The case presented featured the classic "ground-glass" appearance, a hallmark of syphilitic retinitis. This presentation differs from the "chalky white" appearance typically seen in ARN or toxoplasmic retinitis, in which the details underneath the lesion are often obscured. Notably, inflammatory deposits could be related to inflammatory reactions or even spirochetes.

A critical takeaway from this case is that while retinitis due to syphilis can sometimes resemble other conditions, it tends to present with more superficial accumulation, a triangular shape, and distinct hyperfluorescent margins on fluorescein angiography. Vasculitis is often observed alongside the retinitis.

- *Always consider syphilis as a possible diagnosis*: In terms of management, it is critical to think broadly and cover possible infections, such as viral or toxoplasmic causes, while waiting for diagnostic confirmation. Initially, this treatment included broad-spectrum antimicrobials such as trimethoprim–sulfamethoxazole and valacyclovir. Once syphilis was confirmed, therapy was shifted to intravenous penicillin.

Regarding treatment response, there was a discussion on the persistence of high RPR titers despite treatment. In this particular case, after 2 weeks of penicillin, the RPR titer remained elevated at 1:64. The patient was then discharged on doxycycline, and the RPR normalized over time. This approach demonstrates the importance of individualized treatment decisions and ongoing collaboration with infectious disease specialists.

Additionally, the use of corticosteroids was debated. While typically avoided in the "chalky white" forms of syphilitic retinitis, in this case, steroids were used after 48 hours of antibiotic treatment due to the significant vitreous reaction to prevent long-term visual impairment.

This case emphasizes that syphilis should always be considered in the differential diagnosis of uveitis. Multimodal imaging can aid in recognizing specific patterns associated with syphilis, guiding both diagnosis and laboratory testing. Treatment should be tailored based on clinical presentation to address the infection and any accompanying inflammation.

ATYPICAL CASE OF SYPHILIS

Case Presentation

Personal Data

- 23 years old
- Male
- No previous systemic symptoms or prior medical history
- Native of India

History of Present Illness

The patient presented with a 3-day history of acute-onset, painless, and progressively worsening vision in the OD. The vision loss was sudden, and the OS remained unaffected.

Physical Examination (Fig. 13)

The patient presented with a BCVA of 20/160 in OD and 20/20 in OS. Slit-lamp examination revealed a quiet anterior chamber in OU, with no significant findings in either eye. Fundus examination of the OD showed clear media and a cup-to-disc ratio of 0.3:1. Two large granulomas were noted in the peripapillary region, one located superior and the other inferior to the optic disc. There were associated dot and blot hemorrhages, as

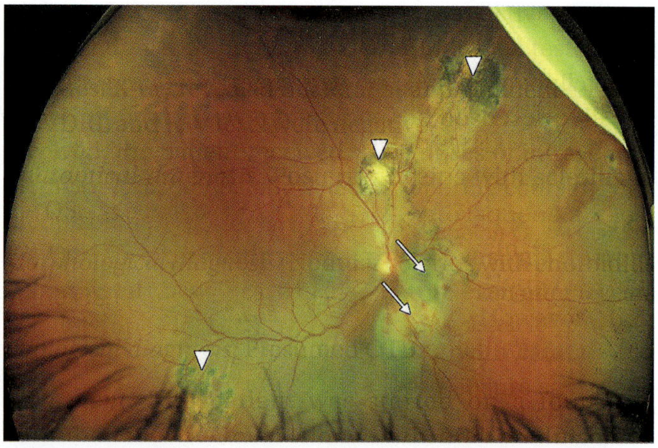

Fig. 13: Baseline fundus examination. The fundus photograph shows two peripapillary granulomas (white arrows) in the OD. Multiple chorioretinal scars can also be observed along the superonasal and inferotemporal arcades (white arrowheads). *Source:* Presented by Shravya Choudhary in the International Uveitis Study Group (IUSG) grand rounds.[5]

TABLE 2: Physical examination of the patient having atypical case of syphilis.

OD	*Parameters*	*OS*
20/160	BCVA	20/20
9 mm Hg	IOP	11 mm Hg
White and quiet	Conjunctiva/sclera	White and quiet
Pigment deposits	Cornea	Normal and clear
3+ cells	Anterior chamber	No cells
Irregular appearance	Iris	No synechiae
Pigment observed on the lens capsule	Lens	Clear
1+	Vitreous	Unremarkable
Two large granulomas; one located superior and the other inferior to the optic disc with some dot and blot hemorrhages, as well as multiple healed chorioretinal scars along the superonasal and inferotemporal arcades	Fundus	Normal

(BCVA: best-corrected visual acuity; IOP: intraocular pressure)

well as multiple healed chorioretinal scars along the superonasal and inferotemporal arcades.[14] The macula exhibited edema with an absent foveal reflex. The fundus examination of the OS was unremarkable **(Table 2)**.

Workup

Optical coherence tomography findings in the OD revealed hyperreflective dots, suggestive of vitreous cells and intraretinal and subretinal fluid consistent with cystoid macular edema **(Fig. 14A)**. Additionally, OCT through the granuloma showed choroidal elevation with subretinal fibrin and involvement of the inner retina **(Fig. 14B)**. Autofluorescence imaging of the OD demonstrated areas of hypoautofluorescence corresponding to healed choroiditis, with active disease noted in the superonasal and inferonasal quadrants **(Fig. 14C)**.

Given the physical examination and multimodal imaging, the initial diagnosis was ocular TB. However, other tests were ordered to identify other possible causes, including:

- Mantoux test, which returned positive (30 × 26 mm)
- Mildly elevated erythrocyte sedimentation rate (ESR) (21 mm/h)
- Human immunodeficiency virus results: Negative

A high-resolution computed tomography revealed small mediastinal lymph nodes and bilateral lower lung lobe opacities, which aligned with a latent history of TB. However, both VDRL and TPHA serology tests returned positive for syphilis, indicating a case of ocular syphilis masquerading as TB.

The patient was started on intravenous benzylpenicillin 14 million IU for 14 days.

The granulomas regressed after 10 days of treatment, and BCVA improved to 20/80. OCT demonstrated resolution of cystoid macular edema and significant regression of the granulomas, with scarring noted **(Figs. 15A and B)**. At the 2-month follow-up, the patient's vision had further improved to 20/30 with no recurrence of symptoms.

The key takeaways from this case highlight that ocular syphilis, often a great masquerader, can present atypically and should always be considered in the differential diagnosis of uveitis. TPHA remains highly sensitive and specific, and ocular syphilis is treated similarly to neurosyphilis, with intravenous penicillin being the treatment of choice.

Discussion

This case presents an interesting example of atypical ocular syphilis, initially misdiagnosed as ocular TB due to its clinical presentation of choroidal granulomas, choroiditis, and a positive Mantoux test. However, as part of the routine protocol in all uveitis cases, the patient was also screened for syphilis serology. Surprisingly, both the TPHA and VDRL tests returned positive, strongly indicating syphilitic etiology. Given syphilis's known ability to masquerade as other conditions, the treatment approach was modified from antitubercular therapy to intravenous penicillin.

The response to penicillin was rapid and remarkable; within 10 days, the patient's visual acuity improved

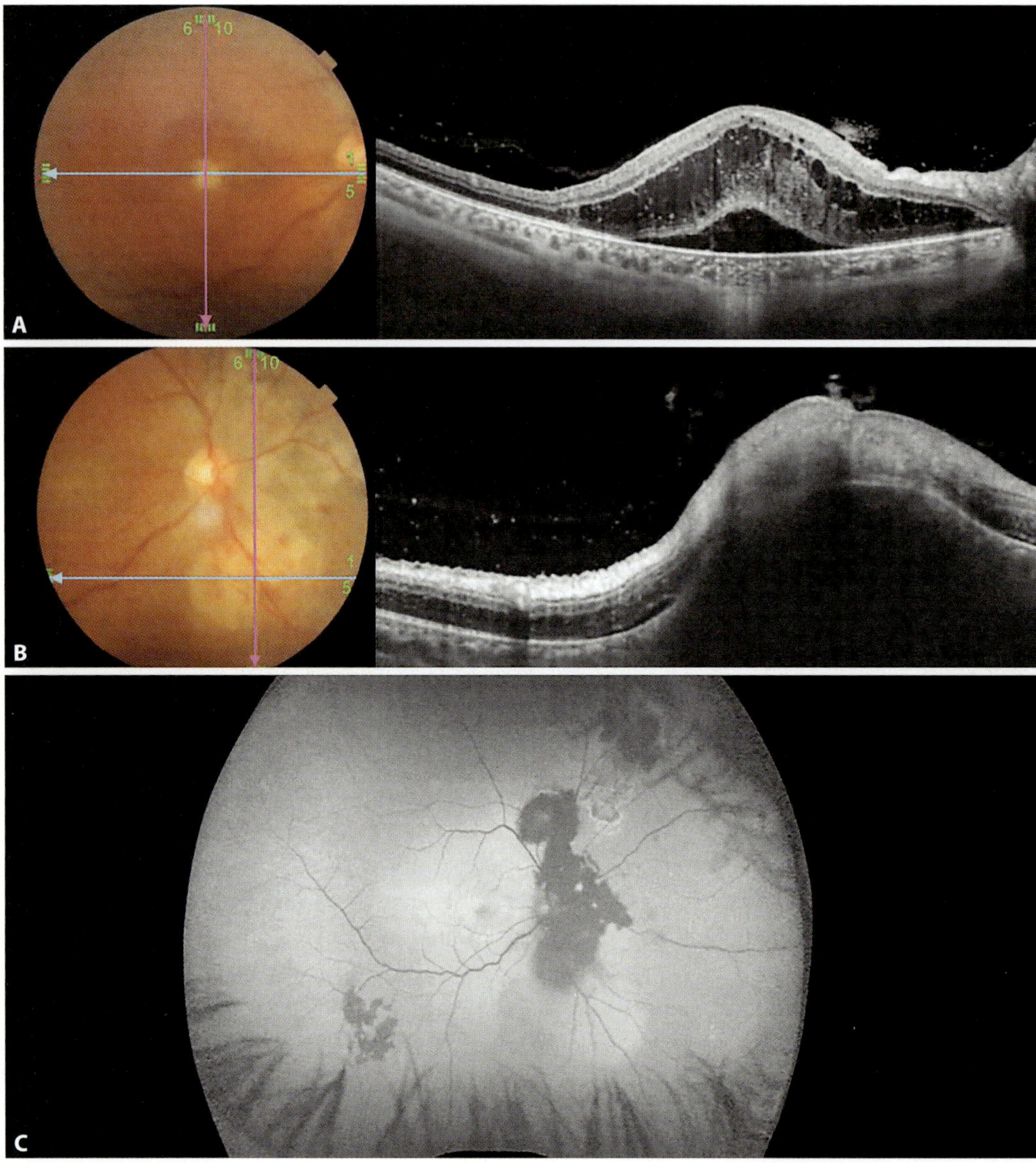

Figs. 14A to C: Multimodal imaging at presentation. (A) A horizontal optical coherence tomography (OCT) scan through the macula showed cystoid macular edema with hyperreflective dots; (B) OCT scan through the peripapillary granuloma demonstrating choroidal elevation and subretinal fibrin; (C) Autofluorescence imaging shows areas of hypoautofluorescence, indicating healed choroiditis, with active lesions in the superonasal and inferonasal quadrants.
Source: Presented by Shravya Choudhary in the International Uveitis Study Group (IUSG) grand rounds.[5]

to 20/80, and OCT showed complete flattening of the granulomas. By the 2-week follow-up, the lesions had completely resolved, and by the 2-month mark, visual acuity had improved to 20/30, with no further treatment required.

The discussion centered around the importance of considering syphilis as a differential diagnosis in all uveitis cases due to its ability to mimic other diseases, including ocular TB. The patient's presentation had all the clinical hallmarks of TB, including strongly positive Mantoux results, but the positive syphilis serology tests ultimately guided the correct diagnosis and treatment. Multimodal imaging, although helpful in characterizing the granulomas and choroidal involvement, was not enough to distinguish between TB and syphilis. It was the blood tests that ultimately provided the definitive diagnosis.

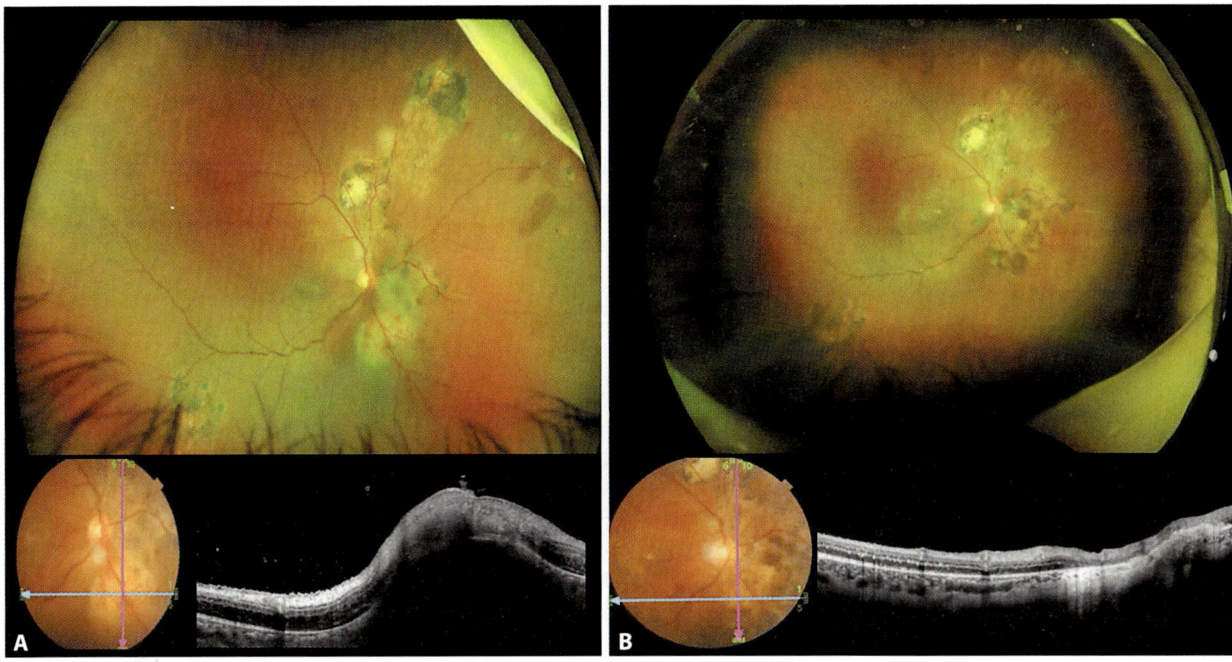

Figs. 15A and B: Comparison of color fundus photograph and optical coherence tomography findings between baseline and 10 days after intravenous penicillin. (A) Baseline; (B) After 10 days of treatment, the granulomas and cystoid macular regressed, and best-corrected visual acuity (BCVA) improved to 20/80.
Source: Presented by Shravya Choudhary in the International Uveitis Study Group (IUSG) grand rounds.[5]

Professor Westcott raised a point about whether OCT imaging might have revealed additional features consistent with syphilitic placoid chorioretinitis, particularly sub-RPE deposits rarely seen in TB. However, further scans through the lesions did not show any placoid features, and all the OCT findings were consistent with granulomas, including choroidal elevation and subretinal fibrin.

In conclusion, this case emphasizes the need to always consider syphilis in the differential diagnosis of uveitis, regardless of how strongly the clinical picture might suggest another etiology, such as TB. Syphilis remains a great masquerader and should be ruled out early through serological testing.

PEARLS FROM THE EXPERTS ON FREQUENTLY ASKED QUESTIONS

1. In cases of anterior uveitis, should syphilis testing be routinely conducted or is it limited to specific cases with recurrent or atypical presentations?

Answer: Syphilis testing should be conducted routinely in all cases of uveitis, including nonspecific anterior uveitis, as surprises can emerge unexpectedly. Testing with TPHA is considered an essential part of the diagnostic process for all forms of uveitis unless the clinical diagnosis is immediately evident.

2. Are there differences in the clinical presentation or outcomes between syphilitic uveitis in HIV-positive and HIV-negative patients?

Answer: One of the key differences is the higher risk of reinfection in HIV-positive patients. In such cases, reinfection must be excluded (by repeat RPR or VDRL testing and assessment of titer levels), and local steroids are recommended only after ensuring that the patient has responded well to antibiotic treatment. For this, it is important to achieve a fourfold reduction in the VDRL from baseline.

3. How often should VDRL titers be monitored in syphilitic patients? Is it done every 4 weeks?

Answer: Monitoring is typically conducted every 4 weeks, though the general/infectious disease physicians often manage this. Ophthalmologists may check titers around the same interval, but the primary focus in eye disease is on clinical improvement rather than solely on titer normalization.

4. What is the current best practice for using steroids in cases of syphilitic uveitis? Should steroids be started concurrently with antibiotics or should they be introduced later?

Answer: There is no single consensus on this matter, but the general rule is to ensure that antibiotics are always administered first or concurrently. Steroids can be introduced cautiously based on the severity of inflammation, mainly if there is significant disc edema or vitritis. The most important principle is that steroids should be used under the cover of antimicrobial therapy.

5. How should persistent inflammation or macular edema be managed if the patient does not respond to initial treatment?

Answer: Before introducing additional treatments, such as steroids or local interventions, it is crucial to confirm that the patient has been adequately treated and that there is no reinfection. Persistent vitritis or macular edema may sometimes be residual debris rather than active inflammation and could be managed with vitrectomy. Assuming that the patient has completed and been compliant with syphilis antimicrobial therapy and reinfection had been excluded, it would be safe to treat macular edema with steroids.

6. Are there specific OCT biomarkers that are characteristic of syphilitic retinitis?

Answer: The most typical OCT findings in syphilitic retinitis include nodularities in the RPE, particularly in the placoid form. These nodularities are highly characteristic and can sometimes be mistaken for lymphoma in older adults. Subretinal fluid may also be seen in the early stages, though it tends to resolve. Combined with clinical and serological data, these findings can guide the diagnosis.

7. Can autofluorescence imaging help confirm the diagnosis of syphilitic retinitis?

Answer: Yes, in cases of placoid syphilis, autofluorescence imaging typically reveals a hyperautofluorescent halo surrounding the lesion. Even when the placoid lesion appears faint on clinical examination, autofluorescence can help locate the lesion and provide diagnostic clarity. The entire lesion often appears as a ground-glass-like hyperautofluorescent area.

8. Should steroids always be added in cases of severe disc edema or vitritis in syphilitic patients?

Answer: The use of steroids in such cases depends on the clinical presentation. While antibiotics alone may be sufficient in many cases, severe disc edema or vitritis may benefit from the addition of steroids. However, steroids should be introduced only under the cover of appropriate antibiotics to prevent exacerbation of the infection.

9. How should persistent cystoid macular edema be managed after syphilis treatment? Is antivascular endothelial growth factor (VEGF) therapy appropriate?

Answer: Anti-VEGF therapy is generally not recommended for managing cystoid macular edema postsyphilis treatment. Instead, systemic steroids may be considered under the cover of antibiotics such as doxycycline. It is also essential to rule out immune recovery uveitis in HIV-positive patients that can sometimes present as cystoid macular edema.

10. Is it possible to misdiagnose syphilis as TB due to similar granulomatous presentations? How should these cases be handled?

Answer: Syphilitic choroidal granulomas are extremely rare, and the first diagnosis you have to consider in patients with granulomas is TB, not syphilis, although treponema must be ruled out.

11. What should be done if an infectious disease specialist refuses to treat ocular syphilis in a patient with no systemic symptoms?

Answer: If the ophthalmologist is confident in the diagnosis and the serology supports the presence of syphilis, treatment should be initiated, regardless of the systemic findings. Collaboration with infectious disease specialists is important, but ocular prognosis takes priority, and treatment should not be delayed.

12. How should syphilis be treated in penicillin-allergic patients, particularly in pregnant women?

Answer: Third-generation cephalosporins, such as ceftriaxone, are recommended for penicillin-allergic patients as the cross-reaction is low. In some cases, desensitization to penicillin can be considered. It is important to consult infectious disease specialists for guidance, but alternatives such as ceftriaxone are usually effective.

13. Should we involve the infectious disease specialist if the partner of a patient with syphilis is asymptomatic and refuses treatment?

Answer: Yes, involving the infectious disease specialist is crucial in these cases to counsel the partner on the importance of testing and treatment. While ocular specialists should initiate treatment for the patient, ensuring that the partner is treated is essential for preventing reinfection.

14. In a case of posterior uveitis with bilateral disc edema, TPHA, and VDRL positive, there was a debate among physicians regarding the need for steroids along with penicillin, as the visual acuity was 20/200 in one eye. Is the use of steroids recommended in this context?
Answer: Steroids would be administered, although no clear evidence of benefit exists.

15. In serological or confirmatory tests with TPHA and high titers, can the prozone phenomenon affect the diagnosis of secondary ocular syphilis?
Answer: It is possible, but it is rare.

16. What is the recommended dose of corticosteroids, and what is the appropriate timing in relation to antibiotics?
Answer: A suggested regimen is oral prednisone 20–60 mg/day for 2 weeks, starting 2 days after penicillin. However, there is a debate about the appropriate time to start. The European guidelines suggest starting corticosteroids 3 days before commencing antitreponemal therapy to prevent the Jarisch–Herxheimer reaction.

17. How common are complications of syphilitic uveitis?
Answer: In early detected cases, complications are not very common. Retinal detachment rates are much lower compared to acute retinal necrosis. Cystoid macular edema can be a problem, and secondary glaucoma is less common.

18. Is there a role for local steroid injections, such as transeptal corticosteroid injections, to manage Jarisch–Herxheimer reactions, especially in cases of panuveitis?
Answer: Local steroids are used for persistent uveitis, especially for cystoid macular edema after syphilis that has not responded to oral and periocular steroids. However, it is crucial to ensure that the patient has been well treated with antibiotics, and there is no reinfection as discussed before.

19. Is there any choroidal involvement in ocular syphilis as observed on OCT imaging?
Answer: In placoid syphilis, hyperreflective dots can be seen in the choroid, though its representation is unclear. Generally, the retina is the main target of syphilis.

20. Should both treponemal and nontreponemal tests always be requested for syphilis, or should one be prioritized over the other?
Answer: The standard approach is to start with syphilis antibody testing, and if positive, proceed to RPR for further evaluation.

21. In cases resembling acute retinal necrosis with syphilitic retinitis, should empirical treatment for herpes, toxoplasmosis, and syphilis be started, along with an anterior chamber tap for PCR testing?
Answer: In such cases, treatment usually begins for acute retinal necrosis and toxoplasmosis but not for syphilis unless specific indicators are present.

FINAL WRAP-UP

This chapter on ocular syphilis provides a comprehensive overview of the clinical presentation, diagnosis, and management of this complex condition. Key takeaways include recognizing the wide variety of clinical manifestations, such as anterior uveitis, posterior uveitis, placoid chorioretinitis, and optic neuritis, which can mimic other conditions. Serological testing, including both treponemal and nontreponemal tests, remains crucial for diagnosis, while multimodal imaging is pivotal in detecting characteristic lesions.

Treatment protocols emphasize high-dose penicillin as the gold standard for syphilitic uveitis, with alternative regimens for penicillin-allergic patients. Steroid use is carefully considered based on the severity of inflammation and is typically administered alongside antibiotics to manage inflammatory reactions such as the Jarisch–Herxheimer reaction. Throughout the chapter, expert commentary underscores the importance of broad differential diagnosis and timely intervention to prevent severe visual outcomes, particularly in populations at high risk, such as those with concurrent HIV infection.

REFERENCES

1. Kojima N, Klausner JD. An update on the global epidemiology of syphilis. Curr Epidemiol Rep. 2018;5(1):24-38.
2. Lasagabaster MA, Guerra LO. Syphilis. Enferm Infecc Microbiol Clin (Engl Ed). 2019;37(6):398-404.
3. UK Health Security Agency. (2010). Sexually transmitted infections (STIs): annual data. [online] Available from https://www.gov.uk/government/statistics/sexually-transmitted-infections-stis-annual-data-tables. [Last accessed February, 2025].

4. Mathew RG, Goh BT, Westcott MC. British ocular syphilis study (BOSS): 2-Year national surveillance study of intraocular inflammation secondary to ocular syphilis. Invest Ophthalmol Vis Sci. 2014;55(8):5394.
5. International Uveitis Study Group (IUSG). (2024). Uveitis Webinar—Grand Round 8. WEBINAR 38: Ocular Syphilis: Case-Based Approach. [online] Available from https://youtu.be/tBbSY3XFCTI?si=TfZ1Eh4zEsmmL-CR.
6. Janier M, Unemo M, Dupin N, Tiplica GS, Potočnik M, Patel R. 2020 European guideline on the management of syphilis. Acad Dermatol Venereol. 2021;35(3):574-88.
7. Centers for Disease Control and Prevention (CDC). (2024). CDC Laboratory Recommendations for Syphilis Testing, United States, 2024. [online] Available from https://www.cdc.gov/mmwr/volumes/73/rr/pdfs/rr7301a1-H.pdf. [Last accessed February, 2025].
8. Soreng K, Levy R, Fakile Y. Serologic testing for syphilis: benefits and challenges of a reverse algorithm. Clin Microbiol Newsl. 2014;36(24):195-202.
9. Pelewicz K, Miśkiewicz P. Glucocorticoid withdrawal—an overview on when and how to diagnose adrenal insufficiency in clinical practice. Diagnostics. 2021;11(4):728.
10. Chauhan K, Fonollosa A, Giralt L, Artaraz J, Randerson EL, Goldstein DA, et al. Demystifying ocular syphilis: a major review. Ocul Immunol Inflammat. 2023;31(7):1425-39.
11. Yusuf IH, Izadi S, Fung THM, Sallam A, Patel CK. Multifocal necrotizing chorioretinitis following phacoemulsification surgery. Ocul Immunol Inflammat. 2015;23(3):261-5.
12. Neri P, Pichi F. Acute syphilitic posterior placoid chorioretinitis: when the great mimicker cannot pretend anymore; new insight of an old acquaintance. J Ophthal Inflamm Infect. 2022;12(1):9.
13. Pichi F, Neri P. Multimodal imaging patterns of posterior syphilitic uveitis: a review of the literature, laboratory evaluation, and treatment. Int Ophthalmol. 2020;40(5):1319-29.
14. Lautredou CC, Hardin JS, Chancellor JR, Uwaydat SH, Ellabban AA, Sallam AB. Repeat intravitreal dexamethasone implant for refractory cystoid macular edema in syphilitic uveitis. Case Rep Ophthalmol Med. 2018;2018:1-3.

CHAPTER

9

Herpetic Anterior Uveitis

Massimo Accorinti, Matteo Menean, Elisabetta Miserocchi, Neofytos Mavris, Radgonde Amer, Daniele de Geronimo, Alejandra de-la-Torre, Germán Mejía-Salgado, Meghan Berkenstock, Reema Bansal, John H Kempen, Vishali Gupta

INTRODUCTION[1]

Anterior uveitis (AU) constitutes approximately 70–93% of all uveitis cases in industrialized countries. Virus-induced uveitis localized in the anterior segment accounts for 54–91% of these cases. Among AU cases, the prevalence of herpetic uveitis ranges from 4.6% to 11.7%.[2] In the United States, herpetic uveitis is more frequently observed in Caucasian individuals compared to the African American population ($p < 0.001$). Regarding age distribution, up to 33% of viral AU occurs in elderly patients (>60 years). The median age at presentation varies by etiological agent: Herpes simplex virus (HSV) is reported between 43 and 56 years, varicella-zoster virus (VZV) between 52 and 67 years, and cytomegalovirus (CMV) between 42 and 54 years.[2,3]

PRACTICAL TIPS IN THE DIAGNOSIS OF OCULAR HERPETIC ANTERIOR UVEITIS[1]

Herpes Simplex Virus

Seroprevalence and Demographics

The prevalence of HSV-1 immunoglobulin G (IgG) seropositivity in individuals over 40 years of age is reported to range from 80 to 90%, while HSV-2 infections are relatively rare on a global scale, although there has been an increasing trend in the last 20 years among the youngest patients. HSV-AU can occur across all age groups. However, the mean age at presentation varies by region, with an average of 50 years in Europe and Japan, compared to 26 years in India.[2] Overall, ocular herpetic infection represents an important cause of ocular morbidity in developed countries and is one of the most common causes of corneal blindness.

Clinical Findings in Herpes Simplex Virus Uveitis

The clinical course of HSV uveitis is acute in 62–72% of cases, chronic in 28–38%, and recurrent in 33% of patients.[4,5] The condition is predominantly unilateral, affecting up to 95% of cases. Bilateral herpetic infections are rare, occurring mainly in atopic and immunosuppressed patients. Common presenting symptoms include pain with severe light sensitivity and blurred vision in 57% of patients. The main clinical features are medium-to-large keratic precipitates (KPs), medium-to-severe anterior chamber inflammation, patchy iris atrophy, mydriasis, pupil distortion, and increased intraocular pressure (IOP). In some very severe cases, fibrin formation, hyphema, posterior synechiae, and vitreous cells can occur.[4] Additional clinical signs include ciliary injection and corneal lesions **(Figs. 1A and B)**.[4,5]

Herpes Zoster Virus

Epidemiology and Clinical Features

Herpes zoster virus (HZV) uveitis has a mean age of presentation of 68 years, with a slight female predominance. Patients with HZV infection are at an increased risk of developing AU within the year following the acute episode. A German study reported that 24% of HZV-associated uveitis cases are bilateral, with the second eye always manifesting keratitis alone.[6-8]

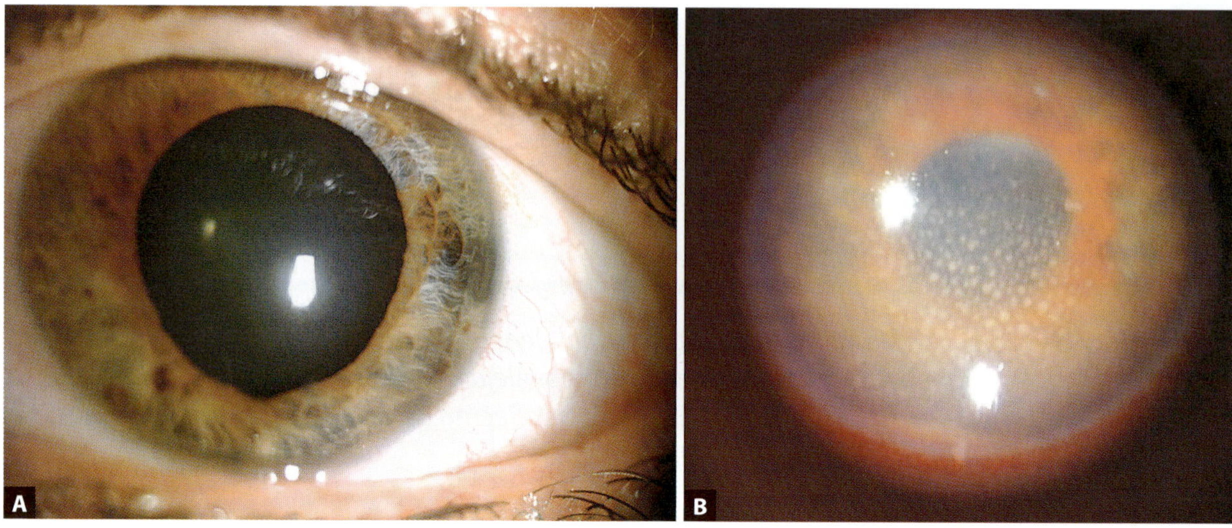

Figs. 1A and B: Clinical finding in herpetic uveitis. (A) Anterior segment photograph of a patient with herpes simplex virus type 1 (HSV-1) herpetic uveitis showing pupil distortion and permanent mydriasis related to the presence of the virus in the iris; (B) Anterior segment photograph of a patient with HSV-1 herpetic uveitis: severe corneal edema, granulomatous precipitates, fibrin, and hyphema.
Source: Presented by Massimo Accorinti in the International Uveitis Study Group (IUSG) grand rounds.[1]

In patients with ophthalmic HZV, the relapse rates are 8% at 1 year, 17% at 3 years, and 25% at 5 years. Ocular hypertension and anterior uveitis significantly increase the likelihood of a relapsing or chronic course of the disease.[9]

Epidemiology of Varicella-zoster Uveitis

Primary VZV infections typically occur in childhood, with ocular involvement seen in up to 20% of cases. Among these, 57% present with AU and 4% with keratouveitis. The condition is generally mild and often self-limiting. Typical findings include fine KPs, small, round, atrophic spots on the iris, pupil distortion, and sectoral iris atrophy.[10]

In adults, AU may develop during the acute phase of the infection, most commonly 2–4 weeks after disease onset. The clinical course is acute in 20–83% of cases, recurrent in 6.4–38%, and chronic in 7–42%.[5,11]

It is important to remember that VZV herpetic uveitis may appear even in the absence of the cutaneous eruption (herpes sine herpete) or when the cutaneous eruption is only confined to the tip of the nose (Hutchinson sign) **(Fig. 2A)**.

Clinical Findings

Varicella-zoster virus-related AU is unilateral in 76–100% of cases. Up to 42% of patients report pain, 70% experience blurred vision, and 71% present with ciliary injection. Corneal lesions are also common. In the anterior chamber, medium-to-large endothelial precipitates, moderate-to-severe inflammation, and focal iris atrophy can be observed. Other findings include pupil distortion, IOP elevation, and posterior synechiae **(Figs. 2A to D)**.[1]

Cytomegalovirus

Epidemiology

Cytomegalovirus-related AU is more commonly reported in Asia, with the Chinese population in Singapore being the most affected. There is a significant male predominance, with males comprising up to 80% of reported cases.[2] CMV-AU can occur across all age groups, with a mean age of presentation of 37 years. The disease manifests in either an acute or a chronic form, with nearly 100% of acute cases unilateral, and up to 20% of chronic cases are bilateral.[12,13]

Clinical Findings

In acute CMV-AU, patients often present with none to mild ciliary injection, coin-shaped KPs, and mild anterior chamber inflammation (<2+ flare and cells). High IOP is a consistent feature, while posterior synechiae are absent. These clinical findings correspond well to the first description of glaucomatocyclitic crisis reported by Posner and Schlossman,[14] which was later defined as Posner-Schlossman syndrome. In 1987, Bloch-Michel, founder and first President of the International Uveitis Study Group

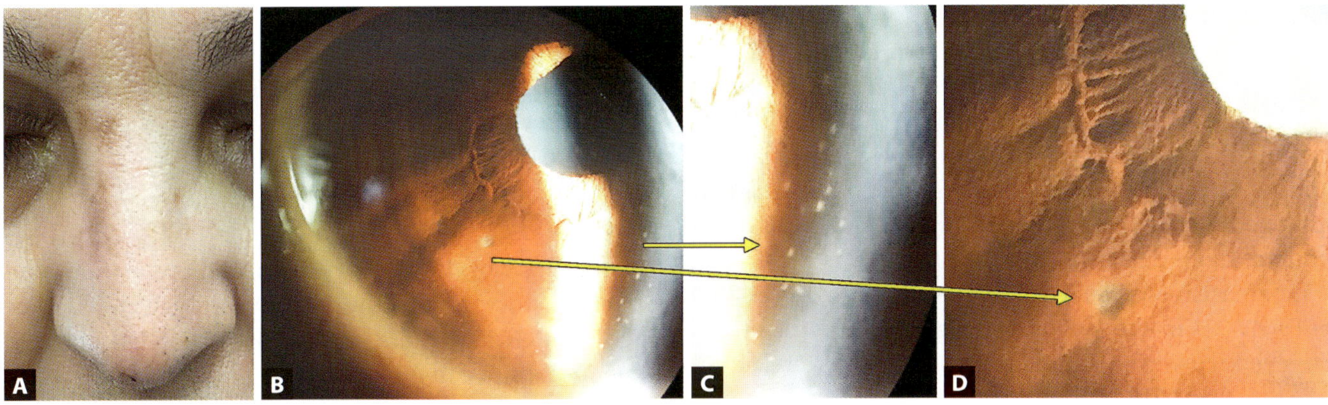

Figs. 2A to D: Varicella-zoster virus (VZV) clinical findings. (A) Typical VZV skin eruption on the nose; (B to D) Photograph of anterior segment evidencing medium-to-large keratic precipitates and focal iris atrophy.
Source: Presented by Massimo Accorinti in the International Uveitis Study Group (IUSG) grand rounds.[1]

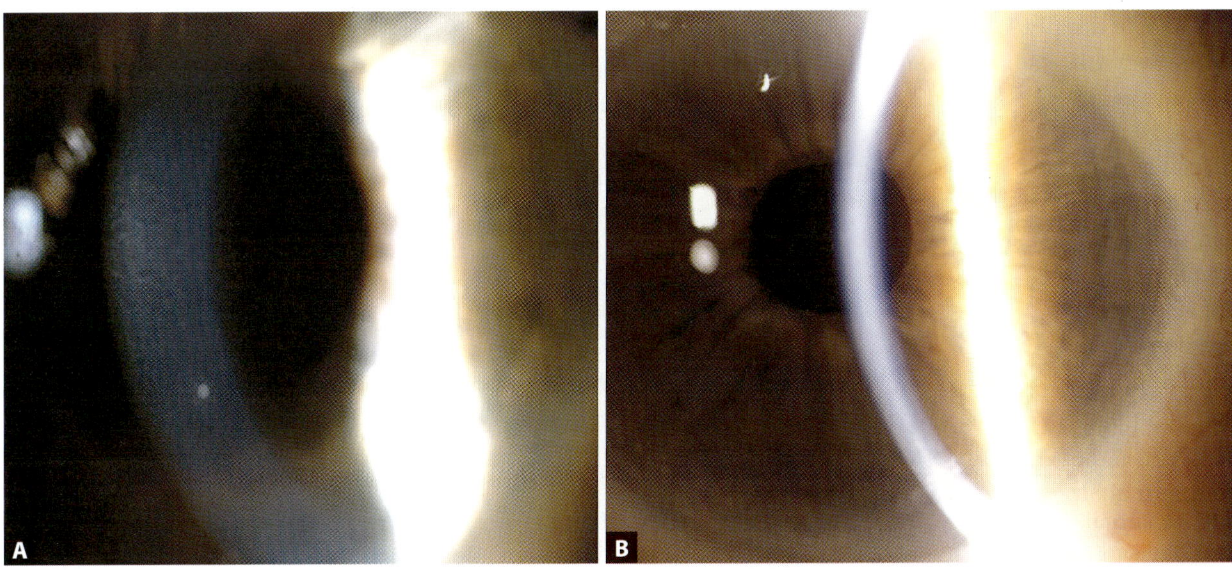

Figs. 3A and B: Typical features of anterior cytomegalovirus (CMV) uveitis. (A) Mild-to-moderate anterior chamber cellularity; (B) Endotheliitis with Descemet folds.
Source: Presented by Massimo Accorinti in the International Uveitis Study Group (IUSG) grand rounds.[1]

(IUSG), for the first time demonstrated the possible role of CMV in the etiology of the Posner–Schlossman syndrome.[15]

The condition typically responds well to anti-inflammatory and hypotensive therapy, leading to rapid resolution. Additional findings include diffuse iris atrophy, endotheliitis, and frequent recurrences (**Figs. 3A and B**).[14]

In chronic cases, CMV-AU can resemble Fuchs-like uveitis. These patients generally lack ciliary injection and present with diffuse stellate or round KPs **(Fig. 4)**, anterior chamber flare and cells, Koeppe's nodules, and no posterior synechiae. Vitreous involvement is variable but can occur.[12]

Differential Diagnosis

Specific clinical features can help differentiate viral from nonviral uveitis. Viral uveitis is commonly characterized by unilaterality, prior keratitis, iris atrophy, and elevated IOP (>24 mm Hg). In contrast, nonviral uveitis is often associated with a limited disease duration, ciliary injection, and fine KPs; Accorinti et al. validated these findings in 2020 **(Table 1)**.[16]

Terada et al.[5] conducted a study to identify distinguishing clinical features of herpetic AU. The study included 259 patients with herpetic AU, comprising polymerase chain reaction (PCR)-confirmed cases of HSV-AU (30 patients), VZV-AU (50 patients), and CMV-AU (147 patients), as well as herpes zoster ophthalmicus (HZO) (32 patients). All HSV-AU and VZV-AU cases were unilateral, whereas 3% of CMV-AU cases were bilateral. HSV-AU and VZV-AU typically presented with a sudden onset and an acute clinical course, whereas CMV-AU had a more insidious onset and chronic course.

There were no significant differences between HSV-AU and VZV-AU in the symptoms, signs, or complications surveyed. However, significant differences were noted between CMV-AU and the other two herpetic AU types. Ocular hyperemia, pain, blurred vision, ciliary injection, medium-to-large KPs, cells, and flare in the anterior chamber, and posterior synechiae were significantly more common in HSV-AU and VZV-AU compared to CMV-AU. Conversely, small KPs, coin-shaped KPs, diffuse iris atrophy, elevated IOP, and a history of glaucoma surgery were significantly more frequent in CMV-AU than in HSV-AU and VZV-AU. These findings underscore the importance of distinguishing clinical characteristics to ensure accurate diagnosis and management of herpetic AU **(Table 2)**.

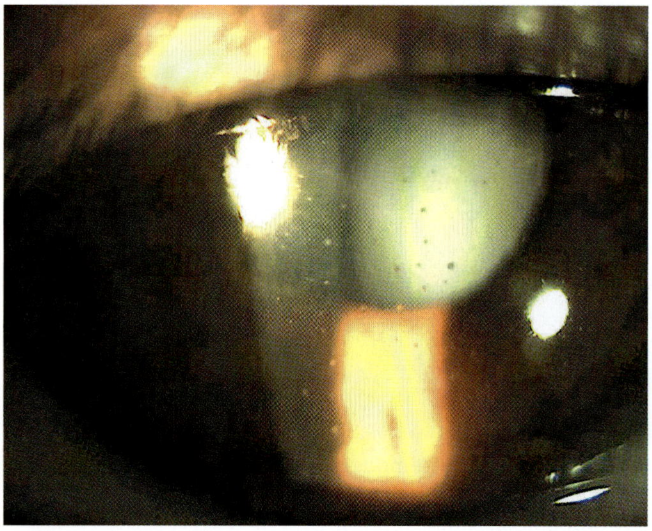

Fig. 4: Round keratic precipitates. Diffuse stellate without posterior synechiae indicative of Fuchs-like uveitis.
Source: Presented by Massimo Accorinti in the International Uveitis Study Group (IUSG) grand rounds.[1]

Diagnosis

The diagnosis of viral AU is based on clinical features and patient history, complemented by serological evidence such as high IgM titers or seroconversion. Analysis of aqueous humor can provide further confirmation through PCR or a Goldmann–Witmer coefficient >3; however, PCR results may become negative after 2 months. Negative PCR results should never be used to exclude viral etiology. The classification criteria by the Standardization of Uveitis Nomenclature (SUN) Working Group for HSV, VZV, and CMV uveitis are found in **Figures 5 to 7**.[17-19] While the exclusion criteria in all of them specify the absence of sarcoidosis evidence on chest imaging or biopsy, there could be rare instances of concomitant herpes infection in patients receiving systemic immunosuppressants for sarcoidosis.

PRACTICAL TIPS IN THE MANAGEMENT OF OCULAR HERPETIC ANTERIOR UVEITIS

Topical and Systemic Therapy for Herpetic Anterior Uveitis

Topical Antiviral Therapy

Topical antivirals could be used to manage herpetic AU, especially in patients with previous or concomitant corneal involvement.[20] Acyclovir ointment is preferred due to its selective antiviral activity and effective penetration into the anterior chamber. Ganciclovir ophthalmic gel also demonstrates selective activity and low toxicity; however, its penetration into the anterior chamber is less effective than acyclovir's.[21]

TABLE 1: Performance of logistic regression model in validation of viral uveitis signs.

Parameters	*AUC (%)*	*p-value*	*Sensitivity (%)*	*Specificity (%)*	*PLR*	*NLR*	*PPV (%)*	*NPV (%)*
Unilaterality + IOP ≥ 24 mm Hg	93.9	<0.0001	87.9	100.0	–	0.12	100.0	89.2
Iris atrophy + Unilaterality + IOP ≥ 24 mm Hg	97.0	<0.0001	93.9	100.0	–	0.061	100.0	94.3

(AUC: area under the curve; IOP: intraocular pressure; NLR: negative likelihood ratio; NPV: negative predictive value; PLR: positive likelihood ratio; PPV: positive predictive value)

TABLE 2: Differences in symptoms and signs regarding herpetic anterior uveitis causes.

Differences in symptoms						
Symptoms	***HSV (30 Patients)***	***VZV (82 Patients)***	***CMV (147 Patients)***	***HSV vs. VZC***	***HSV vs. CMV***	***VZV vs. CMV***
Hyperemia	85%	78%	34%	0.58	<0.001	<0.001
Pain	48%	42%	9%	0.65	<0.001	<0.001
VA reduction	86%	70%	12%	0.13	<0.001	<0.001
Differences in signs						
Signs	***HSV (30 Patients)***	***VZV (82 Patients)***	***CMV (147 Patients)***	***HSV vs. VZC***	***HSV vs. CMV***	***VZV vs. CMV***
Ciliary injections	72%	71%	27%	1	<0.001	<0.001
Fine keratic precipitates	30%	35%	65%	0.82	<0.001	<0.001
Coin-shaped keratic precipitates	4%	0%	38%	0.23	<0.001	<0.001
Cells ≥ 5	97%	96%	74%	1	0.006	<0.001
Flare ≥ 1	91%	78%	30%	0.22	<0.001	<0.001
Diffuse iris atrophy	29%	25%	80%	1	0.02	<0.001
Posterior synechiae	12%	15%	2%	1	0.04	<0.001
IOP > 21 mm Hg	70%	63%	93%	0.51	<0.001	<0.001
Glaucoma surgery	7%	9%	45%	1	<0.001	<0.001

(CMV: cytomegalovirus; HSV: herpes simplex virus; IOP: intraocular pressure; VA: visual acuity; VZV: varicella-zoster virus)
Source: Modified from Terada et al.[5]

Evidence of anterior uveitis
- Anterior chamber cells
- Vitreous cells can be present, but with less severity than anterior chamber cells
- No evidence of retinitis

\+

Unilateral uveitis
Unless there is a positive aqueous PCR for HSV

\+

Evidence of HSV infection in the eye
- Aqueous humor PCR positive for HSV OR
- Sectoral iris atrophy in a patient <50 years old OR
- Herpes simplex keratitis

Exclusions
- Concomitant dermatomal/cutaneous VZV, unless aqueous specimen PCR positive for HSV
- Positive serology for syphilis using a treponemal test
- Evidence of sarcoidosis in chest imaging or tissue biopsy
- Aqueous specimen PCR positive for CMV or VZV

Fig. 5: Classification criteria for herpes simplex virus (HSV) uveitis. (CMV: cytomegalovirus; PCR: polymerase chain reaction; VZV; varicella-zoster virus)
Source: Modified from the Standardization of Uveitis Nomenclature (SUN) Working Group.[17]

Evidence of anterior uveitis
- Anterior chamber cells.
- Vitreous cells can be present, but with less severity than anterior chamber cells
- No evidence of retinitis

\+

Unilateral uveitis
Unless there is a positive aqueous PCR for VZV

\+

Evidence of VZV infection in the eye
- Aqueous humor PCR positive for VZV OR
- Sectoral iris atrophy in a patient > 60 years old OR
- Concurrent or recent dermatomal VZV

Exclusions
- Positive serology for syphilis using a treponemal test
- Evidence of sarcoidosis in chest imaging or tissue biopsy
- Aqueous specimen PCR positive for CMV or HSV

Fig. 6: Classification criteria for varicella-zoster virus (VZV) uveitis. (CMV: cytomegalovirus; HSV: herpes simplex virus; PCR: polymerase chain reaction)
Source: Modified from the Standardization of Uveitis Nomenclature (SUN) Working Group.[18]

Anti-inflammatory Therapy

Corticosteroids are an essential component of anti-inflammatory therapy, but must always be combined with antiviral agents to prevent the onset/exacerbation of herpetic keratitis. Their use should be carefully monitored to ensure no corneal epithelial damage before initiation, as

Evidence of anterior uveitis
- Anterior chamber cells
- If anterior vitreous cells are present, anterior chamber inflammation should be present
- No evidence of retinitis

+

Evidence of CMV infection in the eye
- Aqueous humor PCR positive for CMV

Exclusions
- Positive serology for syphilis using a treponemal test
- Evidence of sarcoidosis in chest imaging or tissue biopsy
- Aqueous specimen PCR positive for VZV or HSV

Fig. 7: Classification criteria for cytomegalovirus (CMV) uveitis. (HSV: herpes simplex virus; PCR: polymerase chain reaction; VZV; varicella-zoster virus)
Source: Modified from the Standardization of Uveitis Nomenclature (SUN) Working Group.[19]

this could favor the onset of keratitis in patients with herpes simplex uveitis. Ensuring an intact ocular surface, referred to as "ocular surface integrity," is crucial when using these therapies; preserving it helps minimize adverse effects and optimize treatment outcomes. In cases where patients become corticosteroid-dependent or resistant, low-dose corticosteroid maintenance therapy may be required to achieve long-term control of intraocular inflammation.[22,23]

Mydriatics

Mydriatics are generally unnecessary in CMV uveitis, but are often employed in HSV and VZV AU to avoid synechiae or to reduce pain from ciliary spasms related to iridocyclitis inflammation. Agents such as tropicamide or atropine can be effective in these cases. However, clinicians should exercise caution due to the potential for postherpetic mydriasis. Notably, postherpetic mydriasis is unrelated to the mydriatic agents and stems from the virus's intrinsic effects on the iris.[23]

Intraocular Pressure Management

Managing IOP spikes is critical in herpetic AU. Preservative-free topical medications should be used as first-line treatment, avoiding prostaglandins, as these have been shown in some cases to increase the risk of herpetic keratitis.[24] Systemic acetazolamide can stabilize the condition during the initial phase of IOP elevation. Close monitoring of IOP and proactive management are vital to prevent long-term complications.

Systemic Therapy

Systemic antiviral therapy is indicated in severe or recurrent cases of herpetic AU. Early initiation of systemic antivirals is essential for effective control of viral replication. Acyclovir and valacyclovir are commonly used, with dosing and duration tailored to the patient's needs. Induction therapy typically lasts between 7 and 21 days, depending on the severity of the disease. For chronic or recurrent cases, long-term prophylaxis with systemic antivirals may be considered, especially in patients with frequent relapses (two or more per year), severe corneal scarring, or those undergoing corticosteroid or immunosuppressive therapy for other conditions[25] **(Table 3)**.

Adverse Events and Monitoring

Although antiviral drugs are generally well tolerated, regular monitoring is necessary, particularly during long-term prophylaxis. Liver and renal functions should be assessed every 3 months. Oral valganciclovir carries a risk of hematological disorders, affecting more than 50% of patients in some reports. In such cases, dose adjustment or discontinuation of therapy may be required.[26] Side effects such as ocular discomfort, mild irritation, and tearing are common but manageable for topical therapy.

Specific Therapy for Cytomegalovirus Uveitis

In CMV-related AU, topical ganciclovir can be used as a gel or an eye drop to achieve higher drug concentrations. Oral valganciclovir is often combined with topical antiviral therapy in acute or chronic cases. For chronic anterior uveitis or CMV endotheliitis, maintaining a higher antiviral dose during the day is recommended to achieve sustained control. In refractory cases, intravitreal ganciclovir injections (two to four injections of 0.2 mL at 2 mg/mL) may be considered during the induction phase **(Table 4)**.

Duration of Antiviral Therapy

A systematic review published in 2021 examined the available evidence on the treatment of AU caused by HSV and VZV. Unfortunately, the review concluded that the current treatment approaches are primarily based on personal and limited clinical experience rather than robust, evidence-based recommendations. This highlights the significant gap in high-quality clinical trials for herpetic AU.[27]

TABLE 3: Systemic therapy.

Drug	***Route of administration***	***Bioavailability***	***Half-life (hours)***	***Dose***	***Duration of induction***	***Prophylaxis***	***Adverse effects***
Acyclovir	Oral	20%	3	400–800 mg × 5 times/day	7–14 days	Up to 800 mg/day	*Common*: Malaise *Less common*: Nausea, vomiting, diarrhea, abdominal pain, transaminitis, rash (including Stevens–Johnson syndrome), renal impairment, vertigo, dizziness, agitation, confusion, alopecia, and thrombocytopenia
Valacyclovir	Oral	54%	8	0.5–1 g × 3 times/day	7–14 days	Up to 500 mg/day	*Common*: Headache, nausea, and vertigo *Less common*: Vomiting, diarrhea, abdominal pain, transaminitis, skin rash, renal impairment, dizziness, agitation, confusion, and thrombocytopenia
Famciclovir	Oral	77%	10	500 mg × 2–3 times/day	7–14 days	Up to 500 mg/day	*Common*: Headache, vertigo, nausea, vomiting, abdominal pain, diarrhea, liver test abnormalities, and cutaneous rash *Less common*: Thrombocytopenia, hallucination, and confusion
Brivudine	Oral	30%	16	125 mg	7–14 days	125 mg twice/week	*Common*: Nausea *Less common*: Malaise, flu-like syndrome, anemia, neutropenia, lymphocytosis, allergic reaction, headache, anxiety, vertigo, paresthesia, systemic hypertension, vomiting, diarrhea, abdominal pain, and transaminitis

Contd...

Contd...

Drug	***Route of administration***	***Bioavailability***	***Half-life (hours)***	***Dose***	***Duration of induction***	***Prophylaxis***	***Adverse effects***
Valganciclovir	Oral	40%	3.5	450 mg × 4 times/day	3 weeks	450 mg twice/week	*Common*: Anemia, diarrhea, neutropenia, and dyspnea *Less common*: Thrombocytopenia, leukopenia, infections, depression, anxiety, headache, confusion, cough, nausea, vomiting, abdominal pain, paresthesia, transaminitis, creatine, and electrolytic changes

TABLE 4: Therapy for CMV uveitis.[26]

	Induction phase*	***Maintenance phase (up to 12 months)***	***Adverse events***
Acute hypertensive CMV-AU	0.15% GCV gel >5×/day for >2 weeks Or Oral VGCV 900 mg 2×/day for 2–3 weeks	0.15% GCV gel >3×/day Or Oral VGCV 450 mg 2×/day	*Topical GCV 0.15% gel*: Ocular discomfort
Chronic CMV-AU	1–2% topical GCV >6×/day for 2–4 weeks And/or Oral VGCV 900 mg 2×/day for 3 weeks	1–2% topical GCV >6×/day And/or Oral VGCV 450 mg 2×/day	*Topical GCV 2% eye drops*: • Mild eye irritation: 27% • Tearing: 18%
CMV endotheliitis	0.5–2% topical GCV >6×/day for 4 weeks And/or Oral VGCV 900–1,800 mg 2×/day for 4 weeks	0.5–2% topical GCV >6×/day (gradually tapered) And/or Oral VGCV 450–900 mg 2×/day	*Oral VGCV 1.8 g/day*: • Hematological disorders: 53% • Creatinine/electrolytic changes: 29% • Gastrointestinal problems: 11.8%

(CMV: cytomegalovirus; GCV: ganciclovir; VGCV: valganciclovir)

*Topical corticosteroids may be added: The duration of the maintenance phase depends on clinical resolution (longer duration is preferred, although inflammation control is being achieved).

Source: Modified from La Distia et al.[26] Some authors also propose intravitreal ganciclovir (2 mg/0.1 mL): Two to four injections.[26]

For herpes simplex virus uveitis:[27] Two studies documented that oral acyclovir for 10 weeks was equal to placebo.

For varicella-zoster virus uveitis:[27]

- Two studies demonstrated that oral acyclovir for 10 days is superior to placebo in managing VZV-associated uveitis.
- One study compared the efficacy of oral acyclovir administered for 7 versus 14 days. The results indicated no significant difference between the two durations, suggesting that a shorter course may be as effective as a longer one for treating VZV uveitis.
- Another study evaluated the effectiveness of topical acyclovir compared to oral acyclovir for 7 days. The findings showed no significant difference between these two routes of administration, indicating that both topical and oral forms may be equally effective in managing the condition.

- One study assessed oral acyclovir versus valacyclovir, administered for 7 days. The results revealed no significant difference in efficacy between the two antiviral agents, suggesting that either drug can effectively treat VZV-associated uveitis.

Indications for Anterior Uveitis Prophylaxis

Long-term prophylaxis should be considered for patients with:

- ≥Two relapses per year
- Severe corneal scarring (keratouveitis)
- Patients submitted to refractive surgery
- Patients on corticosteroids or immunosuppressive therapy

Vaccination[28,29]

Vaccination against herpes zoster offers an additional preventive strategy. Two vaccines are available: (1) an attenuated live virus vaccine and (2) a recombinant vaccine.

Shingrix (Recombinant)[28]

- Two injections, two months apart
- For people >50 years old
- *Reduces postherpetic pain:* Incidence—25.5/100,000/person/year in vaccinated versus 76.7/100,000/person/year in nonvaccinated
- Efficacy changes according to each patient's age:
  - 50–59% (100% efficacy), reducing to 87.6% in 60–69 years
  - 88.9% in 70–79 years
  - 88.8% in ≥80 years

Zostavax (Attenuated Live Virus)[29]

- A single injection
- For people >50 years old
- Efficacy typically decreases over time (10% per year)

COMPLICATIONS OF ANTERIOR HERPETIC UVEITIS

Complications of anterior herpetic uveitis include:

- Recurrences
- Intraocular pressure elevation (75%)
- Keratitis (59%)
- Dry eye (34%)
- Cataracts (32%)
- Glaucoma (15–25%)

These will be treated in the discussion of the last case presentation.

TYPICAL CASE OF HERPES ANTERIOR UVEITIS

Case Presentation

Typical Clinical Case One

Personal data: 37-year-old female.

History of present illness:

- The patient presented with pain, photophobia, redness, and significant visual loss in the right eye (OD).
- She had a history of recurrent oral herpes.

On ocular examination **(Figs. 8A to C)**, the best-corrected visual acuity (BCVA) was 20/80 in the right eye (OD) and 20/20 in the left eye (OS). The IOP was elevated in the OD at 32 mm Hg, while it was 17 mm Hg in the left eye. A slit-lamp examination revealed that scleral

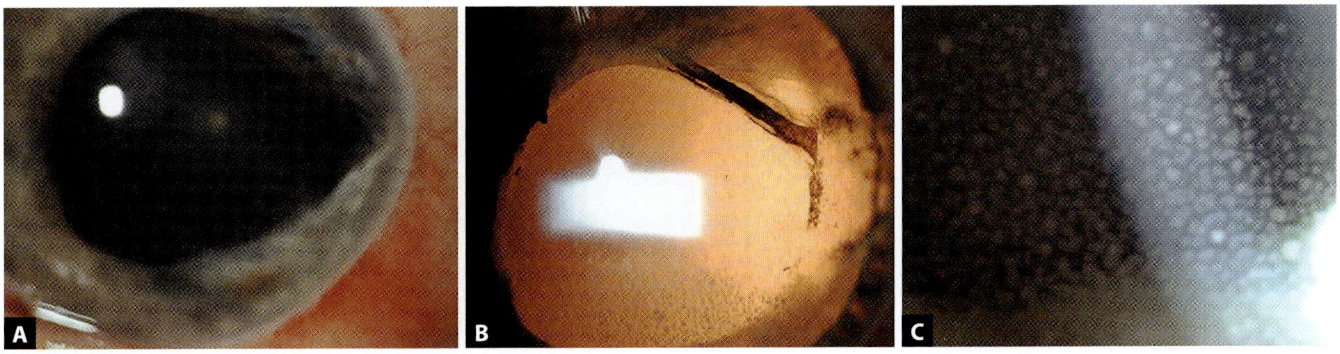

Figs. 8A to C: Clinical characteristics at presentation. (A) Pupillary distortion to a nonreactive pupil secondary to iris atrophy; (B) Posterior synechiae visible upon dilation; (C) Granulomatous keratic precipitates.
Source: Presented by Matteo Menean in the International Uveitis Study Group (IUSG) grand rounds.[1]

and conjunctival injection, granulomatous KPs, and iris atrophy were observed during the transillumination evaluation **(Table 5)**.

Workup: Positive serology for anti-HSV1 IgG confirmed the clinical diagnosis.

Diagnosis: Herpetic AU due to the typical characteristics of acute, unilateral, hypertensive uveitis, with granulomatous KPs and associated iris atrophy.

TABLE 5: Physical examination of the patient having a typical case of herpes anterior uveitis.

OD	*Parameters*	*OS*
20/80	BCVA	20/20
15 mm Hg	IOP	17 mm Hg
Moderate conjunctival hyperemia	Conjunctiva	Quiet
Granulomatous keratic precipitates	Cornea	Normal, clear
No cells ACC: 2+	Anterior chamber	No cells ACC: 0+
Iris atrophy, no reactive pupil	Iris	No synechiae
Clear	Lens	Clear
Unremarkable	Vitreous	Unremarkable
Unremarkable, normal CDR	Fundus	Unremarkable, normal CDR

(ACC: anterior chamber cellularity; BCVA: best-corrected visual acuity; CDR: cup–disc ratio; IOP: intraocular pressure)

Treatment:

- Systemic antiviral therapy: Acyclovir 800 mg thrice daily (TID).
- Topical therapy:
  - Steroids: Prednisolone, four times daily (QID)
  - Mydriatics: Tropicamide, twice daily (BID)
  - Intraocular pressure-lowering agent: Timolol, twice daily (BID)

Outcome: Successful treatment response observed.

Typical Clinical Case Two

Personal data: 53-year-old male.

History of present illness:

- The patient presented with severe pain, photophobia, redness, and significant visual loss in the OD.
- He reported a 3-month history of unilateral uveitis that was initially treated with oral and topical steroids, diagnosed as idiopathic noninfectious uveitis (NIU), but showed no improvement.

Ocular examination: The patient presented with a BCVA of 20/100 in the OD and 20/20 in the OS; the IOP was elevated in the OD (28 mm Hg) and normal in the OS (17 mm Hg). The OD also revealed conjunctival and scleral injection, fine KPs, and stromal edema **(Figs. 9A and B)**.

The second clinical case involves a 53-year-old male who presented with severe pain, severe photophobia, redness, and remarkable visual loss in OD. He had a 3-month history of unilateral uveitis that was treated with oral and topical steroids without benefit after it was diagnosed as idiopathic NIU. The BCVA in OD was 20/100 and in OS

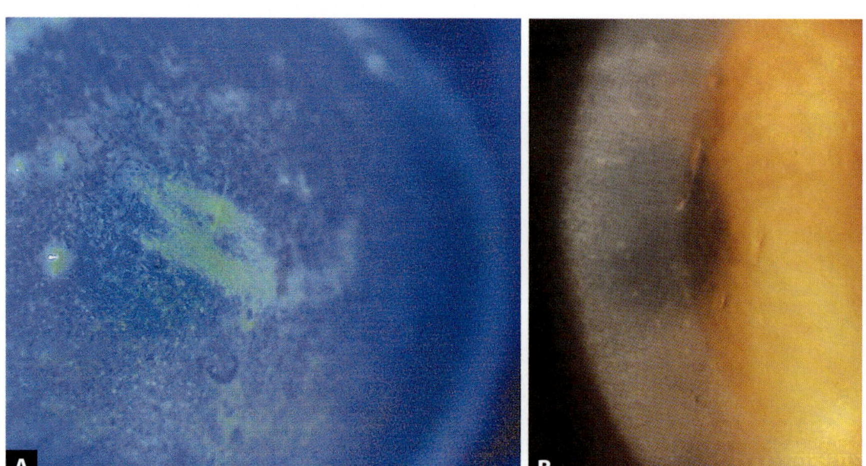

Figs. 9A and B: Typical clinical characteristics at presentation. (A) Epithelial defect; (B) Stromal keratitis, opacity, and fine keratic precipitates. *Source:* Presented by Matteo Menean in the International Uveitis Study Group (IUSG) grand rounds.[1]

TABLE 6: Physical examination of the patient having a typical case of herpes anterior uveitis.

OD	***Parameters***	***OS***
20/100	BCVA	20/20
28 mm Hg	IOP	17 mm Hg
Moderate conjunctival hyperemia	Conjunctiva	Quiet
Fine keratic precipitates	Cornea	Normal, clear
No cells ACC: 2+	Anterior chamber	No cells ACC: 0+
Iris atrophy	Iris	No synechiae
Clear	Lens	Clear
Unremarkable	Vitreous	Unremarkable
Unremarkable, normal CDR	Fundus	Unremarkable, normal CDR

(ACC: anterior chamber cellularity; BCVA: best-corrected visual acuity; CDR: cup–disc ratio; IOP: intraocular pressure)

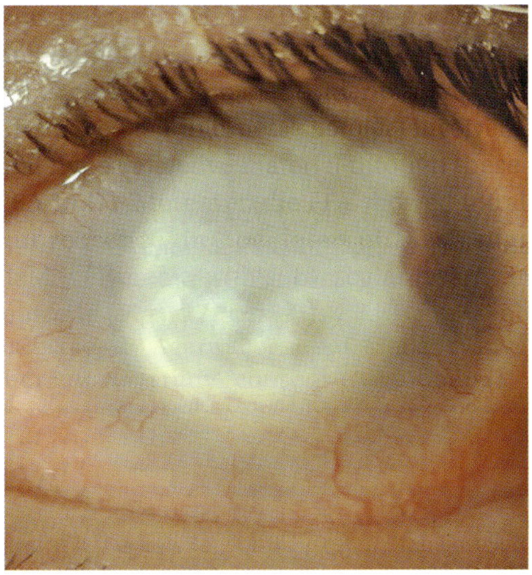

Fig. 10: Ocular morbidity in ocular herpetic disease. Severe chronic stromal keratitis leading to corneal ulcer secondary to neurotrophic keratitis.
Source: Presented by Elisabetta Miserocchi in the International Uveitis Study Group (IUSG) grand rounds.[1]

was 20/20. The IOP in OD was 28 mm Hg, and in OS was 17 mm Hg. The slit-lamp examination exhibited conjunctival and scleral injection, epithelial, fine KPs, and stromal edema **(Table 6 and Fig. 9)**.

Workup: An aqueous tap was performed, given the patient's recent history, revealing a high VZV DNA load and confirming the etiology.

Diagnosis: VZV-AU with associated stromal keratitis.

Treatment:

- *Systemic antiviral therapy:* Acyclovir 800 mg, three times a day (TID)
- *Topical antiviral therapy:* Acyclovir ointment, four times daily (QID)
- *Intraocular pressure-lowering drops:* Timolol, twice daily (BID)
- *Topical steroids:* Prednisolone, four times daily (QID), initiated after epithelial healing (7 days)

Outcome: Treatment response was favorable, with resolution of the epithelial defect and gradual control of intraocular inflammation.

Discussion

Ocular herpetic disease is one of the most common ocular infections in industrialized countries and represents a significant cause of ocular morbidity. Despite its prevalence, the frustrating reality is that current antiviral treatments, which are decades old, cannot eliminate the virus from the body.[30,31] Herpetic disease can affect both the anterior and posterior segments of the eye, leading to severe complications. The management of these patients requires a careful balance between antiviral therapy and corticosteroids, and even with proper treatment, herpetic disease poses significant diagnostic and therapeutic challenges **(Fig. 10)**.[30,31]

Herpetic AU is typically characterized by:[5]

- *Unilateral granulomatous uveitis* ***(Fig. 11)***: Often associated with hypertensive episodes and corneal involvement.
- *Iris atrophy*: Common in both HSV and VZV-associated uveitis **(Fig. 12)**.
- *Corneal involvement*: Ranges from dendritic keratitis to severe stromal keratitis, corneal ulcers, and rare peripheral ulcerative keratitis (PUK) **(Figs. 13A to E)**.

Herpetic uveitis can present bilaterally in rare cases (5–10%), particularly in patients with atopy or immunosuppression. For instance, immunocompromised individuals, such as a young girl with leukemia, may develop anterior uveitis alongside severe retinitis **(Table 7)**.

Differentiating between HSV, VZV, and CMV can be challenging due to overlapping clinical features. Skin

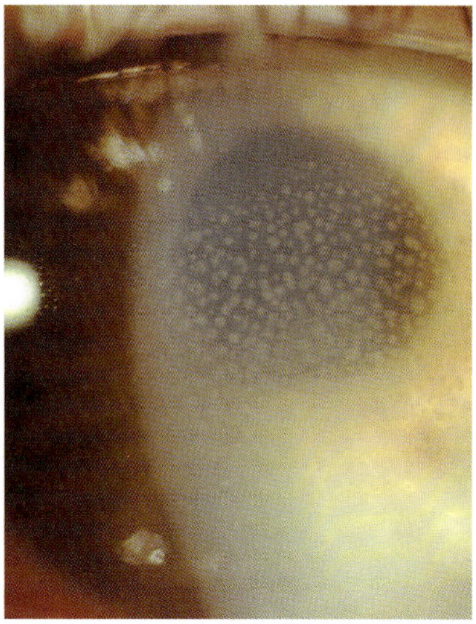

Fig. 11: Clinical picture of herpetic anterior uveitis. Unilateral granulomatous uveitis.
Source: Presented by Elisabetta Miserocchi in the International Uveitis Study Group (IUSG) grand rounds.[1]

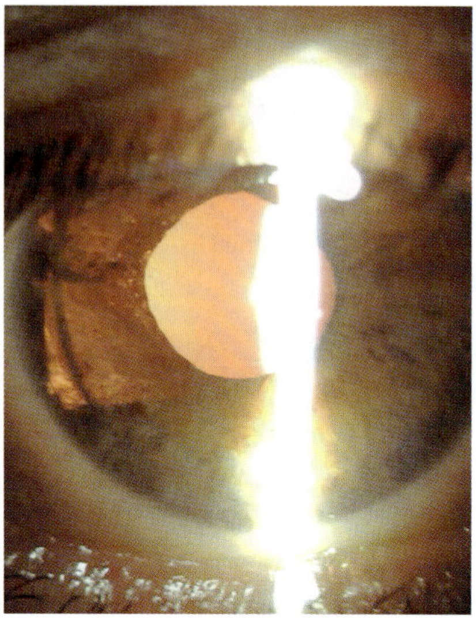

Fig. 12: Iris atrophy. Anterior herpetic uveitis usually produces iris atrophy.
Source: Presented by Elisabetta Miserocchi in the International Uveitis Study Group (IUSG) grand rounds.[1]

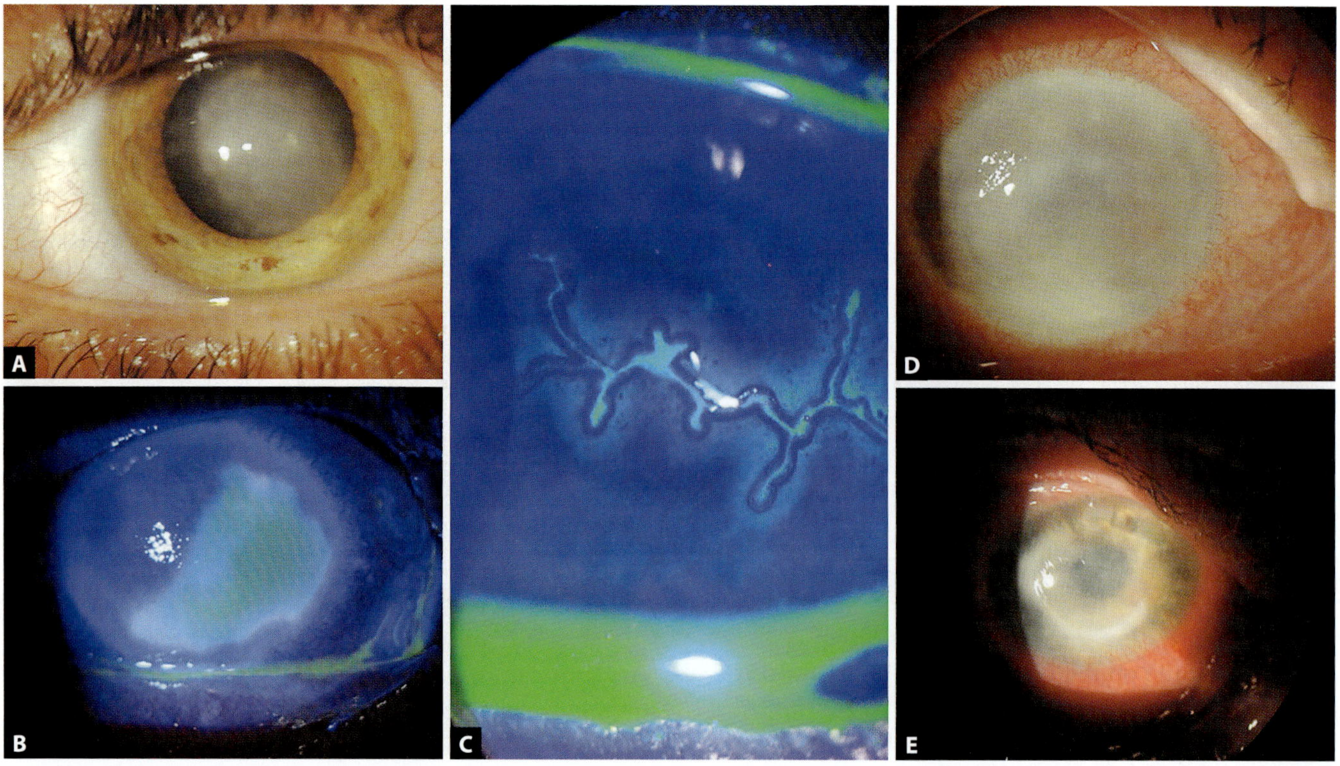

Figs. 13A to E: Different types of keratitis associated with herpetic uveitis caused by HSV and VZV. (A) Stromal disciform keratitis; (B) Large epithelial keratitis with corneal ulcer; (C) Dendritic epithelial keratitis; (D) Severe stromal keratouveitis with hypopyon; (E) Stromal keratitis with immune ring. (HSV: herpes simplex virus; VZV: varicella-zoster virus)
Source: Presented by Elisabetta Miserocchi in the International Uveitis Study Group (IUSG) grand rounds.[1]

TABLE 7: Differences in location and ocular involvement between HSV and VZV.

Location	*HSV (189 Patients)*	*VZV (45 Patients)*
Keratitis		
Stromal	48 (25.4%)	5 (11.1%)
Epithelial	23 (12.2%)	8 (17.8%)
Endotheliitis	4 (2.1%)	1 (2.2%)
Neurotrophic	3 (1.6%)	0
Keratouveitis	63 (33.3%)	13 (28.9%)
Anterior uveitis	35 (18.5%)	5 (11.1%)
Acute retinal necrosis	4 (2.1%)	7 (15.6%)
Scleritis/episcleritis	3 (1.6%)	0
Eyelid involvement	3 (1.6%)	5 (11.1%)
Ocular involvement		
Unilateral	229	95%
Bilateral	12	5%

(HSV: herpes simplex virus; VZV: varicella-zoster virus)
Source: Modified from Miserocchi et al.[30]

involvement, such as the typical zoster vesicular skin eruption, may aid in distinguishing between HSV and VZV **(Figs. 14A and B)**. However, anterior segment findings alone are often insufficient for a definitive diagnosis, as other conditions such as Fuchs' uveitis may present similarly. In atypical cases or in patients with anterior uveitis without suggestive signs of herpetic disease, the definitive etiological diagnosis should be completed with PCR analysis of the aqueous humor.

Key Diagnostic Tools

- *PCR testing of aqueous humor*: Essential for confirming viral DNA and ruling out other alternative diagnoses mimicking herpetic ocular disease, such as Acanthamoeba keratouveitis.
- *Posterior segment examination* is important in cases where AU obscures the view. Herpetic diseases can sometimes involve the retina, leading to acute retinal necrosis (ARN). Consequently, it is crucial to evaluate the peripheral retina in all cases **(Fig. 15)**.

When evaluating a patient with anterior hypertensive unilateral uveitis, it is critical to consider differential diagnoses such as:

- *Fuchs' uveitis*: Distinguished by fine KPs and diffuse iris atrophy, which differ from the findings in herpetic uveitis **(Fig. 16A)**.

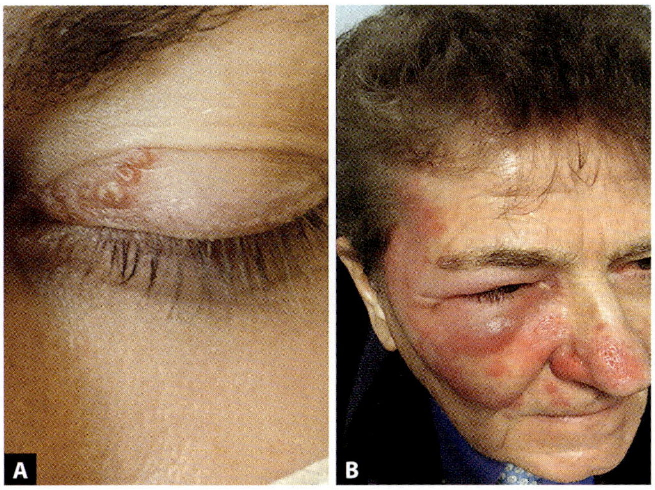

Figs. 14A and B: Skin involvement in different types of herpetic disease. (A) Herpes simplex virus (HSV) typically produces localized vesicular lesions on the eyelids or periorbital skin, often confined to the area directly surrounding the eye. These lesions are generally smaller and limited in distribution; (B) Varicella-zoster virus (VZV) typically causes a dermatomal rash following the distribution of the ophthalmic branch of the trigeminal nerve (herpes zoster ophthalmicus). The rash is often more extensive, with grouped vesicles or pustules that progress to crusting and scarring. It is frequently associated with erythema and swelling of the affected area.
Source: Presented by Elisabetta Miserocchi in the International Uveitis Study Group (IUSG) grand rounds.[1]

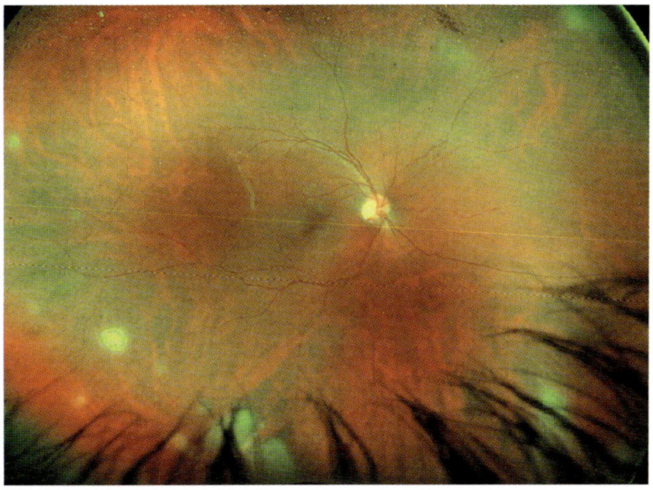

Fig. 15: Acute retinal necrosis associated with anterior herpetic uveitis.
Source: Presented by Elisabetta Miserocchi in the International Uveitis Study Group (IUSG) grand rounds.[1]

- *Acanthamoeba keratouveitis*: Suspected when there is no response to antiviral therapy and confirmed through PCR **(Fig. 16B)**.

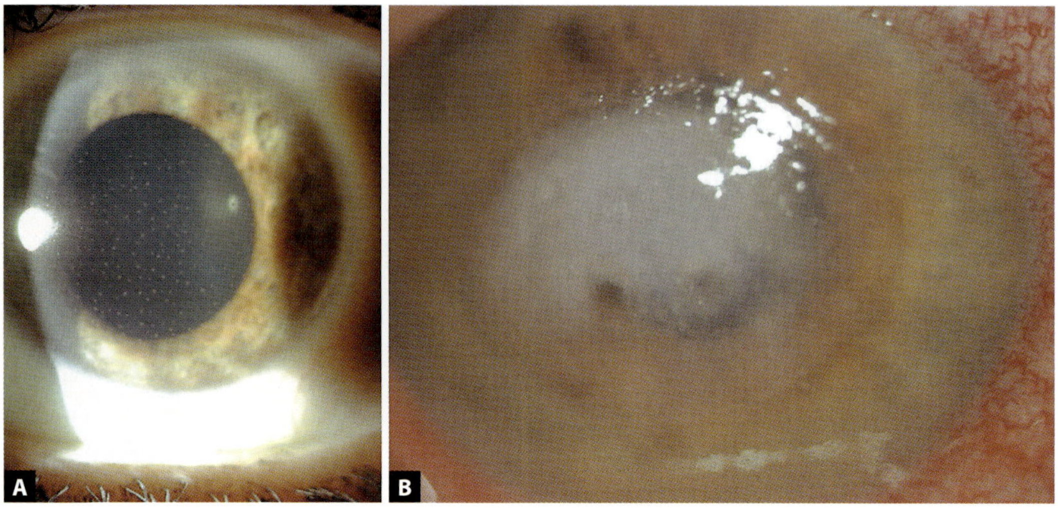

Figs. 16A and B: Differential diagnosis of herpetic (HSV or VZV) anterior uveitis. (A) Fuchs' uveitis; (B) Acanthamoeba keratitis is clinically indistinguishable from stromal herpetic keratouveitis. (HSV: herpes simplex virus; VZV: varicella-zoster virus)
Source: Presented by Elisabetta Miserocchi in the International Uveitis Study Group (IUSG) grand rounds.[1]

Even seemingly simple presentations, such as dendritic keratitis, can progress to catastrophic complications, including corneal ulcers, hypopyon, and severe AU, if not managed promptly and appropriately. Long-term antiviral prophylaxis is critical to preventing such severe outcomes.

ATYPICAL CASE OF HERPES ANTERIOR UVEITIS

Case Presentation

Personal Data

- A 38-year-old man
- Low myopia in both eyes
- Retinal detachment repair in the OS 14 years earlier

History of Present Illness

The patient was referred with a 2-day history of nonspecific blurry vision in his left eye, accompanied by pain and redness. Additionally, the patient reported receiving his second COVID-19 vaccine dose about a month earlier.

Physical Examination

The patient presented with BCVA of 20/20 in each eye and high IOP in the OS with an anterior chamber reaction with dust-like KPs in the inferior cornea and +2 anterior chamber cells **(Table 8)**.

Review of Systems

Negative: No headaches, no fever, no skin rashes, no diarrhea, no arthritis, no ulcers, or auditory symptoms.

Working Diagnosis

Posner–Schlossman syndrome. The patient was treated with topical dexamethasone and timolol–dorzolamide combination for elevated IOP.

Follow-up

One week later, visual acuity was stable, and IOP in the left eye was normalized (20 mm Hg). However, slit-lamp examination revealed medium-sized pigmented KPs and mild atrophy of the temporal iris. Fundus examination of the left eye indicated mild vitritis and perivascular sheathing. The right eye also showed a small area of perivascular sheathing **(Fig. 17)**. Fluorescein angiography revealed diffuse leakage in the left eye, where perivascular sheathing had been observed **(Figs. 18A and B)**.

Serological Blood Tests

- Positive IgG antibodies for HSV-1 and VZV and negative IgM antibodies
- Negative Venereal Disease Research Laboratory (VDRL) and TPHA
- Negative *Toxoplasma* IgM and IgG

TABLE 8: Physical examination of the patient having atypical case of herpes anterior uveitis.

OD	***Parameters***	***OS***
20/20	BCVA	20/20
17 mm Hg	IOP	40 mm Hg
Quiet	Conjunctiva	Quiet
Clear	Cornea	Little dust-like keratic precipitates
• No hypopyon • ACC: 0+ • Wide open angle	Anterior chamber	• No hypopyon • ACC: 2+ C • Wide open angle
Unremarkable	Iris	Unremarkable
Clear	Lens	Clear
Unremarkable	Vitreous	Unremarkable
Optic nerve head sharp margin, normal CDR, normal macula, and retina attached	Fundus	Optic nerve head sharp margin, normal CDR, normal macula, and retina attached

(ACC: anterior chamber cellularity; BCVA: best-corrected visual acuity; CDR: cup–disc ratio; IOP: intraocular pressure)

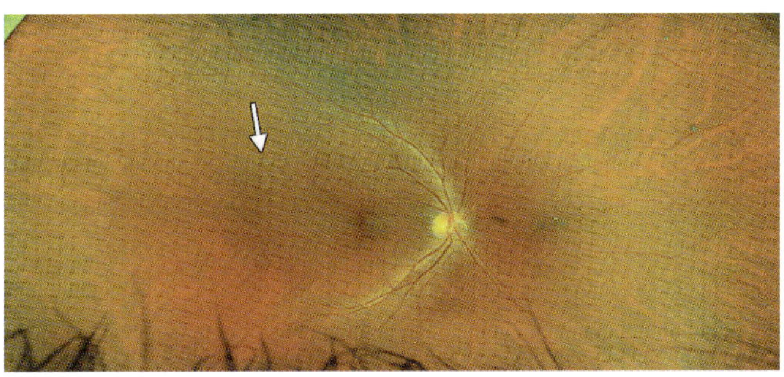

Fig. 17: Pseudocolor wide-angle fundus photograph of the right eye. Localized perivascular sheathing (white arrow) indicative of periphlebitis.
Source: Presented by Neofytos Mavris in the International Uveitis Study Group (IUSG) grand rounds.[1]

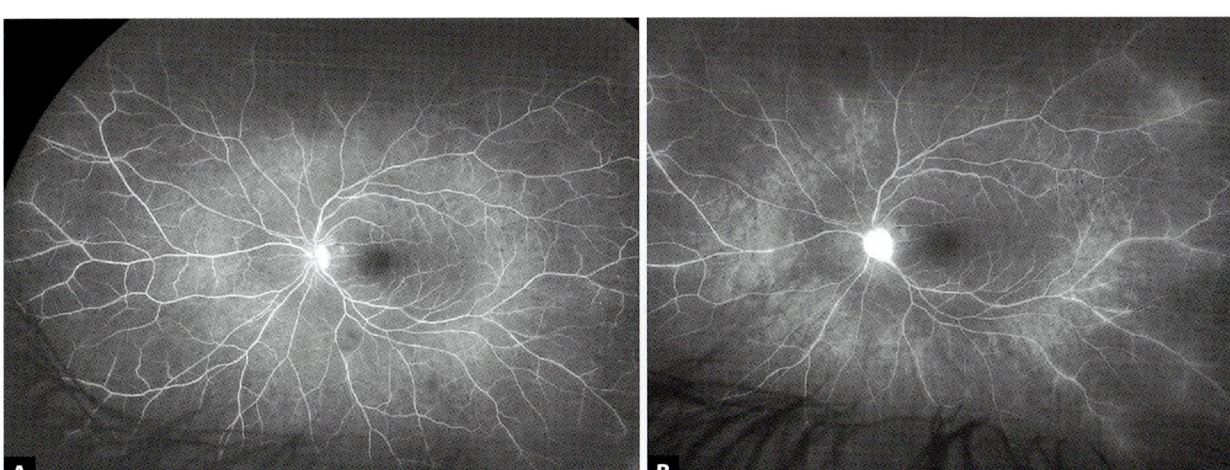

Figs. 18A and B: Fluorescein angiography of the left eye. (A) The arteriovenous phase shows normal filling of arteries and veins; (B) The late phase shows vascular leakage and hot optic disc.
Source: Presented by Neofytos Mavris in the International Uveitis Study Group (IUSG) grand rounds.[1]

Final Diagnosis

Herpetic panuveitis.

Treatment

- Acyclovir 800 mg five times a day orally for 2 weeks and then tapered to 800 mg thrice daily
- Prednisone 60 mg orally for 2 weeks and then tapering
- Dexamethasone eye drops four times daily
- Timolol–dorzolamide drops twice daily

Course

At the 3-week follow-up examination, the patient's BCVA remained stable, and the IOP was within normal limits. There was a complete clearing of KPs and anterior chamber reaction, with resolving perivascular sheathing observed in both eyes. Three months later, we noted the development of sectoral iris atrophy in the temporal part of the left iris, along with the resolution of the perivascular sheathing bilaterally.

It is important to highlight that the patient was monitored for a total of 2 years, during which he discontinued the medication, leading to two relapses characterized by left eye hypertensive AU but without any perivascular sheathing.

Discussion

Herpetic AU is characterized by unilateral granulomatous AU. The presented case discusses (1) the development of retinal periphlebitis and (2) bilaterality.

When HSV and VZV affect the posterior segment of the eye, the resulting phenotype is classic ARN, characterized by the triad of vitritis, occlusive retinal arteriolitis, and necrotizing retinitis.[32] There are, however, case reports and case series that described the occurrence of retinal vasculitis (with no signs of ARN) in patients who suffered from varicella infections and in patients diagnosed with VZV infection in the absence of the classic herpetic skin eruption (zoster sine herpete).[33-35] Noda et al.[33] described two healthy patients who developed hypertensive unilateral AU and retinal periphlebitis, who, by aqueous PCR, were confirmed to be positive for VZV DNA. Both patients were immunocompetent and successfully treated with systemic acyclovir and steroids with marked improvement. Both patients developed, later on, sectoral iris atrophy. The periphlebitis was not associated with retinal hemorrhages, exudates, or periarteritis. Children were also described to develop retinal vasculitis associated with VZV-AU.[34,35] Wimmersberger et al.[35] described unilateral hypertensive AU and marked retinal venous congestion and leakage in an immunocompetent girl who was confirmed to have positive aqueous PCR to VZV DNA. She was diagnosed with a zoster sine herpete. She improved with systemic steroids and acyclovir. Complete resolution of retinal vasculitis was documented by fluorescein angiography 6 weeks later.

Bodaghi et al.[36] reported 37 patients with chronic posterior uveitis who were unresponsive to immunomodulatory therapy (IMT). Five were diagnosed positive aqueous PCR or local antibody production for VZV (three patients) or HSV-1 (two patients). Four of the five patients were women, and four had bilateral posterior uveitis. The authors suggested ruling out a viral etiology in patients with chronic refractory posterior uveitis who have a negative prior workup. Kahloun et al.[37] reported the ocular involvement and visual outcomes of 45 patients with HZO. Six patients (13.3%) had bilateral simultaneous HZO and bilateral eye involvement: two patients had diabetes mellitus, two were on IMT, one had HIV, and one was healthy. Diagnosing bilateral herpetic eye involvement in a patient with bilateral HZO is straightforward. It is, however, much more challenging in a patient who presents with bilateral uveitis in the absence of cutaneous zoster eruption. Nakamura et al.[38] described this scenario in a case report in which a 65-year-old man presented with bilateral hypertensive iridocyclitis and sectoral iris atrophy. Aqueous tap was positive for the VZV genome, thus confirming the diagnosis of zoster sine herpete in this patient.

Bilaterality has also been reported with herpes simplex viral infections. Tugal-Tutkun et al.[11] reported bilateral herpetic keratouveitis in three out of 111 cases. All had atopic disease. Similarly, Miserocchi et al.[39] reported bilateral HSV uveitis in 18% of the cases. de-la-Torre et al. reported three patients with bilateral HSV uveitis, all of whom were under IMT. The authors hypothesized that IMT facilitated the bilateral extension of the infection.[40]

UNCONTROLLED GLAUCOMA IN ANTERIOR HERPETIC UVEITIS CASE

Case Presentation

Personal Data

- Male patient, currently 79 years old.

History of Present Illness

The patient's ocular history began in 1972 at the age of 26 years with blurred vision, mild hyperemia, and ocular discomfort in OD. The episode was characterized by mild intraocular inflammation and elevated IOP, eventually leading to a diagnosis of unilateral hypertensive AU. Two further episodes with the same symptoms occurred in OD between 1972 and 1975, when he was observed for the first time in our department.

Ocular Examination at our Initial Presentation in 1975

- BCVA: OD 20/25, OS 20/20
- OU: High myopia (–9 diopters)
- IOP: OD 38 mm Hg and OS 16 mm Hg
- OD: Mild ciliary injection, rare endothelial precipitates, mild anterior chamber inflammation (flare 1+, rare cells), clear vitreous, and myopic macular dystrophy
- OS: No inflammation in the anterior chamber, clear vitreous, and myopic macular dystrophy

Diagnosis

Posner–Schlossman syndrome.

Over the next decade, the patient experienced *24 relapses* of hypertensive AU in the right eye, with the same clinical findings as previously reported, and with IOP spikes reaching as high as 56 mm Hg. Each episode was managed with topical steroids and hypotensive drops without initiation of chronic IOP-lowering therapy. The visual field in 1985 is reported in **Figure 19**.

By 1986, the OS began to show signs of ocular hypertension without associated inflammation, prompting the initiation of chronic timolol therapy twice daily. The condition of the OD, however, continued to deteriorate, with progressive IOP spikes and relapses of AU.

During the first 4 months of 1987, the patient experienced four relapses of uveitis in OD and a chronic IOP rise >24 mm Hg despite maximum medical topical (timolol, dipivefrin) and systemic (acetazolamide) therapy.

Because of progressive visual field deterioration **(Fig. 20)**, the patient underwent trabeculectomy without mitomycin C in June 1987.

Five months post-trabeculectomy, BCVA was 20/25, IOP was 10 mm Hg without therapy, and the OD visual field is reported in **Figure 21**. No further recurrences of uveitis in OD were detected in the following 37 years of follow-up.

In 1991, symmetric reduction in visual field sensitivity was noted in both eyes, while the IOP was under control [OD: 12 mm Hg (without therapy) and OS: 18 mm Hg (on therapy)] **(Figs. 22A and B)**, attributed to empty sella syndrome diagnosed by imaging (computed tomography evidencing the presence of an arachnoid diverticulum). No surgical intervention was indicated.

In 1998, 11 years post-trabeculectomy, the patient presented an IOP rise in OD (25 mm Hg), which was successfully managed with a combination of timolol and prostaglandins after the exclusion of brimonidine due to an allergic reaction. IOP values over the day were always below 17 mm Hg in both eyes. Pachymetry was 548 μm in OD and 566 μm in OS.

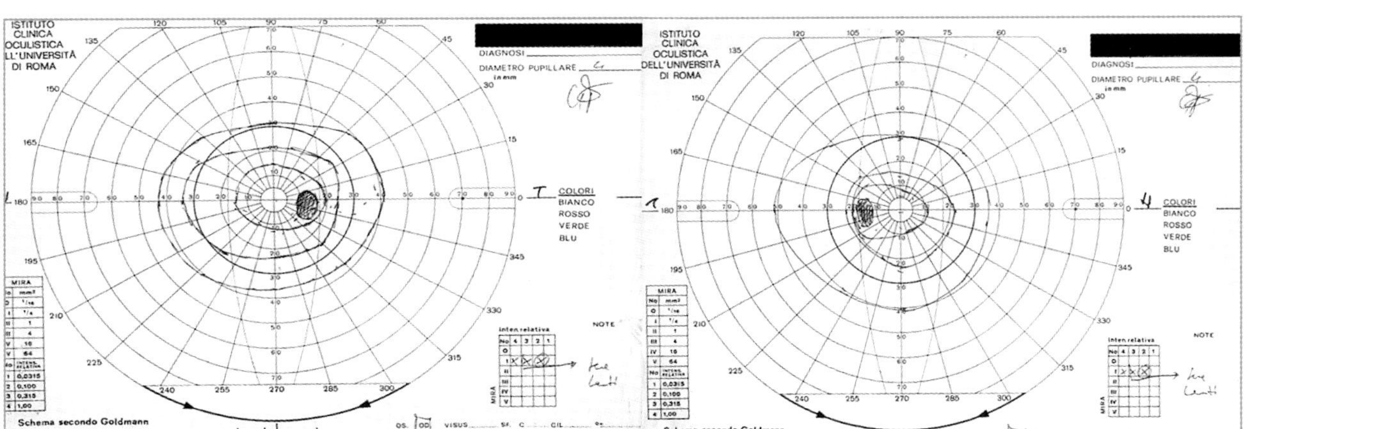

Fig. 19: Visual field of the patient in 1985.
Source: Presented by Daniele de Geronimo in the International Uveitis Study Group (IUSG) grand rounds.[1]

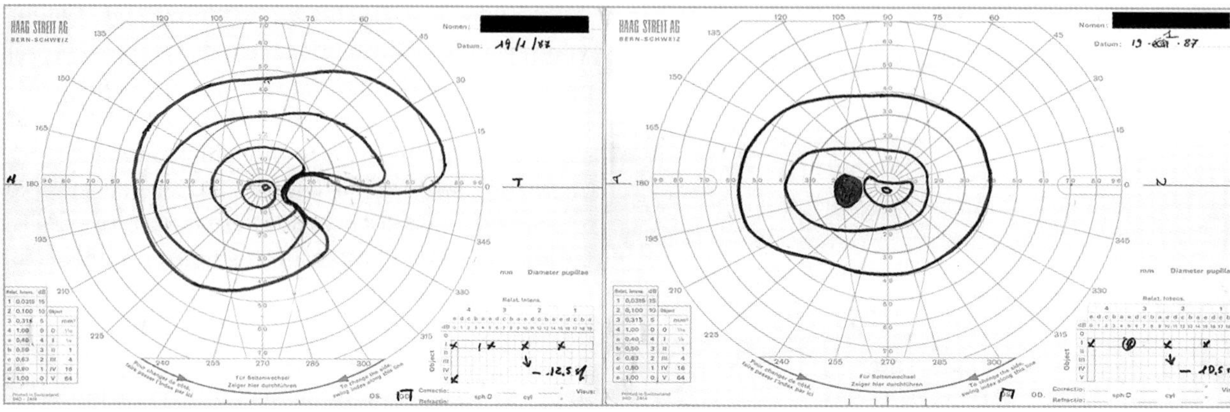

Fig. 20: Visual field in 1987.
Source: Presented by Daniele de Geronimo in the International Uveitis Study Group (IUSG) grand rounds.[1]

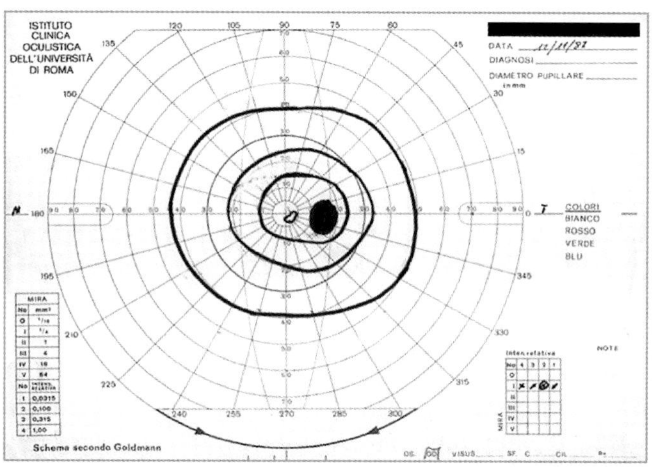

Fig. 21: Visual field 5 months after trabeculectomy.
Source: Presented by Daniele de Geronimo in the International Uveitis Study Group (IUSG) grand rounds.[1]

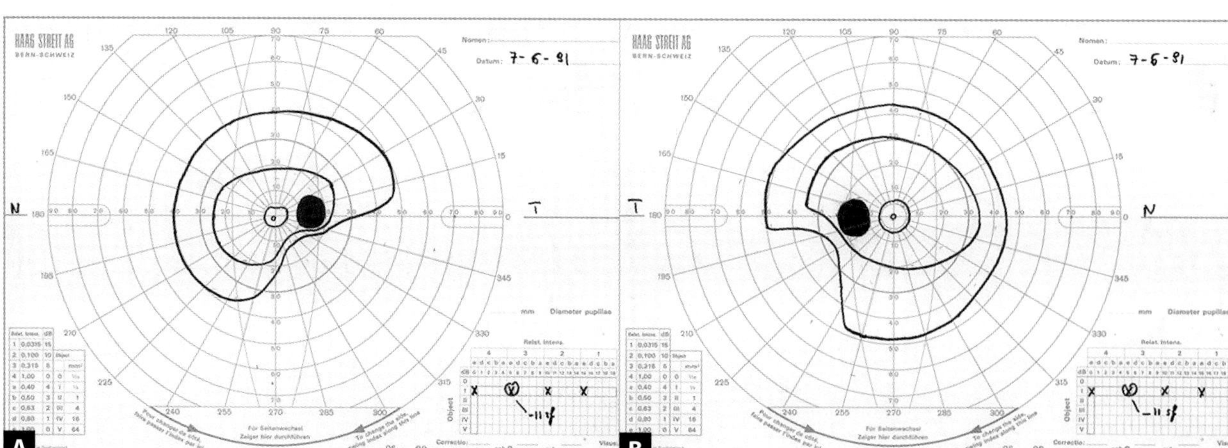

Figs. 22A and B: Visual field performed in 1991. The OD (A) and OS (B) showed a symmetric reduction in visual field sensitivity. Specifically, an inferonasal sector defect was detected in both visual fields. This finding raised concerns about a potential systemic cause, which was later attributed to empty sella syndrome and confirmed by imaging studies.
Source: Presented by Daniele de Geronimo in the International Uveitis Study Group (IUSG) grand rounds.[1]

In 2005, the patient was operated for a cataract in OD. Aqueous tap for viral DNA (HSV-1, HSV-2, VZV, EBV, and CMV) turned out negative.

Nineteen years after trabeculectomy (2006), the patients experienced allergic reactions to all the hypotensive drops, and the maximum tolerated therapy with systemic acetazolamide did not succeed in controlling the IOP in OD, which was constantly raised above 24 mm Hg. Therefore, the patient was submitted to a new trabeculectomy with mitomycin C. IOP after surgery was 13 mm Hg without therapy.

Three years later, the patient presented a blebitis in OD due to a hyperfiltering bleb, successfully managed with topical and systemic antibiotics and systemic corticosteroids but also requiring two appositions of amniotic membrane (which failed) and finally a surgical revision of the bleb that luckily did not negatively affect the IOP for the following 4 years.

In 2013, there was an increase of IOP in OD (21 mm Hg), and the patient was reinitiated with hypotensive therapy (timolol 0.5% BID), while cataract surgery was performed in OS.

Ocular comorbidities were identified during the follow-up: Recurrent chalazion, operated in 1998 and 2002 in OD, and in 1999 in OS, and a retinal tear in OS, treated with laser in 1995.

To summarize, the patient has experienced during a follow-up of 52 years given as follows:

- *In OD:* 32 relapses of uveitis, secondary glaucoma, one blebitis, and recurrent chalazia. He underwent to two trabeculectomies, one cataract extraction with IOL implantation, two amniotic membrane appositions, one bleb revision, and two chalazion removals.
- *In OS:* Ocular hypertension, retinal break, and recurrent chalazia. He underwent to one cataract extraction with IOL implantation, one laser photocoagulation, and one chalazion removal.

Current Management (as of August 2024)

- *Medications*: Timolol twice daily in both eyes
- *Best-corrected visual acuity*: OD 20/25 (with posterior capsular opacity) and OS 20/20
- *Intraocular pressure*: OD 14 mm Hg and OS 16 mm Hg
- *Diurnal IOP variation*: Stable in both eyes

The last visual field done in August 2024 is reported in **Figure 23**.

Figures 24A to D show the anterior segment and fundus photographs of the patient in August 2024.

Discussion

Herpetic AU is a complex condition often complicated by recurrent inflammation, corneal involvement, and

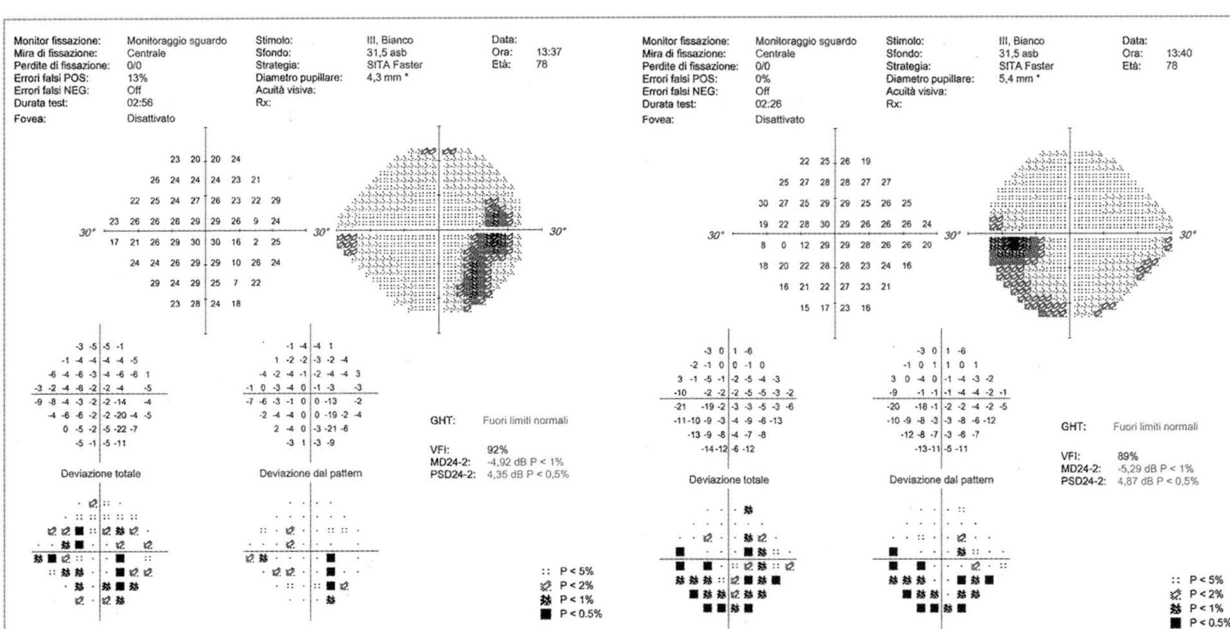

Fig. 23: Visual field of the patient in August 2024. Bilateral blind spot enlargement.
Source: Presented by Daniele de Geronimo in the International Uveitis Study Group (IUSG) grand rounds.[1]

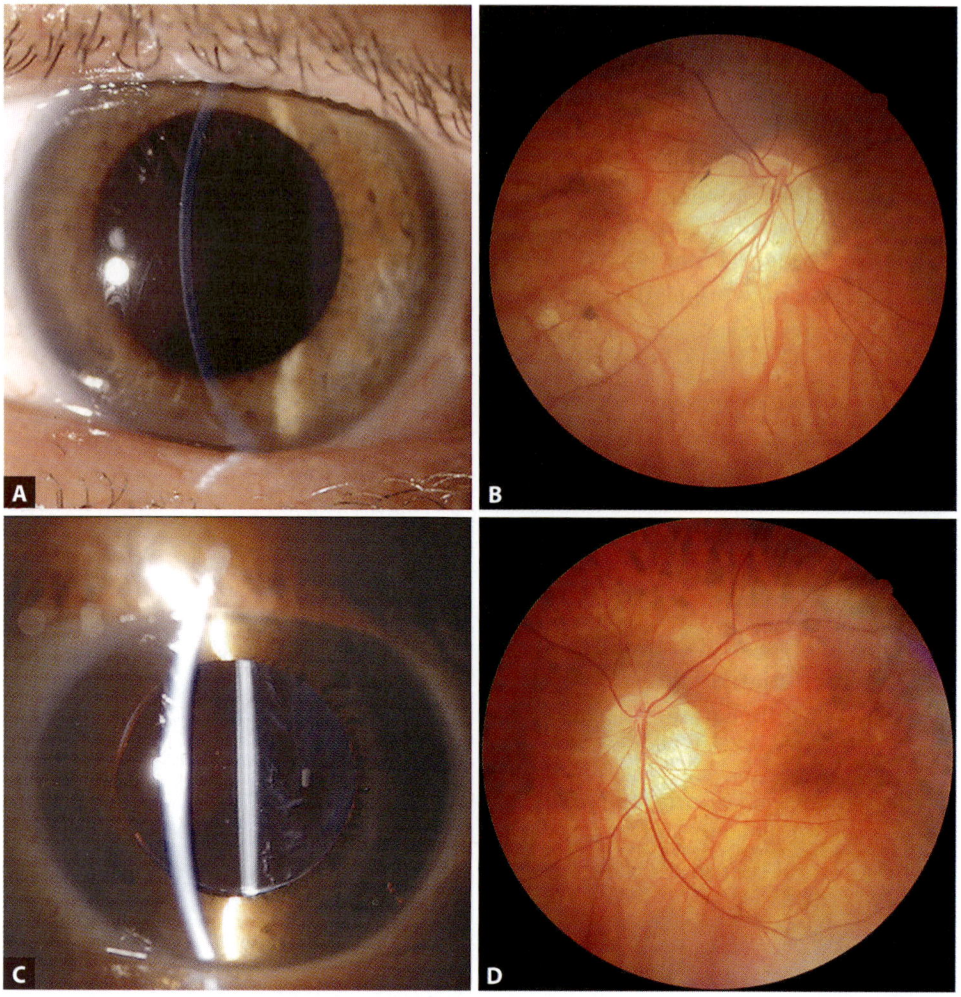

Figs. 24A to D: Anterior segment photographs and color fundus photographs in the last follow-up. Anterior segment photographs of the (A) right eye and (C) left eye of the patient showing no inflammation and the outcomes of cataract surgery. Fundus photographs of the right eye (B), and left eye (D), show no papillary excavation, peripapillary atrophy, mainly due to myopia, and a depigmented fundus. *Source:* Presented by Daniele De Geronimo in the International Uveitis Study Group (IUSG) grand rounds.[1]

IOP elevation, which leads to long-term management challenges. These complications—recurrence, corneal damage, cataract formation, and glaucoma—are interlinked and can significantly impact surgical and medical outcomes **(Figs. 25A to D)**. The presented case and discussion offer a comprehensive view of these challenges and insights into best practices for managing such patients.

Impact of Recurrence and Risk Factors

Recurrent episodes of herpetic uveitis increase the likelihood of secondary glaucoma, with each IOP spike compounding the risk of optic nerve damage. Long-term antiviral prophylaxis has been shown to reduce relapse rates, emphasizing the importance of systemic and topical antiviral therapy.[41,42] While psychological stress, light exposure, and obesity have been suggested as triggers for recurrence, these findings remain inconsistent across studies. Nevertheless, high-risk patients must carefully consider potential triggers and tailored prophylaxis.[43-45]

Corneal Complications

Corneal involvement, such as herpetic dendritic ulcers and stromal keratitis, is a hallmark of HSV and VZV uveitis. Chronic topical therapy with corticosteroids and antivirals can exacerbate ocular surface disease, resulting in severe dry eye. Additionally, blebs from filtering surgeries may disrupt the tear film, worsening dry eye symptoms and

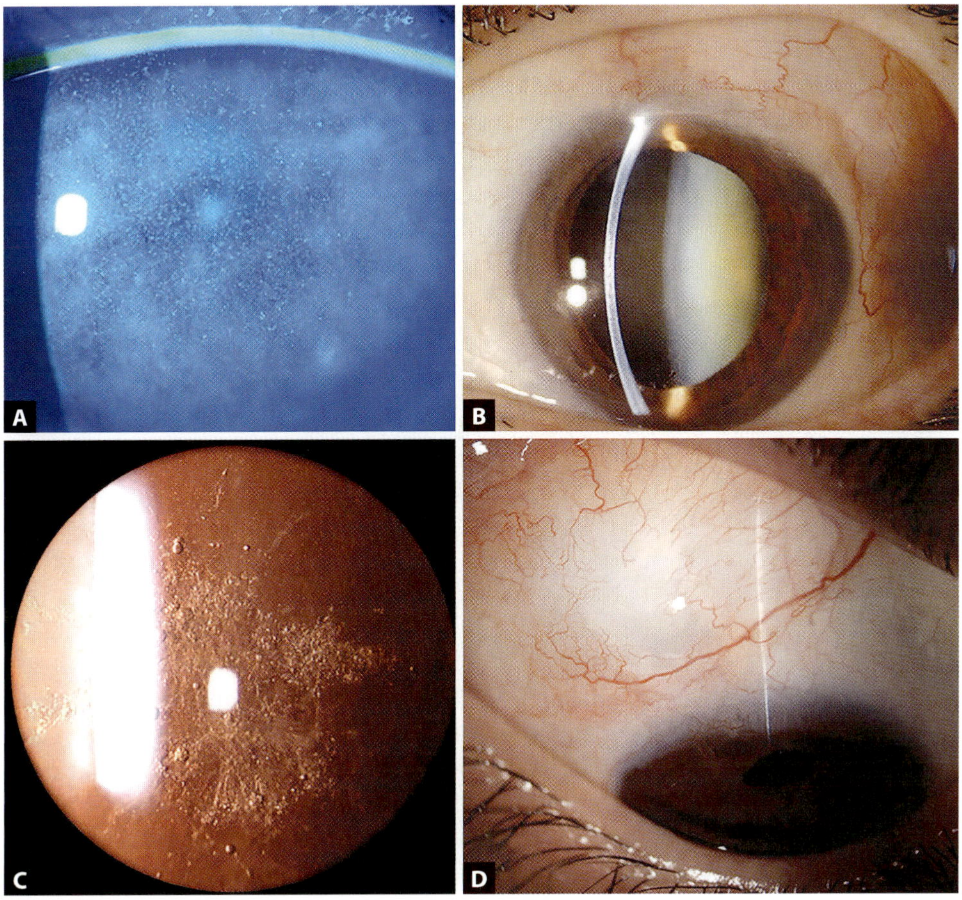

Figs. 25A to D: Common complications of anterior herpetic uveitis. (A) Diffuse superficial punctate keratitis; (B) Nuclear and posterior subcapsular cataract; (C) Posterior capsular cataract; (D) Glaucoma treated with a minimally invasive glaucoma surgery.
Source: Presented by Massimo Accorinti in the International Uveitis Study Group (IUSG) grand rounds.[1]

reducing visual acuity. Surgical approaches may help restore corneal clarity in advanced cases.

Cataract and Surgical Challenges

Cataracts, often nuclear, subcapsular, or mixed, are common in patients with chronic and relapsing uveitis. Furthermore, in patients with herpetic uveitis, the frequent recurrences and, in some cases, the need for chronic corticosteroid therapy to keep uveitis under control can increase the occurrence of cataracts.[22,23]

The presence of a filtering bleb is another important challenge in the surgical approach of the cataract for two main reasons: (1) The possible failure of the bleb after cataract surgery and (2) the impact a bleb can have on the ocular surface, which might also be altered in patients with herpetic uveitis by the chronic administration of eye drops, as previously reported. We suggest that surgeons balance reducing surgical trauma with protecting the ocular surface. Preoperative systemic antiviral prophylaxis is essential to minimize the risk of postoperative relapse. Similarly, postoperative antiviral and corticosteroid therapy for at least 1–2 months reduces inflammation and improves outcomes.

Glaucoma: Pathophysiology and Surgical Risks

In herpetic uveitis, glaucoma arises from multiple mechanisms, including trabeculitis during the acute phase, steroid-induced IOP elevation, and angle closure due to synechiae in chronic cases. The mixed mechanisms of glaucoma demand individualized treatment strategies. Notably, even after a successful trabeculectomy, filtering blebs are at risk of failure, particularly without pre- and postoperative control of inflammation. Long-term bleb maintenance is critical, as complications such as blebitis or hypotony may necessitate additional surgical approaches.[46,47]

TABLE 9: Medical therapy and side effects.

	Timolol	*Dorzolamide*	*Brinzolamide*	*Brimonidine*	*Latanoprost*	*Travoprost*	*Bimatoprost*	*Tafluprost*
Blepharitis	X	X	X	X	X	X	X	X
Conjunctivitis	X	X	X	X	X	X	X	X
Blurred vision	X	X	X	X	X	X	X	X
Reduced corneal sensitivity	X		X					
Corneal edema		X	X				X	
Dry eye	X		X	X	X	X	X	X
Corneal erosion/ulcers	X	X	X		X	X	X	X
Diplopia	X		X					
Ptosis	X							
Iritis/ iridocyclitis		X		X	X	X		X

Regarding medical therapy, all available medications may be utilized, except for pilocarpine, as it has the potential to exacerbate ocular inflammation. However, it is important to consider that these drugs are associated with various local side effects **(Table 9)**.

Management Considerations for Glaucoma Surgery in Herpetic Uveitis[1]

- *Preoperative care*:
  - Use systemic antiviral prophylaxis to prevent relapses
  - Control inflammation meticulously to avoid postoperative complications
- *Surgical approach*:
  - Choose minimally invasive techniques when appropriate
  - Set target IOPs lower than usual for uveitis patients to account for the higher risk of optic nerve damage
  - Prolong postoperative antiviral and corticosteroid therapy to reduce relapse risk
- *Postoperative monitoring*:
  - Protect the ocular surface during and after surgery
  - Regular optical coherence tomography (OCT) and visual field follow-ups should be conducted to monitor progression

Importance of Long-term Follow-up

The presented case illustrates the necessity of long-term care in managing herpetic AU with glaucoma. Over decades, the patient underwent multiple surgeries, including trabeculectomies and cataract extractions, while contending with complications such as blebitis, conjunctival allergic reactions, and recurrent chalazia. Visual field monitoring revealed progressive defects consistent with the cumulative impact of relapses and IOP spikes. Remarkably, despite the chronicity of his condition, the patient retained functional vision in both eyes, underscoring the effectiveness of vigilant follow-up and individualized care.

Addressing the patient's overall health is crucial in addition to ocular management. Conditions such as empty sella syndrome highlight the importance of systemic evaluations in patients with any chronic or relapsing ocular conditions. Moreover, clinicians must remember to always evaluate the contralateral eye, even in cases of unilateral uveitis, as subtle changes can appear, either related or not with the suffered uveitis.

PEARLS FROM THE EXPERTS ON FREQUENTLY ASKED QUESTIONS

1. Is herpetic VZV uveitis in young adults always associated with immunocompromised conditions, or can it also occur in healthy individuals?

Answer: Young patients with HZO should always have their immune status evaluated, including testing for possible HIV seropositivity.

2. Is long-term low-dose antiviral therapy an option for managing recurrent cases of herpetic uveitis?
Answer: Long-term secondary prophylaxis is advisable in recurrent cases, though not indefinitely. Therapy discontinuation may be considered after several years without recurrences.

3. Can prolonged use of local acyclovir ointment (skin or ocular) lead to minimal renal dysfunction, such as systemic acyclovir therapy?
Answer: Prolonged topical acyclovir ointment is not expected to cause renal dysfunction. However, systemic therapy requires regular monitoring of renal and liver function.

4. Are the vaccination results presented specific to reducing ocular inflammation or do they address herpes infections in general?
Answer: The results presented refer to reducing herpes infections in general.

5. Do you recommend the prophylactic use of antiviral therapy before cataract surgery to prevent postoperative recurrences?
Answer: Prophylactic antiviral therapy before cataract surgery is strongly recommended to prevent postoperative recurrences.

6. Can hypopyon be a feature of herpetic uveitis?
Answer: Hypopyon can occur in very severe cases of herpetic uveitis, but it is uncommon.

7. Should acyclovir 400 mg twice daily be continued indefinitely, even in the absence of disease relapses for a prolonged period?
Answer: Acyclovir therapy should not be continued indefinitely. Therapy discontinuation can be attempted cautiously after a long period without relapses, though no published data support this approach.

8. How should one decide between using acyclovir or valacyclovir for systemic prophylaxis, and what is the recommended duration?
Answer: Prophylaxis should typically begin with acyclovir, switching to valacyclovir if resistance is suspected. The duration of therapy depends on the clinical course and recurrence risk.

9. Is metagenomic next-generation sequencing (NGS) widely used to diagnose viral AU?
Answer: There is limited experience with metagenomic NGS in diagnosing viral AU.

10. Can CMV-AU occur in patients without a history of immunosuppression?
Answer: Yes, CMV-AU can occur in immunocompetent individuals, though it is more frequently associated with immunocompromised patients.

11. Does the frequency of herpetic uveitis relapse differ significantly between HSV and VZV etiologies?
Answer: Herpetic AU caused by HSV tends to relapse more frequently compared to VZV.

12. What are the main indicators to differentiate HSV, VZV, and CMV AU clinically?
Answer: Differentiating features include the presence of coin-shaped KPs and diffuse iris atrophy in CMV uveitis, dendritic keratitis in HSV, and associated vesicular skin lesions in VZV.

13. How can one distinguish between Fuchs' uveitis syndrome and herpetic uveitis?
Answer: Key differences include the fine KPs and diffuse iris atrophy typical of Fuchs' uveitis syndrome, whereas herpetic uveitis often presents with granulomatous KPs, sectoral iris atrophy, and elevated IOP.

14. Is there a role for intravitreal antiviral therapy in managing anterior herpetic uveitis?
Answer: Intravitreal antiviral therapy is not typically used for anterior herpetic uveitis but may be considered in severe or refractory cases involving posterior segment involvement.

15. Are there any known predictors of poor visual outcomes in herpetic AU?
Answer: Predictors of poor visual outcomes include recurrent relapses, uncontrolled IOP spikes, severe corneal involvement, and delayed initiation of antiviral therapy.

16. What is the incidence of glaucoma in patients with recurrent herpetic AU?
Answer: Glaucoma develops in a significant proportion of patients with recurrent herpetic AU, particularly those with poorly controlled IOP spikes or frequent relapses.

17. Is there evidence to suggest that early surgical intervention for glaucoma in herpetic uveitis improves long-term outcomes?
Answer: Early surgical intervention, such as trabeculectomy, may improve long-term outcomes in cases of uncontrolled IOP; however, success is contingent on pre-operative control of inflammation.

18. Can herpetic AU be present bilaterally?
Answer: Bilateral presentation is rare but may occur in patients with atopy or severe immunosuppression.

19. Is there a specific role for gonioscopy in the routine follow-up of herpetic uveitis patients?
Answer: Gonioscopy is essential for identifying synechiae, trabeculitis, or angle closure, which may influence management decisions in herpetic uveitis patients.

20. Can herpetic AU occur in the absence of corneal involvement?
Answer: Yes, herpetic AU can occur without corneal involvement, although corneal findings such as dendritic ulcers or stromal keratitis are often present in HSV and VZV infections.

21. What is the role of PCR in confirming the diagnosis of herpetic AU?
Answer: PCR of aqueous humor is a highly sensitive and specific diagnostic tool for confirming herpetic AU by detecting viral DNA.

22. How long after a uveitis relapse should one wait before considering cataract surgery?
Answer: Cataract surgery should generally be delayed until the uveitis is quiescent for at least 3 months to minimize the risk of postoperative complications.

23. Are there specific precautions for performing cataract surgery in patients with herpetic AU?
Answer: Preoperative systemic antiviral prophylaxis, careful control of inflammation, and postoperative antiviral therapy are crucial to prevent relapses and complications.

24. How effective are trabeculectomy and tube shunt procedures in managing glaucoma associated with herpetic AU?
Answer: Both trabeculectomy and tube shunt procedures can effectively control IOP in herpetic uveitis-associated glaucoma, but outcomes depend on adequate preoperative control of inflammation.

25. Can sectoral iris atrophy be present in conditions other than herpetic AU?
Answer: Yes, sectoral iris atrophy can occur in conditions such as trauma or ischemia, but it is a characteristic finding in herpetic AU.

26. Does herpetic AU carry a higher risk of developing macular edema than other uveitis types?
Answer: The risk of macular edema in herpetic AU is lower than in posterior or intermediate uveitis but may occur due to associated inflammation or IOP elevation.

27. What is the recommended approach to managing herpetic uveitis in immunocompromised patients?
Answer: Immunocompromised patients require aggressive antiviral therapy, close monitoring, and tailored immunosuppressive or anti-inflammatory therapy to balance disease control with their systemic condition.

28. Is Fuchs' uveitis syndrome commonly mistaken for herpetic AU, and how can it be differentiated?
Answer: Fuchs' uveitis syndrome is frequently misdiagnosed as herpetic AU. Fine KPs, diffuse iris atrophy, and the absence of significant IOP spikes or corneal involvement can differentiate it.

29. Does herpetic AU require specific laboratory testing apart from PCR?
Answer: In addition to PCR, serologic testing for HSV, VZV, and CMV antibodies may assist in establishing a diagnosis or confirming prior exposure, particularly in atypical presentations.

FINAL WRAP-UP

Herpetic AU is caused primarily by HSV, VZV, and CMV. It presents unilaterally in most cases, often accompanied by localized KPs on the corneal endothelium, sectorial or patchy iris atrophy (HSV, VZV) or diffuse iris atrophy (CMV), and elevated IOP due to trabeculitis. Corneal involvement may occur as stromal inflammation, epithelial dendrites or pseudodendrites (HSV, VZV), or endotheliitis (CMV).

Antiviral therapy in the acute phase, particularly oral antivirals, is useful for reducing viral replication and helping control inflammation. Long-term prophylaxis should also be considered in cases with recurrent episodes or corneal involvement. The treatment also involves topical corticosteroids to control inflammation and, in HSV and VZV-associated uveitis, cycloplegic agents to alleviate pain and prevent posterior synechiae formation.

Intraocular pressure rise is frequent in herpetic uveitis. It can be found both in the acute phase, when it is strictly related to ongoing inflammation, and during follow-up, when various complex mechanisms contribute to altering aqueous humor outflow. Managing IOP is crucial to prevent further sight-threatening complications. Early diagnosis and appropriate treatment are essential to preserve vision and reduce the risk of complications.

REFERENCES

1. International Uveitis Study Group (IUSG). (2024). Uveitis Webinar—Grand Round 09. WEBINAR 39: Herpetic Anterior Uveitis: Case-Based Approach. [online] Available from https://youtu.be/9qbsUAS5y1g?si=knl5Nq43yWGqE0es. [Last accessed March, 2025]
2. Radosavljevic A, Agarwal M, Chee SP, Zierhut M. Epidemiology of viral induced anterior uveitis. Ocul Immunol Inflamm. 2022;30(2):297-309.
3. Bajwa A, Osmanzada D, Osmanzada S, Khan I, Patrie J, Wenjun X, et al. Epidemiology of uveitis in the mid-Atlantic United States. Clin Ophthalmol. 2015;9:889-901.
4. Wensing B, Mochizuki M, De Boer JH. Clinical characteristics of herpes simplex virus associated anterior uveitis. Ocul Immunol Inflammat. 2018;26(3):333-7.
5. Terada Y, Kaburaki T, Takase H, Goto H, Nakano S, Inoue Y, et al. Distinguishing features of anterior uveitis caused by herpes simplex virus, varicella-zoster virus, and cytomegalovirus. Am J Ophthalmol. 2021;227:191-200.
6. Kong CL, Thompson RR, Porco TC, Kim E, Acharya NR. Incidence rate of herpes zoster ophthalmicus. Ophthalmology. 2020;127(3):324-30.
7. Pohlmann D, Schlickeiser S, Metzner S, Lenglinger M, Winterhalter S, Pleyer U. Different composition of intraocular immune mediators in Posner-Schlossman syndrome and Fuchs' uveitis. PLoS ONE. 2018;13(6):e0199301.
8. Yawn BP, Wollan PC, St. Sauver JL, Butterfield LC. Herpes zoster eye complications: rates and trends. Mayo Clin Proc. 2013;88(6):562-70.
9. Tran KD, Falcone MM, Choi DS, Goldhardt R, Karp CL, Davis JL, et al. Epidemiology of herpes zoster ophthalmicus. Ophthalmology. 2016;123(7):1469-75.
10. Tugal-Tutkun I, Cimino L, Akova YA. Review for disease of the year: varicella-zoster virus-induced anterior uveitis. Ocul Immunol Inflammat. 2018;26(2):171-7.
11. Tugal-Tutkun I, Ötük-Yasar B, Altinkurt E. Clinical features and prognosis of herpetic anterior uveitis: a retrospective study of 111 cases. Int Ophthalmol. 2010;30(5):559-65.
12. Chee SP, Bacsal K, Jap A, Se-Thoe SY, Cheng CL, Tan BH. Clinical features of cytomegalovirus anterior uveitis in immunocompetent patients. Am J Ophthalmol. 2008;145(5):834-40.e1.
13. Accorinti M, Gilardi M, Pirraglia MP, Amorelli GM, Nardella C, Abicca I, et al. Cytomegalovirus anterior uveitis: long-term follow-up of immunocompetent patients. Graefes Arch Clin Exp Ophthalmol. 2014;252(11):1817-24.
14. Posner A, Schlossman A. Syndrome of unilateral recurrent attacks of glaucoma with cyclitic symptoms. Arch Ophthalmol. 1948;39(4):517-35.
15. Bloch-Michel E, Dussaix E, Cerqueti P, Patarin D. Possible role of cytomegalovirus infection in the etiology of the Posner-Schlossmann syndrome. Int Ophthalmol. 1987;11(2):95-6.
16. Accorinti M, Saturno MC, Paroli MP, De Geronimo D, Gilardi M. Uveitis-glaucoma-hyphema syndrome: clinical features and differential diagnosis. Ocul Immunol Inflammat. 2022;30(6):1408-13.
17. Standardization of Uveitis Nomenclature (SUN) Working Group. Classification criteria for herpes simplex virus anterior uveitis. Am J Ophthalmol. 2021;228:231-6.
18. Standardization of Uveitis Nomenclature (SUN) Working Group. Classification criteria for varicella zoster virus anterior uveitis. Am J Ophthalmol. 2021;228:165-73.
19. Standardization of Uveitis Nomenclature (SUN) Working Group. Classification criteria for cytomegalovirus anterior uveitis. Am J Ophthalmol. 2021;228:89-95.
20. Balderson DE, Cai G, Fries MA, Kleinman DM, McLaughlin MM, Trivedi TM, et al. A systematic review and meta-analysis to compare the efficacy of acyclovir 3% ophthalmic ointment to idoxuridine in curing herpetic keratitis by day 7 of treatment. BMC Ophthalmol. 2015;15(1):42.
21. Waduthantri S, Zhou L, Chee SP. Intra-cameral level of ganciclovir gel, 0.15% following topical application for cytomegalovirus anterior segment infection: a pilot study. PLoS ONE. 2018;13(1):e0191850.
22. Jones NP. Uveitis: An Illustrated Manual, 2nd edition. London: Jaypee Brothers Medical (P) Pvt. Ltd.; 2013. p. 382.
23. Foster CS, Vitale AT. Diagnosis and Treatment Of Uveitis, 2nd edition. London: Jaypee Brothers Medical (P) Pvt. Ltd.; 2013. p. 1290.
24. Wand M, Gilbert CM, Liesegang TJ. Latanoprost and herpes simplex keratitis. Am J Ophthalmol. 1999;127(5):602-4.
25. Zandi S, Bodaghi B, Garweg JG. Review for disease of the year: treatment of viral anterior uveitis: a perspective. Ocul Immunol Inflammat. 2018;26(7):1135-42.
26. La Distia Nora R, Putera I, Mayasari YD, Hikmahwati W, Pertiwi AM, Ridwan AS, et al. Clinical characteristics and treatment outcomes of cytomegalovirus anterior uveitis and endotheliitis: a systematic review and meta-analysis. Surv Ophthalmol. 2022;67(4):1014-30.
27. Testi I, Aggarwal K, Jaiswal N, Dahiya N, Thng ZX, Agarwal A, et al. Antiviral therapy for varicella zoster virus (VZV) and herpes simplex virus (HSV)-induced anterior uveitis: a systematic review and meta-analysis. Front Med. 2021;8:686427.
28. Lu A, Sun Y, Porco TC, Arnold BF, Acharya NR. Effectiveness of the recombinant zoster vaccine for herpes zoster ophthalmicus in the united states. Ophthalmology. 2021;128(12):1699-707.
29. Litt J, Cunningham AL, Arnalich-Montiel F, Parikh R. Herpes zoster ophthalmicus: presentation, complications, treatment, and prevention. Infect Dis Ther. 2024;13(7):1439-59.
30. Miserocchi E, Fogliato G, Bianchi I, Bandello F, Modorati G. Clinical features of ocular herpetic infection in an italian referral center. Cornea. 2014;33(6):565-70.

31. Feng Y, Garcia R, Rojas-Carabali W, Cifuentes-González C, Putera I, Li J, et al. Viral anterior uveitis: a practical and comprehensive review of diagnosis and treatment. Ocul Immunol Inflammat. 2024;32(8):1804-18.
32. Wong RW, Jumper JM, McDonald HR, Johnson RN, Fu A, Lujan BJ, et al. Emerging concepts in the management of acute retinal necrosis. Br J Ophthalmol. 2013;97(5):545-52.
33. Noda Y, Nakazawa M, Takahashi D, Tsuruya T, Saito M, Sekine M. Retinal periphlebitis as zoster sine herpete. Arch Ophthalmol. 2001;119(10):1550-2.
34. Kuo YH, Yip Y, Chen SN. Retinal vasculitis associated with chickenpox. Am J Ophthalmol. 2001;132(4):584-5.
35. Wimmersberger Y, Gervaix A, Baglivo E. VZV retinal vasculitis without systemic infection: diagnosis and monitoring with quantitative polymerase chain reaction. Int Ophthalmol. 2010;30(1):73-5.
36. Bodaghi B, Rozenberg F, Cassoux N, Fardeau C, LeHoang P. Nonnecrotizing herpetic retinopathies masquerading as severe posterior uveitis. Ophthalmology. 2003;110(9):1737-43.
37. Kahloun R, Attia S, Jelliti B, Attia AZ, Khochtali S, Yahia SB, et al. Ocular involvement and visual outcome of herpes zoster ophthalmicus: review of 45 patients from Tunisia, North Africa. J Ophthal Inflamm Infect. 2014;4(1):25.
38. Nakamura M, Tanabe M, Yamada Y, Azumi A. Zoster sine herpete with bilateral ocular involvement. Am J Ophthalmol. 2000;129(6):809-10.
39. Miserocchi E, Waheed NK, Dios E, Christen W, Merayo J, Roque M, et al. Visual outcome in herpes simplex virus and varicella zoster virus uveitis. Ophthalmology. 2002;109(8):1532-7.
40. de-la-Torre A, Valdes-Camacho J, Foster CS. Bilateral herpes simplex uveitis: review of the literature and own reports. Ocul Immunol Inflammat. 201725(4):497-502.
41. Hoeksema L, Jansonius NM, Los LI. Risk factors for secondary glaucoma in herpetic anterior uveitis. Am J Ophthalmol. 2017;181:55-60.
42. Rojas-Carabali W, Mejía-Salgado G, Cifuentes-González C, Chacón-Zambrano D, Cruz-Reyes DL, Delgado MF, et al. Prevalence and clinical characteristics of uveitic glaucoma: multicentric study in Bogotá, Colombia. Eye. 2024;38(4):714-22.
43. Kardeş E, Bozkurt K, Sezgin Akçay Bİ, Ünlü C, Aydoğan Gezginaslan T, Ergin A. Clinical features and prognosis of herpetic anterior uveitis.Turk J Ophthalmol 2016; 46(3):109-13.
44. Freeman ML, Sheridan BS, Bonneau RH, Hendricks RL. Psychological stress compromises cd8+ t cell control of latent herpes simplex virus type 1 infections. J Immunol. 2007;179(1):322-8.
45. Hsu CJ, Hung JH, Lin IH, Tseng SH, Lin SH, Huang YH. Overweight and obesity as risk factors for recurrent herpetic stromal keratitis during long-term antiviral prophylaxis. Viruses. 2022;14(12):2812.
46. Kwon HJ, Kong YXG, Tao LW, Lim LL, Martin KR, Green C, et al. Surgical outcomes of trabeculectomy and glaucoma drainage implant for uveitic glaucoma and relationship with uveitis activity. Clin Exper Ophthalmol. 2017;45(5):472-80.
47. Kaburaki T, Koshino T, Kawashima H, Numaga J, Tomidokoro A, Shirato S, et al. Initial trabeculectomy with mitomycin C in eyes with uveitic glaucoma with inactive uveitis. Eye. 2009 ;23(7):1509-17.

CHAPTER

10 Acute Retinal Necrosis

Bahram Bodaghi, Sofia Androudi, Athanasios Pappas, J Fernando Arevalo, Jacob S Heng, Carsten Heinz, Charlotte Wortmann, Germán Mejía-Salgado, Meghan Berkenstock, Reema Bansal, John H Kempen, Alejandra de-la-Torre, Vishali Gupta

INTRODUCTION

Acute retinal necrosis (ARN) is a major infectious entity and represents an absolute emergency in uveitis. Due to its high rate of complications and poor visual outcomes, prompt diagnosis and immediate therapy are mandatory.[1,2] This chapter will provide a few practical, day-to-day tips for managing ARN. It is not a conventional textbook chapter.

PRACTICAL TIPS FOR MANAGING A PATIENT WITH ACUTE RETINAL NECROSIS

Historical Background and Clinical Presentation

Acute retinal necrosis was first described in 1971 by Urayama et al. as Kirisawa uveitis, characterized by the following clinical findings:[3]

- Acute uveitis
- Retinal obliterative vasculitis
- Confluent yellow-white lesions at the peripheral retina

Viral Agents

Herpes viruses primarily cause ARN. The most common causative agents include:

- *Herpes simplex virus-1 and 2 (HSV-1 and 2):* Responsible for 6.4% of uveitis cases and 25% of anterior uveitis.
- *Varicella-zoster virus (VZV):* Associated with herpes zoster ophthalmicus (HZO), herpes zoster sine herpete, and chickenpox.
- *Cytomegalovirus (CMV):* Causes retinitis and chronic anterior uveitis.
- *Epstein-Barr virus (EBV):* Associated with retinitis and chronic anterior uveitis.
- *Human herpesvirus 8 (HHV-8):* Linked to conjunctivitis and panuveitis.
- *Nonherpetic viruses:* Include chikungunya, rubella, Zika, Ebola, and coronavirus.

Spectrum of Herpetic Eye Diseases

The clinical manifestations of herpetic eye infections include:

- *Keratitis*
- *Anterior uveitis*
- *Retinopathies:*
  - *Necrotizing:* ARN, progressive outer retinal necrosis (PORN), and CMV retinitis
  - *Nonnecrotizing*

ARN is characterized by its rapid progression of necrotic lesions in the peripheral retina, which may coalesce into larger areas of necrosis.

Diagnostic Criteria

There are three major classifications for ARN, given as follows.

American Uveitis Society (1994)[4]

- One or more foci of retinal necrosis with discrete borders in the peripheral retina
- Rapid progression in the absence of antiviral therapy
- Circumferential spread
- Occlusive vasculopathy with arterial involvement
- Prominent inflammatory reaction in the vitreous and anterior chamber

Japanese Acute Retinal Necrosis Study Group (2015)[5]

1. Ocular findings in the early stage:
    - *1a:* Anterior chamber cells or mutton-fat keratic precipitates (KPs)
    - *1b:* Yellow-white lesion(s) in the peripheral retina (granular or patchy in the early stage and then gradually merging)
    - *1c:* Retinal arteritis
    - *1d:* Hyperemia of the optic disc
    - *1e:* Inflammatory vitreous opacities
    - *1f:* Elevated intraocular pressure (IOP)
2. Clinical courses:
    - *2a:* Rapid expansion of retinal lesion(s) circumferentially
    - *2b:* Development of a retinal break or retinal detachment
    - *2c:* Retinal vascular occlusion
    - *2d:* Optic atrophy
    - *2e:* Response to antiviral agents
3. *Virologic testing of intraocular fluids:* Positive by either polymerase chain reaction (PCR) or Goldmann-Witmer coefficient for HSV-1, HSV-2, or VZV.

Classification:

- *Virus-confirmed ARN*: The presence of ocular findings 1a and 1b, the presence of one of the five clinical courses, and a positive virologic test result.
- *Virus-unconfirmed ARN*: Presence of four of the six ocular findings, including 1a and 1b, the presence of any two of the five clinical courses, and a negative virologic test result, or when virologic testing has not been performed.

Standardization of Uveitis Nomenclature Classification (2021)[6]

1. Necrotizing retinitis involving the peripheral retina and either #2 or #3.
2. Evidence of infection with HSV or VZV:
    a. Positive PCR for either HSV or VZV from either an aqueous or vitreous specimen.
3. Characteristic clinical picture:
    a. Circumferential or confluent retinitis
    b. Retinal vascular sheathing and/or occlusion
    c. More than minimal vitritis

Exclusions

- Positive serology for syphilis using a treponemal test.
- Intraocular specimen PCR positive for CMV or *Toxoplasma gondii* (unless there is an immune compromise, morphologic evidence for more than one infection, the characteristic clinical picture of ARN, and the intraocular fluid specimen has a positive PCR for either HSV or VZV).

Diagnosis Approach

The diagnosis of ARN is primarily confirmed using *PCR* on aqueous humor samples. Real-time PCR is preferred over conventional PCR due to its rapidity, high sensitivity, and ability to quantify the viral load. Monitoring viral load reduction during treatment is critical, particularly in patients under therapy.[7,8]

Monitoring viral load through PCR during intravitreal injections has identified two profiles, given as follows:[9]

1. Rapid responders
2. Slow responders: Persistent high viral loads despite therapy

Variants of Herpetic Retinitis

- *Progressive outer retinal necrosis*:
    - Forster et al., in 1990, described this condition as affecting immunosuppressed patients.[10]
    - Clinical features are as follows:
        - Rapid, full-thickness necrosis of the posterior pole, midretina, and periphery
        - Retinitis progressively spreads outwards and peripherally, often becoming confluent
        - Multiple areas of various sizes
        - Minimal vitritis and non-granulomatous mild anterior uveitis
        - Bilateral in 71% of cases
        - Vasculitis and optic neuritis are rare
        - Visual prognosis remains extremely poor, with a high rate of blindness
- *Cytomegalovirus retinitis*:
    - Associated with peripheral retinitis and vasculitis.[1]
    - Cases have been observed post-Oka strain live zoster vaccination, confirmed via whole-genome sequencing.[11,12]

Management

Antiviral Therapy[13,14]

- *Induction therapy:*
    - *Acyclovir:* 10 mg/kg every 8 hours intravenously
    - *Foscarnet:* 90 mg/kg every 12 hours intravenously for severe cases

- *Maintenance therapy:*
  - *Oral valacyclovir:* 3 g/day, particularly for immunocompetent patients
- *Intravitreal therapy (optional):*
  - *Ganciclovir:* 200–2,000 μg two times per week
  - *Foscarnet:* 1,200 μg two times per week

The duration of therapy is highly variable, ranging from 3 months to lifelong treatment in some cases. Discontinuation may lead to recurrence.

A retrospective, comparative study analyzing the visual outcomes of 62 patients (68 eyes) with ARN treated at Moorfields Eye Hospital between 1992 and 2016 identified no significant difference between 33 patients with intravenous (IV) acyclovir and 29 patients with oral valacyclovir in terms of best-corrected visual acuity (BCVA) improvement over 5 years ($p = 0.16$), rates of severe vision loss ($p = 0.18$), or eyes maintaining good vision ($p = 0.80$). Retinal detachment occurred in 63% of cases, with similar rates in both treatment groups (62% vs. 66%, $p = 0.67$). Adjunctive therapies, including barrier laser and intravitreal injections, did not affect the retinal detachment rate. The study concluded that oral valacyclovir is clinically equivalent to IV acyclovir for ARN management. Oral therapy offers a viable outpatient alternative to inpatient IV treatment, with or without intravitreal foscarnet.[15]

Corticosteroids[13,14]

- *Oral prednisone* may be used after initiation of antiviral therapy
- Local steroid injections and IV pulses are not recommended.
- Immunosuppressive agents are strictly contraindicated.

Additional Considerations[13,14]

- *Aspirin:* May be used adjunctively.
- *Laser photocoagulation:* Unable to halt the spread of retinitis but may prevent retinal detachment.
- *Prophylactic vitrectomy:* Remain controversial. Studies have shown that prophylactic vitrectomy does not significantly reduce recurrent retinal detachments or improve prognosis. Thus, it is not routinely recommended.[16]
- *Interferon (IFN) alfa-2b* has been reported to reduce choroidal involvement and chronic macular edema after the resolution of ARN. Treatment with corticosteroids potentially poses a risk of virus reactivation.[17]

There are three main treatment approaches: (1) Oral antivirals alone, (2) IV antivirals alone, or (3) systemic antivirals + intravitreal antivirals. Clinicians tend to use the combination of systemic and intravitreal antivirals. This combination is believed to achieve better visual acuity (VA) and lower recurrences. However, a systematic review did not identify significant differences between oral antivirals alone or IV antivirals alone.[18]

Given the lack of large randomized clinical trials, an anonymous survey with 22 primary questions (and 10 follow-up questions) was distributed to the American Uveitis Society (AUS) members, focusing on diagnostic testing, antiviral therapy, corticosteroids, and surgical interventions.[19]

The results from 67 responses revealed the following trends:[19]

- *Diagnostic testing:* 87% of respondents frequently or always obtain aqueous fluid for PCR testing to confirm viral etiology.
- *Intravitreal therapy:* 67% administer intravitreal antivirals for unilateral immunocompetent ARN, while 87% do so in bilateral immunosuppressed cases.
- *Corticosteroid use:* Most ophthalmologists prefer systemic corticosteroids over local options, initiating treatment 48 hours after antiviral therapy.
- *Vitrectomy:* 79% avoid vitrectomy unless there is a retinal detachment or tear.
- *Laser barricade:* 63% rarely or never perform prophylactic laser barricade but may consider it for extensive retinal involvement.

The study concluded that the current management practices of AUS members align closely with recommendations from the American Academy of Ophthalmology, which emphasizes a preference for systemic therapies, diagnostic PCR testing, and surgical intervention only when complications arise.[19]

Clinical Outcomes

Despite aggressive treatment, poor outcomes are frequent, with approximately 50% of patients in recent series having low VA. Retinal detachment occurs in 58% of cases (24 out of 41 eyes), with second detachments in six eyes. Additional recurrence of retinitis can also occur in 12% (five out of 41 eyes).[20]

The risk factors for retinal detachment in ARN are low VA at presentation and greater retinitis extent (number of clock hours). Vitrectomy with scleral buckle is performed in around 41% of the cases, with a success rate after a single surgery of 63% with silicone oil used in most cases.[21] Other factors influencing prognosis include the patient's older age, a greater number of intravitreal injections, which indicates disease severity, and VZV infection rather than HSV infection.

Other common complications in ARN include:[18]

- *Retinal detachment:* 43%
- *Cataract:* 17.03%
- *Optic atrophy:* 17.57%
- *Epiretinal membrane:* 27.16%
- *Uveitic macular edema:* 24.12%
- *Phthisis bulbi:* 9.02%
- *Glaucoma:* 6.65%

TYPICAL CASE OF ACUTE RETINAL NECROSIS

Case Presentation

Personal Data

- 32-year-old male

History of Present Illness (November 2011)

- The patient complained of blurred vision and floaters in the right eye (OD) for the past few days.
- Past medical history was noncontributory, with the patient having mild myopia (-3.00 D).

On ocular examination, the patient presented with BCVA of 20/40 in OD and 20/20 in OS. Positive findings in the slit lamp, included papillitis in the OD, accompanied by peripheral whitish infiltrates **(Table 1 and Fig. 1)**.

Multimodal imaging was requested, evidencing hypofluorescence around the optic nerve in the fundus fluorescein angiography (FFA) accompanied by peripheral vasculitis **(Fig. 2)**. In optical coherence tomography (OCT), the hypofluorescence area was related to subretinal fluid. Raised pockets of peripheral fluid were also noted **(Figs. 3A to C)**.

TABLE 1: Ocular examination in a typical case with ARN.

OD	*Parameter*	*OS*
20/40	BCVA	20/20
18	IOP (mm Hg)	18
1+ hyperemia and ciliary injection	Conjunctiva	White and quiet
Clear	Cornea	Clear
+0.5 cells	Anterior chamber	Quiet
Dilated	Iris	Dilated
Clear	Lens	Clear
+2 cells	Vitreous	No cells, no pigment
Optic disc edema with peripheral whitish infiltrates	Fundus	Unremarkable

(BCVA: best-corrected visual acuity; IOP: intraocular pressure)

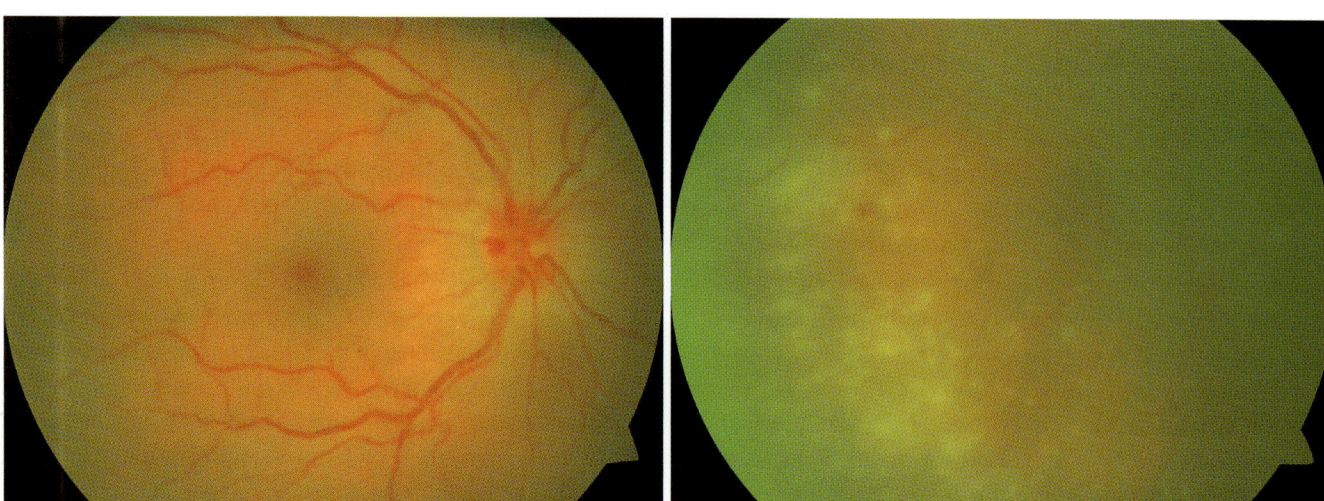

Fig. 1: Clinical picture at presentation. Color fundus photograph of the OD at presentation evidencing optic disc edema, retinal tortuosity, and peripheral whitish infiltrates.
Source: Presented by Athanasios Pappas in the International Uveitis Study Group (IUSG) grand rounds.[1]

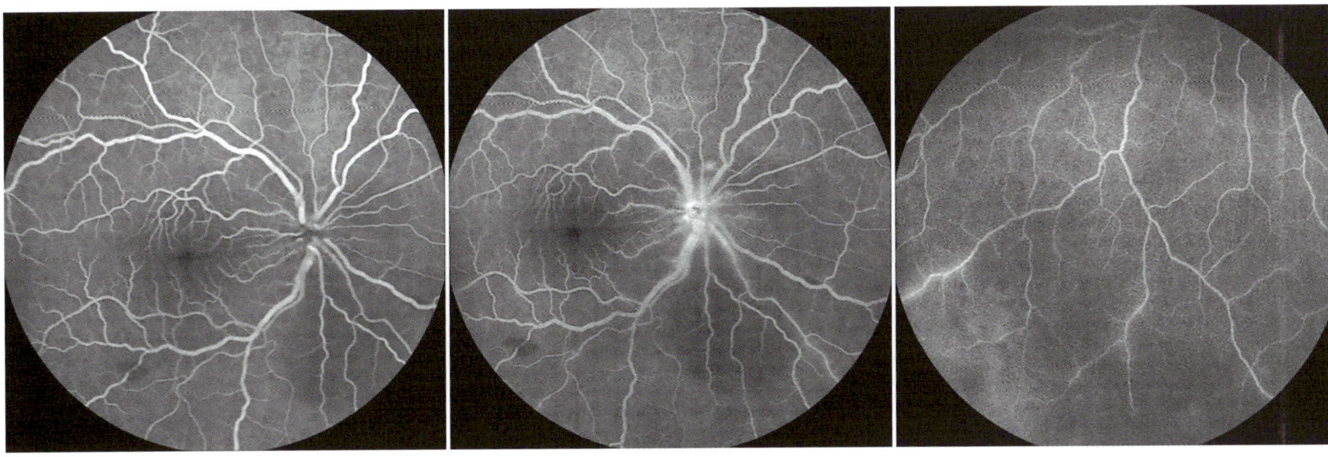

Fig. 2: Fundus fluorescein angiography findings at presentation. Hypofluorescence around the optic nerve at early stages, turning hyperfluorescent in late stages, and vascular leakage was observed in the periphery.
Source: Presented by Athanasios Pappas in the International Uveitis Study Group (IUSG) grand rounds.[1]

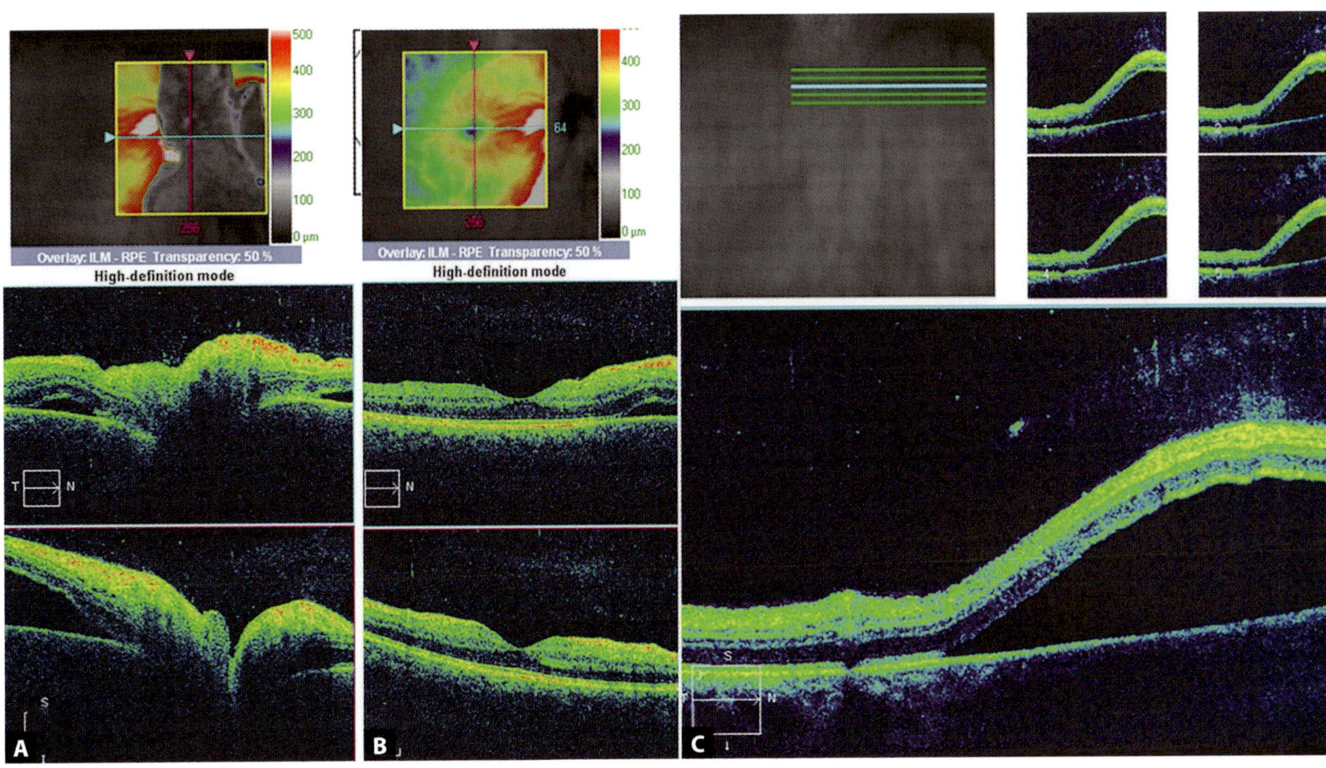

Figs. 3A to C: Optical coherence tomography findings at presentation. (A) optic disc edema; (B) subretinal fluid in the macular area; (C) raised pockets of peripheral fluid.
Source: Presented by Athanasios Pappas in the International Uveitis Study Group (IUSG) grand rounds.[1]

Workup

- Comprehensive uveitis workup, including QuantiFERON-TB Gold, antitreponemal IgG, angiotensin-converting enzyme (ACE) and lysozyme, blood cultures, chest CT, and brain MRI were all negative except for retroperitoneal fluid, which remained unexplained after consultation with infectious disease specialists.
- The anterior chamber tap was positive for VZV.

Diagnosis

- Acute retinal necrosis caused by VZV.

Treatment

- *Hospitalization and initial therapy:*
  - *Intravenous acyclovir:* 10 mg/kg three times daily for 2 weeks
  - *Oral prednisone:* 1 mg/kg initiated on day 3
- *Long-term Therapy*:
  - *Oral valacyclovir:* 1 gram thrice daily, followed by 1 gram daily maintenance
  - *Oral prednisone:* Tapered over 3 months
- *Additional interventions*:
  - Oral steroids and a dexamethasone implant were added to address persistent macular edema.
  - Cataract surgery and vitrectomy with gas tamponade for retinal detachment.

Outcome

Initial response:

- Gradual resolution of optic nerve edema and peripapillary fluid
- Persistent subtle macular edema with epiretinal membrane formation

Long-term follow-up:

- Over 8 years, the patient maintained 20/30 VA on 1-gram daily valacyclovir, Maxidex, and bromfenac drops.
- *Eleven years post-incident:* Discontinuation of therapy resulted in a worsening of macular edema and a drop in VA to 20/40.
- Optical coherence tomography revealed extensive cystic changes in the macular area **(Fig. 4)**.

Current status (December 2024):

- Visual acuity remains 20/40
- The patient continues oral antivirals and bromfenac as needed with no improvement.

Discussion

This case involves a patient with 14 years of follow-up, diagnosed with ARN at a young age and treated promptly on day zero following established protocols. Despite adequate antiviral therapy, the patient developed cystoid macular edema (CME) a few months later, a common

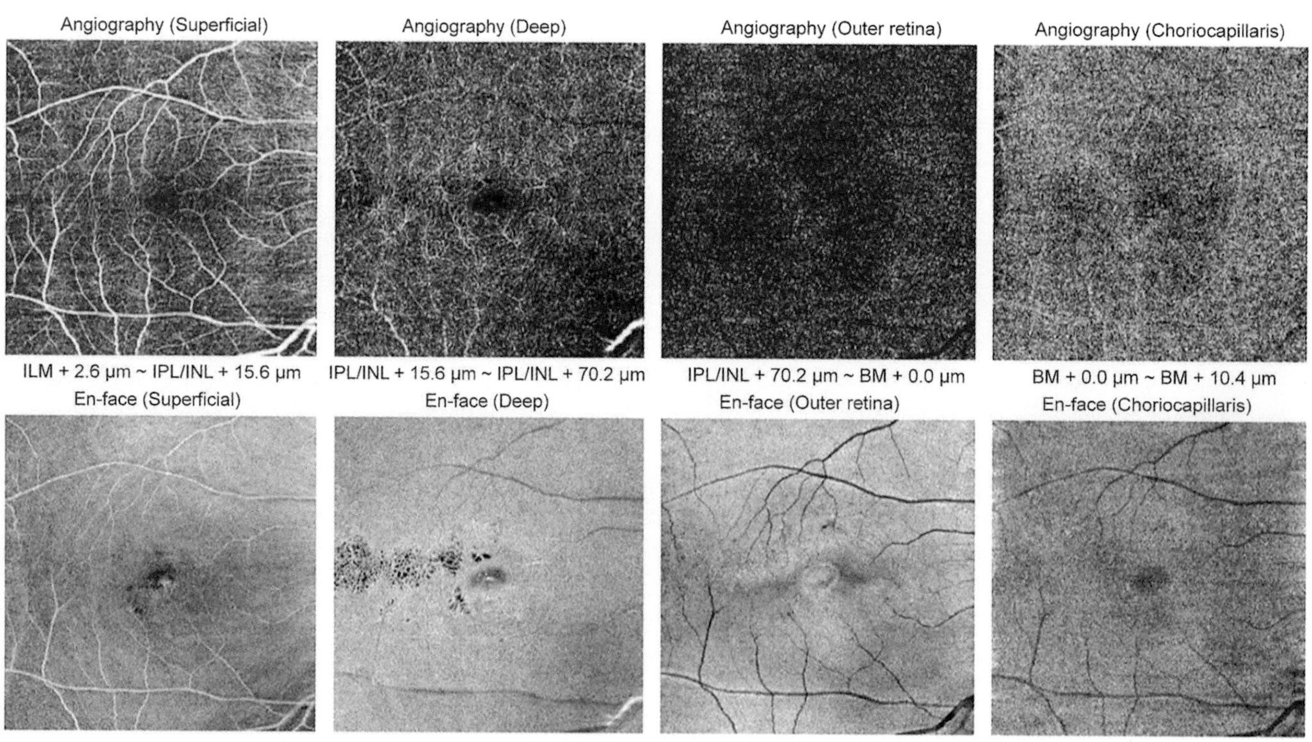

Fig. 4: En face optical coherence tomography 11 years after treatment discontinuation. En face OCT image showing hyporeflective spaces consistent with cystoid macular edema, observed 11 years after the initial incident and subsequent discontinuation of therapy. Presented by Athanasios Pappas in the International Uveitis Study Group (IUSG) grand rounds.[1]

complication of ARN, likely caused by low-grade chronic inflammation.[18] The patient remained on long-term antiviral therapy for over 10 years, as the severity of the condition and risk of recurrence were explained and accepted. However, the macular edema persisted after discontinuing antivirals, highlighting the complexity of managing CME in ARN.[1]

Macular edema in ARN can be challenging to treat. While PCR tests may show negative results, chronic inflammation may persist, potentially driven by elevated cytokine levels reported in the literature.[22] The patient developed a trace epiretinal membrane and band keratopathy, both of which are commonly associated with chronic ARN cases. Characteristic OCT findings revealed persistent cystic changes. Intravitreal therapy with dexamethasone implants was administered to manage the edema, but the condition required continued monitoring, and multiple implants over time became necessary.[23]

Different approaches exist to manage CME in ARN, notably:

- Long-term antivirals are crucial to prevent reactivation, even when intravitreal corticosteroids are administered.
- Prophylactic antiviral dosing typically involves 1 gram of valacyclovir daily. However, some experts opt for 900 mg once daily in low-risk scenarios.
- For patients needing frequent intravitreal injections, fluocinolone acetonide implants may offer a long-lasting effect.

There is a discussion about the role of nonsteroidal anti-inflammatory drugs (NSAIDs) such as bromfenac,[24] which are occasionally used but not part of routine management. Some experts cited evidence of successful outcomes with topical interferon therapy, though this remains experimental.[17] Systemic interferons are no longer widely available, and alternatives such as topical interferon or tocilizumab (an IL-6 inhibitor) may be considered for refractory cases.[25]

The panel of experts in the International Uveitis Study Group (IUSG) during the grand rounds unanimously agreed that intravitreal antiviral therapy is not a preferred treatment, as systemic therapy provides adequate bioavailability, and more efficient alternatives exist for severe cases, such as foscarnet.[1] Moreover, it was underscored that ARN-related complications, including CME, epiretinal membranes, and retinal detachment, require aggressive treatment and close monitoring. While therapies such as dexamethasone implants or fluocinolone provide control, continued prophylactic antivirals are essential to prevent recurrence and preserve vision.[18]

SECOND CASE: "NOT JUST A RETINAL DETACHMENT"

Case Presentation

Personal Data

- 57-year-old female
- History of a deceased donor kidney transplant due to focal segmental glomerulosclerosis secondary to preeclampsia
- Referred to the retina specialists due to a probable diagnosis of ARN

History of Present Illness

- *2.5 months prior:* The patient developed shingles involving the left V1 dermatome, which resolved after 10 days of oral valacyclovir (1 gram daily).
- *Two months prior:* Shingles recurred, involving the tip of her nose (Hutchinson's sign). She was seen by an optometrist and restarted on valacyclovir 1 gram daily. She was subsequently referred to a retina specialist due to concerns about ocular involvement.
- *1.5 months prior:* Development of anterior chamber cells and pseudodendrites in the left eye, prompting the initiation of topical prednisolone.
- *One month prior:* The anterior chamber inflammation resolved, and valacyclovir was reduced to 500 mg daily.
- *One week prior:* The pseudodendrites showed improvement with topical ganciclovir gel.
- *One day prior:* The patient experienced the onset of new floaters in the left eye. She was diagnosed with ARN and associated retinal detachment.

On ocular examination, the patient presented with a BCVA of 20/25 in OD and 20/70 in OS, with an afferent pupillary defect noted in OS. IOP was within normal limits in both eyes (OU). Examination of the anterior segment of the left eye revealed 1+ anterior chamber cells and iris transillumination defects. Fundus examination of the left eye showed peripheral whitish infiltrates adjacent to areas of necrotic and detached retina in all four quadrants **(Table 2 and Figs. 5A and B)**.

OCT showed minor outer retinal changes in OD and macular edema in OS **(Figs. 6A and B)**.

Workup

The patient was admitted to the internal medicine service with input from the nephrology and infectious disease teams.

TABLE 2: Ocular examination of case 2.

OD	*Parameters*	*OS*
20/25	BCVA	20/70
18	IOP (mm Hg)	12
Ptosis	Lids/lashes	Ptosis
White and quiet	Conjunctiva	1+ injection
Clear	Cornea	KPs, subepithelial opacities
Quiet	Anterior chamber	2+ ACC and 1+ flare
Dilated	Iris	Transillumination defects at 3, 4, and 8 hours o'clock
1+ nuclear sclerosis	Lens	1+ nuclear sclerosis
Normal, no cells, no pigment	Vitreous	2+ cell, 1+ haze
CDR: 0.2 unremarkable	Fundus	Peripheral whitish infiltrates adjacent to necrotic and detached retina in all four quadrants, particularly notable in the temporal periphery

(ACC: anterior chamber cellularity; BCVA: best-corrected visual acuity; CDR: cup–disc ratio; IOP: intraocular pressure; KPs: keratic precipitates)

- Intravitreal foscarnet was initiated twice weekly.
- *Systemic therapy:* IV acyclovir 10 mg/kg every 8 hours for 14 days with renal monitoring.
- Surgery and laser were delayed for 5 days while monitoring the retina closely.

Treatment and Surgical Intervention

After 5 days, pars plana vitrectomy was performed as follows:

- Core vitrectomy with careful peripheral vitreous removal
- Debridement of necrotic retina to prevent further detachment
- Injection of perfluorocarbon heavy liquid to stabilize and protect the macula
- Laser photocoagulation and fluid–air exchange
- Silicone oil injection and subconjunctival medications

Outcome

- *Postoperative day 1* ***(Fig. 7):*** The retina was attached with no evidence of whitening posterior to the laser barricade. VA was 20/125 pinhole.
- *Week 3 postoperative* ***(Figs. 8A and B):***
  - Laser scars were stable.
  - No evidence of active vasculitis or inflammation
  - OCT confirmed the resolution of macular edema under silicone oil

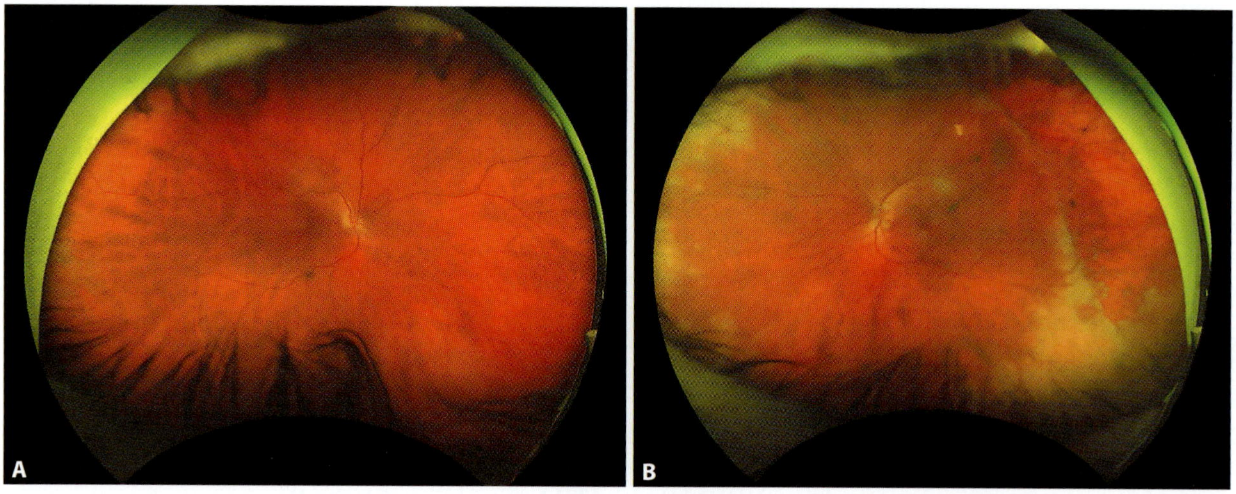

Figs. 5A and B: Clinical picture at presentation. (A) Color fundus photograph of the OD showing a clear vitreous and attached retina without areas of necrosis; (B) Peripheral whitish infiltrates adjacent to the necrotic retina, particularly prominent in the temporal periphery of the OS.

Source: Presented by Jacob Heng in the International Uveitis Study Group (IUSG) grand rounds.[1]

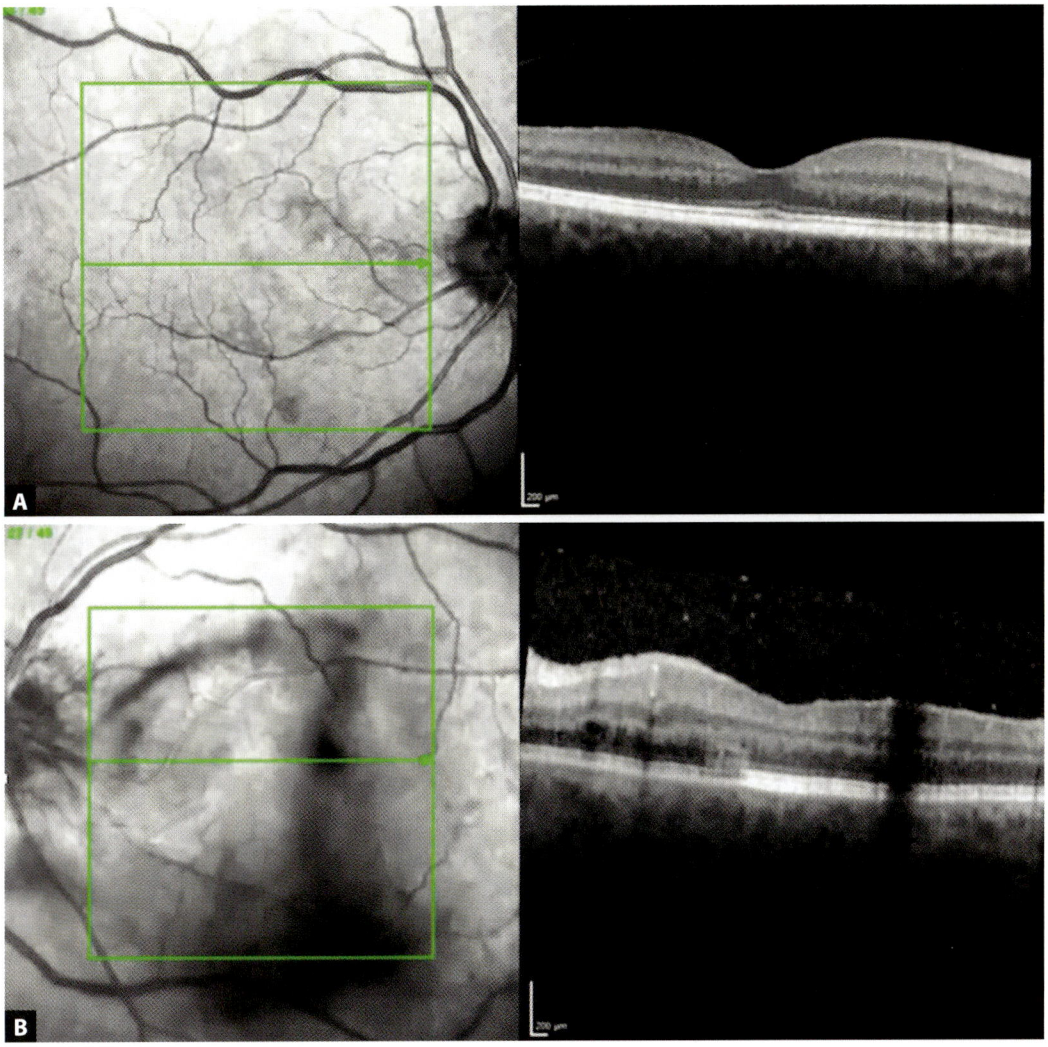

Figs. 6A and B: Optical coherence tomography findings at presentation. (A) Outer retinal changes in OD; (B) Retinal necrosis extending in temporal periphery with macular edema.
Source: Presented by Jacob Heng in the International Uveitis Study Group (IUSG) grand rounds.[1]

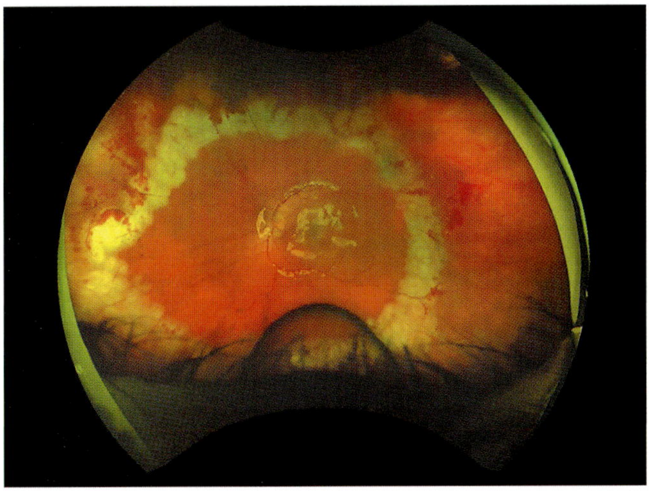

Fig. 7: Postoperative day 1 color fundus photography evidencing attached retina with no evidence of whitening posterior to the laser barricade or new necrosis areas.
Source: Presented by Jacob Heng in the International Uveitis Study Group (IUSG) grand rounds.[1]

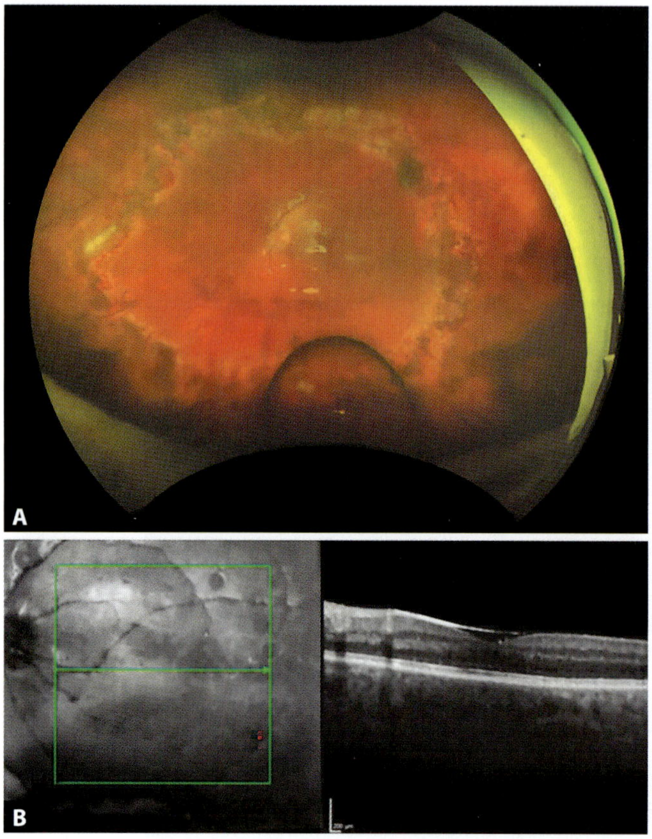

Figs. 8A and B: Postoperative week 3 clinical picture. (A) Color fundus photograph at postoperative week 3 showing stable laser scars with no signs of active vasculitis or inflammation; (B) Optical coherence tomography (OCT) demonstrates the absence of macular edema but reveals the presence of an epiretinal membrane.
Source: Presented by Jacob Heng in the International Uveitis Study Group (IUSG) grand rounds.[1]

Complications and Further Course

- *Six months postvitrectomy*: Silicone oil was removed, and cataract surgery was performed with stable findings and no recurrence of retinitis.
- *Six weeks postoil removal*: The patient developed a total tractional retinal detachment with vision dropping to light perception **(Fig. 9)**.

A repeat vitrectomy with silicone oil was performed to repair the retinal detachment. Additionally, weekly intravitreal methotrexate (six doses) was administered postoperatively for proliferative vitreoretinopathy (PVR). Despite these interventions, the patient developed progressive superonasal traction, which led to localized shallow retinal detachment. Given the poor visual prognosis, the patient opted for observation **(Fig. 10)**.

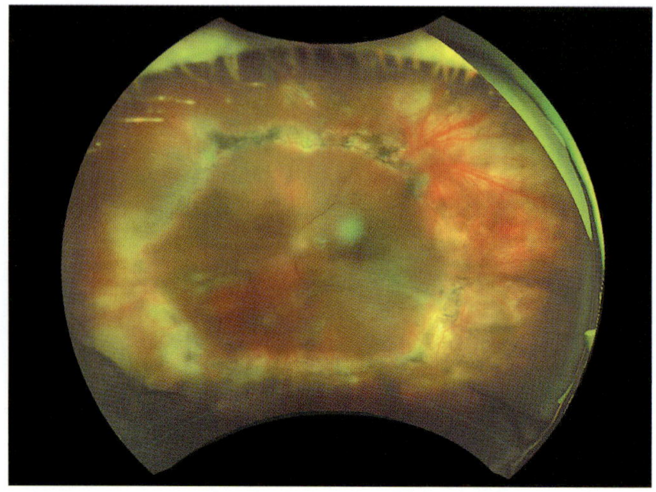

Fig. 9: Recurrence of retinal detachment after 6 weeks postoil removal. Recurrence of tractional retinal detachment in the OS.
Source: Presented by Jacob Heng in the International Uveitis Study Group (IUSG) grand rounds.[1]

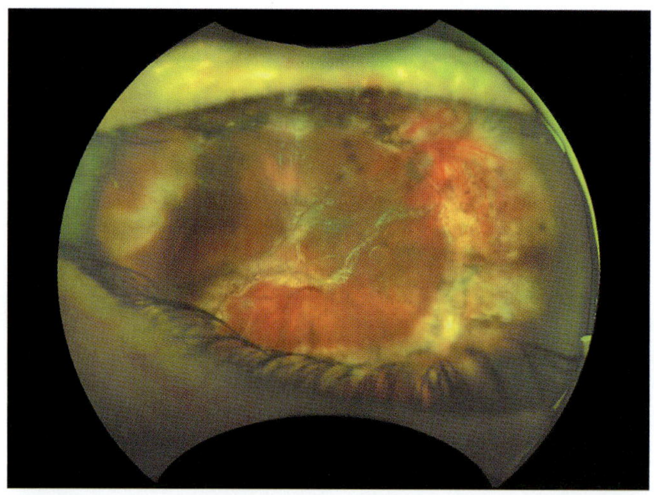

Fig. 10: Four months post-repeat vitrectomy with silicon oil. Color fundus photograph evidencing progressive superonasal traction in the OS with a final best-corrected visual acuity (BCVA) of hand motion.
Source: Presented by Jacob Heng in the International Uveitis Study Group (IUSG) grand rounds.[1]

Final Status

- The superonasal detachment has remained stable under silicone oil.
- Visual acuity in the OS is reduced to hand motions.
- The right eye remains unaffected.

Discussion

This case highlights the challenges and complexities of managing ARN, particularly in an immunocompromised patient with a history of a kidney transplant. The patient presented with a macula-on retinal detachment secondary to active ARN, requiring an urgent yet carefully balanced approach to treatment.

Medical Therapy in Acute Retinal Necrosis

Medical therapy remains the cornerstone of ARN management, with a combination of intravitreal foscarnet and systemic antiviral therapy playing a critical role. This approach has been shown to significantly reduce the risk of retinal detachment by up to 67%.[26,27] To maintain this reduced risk, it is essential to continue systemic antiviral therapy to prevent disease progression and contralateral eye involvement. Without appropriate systemic antiviral treatment, the risk of contralateral eye involvement is as high as 65% within 2 years compared to 25% with proper antiviral management.[28]

The use of systemic corticosteroids remains controversial in ARN. Initiating corticosteroids before antiviral therapy can exacerbate the condition, as extensive retinitis and vascular occlusion may occur in the absence of adequate viral suppression. Therefore, corticosteroids should be introduced only after systemic antiviral therapy to mitigate inflammation and minimize complications.[29]

In this case, IV acyclovir (10 mg/kg every 8 hours) was administered for 14 days under close monitoring of renal function, given the patient's decreased creatinine clearance (estimated glomerular filtration rate [eGFR]: 37 mL/min/1.73 m^2). It is important to note that achieving adequate dosing of oral valacyclovir is critical, as pharmacological studies suggest that at least 1.5 grams every 8 hours are required to meet the IC50 for VZV in the vitreous.[28,30] Underdosing during initial presentation may contribute to disease progression or complications.

The panel also addressed potential adverse effects of antiviral therapy, including nephrotoxicity, neurotoxicity, and thrombotic thrombocytopenic purpura, which require careful monitoring, particularly in patients with renal impairment.

Role of Laser Retinopexy

The role of prophylactic laser retinopexy in ARN remains controversial. While some studies suggest a reduced risk of retinal detachment,[31] others have shown no benefit[32] or even increased risk,[33] likely due to iatrogenic breaks over the necrotic retina. Furthermore, significant inflammation and vitreous debris often limit visibility, making laser treatment challenging for the patient and surgeon. Given the lack of robust randomized trials, the panel agreed that laser retinopexy should be considered on a case-by-case basis, primarily when extensive peripheral involvement is present.

Surgical Considerations

Retinal detachment remains a significant complication in ARN, with redetachment rates reaching 58% following vitrectomy.[27] While prophylactic vitrectomy is controversial, it has been explored in selected cases with mixed results.[16,33] Some panelists agree that reducing inflammatory cytokines through vitrectomy may help control active lesions and prevent tractional complications. However, the panel emphasized the need for aggressive antiviral therapy before considering surgery, as uncontrolled retinitis may compromise outcomes.[26,27]

The choice of tamponade, particularly silicone oil, is favored over gas due to its ability to address high rates of redetachment and prolonged tamponade effect. Techniques such as perfluorocarbon liquid were highlighted as useful for viscodissecting the peripheral vitreous and for facilitating safer and more complete shaving of the vitreous without exacerbating retinal damage.[34,35] Advanced surgical tools such as high-performance instruments used in pars plana vitrectomy procedures with a dual-blade mechanism that allows them to cut the vitreous humor more efficiently and at significantly higher cut rates, have also been noted for their precision in managing vitreoretinal pathology near necrotic lesions.[36]

It is important to balance addressing active retinitis and managing a macula-on-retinal detachment as an emergency. To reduce the risk of surgical complications, surgery is often delayed until antiviral therapy is underway. However, in cases with imminent macular involvement, early surgical intervention with concurrent aggressive antiviral therapy and intravitreal injections is warranted.[36]

Management of Proliferative Vitreoretinopathy

The patient ultimately developed tractional retinal detachment with PVR, requiring repeat vitrectomy and adjunctive intravitreal methotrexate. Methotrexate has shown promise in preventing PVR recurrence when administered weekly post-surgery.[37-40]

THIRD CASE: "IT LOOKS LIKE RETINAL NECROSIS"

Case Presentation

Personal Data

- 81-year-old female

History of Present Illness

The patient presented with a complaint of unilateral vision impairment in the OS that had persisted for 6 weeks and worsened 1 week before the consultation. She was referred to our clinic by her local ophthalmologist due to a vitreous hemorrhage. Her ophthalmologic history included bilateral cataract surgery performed 4 years prior, and her general medical history revealed arterial hypertension, which was managed with oral medication.

On ocular examination, the patient presented with a BCVA of 20/20 in the OD and no light perception in the OS. In the OD, both slit-lamp examination and fundoscopy were unremarkable. In the OS, slit-lamp examination revealed KPs, rubeosis iridis, and dense vitreous opacities. Fundus examination was not performed due to media opacity, with only a mild red reflex observed **(Table 3, Fig. 11)**.

An ocular ultrasound showed a hyperreflective membrane suggestive of an old retinal detachment **(Fig. 12)**. Based on these findings, an immediate vitrectomy was indicated. A 23-gauge vitrectomy was performed

TABLE 3: Ocular examination of case 3.

OD	*Parameters*	*OS*
20/20	BCVA	No light perception
16	IOP (mm Hg)	28
White and quiet	Conjunctiva	Mild hyperemia
Clear	Cornea	Mutton-fat KPs
Deep and quiet	Anterior chamber	AC cells+
Normal	Iris	Rubeosis iridis
IOL in place	Lens	IOL in place
Normal, no cells, and no pigment	Vitreous	Dense vitreous opacities, blood cells
CDR: 0.3 unremarkable	Fundus	No view due to vitreous hemorrhage

(BCVA: best-corrected visual acuity, KPs: keratic precipitates; CDR: cup-disc ratio; IOL: intraocular lens; IOP: intraocular pressure)

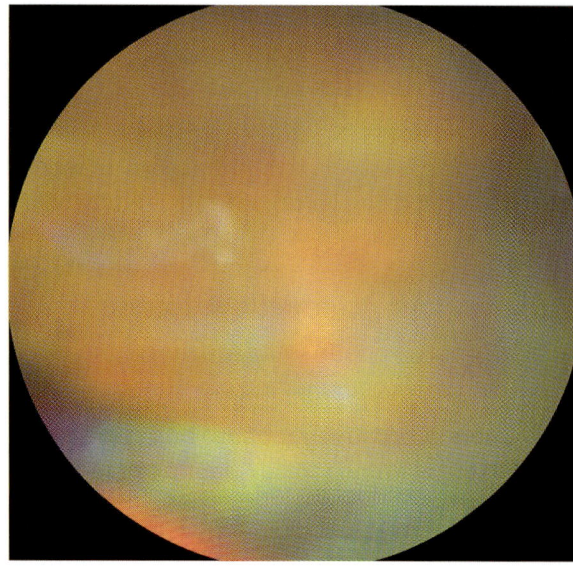

Fig. 11: Clinical picture at presentation. Color fundus photograph (Zeiss Clarus 700, Zeiss, Oberkochen, Germany) of the OS showing dense vitreous opacities, obscuring clear visualization of the fundus details.
Source: Presented by Charlotte Wortmann in the International Uveitis Study Group (IUSG) grand rounds.[1]

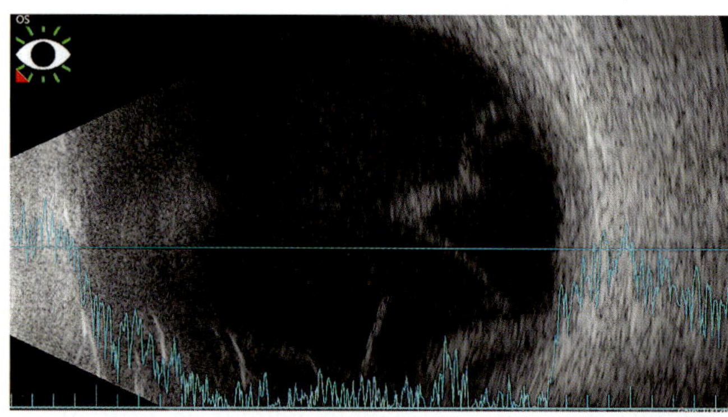

Fig. 12: Ocular ultrasound performed on the left eye. B-scan ocular ultrasound (Ellex Eye Cubed, Ellex, Mawson Lakes, Australia) evidencing a hyperreflective membrane suggestive of an old retinal detachment.
Source: Presented by Charlotte Wortmann in the International Uveitis Study Group (IUSG) grand rounds.[1]

under general anesthesia. Intraoperatively, the following findings were noted: cord-like preretinal thickening, extensive retinal necrosis, and old retinal detachment in the inferior retina **(Fig. 13)**.

The procedure included:

- Endolaser coagulation
- Retinal biopsy
- Silicone oil tamponade

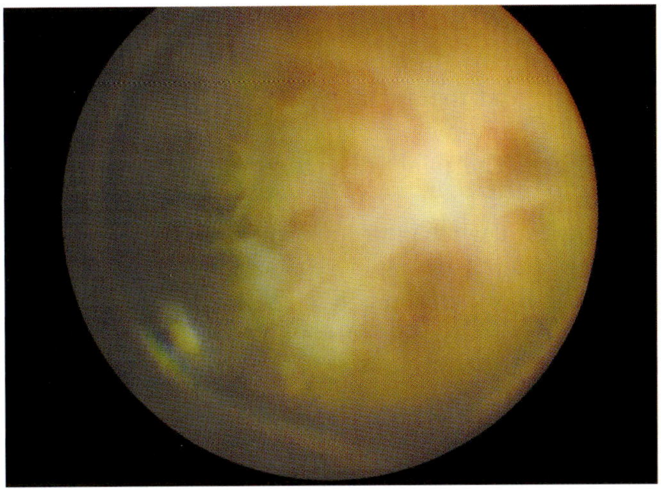

Fig. 13: Intraoperative findings. During the vitrectomy, the following findings were noted: cord-like preretinal thickening, extensive retinal necrosis, and old retinal detachment in the inferior retina (intraoperative picture with Zeiss OPMI Lumera 300, Zeiss, Oberkochen, Germany).
Source: Presented by Charlotte Wortmann in the International Uveitis Study Group (IUSG) grand rounds.[1]

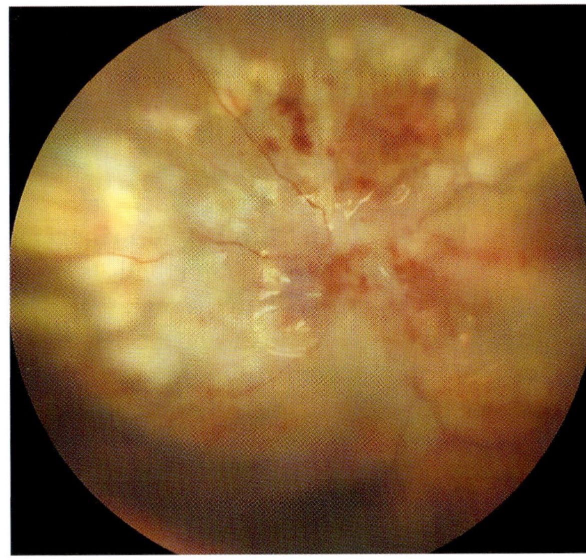

Fig. 14: Color fundus photograph 2 weeks after vitrectomy. Color fundus photograph (Zeiss Clarus 700, Zeiss, Oberkochen, Germany) evidencing new retinal hemorrhages in the necrotic areas.
Source: Presented by Charlotte Wortmann in the International Uveitis Study Group (IUSG) grand rounds.[1]

Notably, no undiluted vitreous sample was obtained at the start of surgery.

Immediately after vitrectomy, antiviral therapy with acyclovir 500 mg three times daily intravenously, prednisolone 30 mg orally, topical prednisolone acetate 1% QID, atropine 0.5% BID, and antiglaucomatous therapy were initiated.

On postoperative day 1, the examination revealed 3+ anterior chamber cells and 2+ flare, with a prelenticular fibrin plaque. Visualization of the necrotic retinal areas remained limited due to residual media opacity. After 2 weeks of the vitrectomy, new retinal hemorrhages in the necrotic areas were noted **(Fig. 14)**.

Further Workup

- An anterior chamber tap was performed on postoperative day 1 due to the absence of vitreous sampling, and a viral PCR was ordered, which returned negative for herpes virus.
- The uveitis workup, including differential blood count, C-reactive protein (CRP), liver and kidney function tests, syphilis serology, ACE, and the soluble interleukin-2 receptor (sIL2R), returned unremarkable findings.
- The patient reported a headache and a subjective feeling of confusion, prompting a neurological evaluation. The electroencephalogram and neurological examination were normal. Furthermore, the cerebral MRI showed multifocal asymmetrical diffusion disturbances in both hemispheres, raising suspicion of herpetic encephalitis. Consequently, the patient was transferred to the neurology department for cerebrospinal fluid (CSF) analysis, which returned negative for the herpes virus and malignancy.
- The retinal biopsy showed no evidence of vitreoretinal lymphoma.

Differential Diagnosis

Given the MRI findings, the differential diagnosis included:

- Posterior reversible encephalopathy syndrome (PRES)
- Cerebral lymphoma

A follow-up cerebral MRI performed 10 days postoperatively ruled out PRES and increased suspicion of cerebral lymphoma.

Final Diagnosis

A subsequent cerebral biopsy confirmed a diagnosis of large B-cell lymphoma. Additionally, a MYD88 mutation was detected on further analysis of the retinal biopsy, and histological re-evaluation revealed clusters of large B-cell lymphocytes. These findings were consistent with vitreoretinal lymphoma.

The patient was transferred to the oncology department, where she started chemotherapy. Unfortunately, despite intervention, the patient's condition deteriorated, and she passed away a few weeks after initiating treatment.

Discussion

This case highlights the diagnostic and management challenges in vitreoretinal lymphoma and its overlap with conditions such as ARN. The patient, an 81-year-old woman, presented with vitreous hemorrhage, severe vision loss, and intraoperative findings suggestive of extensive retinal necrosis. However, the subsequent clinical course, imaging, and biopsies revealed a diagnosis of central nervous system (CNS) lymphoma.

Key Points of Discussion

Diagnostic challenges: Initially, the clinical suspicion was long-standing retinal necrosis, given the findings of retinal thickening, extensive necrosis, and poor visualization of the posterior pole. An immediate vitrectomy was justified to improve visualization and obtain a retinal biopsy. This biopsy and imaging ultimately played a critical role in the identification of vitreoretinal lymphoma. Notably, immunocompromised patients are at higher risk for infectious uveitis and malignancies, which often coexist or present with overlapping features.

However, as the panel of experts in the grand round emphasized, the timing and accuracy of diagnostics such as PCR can vary. PCR is highly effective in the early phase of viral replication but may yield false negatives later.[8] Goldmann-Witmer coefficients could provide additional information but are rarely performed due to logistical challenges. In immunocompromised patients, clinicians must also consider infectious etiologies, such as herpetic retinitis or toxoplasmosis, which can mimic vitreoretinal lymphoma.[41] Multiplex PCR for herpes viruses, CMV, and *T. gondii* can help differentiate between these conditions.[42]

Role of imaging and systemic workup: The cerebral MRI findings, showing multifocal diffusion disturbances, initially raised suspicion for herpetic encephalitis. However, the subsequent CSF PCR was negative for herpes as systemic antiviral treatment was started directly after vitrectomy, further complicating the diagnosis. This case demonstrates the importance of neurological evaluations in atypical posterior segment presentations, particularly in immunocompromised patients. The eventual diagnosis of CNS lymphoma was confirmed via cerebral biopsy.[1]

Management Decisions

Immediate vitrectomy was the appropriate step for diagnostic and therapeutic purposes, as retinal tissue samples are often essential for diagnosing masquerade syndromes. The panel discussed the role of systemic therapy in such cases. In ARN, systemic IV acyclovir is the gold standard, while intravitreal antivirals (e.g., foscarnet) are often added for rapid viral suppression. However, in this case, the absence of viral markers and MYD88 mutation on biopsy shifted the diagnosis to vitreoretinal lymphoma, which required prompt referral to oncology for systemic chemotherapy.[1]

Role of Corticosteroids

The use of corticosteroids remains controversial in ARN due to concerns that they may exacerbate active viral replication. Steroids may be employed cautiously after systemic malignancy has been confirmed and adequately addressed in vitreoretinal lymphoma.[1]

Take Home Messages from this Case

- Immediate intervention is critical in cases of severe vision loss with vitreous opacity, but clinicians must maintain a broad differential diagnosis, particularly in immunocompromised patients.
- Diagnostic tools, including PCR, cytokine analysis (IL-10/IL-6 ratios), and retinal biopsies, are essential for differentiating infectious retinitis and malignancy.
- Retinal biopsy is a valuable diagnostic tool, but tissue adequacy is critical for accurate interpretation. If findings are inconclusive, repeating a biopsy or pursuing a CNS biopsy may be necessary.
- Collaboration between uveitis specialists, retina surgeons, and neurologists is essential for managing complex masquerade syndromes.

PEARLS FROM THE EXPERTS ON FREQUENTLY ASKED QUESTIONS

1. Why do we classify CMV retinitis as a separate entity and not include it under ARN?

Answer: CMV retinitis exhibits a distinct clinical pattern compared to ARN. CMV presents as focal or paucifocal lesions, whereas ARN typically demonstrates circumferential necrosis. Additionally, CMV progresses more slowly and generally has a better prognosis. It is also almost exclusively associated with severe immunocompromise, whereas ARN often occurs in immunocompetent patients.

2. After 3 months of antiviral treatment, what is your principle for tapering antivirals, including duration and dosage?
Answer: There is currently an inconsistency in practice regarding antiviral tapering. However, the trend is moving toward long-term treatment, often extending for years. The rationale is that patients may have an underlying immune deficiency against the virus, placing them at risk for recurrence if treatment is stopped too soon.

3. Regarding intravitreal foscarnet and ganciclovir, would you recommend using both for CMV retinitis?
Answer: For CMV retinitis, using one intravitreal agent (either foscarnet or ganciclovir) combined with highly active antiretroviral therapy (HAART) or reduced immunosuppression is typically sufficient. However, in rapidly progressive outer retinal necrosis, both agents have been proposed due to the poor outcomes associated with this condition.

4. Is photocoagulation performed before the implantation of a dexamethasone implant?
Answer: No, photocoagulation is not routinely performed before dexamethasone implant placement.

5. We observed inflammation in the ciliary body (histologically) in ARN syndrome. According to your data, how often does this occur?
Answer: Thank you for the question. I do not believe this has been published. Clinically, we are unable to directly observe the ciliary body. An ultrasound biomicroscopy (UBM) study might provide insights, but to date, I have not heard of any studies addressing this specifically.

6. In which cases do you consider prophylactic photocoagulation?
Answer: Prophylactic laser has no role in ARN. Historically, it was performed in the belief that it could prevent retinal detachment, but evidence has shown it lacks long-term efficacy.

7. Do you consider prophylactic vitrectomy for patients with severe CMV retinitis?
Answer: Prophylactic vitrectomy in severe CMV retinitis remains *highly controversial*, especially when dealing with an *active (hot) eye* where the vitreous is still attached. Entering the eye prematurely can exacerbate inflammation or complications.

8. In bilateral CMV retinitis, should we proceed with intravitreal injections in both eyes or use oral valganciclovir in a human immunodeficiency virus (HIV) patient with a CD4 count below 50?
Answer: Intravitreal injections should be administered promptly upon initiation of HAART if the condition is vision-threatening.

If the retinitis is peripheral, oral valganciclovir combined with HAART may be sufficient.

Some clinicians delay HAART initiation until the opportunistic infection has been treated to avoid immune recovery inflammatory syndrome (IRIS). However, in CMV retinitis with very low CD4 counts (e.g., <50), delaying HAART increases the risk of high mortality, so HAART should not be postponed.

9. Would you recommend reducing the volume or concentration of antibiotics in eyes with silicone oil?
Answer: Dr. Arevalo recommended halving the antibiotic dose in eyes with silicone oil to minimize the risk of toxicity.

FINAL WRAP-UP

Acute retinal necrosis remains a sight-threatening infectious emergency that requires prompt recognition and immediate intervention to preserve vision. The hallmark features—peripheral retinal necrosis, rapid progression, dense vitritis, and occlusive vasculopathy—underscore the importance of early diagnosis through clinical findings and confirmatory testing, such as PCR of ocular fluids. Systemic antiviral therapy, particularly IV acyclovir, remains the cornerstone of treatment, with intravitreal antivirals such as foscarnet or ganciclovir serving as critical adjuncts in severe or vision-threatening cases. Oral valacyclovir has been documented to be clinically equivalent to IV acyclovir for ARN management. The role of systemic corticosteroids remains controversial and should only be initiated after effective antiviral therapy to mitigate inflammation without exacerbating viral replication. Prophylactic laser retinopexy and vitrectomy remain debated, with no definitive evidence supporting their routine use, though careful consideration may be warranted in selected cases to manage complications such as retinal detachment.

Differentiating ARN from masquerade syndromes such as vitreoretinal lymphoma or CMV retinitis is crucial, especially in immunocompromised patients, where overlapping clinical presentations can complicate diagnosis. Tools such as retinal biopsy, MYD88 mutation testing, and cytokine analysis (IL-10/IL-6 ratios) may aid in identifying malignancies when ARN is suspected but unconfirmed. Long-term antiviral prophylaxis is essential to reduce the risk of recurrence and contralateral eye involvement, particularly within the first 6 months, when the risk is highest. Multidisciplinary collaboration among uveitis specialists, vitreoretinal surgeons, neurologists, and oncologists is vital for managing complex presentations, ensuring diagnostic precision, and tailoring therapeutic strategies. As ARN remains a condition with high morbidity despite advances in therapy, ongoing research is needed to refine treatment protocols, minimize complications, and improve long-term visual outcomes.

REFERENCES

1. International Uveitis Study Group (IUSG). (2025). Uveitis grand round 10: acute retinal necrosis. [online] Available from https://www.youtube.com/@uveitiswebinar9194/videos. [Last accessed February, 2025].
2. Rangel CM, Restrepo-Arango M, Mejía-Salgado G, Gómez-Rocha MA, Gómez Velasco M, García MF, et al. Acute retinal necrosis: experience in a reference center in Santander–Colombia. Ocul Immunol Inflamm. 2023;1-9.
3. Urayama A, Yamada N, Sasaki T. Unilateral acute uveitis with retinal periarteritis and detachment. Jpn J Clin Ophthalmol. 1971;607-19.
4. Holland GN. Standard diagnostic criteria for the acute retinal necrosis syndrome. Am J Ophthalmol. 1994;117(5): 663-6.
5. Takase H, Okada AA, Goto H, Mizuki N, Namba K, Ohguro N, et al. Development and validation of new diagnostic criteria for acute retinal necrosis. Jpn J Ophthalmol. 2015;59(1):14-20.
6. Classification criteria for acute retinal necrosis syndrome. Am J Ophthalmol. 2021;228:237-44.
7. Dworkin LL. Real-time quantitative polymerase chain reaction diagnosis of infectious posterior uveitis. Arch Ophthalmol. 2002;120(11):1534.
8. Rothova A, De Boer JH, Ten Dam-van Loon NH, Postma G, De Visser L, Zuurveen SJ, et al. Usefulness of aqueous humor analysis for the diagnosis of posterior uveitis. Ophthalmology. 2008;115(2):306-11.
9. Fitoussi L, Baptiste A, Mainguy A, L'Honneur AS, Bojanova M, Dechartres A, et al. Clinical and virological characteristics and prognostic factors in viral necrotizing retinitis. J Pers Med. 2022;12(11):1785.
10. Forster DJ, Dugel PU, Frangieh GT, Liggett PE, Rao NA. Rapidly progressive outer retinal necrosis in the acquired immunodeficiency syndrome. Am J Ophthalmol. 1990;110(4):341-8.
11. Charkoudian LD. Acute retinal necrosis after herpes zoster vaccination. Arch Ophthalmol. 2011;129(11):1495.
12. Heath G, Depledge DP, Brown JR, Hale AD, Tutil H, Williams R, et al. Acute retinal necrosis caused by the zoster vaccine virus. Clin Infect Dis. 2017;65(12):2122-5.
13. Kawaguchi T, Spencer DB, Mochizuki M. Therapy for acute retinal necrosis. Semin Ophthalmol. 2008;23(4):285-90.
14. Hillenkamp J, Nölle B, Bruns C, Rautenberg P, Fickenscher H, Roider J. Acute retinal necrosis: clinical features, early vitrectomy, and outcomes. Ophthalmology. 2009;116(10):1971-5.e2.
15. Baltinas J, Lightman S, Tomkins-Netzer O. Comparing treatment of acute retinal necrosis with either oral valacyclovir or intravenous acyclovir. Am J Ophthalmol. 2018;188:173-80.
16. Liu S, Wang D, Zhang X. The necessity and optimal time for performing pars plana vitrectomy in acute retinal necrosis patients. BMC Ophthalmol. 2018;18(1):15.
17. Kawali A, Patil A, Mishra SB, Mahendradas P, Shetty R. Choroidal involvement and chronic macular edema in acute retinal necrosis: a novel finding and a novel treatment. Ocul Immunol Inflamm. 2024;32(7):1457-61.
18. Putera I, Ridwan AS, Dewi M, Cifuentes-González C, Rojas-Carabali W, Sitompul R, et al. Antiviral treatment for acute retinal necrosis: a systematic review and meta-analysis. Surv Ophthalmol. 2024;69(1):67-84.
19. Ray IK, Sobrin L, Moorthy R, Yeh S, Thorne JE, Shantha JG. Common practice patterns in the diagnosis and management of acute retinal necrosis: a survey study of uveitis specialists. Ocul Immunol Inflamm. 2024;1-7.
20. Butler NJ, Moradi A, Salek SS, Burkholder BM, Leung TG, Dunn JP, et al. Acute retinal necrosis: presenting characteristics and clinical outcomes in a cohort of polymerase chain reaction-positive patients. Am J Ophthalmol. 2017;179:179-89.
21. Wu CY, Fan J, Davis JL, Berrocal AM, Haddock LJ, Yannuzzi NA, et al. Surgical outcomes of acute retinal necrosis-related retinal detachment in polymerase chain reaction-positive patients. Ophthalmol Retina. 2022;6(11):992-1000.
22. de Visser L, de Boer JH, T Rijkers G, Wiertz K, van den Ham HJ, de Boer R, et al. Cytokines and chemokines involved in acute retinal necrosis. Invest Ophthalmol Vis Sci. 2017;58(4):2139-51.
23. Sørland RØ, Erichsen AK, Jonsdottir TE, Bromnes MN, Lauritzen PM, Eidet JR. Successful treatment with repeated dexamethasone implant injections for recurrent macular edema after acute retinal necrosis. J Ophthalmic Inflamm Infect. 2022;12(1):33.
24. Saade JS, Istambouli R, AbdulAal M, Antonios R, Hamam RN. Bromfenac 0.09% for the treatment of macular edema secondary to noninfectious uveitis. Middle East Afr J Ophthalmol. 2021;28(2):98-103.
25. Nguyen BT, Hung JH, Thng ZX, El Feky D, Mobasserian A, Saengsirinavin AO, et al. Tocilizumab for cystoid

macular edema secondary to immune recovery uveitis in a patient with contraindications to long-term systemic corticosteroid. Yale J Biol Med. 2024;97(4):423-30.
26. Flaxel CJ, Yeh S, Lauer AK. Combination systemic and intravitreal antiviral therapy in the management of acute retinal necrosis syndrome (an American Ophthalmological Society thesis). Trans Am Ophthalmol Soc. 2013;111:133-44.
27. Wong RW, Jumper JM, McDonald HR, Johnson RN, Fu A, Lujan BJ, et al. Emerging concepts in the management of acute retinal necrosis. Br J Ophthalmol. 2013;97(5):545-52.
28. Palay DA, Sternberg P, Davis J, Lewis H, Holland GN, Mieler WF, et al. Decrease in the risk of bilateral acute retinal necrosis by acyclovir therapy. Am J Ophthalmol. 1991;112(3):250-5.
29. Fahle G. Central retinal vascular occlusion associated with acute retinal necrosis. Arch Ophthalmol. 2012;130(4):514.
30. Liu T, Jain A, Fung M, Vinnard C, Ivaturi V. Valacyclovir as initial treatment for acute retinal necrosis: a pharmacokinetic modeling and simulation study. Curr Eye Res. 2017;42(7):1035-8.
31. Chen M, Zhang M, Chen H. Efficiency of laser photocoagulation on the prevention of retinal detachment in acute retinal necrosis: a systematic review and meta-analysis. Retina. 2022;42(9):1702-8.
32. Sims JL, Yeoh J, Stawell RJ. Acute retinal necrosis: a case series with clinical features and treatment outcomes. Clin Exp Ophthalmol. 2009;37(5):473-7.
33. Risseeuw S, De Boer JH, Ten Dam-Van Loon NH, Van Leeuwen R. Risk of rhegmatogenous retinal detachment in acute retinal necrosis with and without prophylactic intervention. Am J Ophthalmol. 2019;206:140-8.
34. Arevalo JF. En bloc perfluorodissection in vitreoretinal surgery: a new surgical technique. Retina. 2008;28(4):653-6.
35. Arevalo JF. En bloc perfluorodissection for tractional retinal detachment in proliferative diabetic retinopathy. Ophthalmol. 2008 Jun;115(6):e21-5.
36. MyAlconProfessionals. (2025). Hypervit Dual Blade Vitrectomy Probe. [online] Available from https://www.myalcon.com/professional/vitreoretinal-surgery/platforms-and-probes/hypervit-dual-blade/. [Last accessed February, 2025].
37. Toh VTR, Gerard G, Tay ZQ, Chen J, Chew GWM, Teoh CS. Efficacy and safety of methotrexate in the treatment of proliferative vitreoretinopathy: a systematic review. Eye Lond Engl. 2024;1:460-7.
38. Nourinia R, Safi S, Mohammadpour M, Riazi-Esfahani H, Ansari Astaneh MR, Falavarjani KG, et al. Effects of repeated intra-silicone oil injections of methotrexate on proliferative vitreoretinopathy grade C: a multicenter randomized controlled trial. Sci Rep. 2024;14(1):28842.
39. Rajan RP, Babu KN, Arumugam KK, Muraleedharan S, Ramachandran O, Jena S, et al. Intravitreal methotrexate as an adjuvant in vitrectomy in cases of retinal detachment with proliferative vitreoretinopathy. Graefes Arch Clin Exp Ophthalmol. 2024. [Online ahead of print].
40. Balas M, Abdelaal A, Popovic MM, Kertes PJ, Muni RH. Intravitreal methotrexate for the prevention and treatment of proliferative vitreoretinopathy in rhegmatogenous retinal detachment: a systematic review. Ophthalmic Surg Lasers Imaging Retina. 2022;53(10):561-8.
41. Rothova A, Hajjaj A, De Hoog J, Thiadens AAHJ, Dalm VASH. Uveitis causes according to immune status of patients. Acta Ophthalmol (Copenh). 2019;97(1):53-9.
42. Nakano S, Sugita S, Tomaru Y, Hono A, Nakamuro T, Kubota T, et al. Establishment of multiplex solid-phase strip pcr test for detection of 24 ocular infectious disease pathogens. Investig Ophthalmology Vis Sci. 2017;58(3):1553.

CHAPTER 11

RNA Viruses and Uveitis

Piergiorgio Neri, Shravya Choudhary Bala, Mudit Tyagi, Pallavi Goel, Manisha Agarwal, Radhika Sriram, Padmamalini Mahendradas, Sara Prischak, Vishali Gupta, Germán Mejía-Salgado, Alejandra de-la-Torre, Reema Bansal, John H Kempen, Meghan Berkenstock

INTRODUCTION

Though rare, RNA viruses can cause uveitis, leading to significant ocular morbidity, and should be looked for, especially during disease outbreaks. The clinical spectrum is extremely wide, but some of the viruses may have typical ocular features. Any structure of the eye may be involved ranging from the conjunctiva to the optic nerve. However, the retina is affected most commonly by coronavirus, mumps, measles, dengue, chikungunya, rickettsia, influenza, and the human immunodeficiency virus (HIV). Conversely, rubella primarily affects the anterior segment. More than one virus may be present simultaneously in the eye requiring identification by polymerase chain reaction (PCR) of intraocular samples. Besides serological or molecular testing, it is important to recognize systemic symptoms for etiological association.

THEMATIC LECTURE: RNA VIRUSES

The spectrum of diseases caused by RNA viruses is very diverse. The diagnosis is sometimes challenging and treatment is limited by a lack of antiviral medications for most of the viruses. We will focus on the taxonomy, presentation, and treatments of several RNA viruses that cause ocular inflammation: Mumps, measles, rubella, dengue, chikungunya, HIV, Zika, influenza, hepatitis C, West Nile, Lassa, Ebola, Marburg, Rift Valley fever, human T-lymphotropic virus (HTLV-1), and severe acute respiratory syndrome coronavirus 2 (SARS-CoV-2).

Mumps is a ubiquitous virus in the Paramyxoviridae family (Rubelavirus genus) that is transmitted through respiratory (Flugge's) droplets. The spectrum of ocular diseases includes anterior uveitis, vitritis, retinitis, chorioretinitis, or acute posterior multifocal placoid pigment epitheliopathy (APMPPE) lesions.[1] Complications can include macular edema. Given these non-specific ocular findings, diagnosis is based on systemic medical findings including parotitis, orchitis, and in rare cases encephalitis or meningitis with an accompanying positive IgM and IgG serologic titers for mumps. On optical coherence tomography (OCT), disruption of the ellipsoid zone and the presence of intra- and subretinal fluid can be seen. On fluorescein angiography, placoid lesions block early and stain late. Management includes observation for mild cases or the use of oral corticosteroids for inflammation involving the posterior pole. Vaccination plays an important role in disease prevention.

Measles is single-stranded RNA virus that is universal and highly contagious belonging to the Paramyxoviridae family (Morbillivirus genus) that is spread through respiratory droplets. The ophthalmic presentation can include retinitis, chorioretinitis, or panuveitis due to anterior chamber spillover.[1] Posterior pole findings include a typical "salt and pepper" appearance of the retinal pigment epithelium (RPE). These changes can be highlighted with a granular alternating hyper- and hypoautofluorescence on fundus autofluorescence imaging or seen as window defects in areas of RPE loss in late fluorescein angiogram imaging. A medical history of fever, a diffuse sandpaper-like rash, Koplik's spots in the mouth, and positive immunoglobulin M (IgM) and IgG titers can aid in the diagnosis. Supportive care with use of oral corticosteroids to treat posterior pole inflammation can be initiated for treatment. Similar to mumps, vaccination is preventative.

Rubella is a single-stranded RNA virus that was reclassified in 2018 into the Matonaviridae family (Rubivirus genus). In addition to respiratory droplets, maternal-fetal transmission can occur. The ocular presentation can include a pseudo-Fuch's heterochromic iridocyclitis or a hypertensive, chronic anterior uveitis. In this clinical scenario, it is important to not only think of the herpes viruses as a cause, but include PCR testing for rubella in aqueous humor removed from an anterior chamber tap.[1] Management includes antiglaucoma medications to treat the hypertensive crisis with concurrent use of topical corticosteroids to treat anterior chamber inflammation. Complications can include cataract formation.

Dengue is a single-stranded RNA virus in the Flaviviridae family (Flavivirus genus). It is endemic in tropical and subtropical regions, particularly in Asia, Latin America, Africa, and the Pacific Islands. The mode of transmission is the Aedes mosquito, and the spectrum of ophthalmic disease can be variable. Characteristic retinal hemorrhages with cotton wool spots and macular edema can be seen posteriorly along with an anterior uveitis.[2] Diagnosis relies on a travel history to an endemic region. Systemic symptoms can include fever, muscle and joint pains, rash, and in severe cases, hypotension. Serologic testing for the NS1 antigen and IgM/IgG antibody titers are available. Multimodal imaging using OCT can show nerve fiber layer edema in areas of cotton wool spots, exudates in the superficial retinal plexus in areas of intraretinal hemorrhage, and areas of subretinal fluid. Management is limited to supportive care with judicious use of oral corticosteroids depending on the disease severity.

Chikungunya is a single-stranded RNA Alphavirus (Togaviridae genus). It is endemic in tropical and subtropical regions and transmitted by Aedes mosquitoes. Ophthalmically, infection can present as anterior uveitis, retinitis, and optic neuritis.[3] Sequelae can lead to vision loss due to retinal atrophy, highlighting the need to acutely elicit a recent travel history to endemic regions and obtain serologic PCR testing for chikungunya. The management is administration of supportive care with oral corticosteroids for posterior pole and optic nerve inflammation. Follow-up testing with OCT imaging and visual fields are needed to assess for optic nerve damage.

HIV is a single-stranded RNA virus and a member of the Retroviridae family (Lentivirus genus). Transmission can occur with mucous membrane contact with infected body fluids, blood transfusions, and the maternofetal route. Transmission rates increase with higher viral titers. Given the predilection for the infection of pericytes, cotton wool spots along the retinal vasculature can be seen on fundoscopic examination. Depending on the host immune status, cytomegalovirus (CMV) retinitis may also be seen with low CD 4+ cell counts or an anterior uveitis may be present with macular edema as cell counts rise (immune recovery uveitis).[4] Serologic assessment for HIV antibodies with reflex testing for CD4+ T-cell counts and viral loads are necessary to make the diagnosis. Testing for coinfection with other sexually transmitted diseases is warranted along with start of combined antiretroviral therapy (cART). Corticosteroids are used to treat immune recovery uveitis, and antivirals are the mainstay of CMV treatment including ganciclovir and valganciclovir in addition to intravitreal foscarnet, ganciclovir, or cidofovir.[5]

Zika virus is a single-stranded RNA virus in the Flaviviridae family (Flavivirus genus). It is endemic in tropical and subtropical regions of Central and South America, Southern Asia, and Africa. Transmission is through the Aedes mosquito, blood transfusions, and maternofetal or sexual routes. On examination, the most common presentation is a chorioretinitis or rarely, an optic neuritis. While most cases are asymptomatic, systemic symptoms of rashes, fever, and joint pain can occur. Maternofetal transmission can lead to fetal microcephaly and chorioretinal scars.[6] Fundus examination shows multifocal active, and later atrophic, spots occurring in clusters around the retinal vessels. The diagnosis relies on a recent travel history to an endemic region and serologic PCR testing for Zika. Treatment is supportive care, and prevention is through mosquito control.

Influenza is a single-stranded RNA virus in the Orthomyxoviridae family (Alphainfluenzavirus genus). It is transmitted by respiratory droplets. However, it has been associated with the development of anterior uveitis and APMPPE. A clinical history of flu-like symptoms and nasal swab testing for PCR can make the diagnosis and confirm the strain. Indocyanine green angiography (ICGA) shows blockage in areas of placoid lesions. Antivirals are most effective if taken in the first 48 hours for systemic symptoms: oseltamivir, baloxavir, zanamivir, and peramivir.[7] However, the ocular penetration and effectiveness of these medications are unknown. Oral corticosteroids can be given, with caution, particularly in cases of APMPPE.

Hepatitis C is a ubiquitous, single-stranded RNA virus in the Flaviviridae family (Hepacivirus genus). The transmission is through reused needles, solid organ transplantation, maternofetal transmission, blood transfusions, and sexual intercourse. Similar to HIV, a higher viral load increases the risk of transmission. Ocular complications are not common and can include anterior or intermediate uveitis or, retinal vasculitis that occurs with acute infection. Even rarer is the development of an ischemic optic neuropathy secondary to cryoglobulinemia. In patients with hepatitis C infection that has been treated, use of topical corticosteroids can be used as there is no specific tropism of the virus for the eye. Testing for hepatitis C antibodies and viral titers using PCR testing confirms the diagnosis. Direct-acting antivirals are the current standard of care to achieve a 95% cure rate, whereas cryoglobulinemia is treated with plasmapheresis and immunosuppression.[8] Corticosteroids can be used to treat the ocular inflammation with caution when using oral formulations.

West Nile virus is a single-stranded RNA virus that is in the Flaviviridae family (Flavivirus genus). It is endemic in Africa, Europe, Middle East, North America, and Western Asia with transmission through the Culex mosquito. The ophthalmic spectrum of disease includes retinal vasculitis and chorioretinitis with the distribution of the atrophic spots along the vessels in linear patterns.[7] There is an increased incidence in patients with diabetes. A history of recent travel with positive IgM and IgG antibody testing can make the diagnosis. Treatment is supportive care with vector control.

Lassa virus is a single-stranded RNA virus in the Arenaviridae family (Mammarenavirus genus). Transmission occurs through inhalation or ingestion of the Natal multimammate mouse excrement or contact with contaminated bodily fluids from other humans. Outbreaks occur in areas with poor hygiene. Clinically, conjunctivitis and anterior uveitis have been reported and possibly, posterior uveitis based on the presence of retinal scars in survivors.[9] IgM antibody and serum PCR testing are available to discern this virus from other causes of hemorrhagic fevers. Treatment relies on supportive care with multidisciplinary management in the minority of patients that develop hypotensive shock. Prevention lies in vector control.

Ebola is a single-stranded RNA virus in the Filoviridae family (Ebolavirus genus) and is endemic in Central and Western Africa. Transmission is through contact with infected bodily tissues or fluids, and the natural reservoir is the fruit bat. The most common ophthalmic presentation is anterior uveitis, although intermediate and posterior uveitis have been suspected given retinal scars seen in survivors. The virus has also been isolated from aqueous samples in survivors.[10] A travel history to endemic regions can help diagnostically along with other systemic symptoms of viral hemorrhagic fevers, similar to Lassa virus. Available serologic testing includes viral PCR or ELISA testing for antibody formation.[11] Early diagnosis is critical given the high mortality rate and need for isolation. Supportive care and cautious use of corticosteroids are the mainstays of treatment. Vector control is the only form of prevention.

Marburg virus is a single-stranded RNA virus in the Filoviridae family (Marburgvirus genus) that is endemic in Central and Eastern Africa. Transmission occurs through contact with bat excrement or contaminated bodily fluids. Cases of conjunctivitis, retinitis, and posterior uveitis have been reported.[12] However, tropism for the eye is unknown, as any illness causing a fever can result in vascular congestion of the conjunctiva. While vaccines have been studied, none are commercially available at this time. Serologic testing for viral PCR is available, and a clinical history of recent travel to an endemic area and systemic signs of viral hemorrhagic fever would be present in acute cases. Treatment involves supportive care, and continued public health measures are needed to prevent the disease.

Rift Valley virus is a single-stranded RNA virus in the Phenuiviridae family (Phlebovirus genus) that is endemic in sub-Saharan Africa, with outbreaks in North Africa, the Middle East, and occasionally in other regions. The vector of transmission is the Aedes aegypti mosquito or contact with contaminated livestock tissues. The most common ophthalmic presentation is retinitis and macular edema that can lead to the formation of chorioretinal scars.[13] Serologic testing for viral PCR can confirm the diagnosis. Inflammation can be cautiously treated with corticosteroids and observation for disease resolution. Prevention lies in mosquito control.

Human T-lymphotropic virus-1 is a single-stranded RNA virus in the Retroviridae family (Deltaretrovirus genus) and is endemic in Japan, the Caribbean, parts of South America, sub-Saharan Africa, and the Middle East. Transmission occurs through a maternofetal route or through contact with contaminated bodily fluids.

The most common ocular findings in HTLV-1 carriers is uveitis. Testing for HTLV-1 viral PCR or antibodies and a positive travel history accompanying myelopathy (tropical spastic paraparesis), adult T-cell leukemia, dermatitis, or pneumonitis can aid in the diagnosis. Corticosteroid administration for ocular inflammation and long-term monitoring for neurologic and hematopoietic involvement are crucial.

Severe acute respiratory syndrome coronavirus 2 (SARS-CoV-2) is a single-stranded RNA virus in the Coronaviridae family (Betacoronavirus genus) that is universally spread through respiratory droplets or zoonotic vectors. Conjunctivitis, anterior uveitis, and occlusive retinitis have been reported. Cases of ocular inflammation after vaccination, ranging from anterior scleritis to acute macular neuroretinopathy, have also been published.[14] Testing includes viral antigen or PCR testing of nasal secretions. Treatment includes multidisciplinary management with supportive care and the use of antiviral medications in those at high-risk for severe disease: Molnupiravir, remdesivir, or ritonavir and nirmatrelvir. For ocular inflammation, judicious use of corticosteroids is recommended.

In conclusion, RNA virus cause a variety of ocular inflammatory diseases that can lead to significant morbidity and loss of vision. Early recognition and use of targeted therapies are essential for management. Multidisciplinary care, especially in those with systemic disease manifestations, improves outcomes in addition to prevention through vaccination and vector control.

A TALE OF TWO VIRUSES: ACUTE RETINAL NECROSIS AFTER SARS-CoV-2 INFECTION

Case Presentation

Personal Data

A 31-year-old male with no known comorbidities had a history of acute retinal necrosis (ARN) in May 2016. He received prophylactive barrier laser for the old ARN lesions in the inferonasal quadrant in the right eye.

History of Present Illness

Six years later, in 2022, he presented with floaters and reduced vision in his right eye for 1 week. He had tested positive for SARS-CoV-2 one month before the onset of his ocular symptoms and was treated with oral antibiotics by his general physician.

Physical Examination

Visual acuity was 20/30 in the right eye and 20/20 in the left eye. The anterior chamber was quiet in both eyes. There was an early posterior subcapsular cataract in the right eye. Fundus examination showed new areas of retinitis near the prior laser barricade in the right eye **(Table 1 and Fig. 1)**.

TABLE 1: Physical examination of the patient having acute retinal necrosis after SARS-CoV-2 infection.

OD	*Parameter*	*OS*
20/30	BCVA	20/20
12 mm Hg	IOP	12 mm Hg
Quiet	Conjunctiva	Quiet
Normal, clear	Cornea	Normal, clear
No cells ACC: 0+	Anterior chamber	No cells ACC: 0+
No synechiae	Iris	No synechiae
1+ Posterior subcapsular cataract	Lens	Clear
Unremarkable	Vitreous	Unremarkable
Mid peripheral retinal scars with whitish preretinal exudates and hemorrhages	Fundus	Normal

(ACC: anterior chamber cellularity; BCVA: best-corrected visual acuity; IOP: intraocular pressure; OD: right eye; OS: left eye)
Source: Uveitis Webinar - Grand Round 11. International Uveitis Study Group (IUSG). 2025. https://youtu.be/CliZo0xOKpQ.

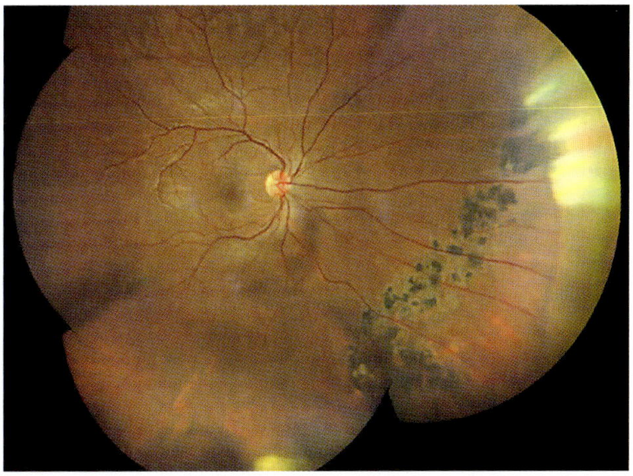

Fig. 1: A color fundus montage of the right eye showing peripheral barricade laser in the inferonasal quadrant with adjacent retinitis. A patch of retinitis is also seen inferiorly at 6 o'clock.
Source: Uveitis Webinar - Grand Round 11. International Uveitis Study Group (IUSG). 2025. https://youtu.be/CliZo0xOKpQ.

Uveitis Work-up

Based on the location of the exudates and hemorrhages in the area of prior ARN, a diagnosis of ARN reactivation was made. A prior work-up in 2016 included negative HIV and treponema pallidum hemagglutination (TPHA) results.

Initial Treatment

He was started on oral valacyclovir 2 g three times a day and tapering doses of oral corticosteroids over 6 weeks.

Follow-up

The patient followed up weekly until resolution of the retinitis, as seen in **Figure 2**, and vision improved to 20/20. The patient was started on a maintenance dose of 1 g of valacyclovir daily. The patient developed macular edema 13 weeks later that recurred with the taper of prednisone to 5 mg daily. The daily prednisone dose was increased back to 7.5 mg/day with resolution, and he was also kept on a maintenance dose of systemic antivirals (500 mg of oral valacyclovir).

In December 2024, he presented again with reduced vision in his right eye for 2 weeks, while being maintained on oral valacyclovir 500 mg daily and prednisone 5 mg daily. Three months prior, he had another episode of fever, for which he had received oral antibiotics. No blood or nasal swab testing was performed, but the fundus examination showed a bright yellow area of retinitis in the periphery with preretinal exudates near the prior ARN lesions **(Figs. 3A and B)**. A recurrence of ARN was diagnosed, and he was restarted on 2 g of oral valacyclovir three times a day, along with an oral prednisone taper.

Discussion

As of December 2024, there have been 717 million cases of SARS-CoV-2, which have resulted in over 7 million reported deaths. SARS-CoV-2 virus is known to cause respiratory distress syndrome and secondary infections. The clinical manifestations can range from asymptomatic or mild flu-like symptoms to severe respiratory distress. Various ocular manifestations have been reported and are

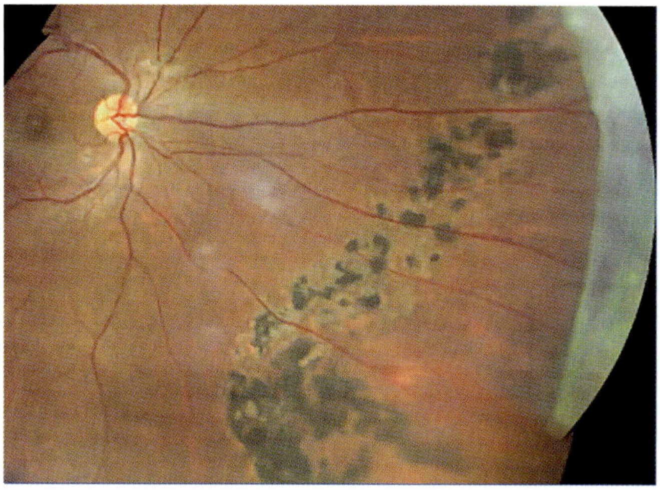

Fig. 2: A color fundus photo of the nasal right eye showing the resolution of the retinitis abutting the laser barricade. *Source:* Uveitis Webinar - Grand Round 11. International Uveitis Study Group (IUSG). 2025. https://youtu.be/CIiZo0xOKpQ.

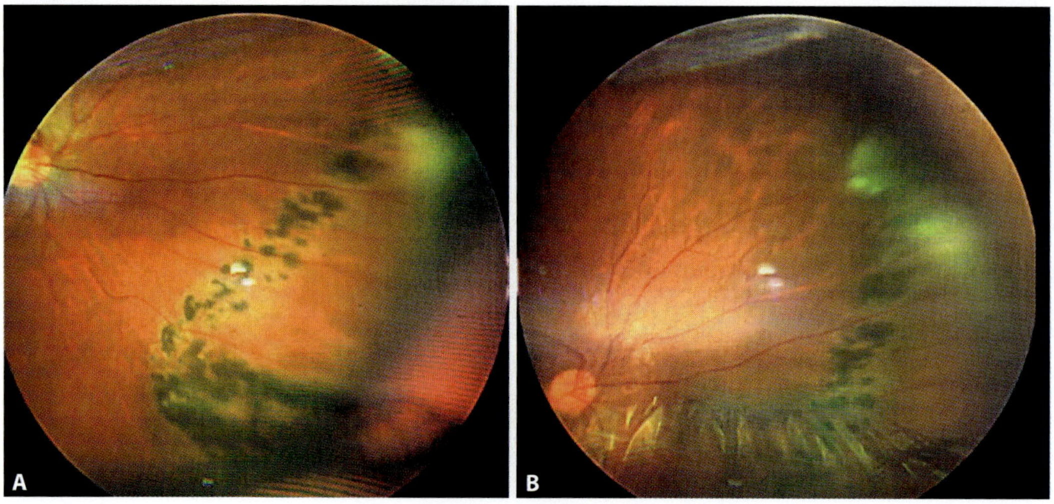

Figs. 3A and B: Color fundus photos of the nasal right eye showing reactivation of the retinitis abutting the laser barricade. *Source:* Uveitis Webinar - Grand Round 11. International Uveitis Study Group (IUSG). 2025. https://youtu.be/CIiZo0xOKpQ.

more common in patients with severe systemic disease. In the initial phase of the disease, viral replication triggers a strong immune response by both innate and adaptive immunity. The first line of defense is innate immunity, which starts immediately by secreting interferons to decrease with viral replication. The adaptive immune response starts 6–8 days later through antigen-specific T- and B-cell responses. Once the SARS-CoV-2 virus binds to angiotensin-converting enzyme (ACE) receptors on the lung epithelium, entry into the host cells occurs. The viral replication cycle and subsequent release then begins. This activates the host immune system, and an exuberant release of inflammatory cytokines can lead to the development of a cytokine storm. The result is an elevated number of macrophages, hyperactivation of T-cells, and an increase in plasma levels of proinflammatory cytokines, such as interleukin 1 (IL-1), IL-1β IL-6, and tumor necrosis factor alpha (TNF-α). SARS-CoV-2 infection is also associated with developing biological and clinical markers of acquired immunosuppression, such as lymphopenia, eosinopenia, and multiorgan failure. This dysfunctional immune response can further lead to the development of secondary bacterial, viral, and fungal infections, especially in those who have been hospitalized. The state of immunodeficiency and immune dysfunction can also result in reactivation of prior herpes virus infections. After primary herpetic viral infection, a lifelong latency in the sensory ganglia is established via the retrograde transport to peripheral neurons. Conditions of immune dysregulation, fever, or stress can result in the upregulation of the herpes simplex virus (HSV) lytic genes, which cause reactivation and viral replication. During active SARS-CoV-2 infection, the upregulation of the host adaptive immunity through activation of CD8+ T-cells concurrently impairs suppression of the HSV viral lytic genes. Atypical, bilateral, ARN has been reported previously during or after SARS-CoV-2 infection. In summary, clinicians should be aware that SARS-CoV-2 infection can lead to immune dysregulation and reactivation of a latent herpes viral infection.

POST-FEVER RETINITIS

Case Presentation

Personal Data

A 66-year-old female without a past ophthalmic history presented with 10-days of a bilateral, sudden, painless decrease in vision preceded by fever and myalgia.

History of Present Illness

She had a history of chronic cystitis, but no other systemic symptoms or rashes were reported. On presentation, the vision was 6/36, N24 in the right eye and 3/60, N36 in the left eye. The anterior segment examination was unremarkable in both eyes. Fundus examination showed white retinitis patches with interspersed intraretinal hemorrhages in both eyes, with a macular star in the right eye and retinitis involving the macula in the left eye **(Figs. 4A and B)**.

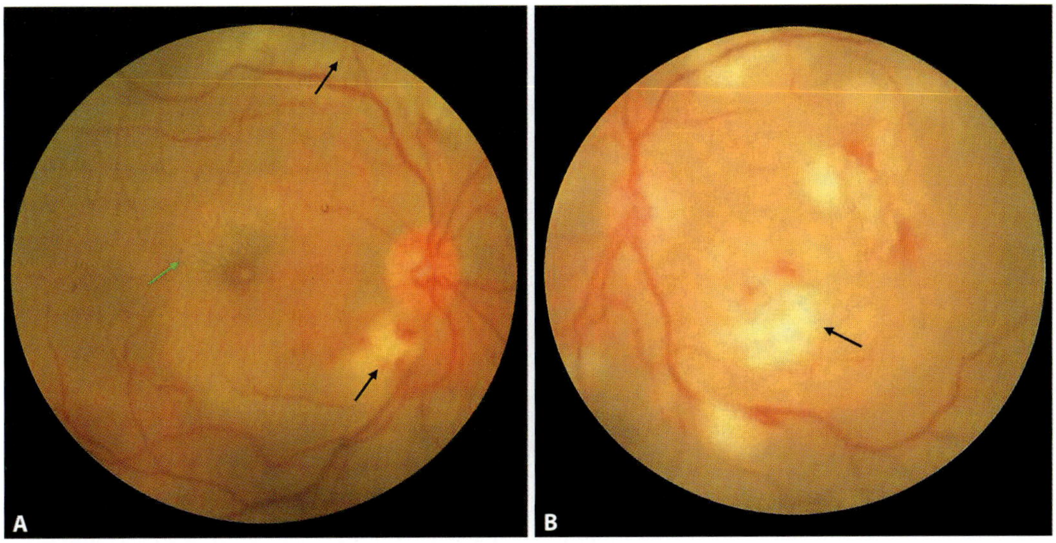

Figs. 4A and B: Color fundus photographs showing bilateral retinitis patches (black arrows) with a macular star (green arrow) in the right eye and retinitis involving macula in the left eye.
Source: Uveitis Webinar - Grand Round 11. International Uveitis Study Group (IUSG). 2025. https://youtu.be/CIiZo0xOKpQ.

Physical Examination

Slit lamp examination is shown in **Table 2**.

Ancillary Testing

An OCT scan through retinitis lesions in the right eye showed inner retinal hyperreflectivity with back shadowing and associated subretinal and intraretinal fluid **(Fig. 5a1 and a2)**. OCT scan through the macula in left eye showed an elevated foveal contour with multiple hyperreflective dots in the outer retinal layer and the presence of subfoveal fluid **(Fig. 5b1 and b2)**.

Uveitis Work-up

Prior to presentation, a complete blood count (CBC) showed leukocytosis (total leukocyte count: 13,500), CRP (15 mg/dL) was elevated, and a TPHA was nonreactive. In addition, an erythrocyte sedimentation rate (ESR) (42 mm/h) was borderline elevated, and NS1 antigen testing was negative. Based on the clinical presentation, the patient was advised to obtain a Weil–Felix Test.

TABLE 2: Physical examination of the patient having post-fever retinitis.

OD	*Parameter*	*OS*
6/36, N24	BCVA	3/60, N36
12 mm Hg	IOP	14 mm Hg
Quiet	Conjunctiva	Quiet
Normal, clear	Cornea	Normal, clear
No cells ACC: 0+	Anterior chamber	No cells ACC: 0+
No synechiae	Iris	No synechiae
Clear	Lens	Clear
Unremarkable	Vitreous	Unremarkable
White, fluffy retinitis patches with interspersed intraretinal hemorrhages and a macular star	Fundus	White fluffy retinitis with interspersed hemorrhages involving the macula

(ACC: anterior chamber cellularity; BCVA: best-corrected visual acuity; IOP: intraocular pressure; OD: right eye; OS: left eye)

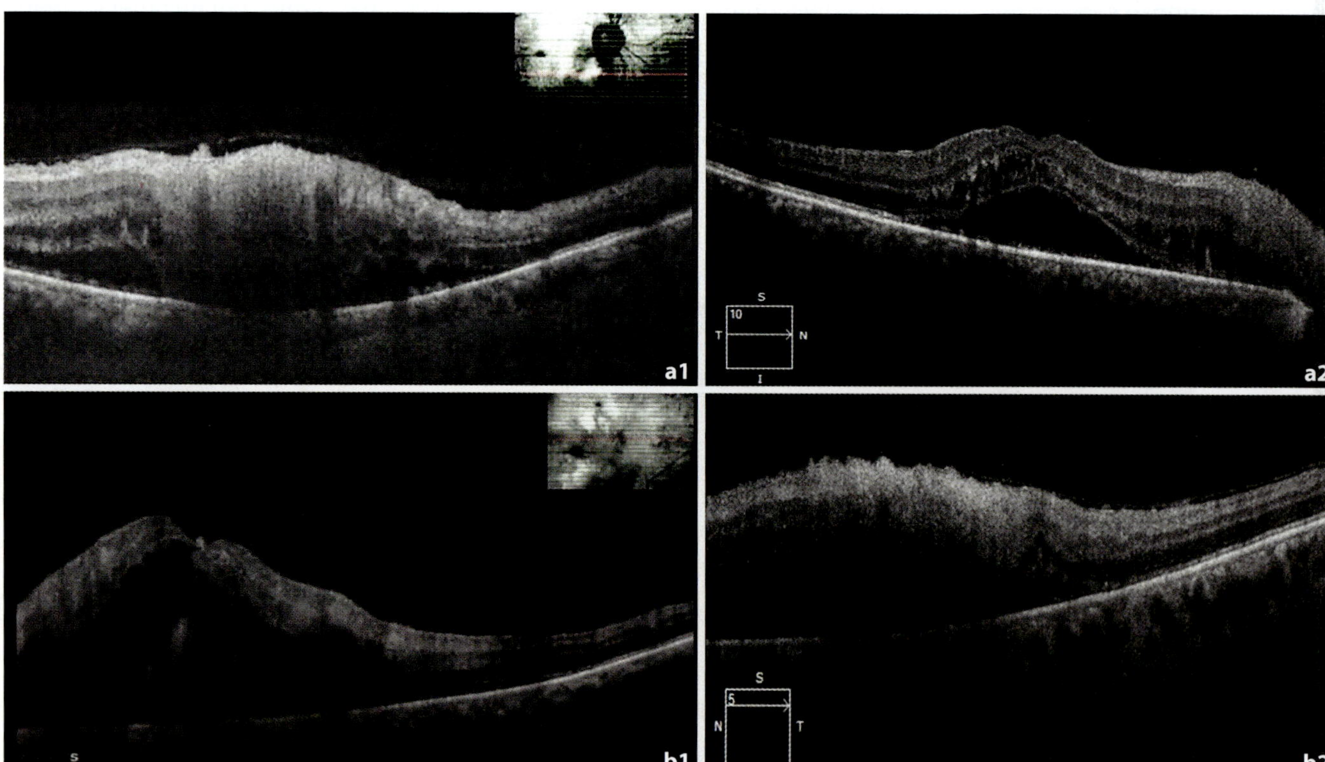

Figs. 5A and B: OCT scans through retinitis lesions in the right eye (a1) and left eye (b2) showed inner retinal hyperreflectivity with after shadowing and associated subretinal fluid. Another scan through the macula in right eye (a2) showed an elevated foveal contour with multiple hyperreflective dots in outer retinal layer and the presence of subfoveal fluid. An OCT scan through the macula of left eye (b1) showed elevated foveal contour with hyperreflectivity of retinal layers and the presence of intraretinal and subretinal fluid.
Source: Uveitis Webinar - Grand Round 11. International Uveitis Study Group (IUSG). 2025. https://youtu.be/CliZo0xOKpQ.

Anatomic Diagnosis

With a history of fever preceding the diminution of vision, a provisional diagnosis of bilateral post-fever retinitis was made.

Initial Treatment

The patient was started empirically on oral prednisolone (1 mg/kg/day) with a weekly taper with oral valacyclovir 500 mg twice a day and doxycycline 100 mg twice a day. The macula-threatening nature of the disease warranted early treatment.

Follow-up

The Weil–Felix test was positive for OX 19, OX K, and OX 2, and the diagnosis of rickettsial retinitis was made. Valacyclovir was discontinued. After 3 weeks of treatment, the retinitis resolved in both eyes **(Figs. 6A and B)**. On OCT scans, the hyperreflective dots and subretinal fluid resolved. The normal reflectivity of the inner retinal layers returned with the restoration of the foveal contour in the right eye **(Fig. 7A)**. The distortion of the ellipsoid zone and the loss of continuity of the external limiting membrane remained in the areas of prior retinitis in the left eye **(Fig. 7B)**. The final best-corrected visual acuity was 6/6, N6 in the right eye and 6/12, N8 in the left eye.

Discussion

Post-fever retinitis is characterized by multifocal or unifocal cotton wool spots predominantly found at the posterior pole. The retinal changes occur about 2–4 weeks following the onset of the fever. The condition has a seasonal variation and is often known as epidemic retinitis. Etiologies include a heterogeneous group

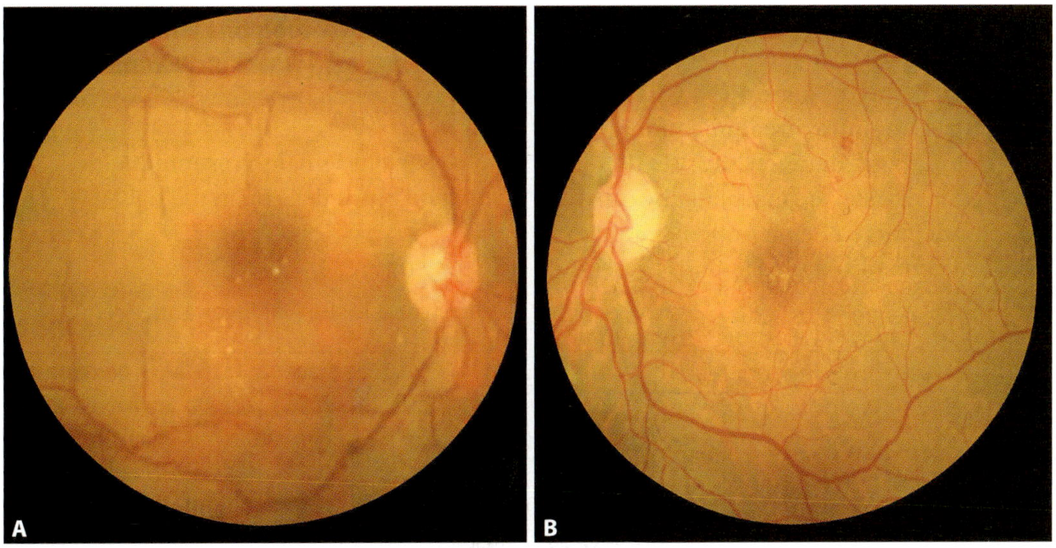

Figs. 6A and B: Fundus photos of the right (A) and left eyes (B) after 6 weeks of follow-up shows resolution of the retinitis.
Source: Uveitis Webinar - Grand Round 11. International Uveitis Study Group (IUSG). 2025. https://youtu.be/CliZo0xOKpQ.

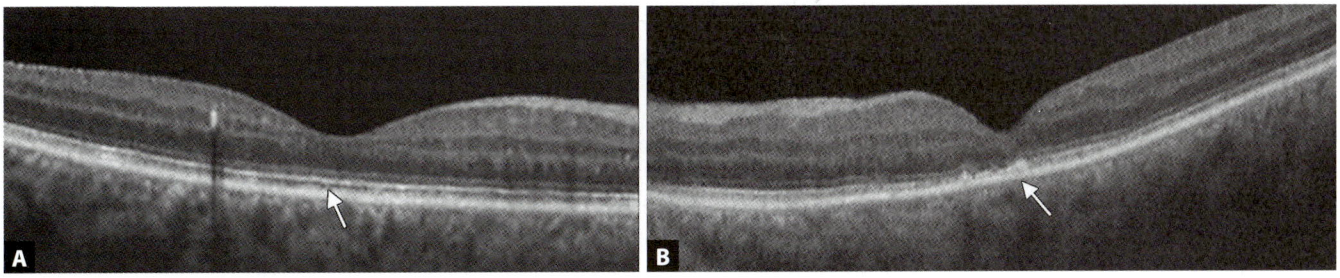

Figs 7A and B: OCT scans of the right eye (A) showing resolution of hyperreflective dots and subretinal fluid. The normal foveal contour was restored. The normal reflectivity of inner and outer retinal layers (arrow) were also seen at 6 weeks. The macular scan in the left eye (B) showed resolution of retinal hyperreflectivity but distortion of the subfoveal ellipsoid zone remained (arrow).
Source: Uveitis Webinar - Grand Round 11. International Uveitis Study Group (IUSG). 2025. https://youtu.be/CliZo0xOKpQ.

of infectious diseases, including rickettsial and other bacterial infections, such as typhoid. In addition, various viral infections could be the underlying etiology, including dengue, West Nile, chikungunya, Zika, or SARS-CoV-2.[15] The post-fever retinitis phenotype could also be secondary to protozoal infections. The exact pathophysiology is unknown but has been speculated to be either a direct infection of the retina by an organism or secondary to an immune-mediated response. The latter is more likely as the ocular symptoms often occur several weeks after the subsidence of the febrile illness. A good clinical response to corticosteroids also suggests an underlying immune-mediated response mechanism.[16] The presentation is commonly bilateral, symmetric, and occurs in immunocompetent patients. There could be evidence of occlusive vasculitis on fundoscopic examination, which may lead to the appearance of intraretinal hemorrhages with venous occlusions and cotton wool spots. Other rare complications from retinal vasculitis include exudative detachments and neovascularization due to elevated vascular endothelial growth factor (VEGF) levels. Treatment with anti-VEGF intravitreal injections helps reduce macular edema and dampen the VEGF surge during the disease course. A stellate maculopathy can also be present due to optic nerve edema or neuroretinitis.[17] Any optic nerve involvement requires a more aggressive and prompt treatment.

On multimodal imaging, OCT shows involvement limited to the inner retinal layers, leading to the appearance of hyperreflective dots, intraretinal fluid, or subretinal fluid. A clue to differentiate these findings from viral etiologies is the lack of full retinal involvement by the inflammation.[18] Using OCT angiography, areas with active retinitis lesions will show flow voids in the superficial and deep capillary plexi, which correspond to the small areas of venous blockages.[19] On fluorescein angiography, occlusive vasculitis with secondary vascular dropout and choroidal ischemia can be seen.

The key points for diagnosis are that rickettsial infections are common in many geographic areas, and only 1% of the patients present with systemic symptoms, such as joint pain with rashes. Therefore, with only ocular manifestations, a high index of suspicion is needed to include rickettsiae into the differential diagnosis, especially in non-endemic areas. The Weil–Felix test, although it is a non-specific agglutination test with a low sensitivity and specificity, is affordable and can assist in making a diagnosis.[20]

Management considerations should include oral corticosteroids to hasten the recovery. Post-fever retinitis is non-necrotizing and follows a febrile illness with some cases requiring observation alone until resolution. However, any optic nerve involvement necessitates treatment with oral corticosteroids. All cases require further investigation into the underlying etiology and treatment with antiviral, antibiotic, or antihelminthic medications. The medical literature advocates for treatment with doxycycline to lessen macular ischemia and improve visual recovery. Detection of neovascularization on fundoscopic examination or on multimodal imaging requires use of anti-VEGF injections. Treatment includes a-2–3-week course of doxycycline, or alternatively a fluoroquinolone or azithromycin, along with tapering doses of an oral corticosteroid, which can be commenced 4–5 days after the start of antibiotic therapy.

MUMPS RETINITIS

Case Presentation

Personal Data

A 35-year-old female presented with 4 days of redness, pain, and blurred vision in the right eye.

History of Present Illness

There was a history of fever and swelling around her neck 2 weeks prior.

Physical Examination

Both pupils were mid-dilated and sluggishly reactive. There was anisocoria more in the right eye than the left eye without light near dissociation. Corneal sensation was normal in both eyes, but pigment, corneal edema, and Descemet folds were present in the right eye **(Fig. 8)**. Gonioscopy in the right eye revealed occludable angles. In the left eye, there was a positional closure which opened on compression **(Table 3)**.

Ancillary Testing

Visual field testing and an MRI of the brain and optic nerves were normal.

Uveitis Work-up

Ancillary blood investigations were negative for HIV and syphilis, but she had raised serum mumps IgM and IgG levels.

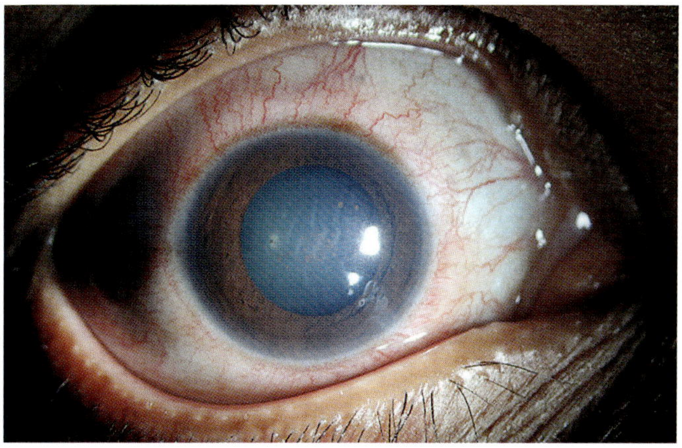

Fig. 8: Slit lamp photography of the right eye showing Descemet folds, endothelial pigment, ciliary flush, and a mid-dilated pupil. The anterior chamber was peripherally narrow and graded as van Herrick 2 (VH-2).
Source: Uveitis Webinar - Grand Round 11. International Uveitis Study Group (IUSG). 2025. https://youtu.be/CIiZo0xOKpQ.

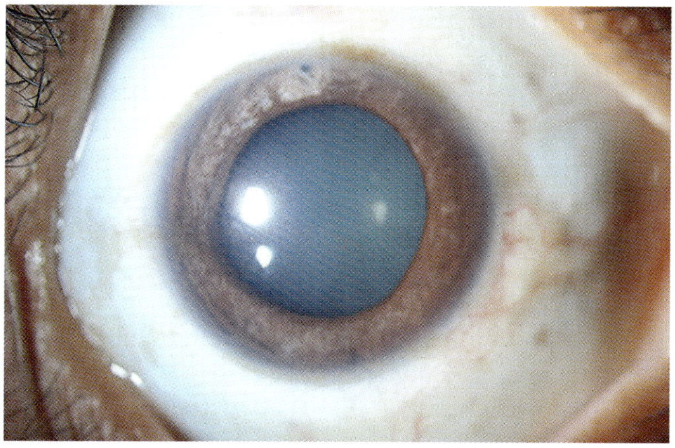

Fig. 9: Anterior segment photo showing iris atrophy in the right eye along with a patent laser peripheral iridotomy superiorly.
Source: Uveitis Webinar - Grand Round 11. International Uveitis Study Group (IUSG). 2025. https://youtu.be/CIiZo0xOKpQ.

TABLE 3: Physical examination of the patient having mumps anterior uveitis.

OD	*Parameter*	*OS*
6/9	BCVA	6/6
24 mm Hg	IOP	16 mm Hg
Ciliary flush	Conjunctiva	White and quiet
Fine keratic precipitates, pigment, and Descemet folds	Cornea	Clear
1+ cell and 1+ flare	Anterior chamber	No cells ACC: 0+
No synechiae	Iris	No synechiae
Clear	Lens	Clear
Unremarkable	Vitreous	Unremarkable
Normal	Fundus	Normal

(ACC: anterior chamber cellularity; BCVA: best-corrected visual acuity, IOP: intraocular pressure; OD: right eye; OS: left eye)

Anatomic Diagnosis

Considering the clinical history and findings, a diagnosis of acute anterior uveitis in the right eye secondary to the mumps virus was made along with suspected primary angle closure.

Initial Treatment

She was started on a topical corticosteroid four times a day and a topical anti-glaucoma medication twice a day in the right eye. She subsequently underwent a laser peripheral iridotomy (LPI) in both eyes, after which topical cycloplegics were added.

Clinical Course

Three weeks post-treatment, visual acuity improved to 6/6 in both eyes. Intraocular pressures were controlled, and pigment remained on the corneal endothelium of the right eye. The Descemet folds had resolved, but the pupils remained sluggishly reactive with anisocoria in the right eye. The right iris showed atrophy, and the LPI was patent in both eyes **(Fig. 9)**. Gonioscopy showed persistent appositional closure with peripheral anterior synechiae in the temporal quadrant. In the left eye, there was appositional closure but opening on compression.

Final Follow-up

Three months later, she maintained 6/6 visual acuity in both eyes with controlled intraocular pressures.

Discussion

The mumps virus is RNA virus of Paramyxovirus family with humans as the natural host. Transmission of the virus occurs via respiratory droplets. Patients can have a history of fever and parotitis or salivary gland swelling for several weeks prior to the ocular presentation. Central nervous system (CNS) manifestations, such as aseptic meningitis, encephalitis, and rarely, sensorineural hearing loss may occur. The reproductive tract can also be affected with orchitis or oophoritis. Other manifestations can include myocarditis, pancreatitis, or nephritis. Ophthalmically, mumps can affect both the anterior and posterior segments of the eye.[21] Anterior involvement is characterized by anterior uveitis or keratouveitis, corneal endotheliitis, conjunctivitis, or dacryodenitis.[22-26] Posterior segment manifestations include APMPPE, retinitis, neuroretinitis, or optic neuritis.[27-31] Administration of the measles, mumps, and rubella (MMR) vaccine has been associated with developing acute, idiopathic blind spot enlargement and non-granulomatous anterior uveitis. Publications regarding mumps retinitis show all cases have occurred in the pediatric age group **(Table 4)**.

The presentation includes a sudden, painless decrease in vision in children who have not received vaccination for mumps. Vision on presentation is generally poor; either light perception or hand motions. Fundus examination findings have been described as a cerebriform pattern of retinitis. A case report of frosted branch angiitis has also been reported. On OCT, there is predominantly outer retinal involvement. Serological investigations require ruling out other infections, such as syphilis and HIV, and the diagnosis is made with positive serum mumps IgM and IgG antibodies. When we look at necrotizing retinitis, treatment empirically with antivirals is encouraged until

TABLE 4: Mumps retinitis publications showing a pediatric age of onset.

	Trehan et al.	*Sayadi et al.*	*Kahloun et al.*	*Babu et al.*	*Sriram et al. (Our Case)*
Age/Gender	An 8-year-old male	A 4-year-old male	A 12-year-old male	A 9-year-old female	An 8-year-old male
Presentation	Bilateral, sudden, painless vision loss for 3 days	Bilateral, sudden, painless vision loss for 2 days	Bilateral, sudden, painless vision loss for 5 days	Bilateral, sudden, painless vision loss for 4 days	Bilateral, sudden, painless vision loss for 3 days
Vaccination status	Not known	Not vaccinated against mumps	Not vaccinated against mumps	Not known	Up-to-date
Visual acuity	OD-CF 1 m; OS-CF 0.5 m	Light perception OU	Hand motions OU	Light perception OU	Hand motions OU
Fundus examination	Bilateral cerebriform retinitis	Frosted branch angiitis with disc hyperemia OU	Bilateral cerebriform retinitis	Bilateral retinal necrosis	Bilateral cerebriform retinitis
OCT at presentation	Outer retinitis	Disruption of the ellipsoid zone and external limiting membrane OU, outer nuclear layer loss in OS	Disorganized outer retinal layers OU	Hyperreflectivity of outer retinal layers OU	Disorganized outer retinal layers OU
Investigation	• Serology for HIV was negative • AC tap was negative for HSV, VZV, and mumps • Serology was positive for mumps IgG	• AC tap was negative for HSV, VZV, and mumps • Serology was positive for mumps IgM and IgG	Serology for syphilis, EBV, Parvovirus B19 was negative. Serology was positive for mumps IgM and IgG	• AC tap was negative for HSV, VZV, CMV, rubella, TB, and toxoplasmosis. • Serology was positive for mumps IgG	Serology for syphilis and HIV was negative. Serology was positive for mumps IgM and IgG
Treatment	IV acyclovir 200 mg every 8 hours followed by oral prednisone 20 mg/day	IV acyclovir 200 mg every 8 hours, IV methylprednisolone followed by oral corticosteroids and hyperbaric oxygen	IV acyclovir 10 mg/kg for 3 days followed by oral prednisone	IV acyclovir 315 mg every 8 hours with transition to oral corticosteroids and oral acyclovir	Oral acyclovir 400 mg with IV methylprednisolone, with transition to oral corticosteroids and hyperbaric oxygen

(AC: anterior chamber; CMV: cytomegalovirus; EBV: Epstein Barr virus; HIV: human immunodeficiency virus; HSV: herpes simplex virus; IV: intravenous; IgM: immunoglobulin M; OD: right eye; OS: left eye; OU: both eyes; TB: tuberculosis; VZV: varicella zoster virus)

Source: Uveitis Webinar - Grand Round 11. International Uveitis Study Group (IUSG). 2025. https://youtu.be/CIiZo0xOKpQ.

serologic testing results are available. Management then shifts to intravenous, followed by oral corticosteroids. While more commonly used for other systemic medical conditions, two reports in the literature support the use of hyperbaric oxygen therapy.[32-35] No specific antiviral therapy is available for Mumps or other single-stranded RNA viruses. Symptomatic and supportive treatments include analgesics for parotitis and arthritis. Alternatively, intravenous immunoglobulins or intravenous interferon-α can be administered for CNS manifestations. Prevention with the live, attenuated mumps vaccine administered in combination as the MMR vaccine is recommended, with the first dose usually given at 12–15 months of age. The second dose can be given anytime between 13 months to 13 years. A booster dose is required if the first dose is given at less than 1 year of age.

In summary, it is important to rule out other causes of necrotizing retinitis. Mumps can form patchy iris atrophy similar to other causes of viral anterior uveitis. An anterior chamber tap to test aqueous fluid for mumps PCR can also be done to improve diagnostic certainty. As opposed to herpetic viral anterior uveitis cases, mumps-associated anterior uveitis will not remain hypertensive after corticosteroid treatment.

PEARLS FROM THE EXPERTS ON FREQUENTLY ASKED QUESTIONS

1. What is the role of intravitreal corticosteroids in viral retinitis or infectious uveitis?

Answer: The decision to give intravitreal corticosteroid implants should be made with extreme caution, as there are no antivirals for single-stranded RNA viruses. Difluprednate eyedrops or oral corticosteroids can be given until the inflammation is resolved, which in most cases, is within 8–10 weeks. Additionally, when administered as eye drops or orally, the corticosteroid dose can easily be adjusted or discontinued if the disease worsens. Any route of corticosteroid administration in the setting of an infectious disease should only be given under the continued cover of an antiviral or antibiotic medication specific to the underlying infection.

2. What is the role of vaccination after the resolution of ocular inflammation due to an RNA virus?

Answer: Vaccination is designed to prevent or lead to a milder disease presentation. After the development of the disease, vaccination is not therapeutic. The adaptive immune response of antibody formation occurs due to exposure to the virus, leading to post-infection immunity similar to the response generated by vaccines. Vaccination after infection may carry the risk of worsening the ocular inflammation and it is not advised.

3. Has there been an increase in ARN recurrences after SARS-CoV-2 infections?

Answer: Acute retinal necrosis following SARS-CoV-2 infection has increased with posterior pole involvement, more occlusions, and peripheral retinal hemorrhages on a regional basis. This differential presentation may result from variable expression of the virus and the host immune response from both genetic and post-vaccination standpoints. An interplay between the host and viral phenotypes plays a role in any disease presentation and aggressiveness.

FINAL WRAP-UP

RNA viruses can cause a wide range of ocular inflammatory conditions, and without specific antiviral medications to treat each virus, vaccination is the key to prevention. Once ocular inflammation is diagnosed, serologic testing and early targeted therapies are needed to prevent vision loss. Multidisciplinary management helps decrease both morbidity and mortality with systemic involvement.

REFERENCES

1. Neri P, Piriani V, Gresti G, Arapi I. "Measles." Intraocular Inflammation. Springer Nature: London; 2016. pp. 1203-7.
2. Xie Cen A, Ng AWW, Rojas-Carabali W, Cifuentes-González C, de-la-Torre A, Mahendradas P, et al. Dengue Uveitis - A Major Review. Ocul Immunol Inflamm. 2023;31(7):1440-53.
3. Lee JH, Agarwal A, Mahendradas P, Lee CS, Gupta V, Pavesio CE, et al. Viral posterior uveitis. Surv Ophthalmol. 2017;62(4):404-45.
4. Yeo TH, Yeo TK, Wong EP, Agrawal R, Teoh SC. Immune recovery uveitis in HIV patients with cytomegalovirus retinitis in the era of HAART therapy-a 5-year study from Singapore. J Ophthalmic Inflamm Infect. 2016;6(1):41.
5. Pepose JS, Newman C, Bach MC, Quinn TC, Ambinder RF, Holland GN, et al. Pathologic features of cytomegalovirus retinopathy after treatment with the antiviral agent ganciclovir. Ophthalmology. 1987;94:414-24.
6. Manangeeswaran M, Kielczewski JL, Sen HN, Xu BC, Ireland DDC, McWilliams IL, et al. ZIKA virus infection causes persistent chorioretinal lesions. Emerg Microbes Infect. 2018;7(1):96.

7. Pleyer U, Alio JL, Barisani-Asenbauer T, LeHoang P, Rao NA (Eds). Immune Modulation and Anti-Inflammatory Therapy in Ocular Disorders: IOIS Guidelines. Springer Nature; 2014.
8. Kridin M, Zloto O, Kridin K, Cohen AD, Mann O, Weinstein O. The association of uveitis with hepatitis B and hepatitis C viruses: a large-scale population-based study. Eye (Lond). 2023;37(4):720-4.
9. Li A, Grant D, Gbakie M, Kanneh L, Mustafa I, Bond N, et al. Ophthalmic manifestations and vision impairment in Lassa fever survivors. PLoS ONE. 2020;15(12):e0243766.
10. Varkey JB, Shantha JG, Crozier I, Kraft CS, Lyon GM, Mehta AK, et al. Persistence of Ebola Virus in Ocular Fluid during Convalescence. N Engl J Med. 2015;372(25):2423-7.
11. Chancellor JR, Padmanabhan SP, Greenough TC, Sacra R, Ellison RT 3rd, Madoff LC, et al. Uveitis and Systemic Inflammatory Markers in Convalescent Phase of Ebola Virus Disease. Emerg Infect Dis. 2016;22(2):295-7.
12. Kuming BS, Kokoris N. Uveal involvement in Marburg virus disease. Br J Ophthalmol. 1977;61(4):265-6.
13. Agarwal A, Kumar A, Khairallah M, Abboud E. Rift valley fever uveitis. In: Gupta V, Nguyen Q, LeHoang P, Herbort Jr C (Eds). The Uveitis Atlas. New Delhi: Springer; 2018.
14. Pichi F, Aljinebi A, Neri P, Hay S, Dackiw C, Ghazi NG. Association of ocular adverse events with inactivated COVID-19 vaccination in patients in Abu Dhabi. JAMA Ophthalmol. 2021;139(10):1131-5.
15. Mahendradas P, Kawali A, Luthra S, Srinivasan S, Curi AL, Maheswari S, et al. Post-fever retinitis - Newer concepts. Indian J Ophthalmol. 2020;68(9):1775-86.
16. Kawali A, Mahendradas P, Srinivasan P, Yadav NK, Avadhani K, Gupta K, et al. Rickettsial retinitis—an Indian perspective. J Ophthal Inflamm Infect. 2015;5:37.
17. Kawali A, Mahendradas P, Mohan A, Mallavarapu M, Shetty B. Epidemic Retinitis. Ocul Immunol Inflamm. 2019;27(4):571-7.
18. Sundar D, Chawla R, Balaji A, Garg I, Kalathil R, Hasan N, et. al. Clinical features, optical coherence tomography findings and treatment outcomes of post-fever retinitis. Ther Adv Ophthalmol. 2020;12:2515841420979111.
19. Baharani A, Reddy RRP. Treatment Outcomes of Presumed Rickettsial Retinitis: Evidence from OCTA Based Quantitative Analysis. Ocul Immunol Inflamm. 2024;32(7):1197-204.
20. Ajantha GS, Patil SS, Chitharagi VB, Kulkarni RD. Rickettsiosis: a cause of acute febrile illness and value of Weil-Felix test. Indian J Public Health. 2013;57:182-3.
21. Riffenburgh RS. Ocular manifestations of mumps. Arch Ophthalmol. 1961;66(5):739-43.
22. Meyer RF, Sullivan JH, Oh JO. Mumps conjunctivitis. Am J Ophthalmol. 1974;78(6):1022-4.
23. Fields J. Ocular manifestations of mumps: a case of mumps keratitis. Am J Ophthalmol. 1947;30(5):591-5.
24. Khubchandani R, Rane T, Agarwal P, Nabi F, Patel P, Shetty AK. Bilateral neuroretinitis associated with mumps. Arch Neurol. 2002;59(10):1633-6.
25. Ando K, Ishihara M, Kusumoto Y, Shibuya E, Nakamura S, Mizuki N. A case of corneal endotheliitis with mumps virus RNA in aqueous humor detected by rt-PCR. Ocul Immunol Inflamm. 201;21(2):150-2.
26. Onal S, Toker E. A rare ocular complication of mumps: kerato-uveitis. Ocul Immunol Inflamm. 2005;13(5):395-7.
27. Trehan HS, Sheth SS, Mathai A, Reddy RK, Moorthy RS. Diagnostic and therapeutic challenge. Retina. 2010;30(1):180-3.
28. Babu K, De C, Sampangi R. Bilateral outer retinal necrosis following mumps infection. Ocul Immunol Inflamm. 2018;26(1):130-2.
29. Kahloun R, Ben Amor H, Ksiaa I, Zina S, Jelliti B, Ben Yahia S, et al. Multimodal imaging in a case of bilateral outer retinitis associated with mumps infection. Int Ophthalmol. 2018;38:339-43.
30. Borruat FX, Piguet B, Herbort CP. Acute posterior multifocal placoid pigment epitheliopathy following mumps. Ocul Immunol Inflamm. 1998;6(3):189-93.
31. Sriram R, Sethu S, Ghosh A, Shetty R, Rizvi S, Dave N, et al. Vision Crisis-Bilateral Outer Retinitis Due to Mumps Virus. Ocul Immunol Inflamm. 2025;33(7):1436-43.
32. Sayadi J, Ksiaa I, Malek I, Ben Sassi R, Essaddam L, Khairallah M, et al. Hyperbaric oxygen therapy for mumps-associated outer retinitis with frosted branch angiitis. Ocul Immunol Inflamm. 2022;30(4):1001-4.
33. Oguz H, Sobaci G. The use of hyperbaric oxygen therapy in ophthalmology. Surv Ophthalmol. 2008;53(2):112-20.
34. Shroff D, Kothari A, Gupta P, Sahni TK, Narain S. Hyperbaric Oxygen Therapy Combined with Immunosuppression for Acute Macular Neuroretinopathy in Systemic Lupus Erythematosus. Ocul Immunol Inflamm. 2023;31(2):355-61.
35. Celebi AR. Hyperbaric oxygen therapy for central retinal artery occlusion: patient selection and perspectives. Clin Ophthalmol. 2021;15:3443-57.

CHAPTER 12

Ocular Complications of HIV and AIDS

Derrick Smit, Israel Mendez, Jennifer Thorne, Maria Carolina Kuba, Andre Luiz Land Curi, Linda Visser, Sara Prischak, Vishali Gupta, Reema Bansal, John H Kempen, Alejandra de-la-Torre, Meghan Berkenstock

INTRODUCTION

Ocular complications of the human immunodeficiency virus (HIV) and acquired immunodeficiency syndrome (AIDS) are less common in the era of combined antiretroviral treatment (cART), but new cases still occur worldwide. The immunocompromised host can develop multiple simultaneous infections or a singular AIDS defining illness. The lessons learned from the HIV and AIDS epidemic can be generalized to treat the ocular complications in other types of immunodeficient states, including iatrogenic immunosuppression for organ transplantation and in the treatment of rheumatic diseases.

THEMATIC LECTURE: OCULAR COMPLICATIONS OF HIV INFECTION IN SOUTH AFRICA: MULTIPLE FACES

Introduction

HIV is a viral infection that affects nearly 39.9 million people worldwide. In South Africa, there are nearly 8 million people living with HIV, of whom 77% are receiving cART and 71% have suppressed viral loads.[1] According to the United Nations AIDS figures from 2023, more than half of the 40 million cases worldwide occur in Eastern and Southern Africa.[2] Complications of HIV span all of the ocular and adnexal structures, and we will review each of these ocular opportunistic infections by location.

Orbital complications can include preseptal and orbital cellulitis, orbital lymphoma, and keratinocyte carcinomas. Preseptal and orbital cellulitis is polymicrobial in 40% of cases and a quarter of cases result from hematogenous spread. Risk factors include a low CD4+ count or neutropenia. Treatment requires the use of antibiotics and neuroimaging with a CT or MRI in cases concerning for orbital extension. Orbital cellulitis increases the risk of the development of panophthalmitis and requires a systemic examination and laboratory testing for the source. In acutely ill patients or those non-responsive to therapy, antibiotic resistance or fungal infection should be considered, including mucormycosis and aspergillosis. The presence of an orbital or subperiosteal abscess requires surgical drainage. Orbital lymphoma is a rare complication occurring in <1% of patients with HIV with extranodal or marginal B cell lymphoma as the most common subtypes. Lesions are salmon colored and progress slowly. Early detection via neuroimaging and tissue biopsy can confirm the diagnosis and warrant prompt referral to oncology for management. Keratinocyte carcinomas are uncommon in dark skinned individuals, but squamous cell carcinoma can develop from squamous ocular surface neoplasia in patients with HIV infection. Also commonly seen is basal cell carcinoma, which can be difficult to treat. Prior publications have shown that a basal cell carcinoma lesion in the medial canthus can be treated with intralesional bleomycin injections, leading to clinical resolution.[3]

Eyelid complications include herpes zoster ophthalmicus (HZO), molluscum contagiosum, and Kaposi sarcoma. Patients with HIV have a 15–25 times greater chance of developing HZO, and the presentation of the condition in those under 50 years old has been a reason to screen for the disease. The presence of Hutchinson's sign **(Fig. 1)** has a high positive predictive value for intraocular involvement and requires a referral to ophthalmology for a thorough examination. Treatment involves intravenous acyclovir for induction with a transition to oral acyclovir, famciclovir, or valacyclovir. There is a decreased risk

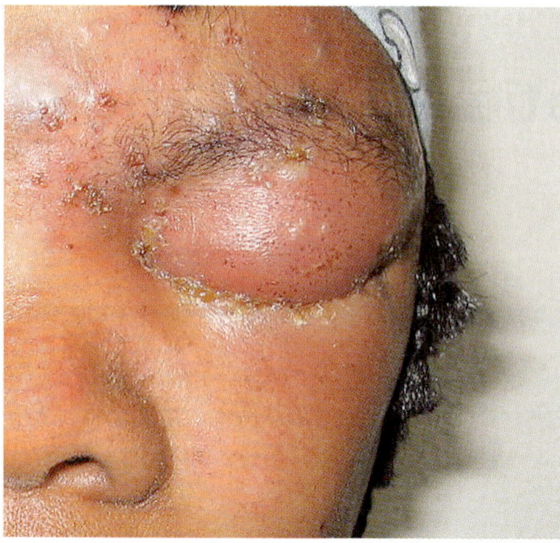

Fig. 1: The presence of vesicles on the distal nose (Hutchinson's sign) is associated with and increased risk of intraocular inflammation in cases of herpes zoster ophthalmicus.
Source: Uveitis Webinar - Grand Round 12. International Uveitis Study Group (IUSG). 2025. https://youtu.be/1P4dx4lHwUc.[4]

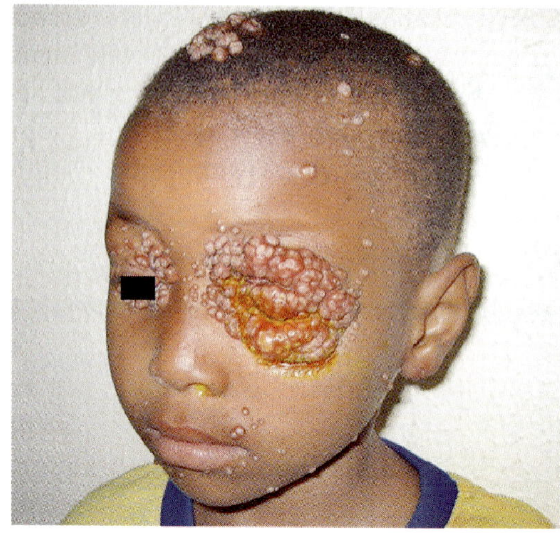

Fig. 2: Multifocal, large molluscum contagiosum lesions predominately affect the face in patients with human immunodeficiency virus (HIV) infection.
Source: Uveitis Webinar - Grand Round 12. International Uveitis Study Group (IUSG). 2025. https://youtu.be/1P4dx4lHwUc.[4]

of post-herpetic neuralgia if antivirals are started within 72 hours of vesicular eruption. Common sequelae of the disease include corneal scarring, exposure keratopathy, trichiasis, ptosis, and cicatricial ectropion. Sporotrichosis should be included in the differential diagnosis of HZO as it may present similarly; however, it will not respect the anatomic midline. Treatment also differs, as long-term use of antifungals is required. Another condition in the differential diagnosis is molluscum contagiosum, which belongs to the Poxviridae family. The presentation in patients with HIV differs due to the numerous, disseminated lesions that are 10 mm or larger and multifocal **(Fig. 2)**. The lesions are more commonly found on the face. Medical treatments include topical salicylic acid or tretinoin; whereas curettage, electrodessication or cryotherapy are surgical options. Finally, Kaposi sarcoma is due to human herpes virus 8 (HHV-8) and presents as painless, violaceous, or brown eyelid nodules. If present on the conjunctiva, these lesions can appear as reddish-blue, and have a nodular or diffuse bulbar appearance. Treatment includes radiotherapy and cART, as this combination has been shown to be as effective as cART plus chemotherapy. Alternatively, intralesional bleomycin has shown efficacy in localized tumors.[3]

Conjunctival complications include ocular surface squamous neoplasia (OSSN), which more commonly affects Caucasian men in their seventh and eighth decades in the West. However, in Africa, young patients are at greater risk with known risk factors including ultraviolet light exposure, coinfection with the human papilloma virus, and HIV infection. OSSN is the third most common neoplasm in patients with HIV after Kaposi sarcoma and lymphoma. In a study in Zimbabwe, 92% of patients had corneal involvement with OSSN and 50% of patients with previously undiagnosed HIV or AIDS presented with a conjunctival malignancy.[5] This reinforces the need to test a younger patient presenting with a conjunctival malignancy for HIV infection. This presentation includes papilliform, gelatinous, or leukoplakic lesions. In addition to no touch excision with double freeze-thaw cryotherapy to the surgical margins, medical treatment includes topical or subconjunctival interferon A2b, 5-fluorouracil, mitomycin-C, antivascular endothelial growth factor (anti-VEGF), or bleomycin.

Scleral involvement can include the development of cryptococcal nodular scleritis with immune reconstitution syndrome (IRIS). Our group has published a case of a 32-year-old female who presented with granulomatous panuveitis of the right eye with dense vitritis precluding a view to the fundus. She was initially started on cART with a CD4+ count nadir of 84 cells/mL. All laboratories were initially negative, and her CD4+ count rose to 325, which is when a scleral nodule was noted on slit lamp examination. The biopsy was positive for *Cryptococcus neoformans*, and the patient was subsequently treated with oral fluconazole with rapid improvement.[6]

Corneal complications can be subdivided into infectious (viral, bacteria, fungal, or protozoal) and non-infectious categories [peripheral ulcerative keratitis (PUK), keratoconjunctivitis sicca (KCS), or neoplastic].[7] Viral involvement includes the aforementioned HZO and herpes simplex keratitis. The latter has a more severe clinical course and is often bilateral with bacterial superinfection in half of the cases. The difficulty in determining the cause of stromal necrosis in these cases reinforces the need for culturing of the ulcer with polymerase chain reaction (PCR) testing for herpes viruses. Metagenomic next-generation sequencing may play a role in future to determine the causative agents in polymicrobial infections. There is a ten-fold increased risk of bacterial keratitis in patients with HIV. Risk factors include HIV-induced KCS, blepharitis, herpetic eye disease, atopy, and more virulent flora. The most common ocular surface bacteria include *Staphylococcus epidermidis, Staphylococcus aureus, Pseudomonas aeruginosa, alpha hemolytic Streptococcus,* and *Bacillus* species. These manifestations are often severe, bilateral, and polymicrobial with resistance to treatment and a higher risk of endophthalmitis. Similar to bacterial infections, fungal keratitis is more commonly bilateral and due to filamentous fungi, including *Aspergillus* and *Fusarium* species **(Fig. 3)**. Treatment includes 5% natamycin for filamentous fungi, and amphotericin B is preferred for yeast infections. Often a therapeutic or tectonic keratoplasty is needed. Protozoal involvement can develop as a result of acanthamoeba and microsporidial infection with the latter being more common in patients with HIV. Patients present with a chronic follicular conjunctivitis and a coarse punctate epithelial keratopathy. Diagnosis is achieved using calcofluor white or gram staining or with confocal microscopy. In a prospective study, patients treated with placebo, and those treated with polyhexamethyline biguanide showed no difference in the time to clinical resolution.

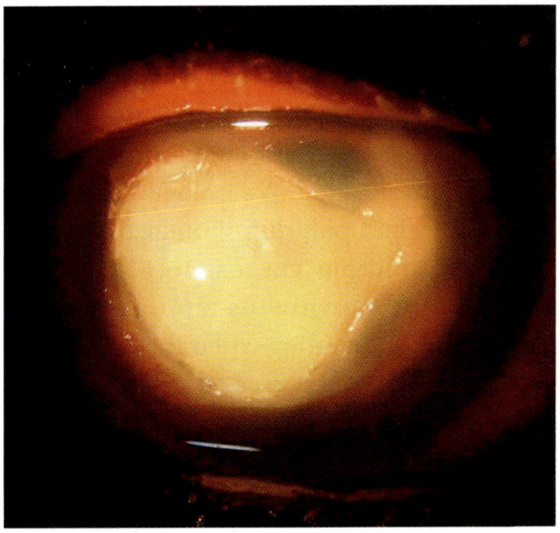

Fig. 3: A slit lamp photograph of a large central corneal ulcer with fungal stromal infiltrates.
Source: Uveitis Webinar - Grand Round 12. International Uveitis Study Group (IUSG). 2025. https://youtu.be/1P4dx4lHwUc.[4]

Switching to non-infectious corneal conditions, the pathophysiology of PUK in patients with HIV is not completely understood. Patients can present with bilateral cornea ulceration (Mooren's ulcer) after the start of cART. Diagnosis is based on ruling out infectious and autoimmune causes through corneal cultures and PCR, in addition to serologic and radiographic testing. Rapid resolution was achieved in a case report, using a taper of 0.1% dexamethasone drops and aggressive lubrication.[8] KCS affects 39% of men and 17% of women with HIV compared to 1% of the general population. Clinical presentations can range from severe, bilateral dry eyes to central sterile perforations. Treatment requires frequent use of preservative free artificial tears and ointments with escalation to punctal plugs and anti-inflammatory drops as needed.

Uveal complications include infectious [tuberculosis, syphilis, and cytomegalovirus (CMV) retinitis] as well as HIV-associated uveitis. Our understanding of the pathophysiology of HIV-associated uveitis has increased over time.[9] The HIV virus was first cultured from the eye in 1998, and later studies showed higher viral loads in the eye than in the plasma, suggesting active viral replication within ocular structures.[9] Patients with HIV-associated uveitis present with decreased vision and are typically cART naïve. On slit lamp examination, large keratic precipitates and anterior chamber cells are present without retinal lesions or other stigmata of opportunistic infections. Aqueous humor PCR testing for the HIV virus shows much higher intraocular titers than in the serum. As opposed to other forms of uveitis, the inflammation is not corticosteroid responsive.[10] Complete resolution is often seen in patients with the induction of cART.[11,12]

There have been several papers on the incidence of ocular tuberculosis (OTB) in patients with HIV. Our group in South Africa found that 33% of patients were diagnosed with OTB. Of those with OTB, 31% were HIV positive. Patients with a systemic tuberculosis infection (diagnosed in another organ) were more commonly young, male, and HIV positive.[4] The role of QuantiFERON-TB Gold (QFT-TB Gold and tuberculin skin test (TST) as diagnostic tools to assess for OTB was negative in both HIV positive and negative patients in equal amounts.[13] However, less patients with HIV tested positive with both tests. The QFT-TB Gold and TST are immunological tests that can lead to false negative results in immunocompromised population.

Other testing with diagnostic implications for uveitis in patients with HIV include PCR and the Goldmann Witmer coefficient (GWC). In patients with and without HIV infection in the same cohort from South Africa, 27 patients had a positive PCR and/or a GWC result.[14] Of those with positive results, more than half were HIV positive and had intermediate, posterior, or panuveitis. In cases of herpetic anterior uveitis, patients tested PCR negative but GWC positive, whereas patients with herpetic non-anterior uveitis, of which the vast majority were HIV positive, tested PCR positive and GWC negative. Thus, there was a clear divide between test results depending on HIV status and the anatomic location of the uveitis. In addition, rubella cases tested positive for both PCR and GWC. Therefore, one can deduce that PCR is useful for patients with herpetic, non-anterior uveitis if HIV positive, whereas the GWC is useful for patients with herpetic anterior uveitis.

Causes of uveitis in HIV positive and negative patients have also been assessed in South Africa.[15] Of the cohort of 106 patients, 37.7% were HIV positive. Infectious uveitis was diagnosed in 80% of HIV positive patients compared to 66% overall. The most common infections were tuberculosis, herpes viruses, and syphilis. The remaining cases were non-infectious (17%), which included sarcoidosis and human leukocyte antigen (HLA)-B27, and 17% were idiopathic. Anterior uveitis in those with HIV infection was idiopathic or most often caused by tuberculosis or syphilis. Similarly, panuveitis in the same population was most commonly caused by syphilis, tuberculosis, toxoplasmosis, and herpes zoster retinitis.

Focusing on ocular syphilis, we found that of the 146 patients studied, 52.1% were coinfected with HIV and 23.7% were newly diagnosed with HIV.[16] Forty percent of HIV positive patients had a presenting vision of <20/200 and with posterior or panuveitis. Ocular manifestations were bilateral in 47.3%, and of these, 68% were HIV positive. There was a stronger association between the codevelopment of neurosyphilis in HIV positive patients. Bear in mind that patients may have multiple ocular infections depending on the level of the immunosuppression.[17]

TABLE 1: Slit lamp examination of the patient having ocular complications of HIV infection in South Africa.

OD	Parameter	OS
0.1	BCVA	CF at 2 m
No injection	Conjunctiva	No injection
Pigmented KP	Cornea	Pigmented KP
2+ cells	AC	3+ cells
Reactive and round	Pupil	Reactive and round
Clear	Lens	Clear
1+ haze	Vitreous	2+ haze
11	IOP	13
Retinitis involving the posterior pole with scattered retinal hemorrhages	Fundus	Retinitis involving the posterior pole with scattered retinal hemorrhages

(AC: anterior chamber; BCVA: best-corrected visual acuity; CF: counting fingers; IOP: intraocular pressure; KP: keratic precipitates; OD: right eye; OS: left eye)

The following two cases illustrate the concepts mentioned above. The first case was of a 35-year-old male with a 2-week history of painless vision loss in the left more than the right eye. He had no past ocular history and had been on cART for 3 years with a chronically low CD4+ count of 24 cells per cubic millimeter. Slit lamp examination for ocular complications of HIV infection in South Africa is shown in **Table 1**.

An initial diagnosis of bilateral viral retinitis due to presumed CMV was made given his HIV status. A vitreous tap and intravitreal injection of ganciclovir in the left eye was performed. A serologic work-up showed a reactive treponema pallidum hemagglutination assay (TPHA) with a rapid plasma reagin (RPR) titer of 1:32. A gram stain from the vitreous tap was negative. Viral PCR testing was still pending when the lumbar puncture showed elevated lymphocytes and a positive fluorescent treponemal antibody-absorption (FTA-ABS). No bacteria were identified on a gram stain from the CSF and the cryptococcal antigen was negative. He was started on intravenous penicillin G for a 2-week course. By days 2 and 4 post-presentation, the retinal hemorrhages showed improvement **(Figs. 4A and B)**, and there was less macular

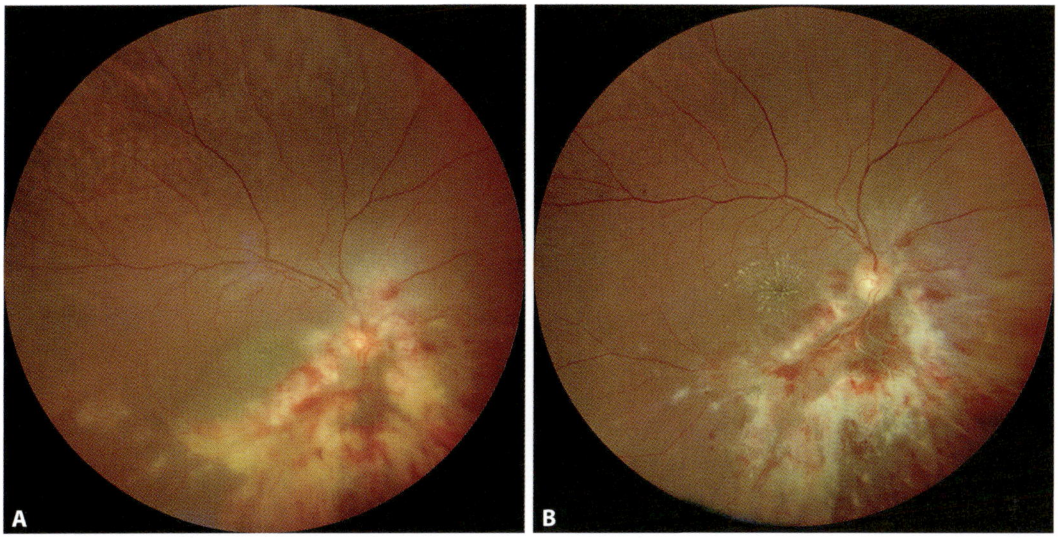

Figs. 4A and B: Color fundus photos of the right eye showing retinitis adjacent to the optic nerve with extension into the inferior arcade and the macula at clinical presentation (A) with consolidation and macular star formation 8 days later (B).
Source: Uveitis Webinar - Grand Round 12. International Uveitis Study Group (IUSG). 2025. https://youtu.be/1P4dx4IHwUc.[4]

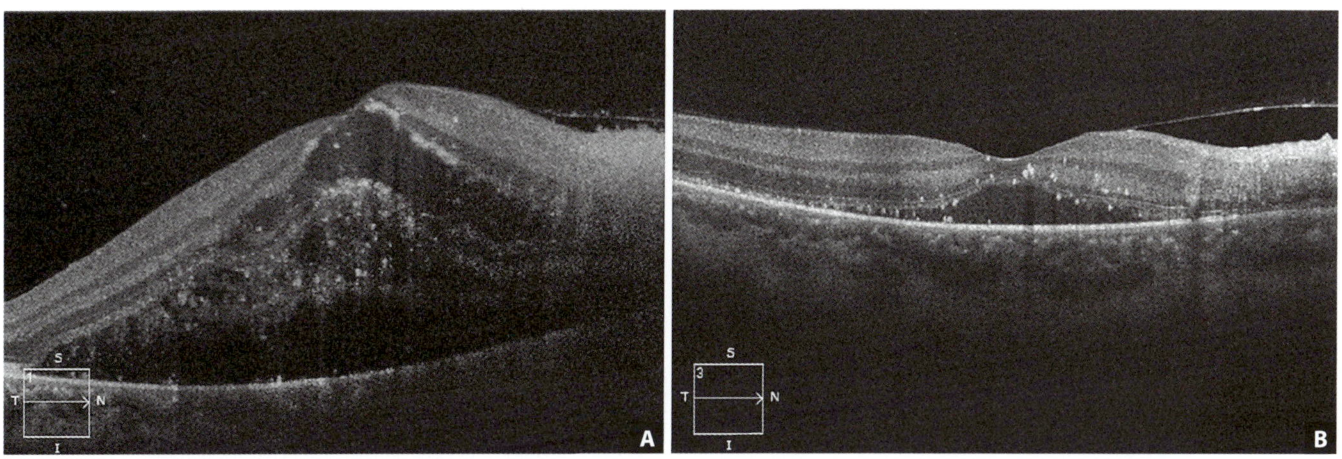

Figs. 5A and B: Optical coherence tomography (OCT) scans through the macula of the right eye showing intraretinal exudates and subretinal fluid on clinical presentation (A) that decreased by day 8 of follow-up (B).
Source: Uveitis Webinar - Grand Round 12. International Uveitis Study Group (IUSG). 2025. https://youtu.be/1P4dx4IHwUc.[4]

edema noted on OCT **(Figs. 4A and B)** with macular star formation in the right eye greater than the left **(Figs. 5A and B)**.

Case 2 is of a 29-year-old female with a 2–3-week history of pain and progressive vision loss. She was seen 4 days prior at another hospital where she was diagnosed with panuveitis presumed to be due to CMV. She underwent a vitreous tap and intravitreal injection of ganciclovir prior to referral to our hospital. She was diagnosed with HIV 5 months prior with a CD4+ count nadir of 34 cells per cubic millimeter with one episode of prior visual symptoms that were treated with eyedrops and unknown oral medications elsewhere **(Table 2)**.

Optical coherence tomography scans of the macula were within normal limits bilaterally. The results of the vitreous tap were negative for HSV subtypes 1 and 2, CMV, varicella zoster virus, and toxoplasmosis. However, a lumbar puncture was performed with a positive FTA-abs and the RPR in the serum was also positive with a titer of 1:8. She was treated with intravenous penicillin G for 14 days. On day 6, the retinal imaging showed marked improvement **(Figs. 6A and B)**.

Despite advancements in therapy, there is still an HIV disease burden in sub-Saharan Africa. Ocular complications of HIV can involve any ocular structure and can result in irreversible vision loss. It is possible that HIV infection alone can incite uveitis in patients, especially in those who are cART naïve. In your clinical assessment, it is important to consider the HIV status. If the HIV status is unknown, determine if the ophthalmic presentation warrants concomitant testing for HIV with a high suspicion in cases with multiple infections.

TABLE 2: Physical examination of the patient having HIV 5 months prior with a CD4+ count nadir of 34 cells per cubic millimeter with one episode of prior visual symptoms.

OD	*Parameter*	*OS*
0.15	BCVA	0.2
Mild injection	Conjunctiva	Normal
Endothelial dusting	Cornea	Pigmented KP
1+ cells	AC	0.5+ cells
Pharmacologically dilated	Pupil	Pharmacologically dilated
Clear	Lens	Clear
2+ haze, veils	Vitreous	2+ haze, veils
Retinal whitening	Fundus	Retinal whitening

(AC: anterior chamber; BCVA: best-corrected visual acuity; IOP: intraocular pressure; KP: keratic precipitates; OD: right eye; OS: left eye)

VIRAL EXPLOSION

Case Presentation

Personal Data

A 36-year-old female presented with a 1-month history of bilateral, painless vision loss and floaters.

History of Present Illness

The symptoms initially started in the right eye with progression to the left eye 2 weeks later. She was diagnosed with HIV 12 years prior and reported intermittent adherence to cART. She had completely stopped the medications for the 5 months prior to presentation. She also had a past medical history of diabetes mellitus with a recent hemoglobin A1c of 8.1%. On review of systems, she had oral thrush and a dry cough.

Physical Examination

The best-corrected visual acuity was 20/200 in the right eye and counting fingers in the left eye. Retinitis with hemorrhages was noted in zone 1 in both eyes. Both eyes showed multifocal hemorrhagic retinitis involving the optic nerves with macular extension in the left eye. **(Figs. 7A and B)**.

Slit Lamp Examination

Slit lamp examination is shown in **Table 3**.

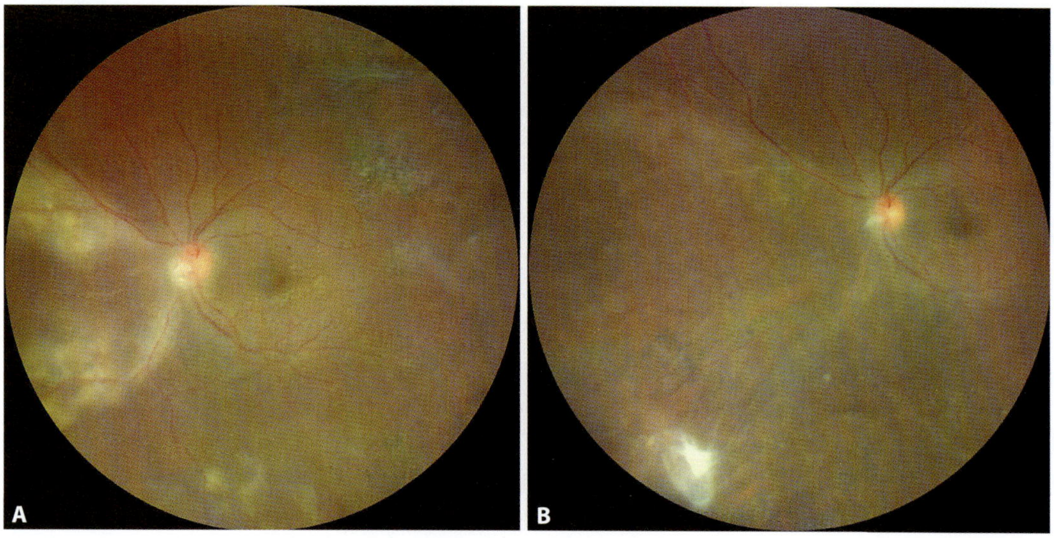

Figs. 6A and B: Color fundus photos of the left eye showing perivascular retinitis nasal to the optic nerve at clinical presentation (A) with regression 6 days after the start of intravenous penicillin G treatment (B).
Source: Uveitis Webinar - Grand Round 12. International Uveitis Study Group (IUSG). 2025. https://youtu.be/1P4dx4lHwUc.[4]

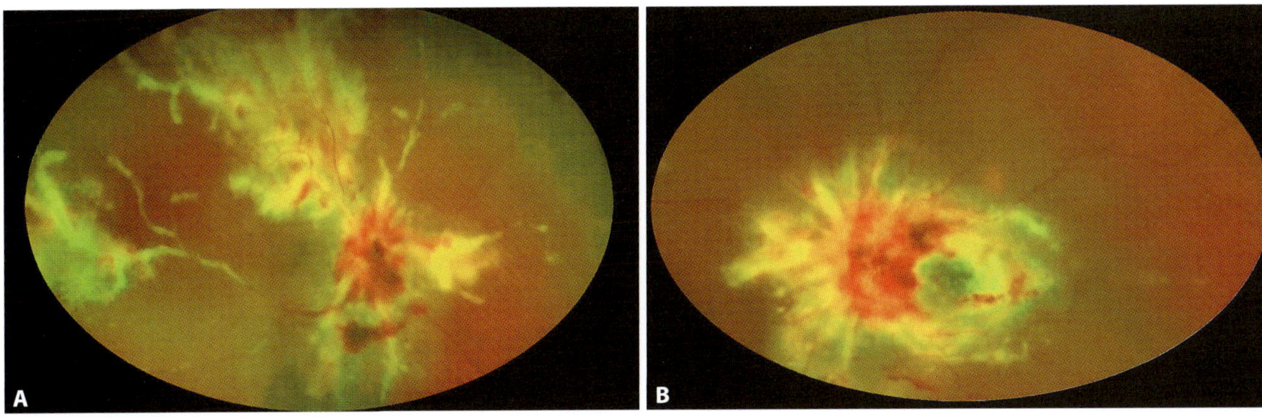

Figs. 7A and B: Color fundus photos of both eyes showing multifocal hemorrhagic retinitis involving the optic nerves with macular extension in the left eye.
Source: Uveitis Webinar - Grand Round 12. International Uveitis Study Group (IUSG). 2025. https://youtu.be/1P4dx4lHwUc.[4]

TABLE 3: Slit lamp examination of the patient having viral explosion.

OD	*Parameter*	*OS*
20/100	BCVA	CF at face
16	IOP	17
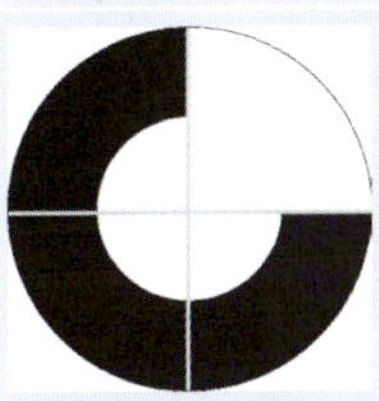	Visual field	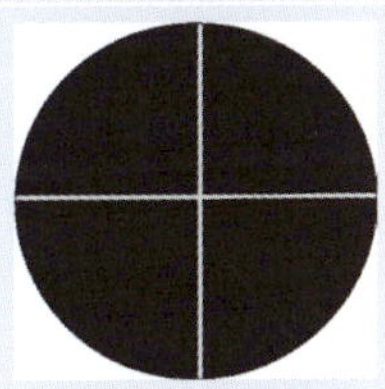
Normal	Exernal	Normal
Normal	Lids/lashes	Normal
White and quiet	Conjunctiva/sclera	White and quiet
1+ punctate epithelial erosions, pigment on the endothelium	Cornea	1+ punctate epithelial erosions, pigment on the endothelium
Normal	Iris	Normal
1+ flare, no cells	AC	1+ flare, no cells
Pigment deposits	Lens	Clear
Trace cell	Anterior vitreous	1+ cell
No view to the optic nerve due to preretinal hemorrhages, retinitis in zones 1, 2, and 3 with granular borders along vessels, perivascular sheathing	Fundus	Zone 1 retinitis with scattered mid peripheral punctate, hypopigmented lesions corresponding to smaller areas of retinitis

(AC: anterior chamber; BCVA: best-corrected visual acuity; CF: counting fingers; IOP: intraocular pressure; OD: right eye; OS: left eye)

Uveitis Work-up

The serologic work-up included a complete blood count (CBC), which showed a decreased lymphocyte count, and a CMP showed increased glucose levels. TPHA and RPR testing were negative. HIV testing was positive with a viral load of 135,000 copies per milliliter and a CD4+ count of 3 cells per cubic millimeter. An aqueous tap was performed. The PCR from the tap was negative for HSV 1 and 2 and varicella zoster viruses; however, the PCR was positive for CMV.

Initial Treatment

Given the bilateral retinitis on examination, the differential diagnosis included CMV retinitis, progressive outer retinal necrosis, bilateral acute retinal necrosis, and syphilitic retinitis. Initial treatments included bilateral intravitreal injections of foscarnet and admission to the hospital for induction with intravenous ganciclovir 5 mg/kg twice a day. A consult to the infectious disease specialists was placed due to the concern for concomitant AIDS defining illnesses, monitoring for drug-associated side effects, and to restart cART.

Follow-up

A second set of bilateral intravitreal injections of foscarnet were given 2 days after initial presentation due to zone 1 retinal involvement. Ten days after presentation, the retinitis patches had not increased in size and the peripheral, punctate lesions began to resolve **(Figs. 8A and B)**. Perivascular leakage improved on repeat fluorescein angiogram, and OCT scans showed improvement in the subretinal fluid with retinal pigment epithelium (RPE)

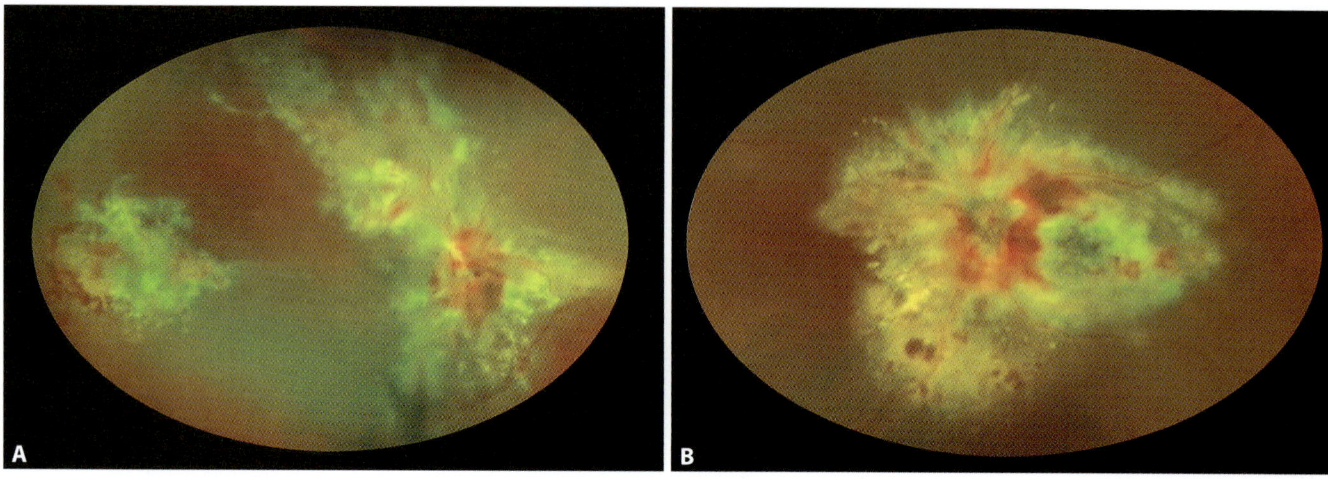

Figs. 8A and B: Color fundus photos of both eyes showing more defined, regressing areas of retinitis 10 days after presentation.
Source: Uveitis Webinar - Grand Round 12. International Uveitis Study Group (IUSG). 2025. https://youtu.be/1P4dx4lHwUc.[4]

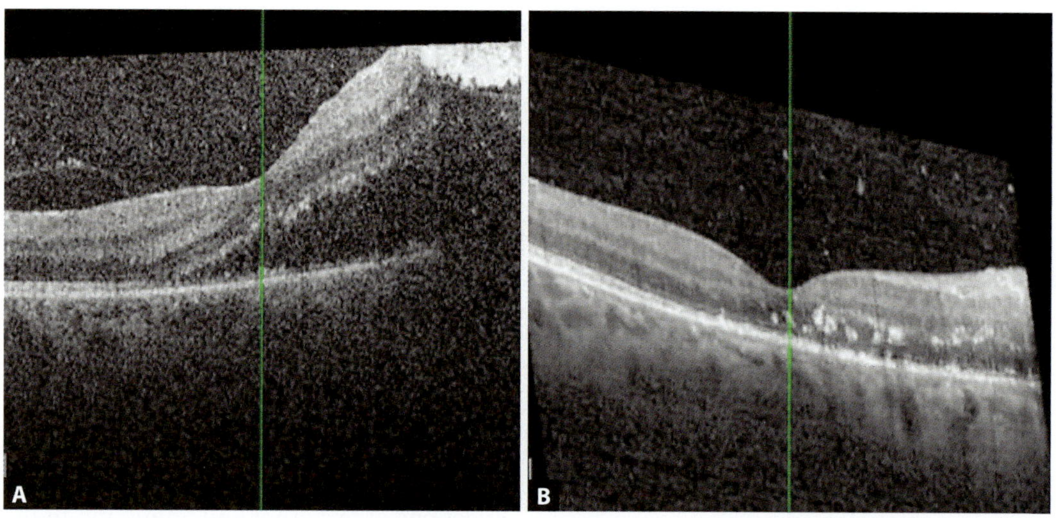

Figs. 9A and B: Optical coherence tomography (OCT) scans through the macula of the right eye showing nasal subretinal fluid at presentation (A) that resolved with residual intraretinal exudates and disruption of the ellipsoid zone in the same area 28 days later (B).
Source: Uveitis Webinar - Grand Round 12. International Uveitis Study Group (IUSG). 2025. https://youtu.be/1P4dx4lHwUc.[4]

stippling in the right eye. Due to the macular involving retinitis, the OCT scan of the left eye showed persistent hyperreflectivity and early signs of central atrophy. The patient was eventually transitioned to an oral valganciclovir maintenance dose of 450 mg twice a day. The vision in right eye continued to improve through her last follow-up at day 28 with a best-corrected vision of 20/70; however, the left eye remained with counting fingers vision. On repeat examination, the retinal lesions showed both a stable size and early pigmentation. OCT scans of the macula showed continued exudates in the right eye, resolved subretinal fluid, and disruption of the ellipsoid zone nasally **(Figs. 9A and B)**. In the left eye, there was a dense epiretinal membrane with diffuse retinal atrophy and disruption of the retinal anatomy **(Figs. 10A and B)**. The patient continued on valganciclovir maintenance dosing through immune system recovery. She was referred to a low-vision specialist given the reduced vision in both eyes. The infectious disease clinic continues to monitor her CD4+ cell count and for possible antiviral resistance over time.

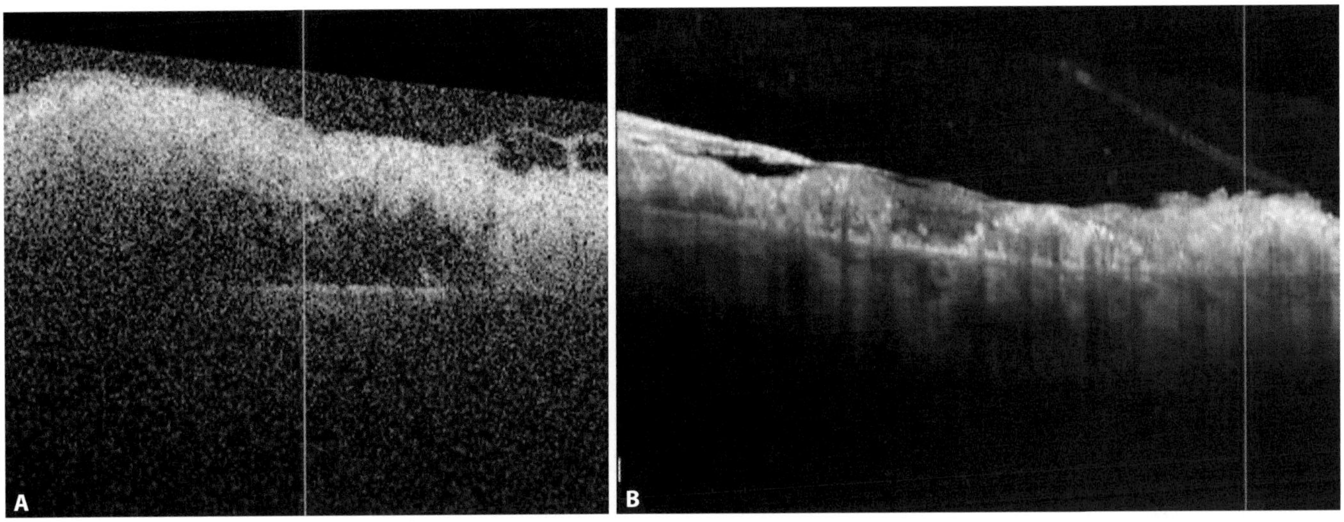

Figs. 10A and B: Optical coherence tomography (OCT) scans through the macula of the left eye showing retinal edema with loss of retinal architecture on presentation (A) and a dense epiretinal membrane with diffuse retinal atrophy and continued anatomic disruption on day 28 of follow-up (B).
Source: Uveitis Webinar - Grand Round 12. International Uveitis Study Group (IUSG). 2025. https://youtu.be/1P4dx4lHwUc.[4]

Discussion

This is a typical case that we would have seen in the early days of the HIV pandemic, and it is unfortunate that we still see this presentation. It is largely due to the struggle either to access health care or with compliance with cART due to side effects or cost. Additionally, patients may have difficulties with substance abuse, mental health disorders, and transportation issues. These socioeconomic struggles make this type of CMV retinitis with the low CD4+ counts challenging to treat.

The patient had bilateral CMV retinitis in Zone 1. To review, Zone 1 disease is within a disc diameter around the optic nerve and the macula. Zone 2 is anterior to Zone 1 out to the vortex veins. Zone 3 extends anteriorly to the ora serrata from the vortex veins. There is a large, Zone 1 lesion involving the center of the macula in the left eye, which explains the full-thickness retinal necrosis of the fovea and the uncorrectable count fingers vision. Fortunately, in the right eye, although there are larger patches of retinitis, none involve the central macula leading to partial visual recovery. In the future, the right eye will be particularly vulnerable for recurrence of the retinitis if her CD4+ count remains low. As the CD4+ count rises, the eye is also at risk to develop macular edema secondary to immune recovery uveitis. The peripheral lesion in the right eye is located in Zone 2, but may stretch to Zone 3, which increases the risk of retinal detachment.[18]

If a patient with Zone 1 disease is hospitalized, we start intravenous ganciclovir therapy with transition to oral maintenance dosing with valganciclovir. As was done in this patient, intravitreal foscarnet injections are highly recommended for Zone 1 disease due to the faster antiviral efficacy and drug delivery to the site of the infection. It can often halt the progression of the retinitis and avoid more damage to the adjacent retina. Unfortunately, the leading edges of the retinitis are already undergoing necrosis, which requires prompt treatment to salvage vision. The CD4 count of 3 cells per cubic millimeter in this patient is not uncommon at presentation. We increase our screening for CMV retinitis at CD4+ counts of ≤50 cells to every 3 months. The risk of CMV retinitis increases as the CD4+ count drops. In this case, the presentation of this patient with oral thrush is a sign of profound immunosuppression with an elevated concern for Pneumocystis jirovecii infection as the cause of the dry cough. Given the low CD4+ count on presentation, the prior history of medication non-compliance, and the macular involving or threatening retinitis lesions, this patient should be followed every 2 weeks after discharge. A low threshold for reinjection of intravitreal foscarnet in the office should be maintained if the patient returns with any evidence of worsening retinitis. Both clinically and in trials treating CMV retinitis, fundus photographs were used to monitor the lesion size and location. Ultra-wide field imaging gives a more complete view of the fundus in a single image. Side-by-side photos for comparison, as opposed to a clinical exam alone, can be helpful for management.

Antiviral resistance to ganciclovir should be considered if the medication is taken as prescribed yet new or extending areas of retinitis are noted on examination. There are a limited number of cases of foscarnet resistance. Treatment with oral valganciclovir requires laboratory monitoring of the creatinine clearance with a CMP and also a CBC to assess for neutropenia. These laboratory studies should be repeated every 3 months. If you are not comfortable monitoring for drug-associated toxicities, then working with an infectious disease specialist is recommended. Monitoring of the CD4+ count is followed in our infectious disease clinic. When it rises to above 200 cells/mm^3 for over 4 months, there are data that suggest there is reconstituted immunity against CMV, and antiviral treatment can be stopped. This should be done under close observation, as not all patients that have immune reconstitution develop CMV-specific immunity. Given the CMV virus remains dormant inside the body, the virus has the potential to reactivate off therapy.[19,20]

Lastly, a patient with a CD4+ count of three is at risk of imminent death. Prior to the availability of cART, studies showed that 20% of patients died within 2 months with profoundly low CD4+ counts.[21] These patients urgently need to be started on cART. Unlike other opportunistic infections, you should not wait and treat with anti-CMV treatment for awhile in hopes of avoiding an immune recovery inflammatory syndrome as the patient may die during that time. Coinfection with CMV and HIV leads to a symbiotic state where each is more virulent.[22]

A COMPLEX CASE

Case Presentation

Case 1

Personal data: A 36-year-old male admitted in the National Institute of Infectious Diseases presented with a headache, vomiting, nausea, and upper and lower limb paresthesias.

History of present illness: He had tested positive for HIV in 2015 and was untreated in last 2 years. He also had a history of illicit drug use. He was sent for ophthalmic examination to clarify the systemic diagnosis given bilateral blurred vision without pain.

Physical examination: The best-corrected visual acuity was 20/60 in both eyes, and the fundus examination was remarkable for bilateral, deep, yellow lesions throughout the retina.

TABLE 4: Slit lamp examination of the patient with choroiditis.

OD	*Parameter*	*OS*
20/60	BCVA	20/60
15	IOP	14
Normal	Exernal	Normal
Normal	Lids/lashes	Normal
White and quiet	Conjunctiva/sclera	White and quiet
Clear	Cornea	Clear
Normal	Iris	Normal
No cell or flare	AC	No cell or flare
Pigment deposits	Lens	Clear
Clear	Anterior vitreous	Clear
Deep yellow lesions throughout the retina	Fundus	Deep yellow lesions throughout the retina

(AC: anterior chamber; BCVA: best-corrected visual acuity; IOP: intraocular pressure; KP: keratic precipitates; OD: right eye; OS: left eye)

Slit lamp examination: Slit lamp examination is shown in **Table 4**.

Uveitis work-up: The CD4+ count was 1 cell per cubic millimeter with a viral load of 205,418 copies. Lumbar puncture was positive for *Cryptococcal* culture and India ink staining. Further testing was negative for JC virus, venereal disease research laboratory (VDRL), and GeneXpert.

Ancillary testing: Indocyanine green angiography revealed more hypocyanescent choroidal lesions than seen on fundus examination **(Fig. 11)**.

Treatment: The patient was started on intravenous amphotericin B for 10 days with slow clinical resolution of the headache and the choroidal lesions in both eyes **(Fig. 11)**. Treatment was then transitioned to fluconazole 800 mg/day for the following 30 days. Testing of CSF fluid obtained during a repeated lumbar puncture was negative for cryptococcal infection on both culture and India ink staining.

Follow-up: The patient was sent for re-evaluation after completion of antifungal medications. On examination, visual acuity was 20/30 in the right eye and 20/60 in the left eye. Fundoscopy showed optic nerve pallor in both eyes and resolution of the choroidal lesions.

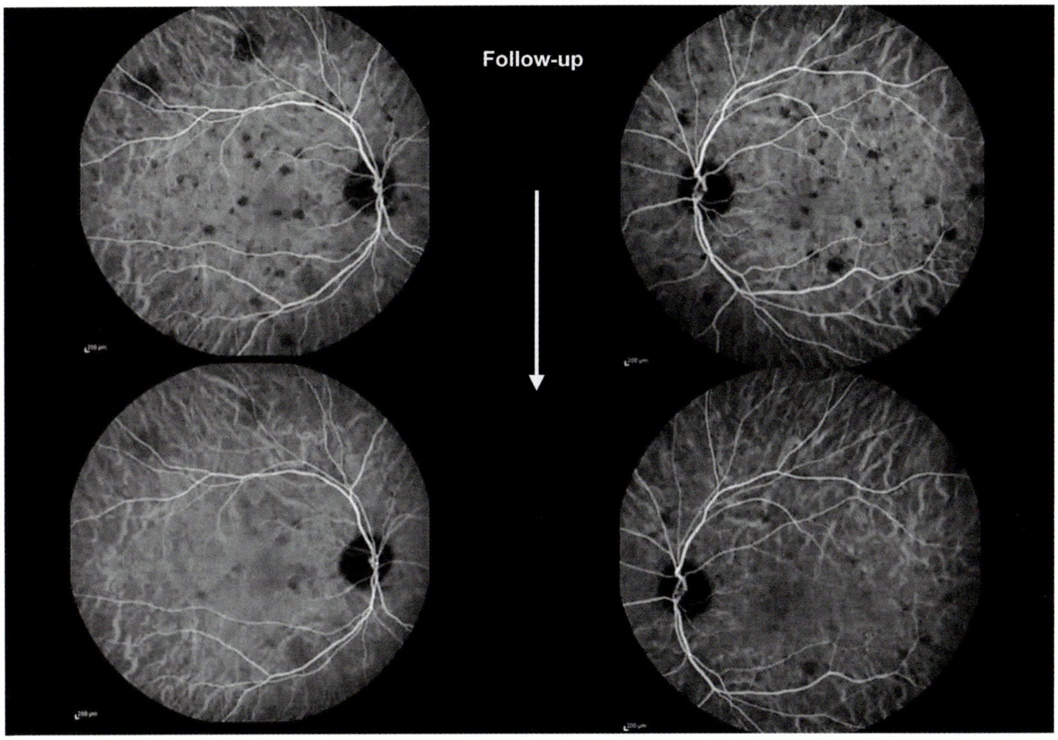

Fig. 11: ICGA imaging showing blockage in areas of choroidal lesions in both eyes at presentation (top) that resolved with administration of amphotericin B (bottom).
Source: Uveitis Webinar - Grand Round 12. International Uveitis Study Group (IUSG). 2025. https://youtu.be/1P4dx4IHwUc.[4]

Case 2

Personal data: A 27-year-old female patient presented with new skin lesions, a headache, and diplopia.

History of present illness: The duration of the new symptoms was not known, but she had a history of HIV positivity with an unknown CD4+ count. A skin rash was present on the face.

Physical examination: The best-corrected vision was 20/20 despite the presence of papilledema and retinal hemorrhages surrounding the optic nerves bilaterally. Choroidal lesions were also noted on dilated fundus examination **(Figs. 12A and B)**.

Slit lamp examination: Slit lamp examination is shown in **Table 5**.

Work-up: Pathologic testing of a skin biopsy was positive for *Cryptococcus* spp. **(Figs. 13A and B)**. Lumbar puncture was positive for *Cryptococcus neoformans* on both direct examination and on culture.

Treatment: The patient was started on intravenous amphotericin B for 10 days with slow resolution of the optic nerve edema and choroidal lesions.

TABLE 5: Slit lamp examination of the patient with optic nerve edema and choroiditis.

OD	*Parameter*	*OS*
20/20	BCVA	20/20
10	IOP	10
Normal	Exernal	Normal
Normal	Lids/lashes	Normal
White and quiet	Conjunctiva/ sclera	White and quiet
Clear	Cornea	Clear
Normal	Iris	Normal
No cell or flare	AC	No cell or flare
Pigment deposits	Lens	Clear
Clear	Anterior vitreous	Clear
Papilledema, retinal hemorrhages, and choroidal lesions under the posterior pole	Fundus	Papilledema, retinal hemorrhages, and choroidal lesions under the posterior pole

(AC: anterior chamber; BCVA: best-corrected visual acuity; IOP: intraocular pressure; KP: keratic precipitates; OD: right eye; OS: left eye)

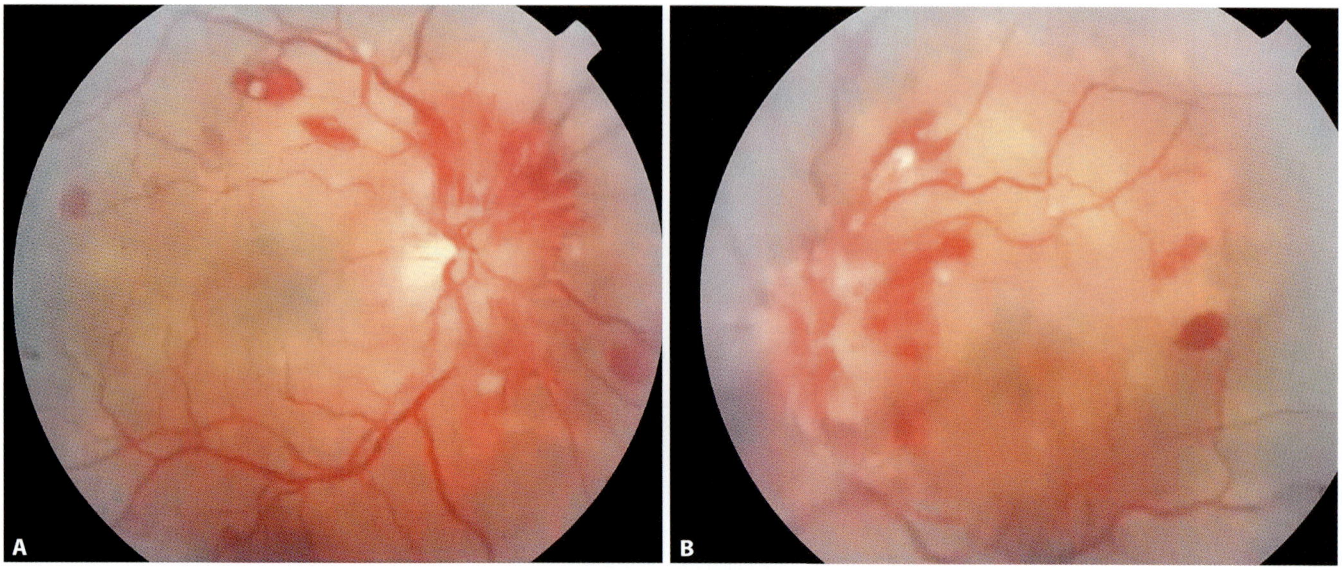

Figs. 12A and B: Color fundus photos of both eyes showing optic nerve edema with surrounding hemorrhages and multifocal choroidal lesions.
Source: Uveitis Webinar - Grand Round 12. International Uveitis Study Group (IUSG). 2025. https://youtu.be/1P4dx4IHwUc.[4]

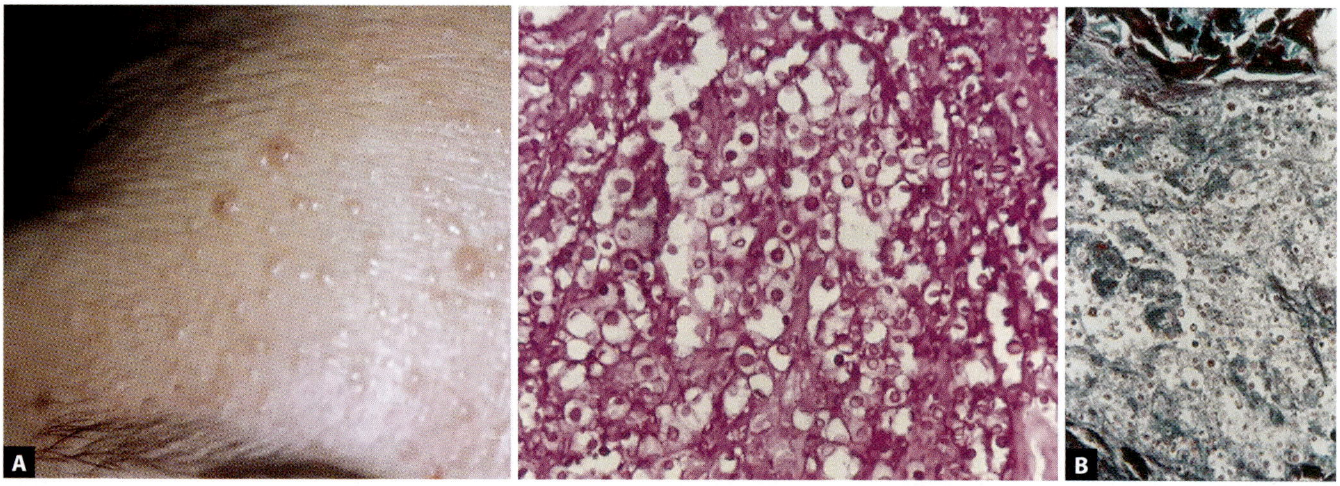

Figs. 13A and B: A diffuse, tan, macular rash on the forehead at presentation (left) and dermatopathologic stains highlighting the presence of *Cryptococcus neoformans* (right).
Source: Uveitis Webinar - Grand Round 12. International Uveitis Study Group (IUSG). 2025. https://youtu.be/1P4dx4IHwUc.[4]

Case 3

Personal data: A 32-year-old male was referred for an ophthalmologic examination.

History of present illness: He had a history of HIV positivity and was diagnosed with a disseminated cryptococcal infection leading to the current hospital admission. He reported no visual symptoms.

Physical examination: The best-corrected vision was 20/20 in both eyes, and deep, yellow choroidal lesions were noted bilaterally under the posterior pole without optic nerve edema **(Fig. 14)**.

Slit lamp examination: Slit lamp examination is shown in **Table 6**.

TABLE 6: Slit lamp examination of the patient with cotton wool spots and retinal hemorrhages.

OD	***Parameter***	***OS***
20/20	BCVA	20/20
11	IOP	13
Normal	Exernal	Normal
Normal	Lids/lashes	Normal
White and quiet	Conjunctiva/sclera	White and quiet
Clear	Cornea	Clear
Normal	Iris	Normal
No cell or flare	AC	No cell or flare
Pigment deposits	Lens	Clear
Clear	Anterior vitreous	Clear
Deep, yellow, choroidal lesions under the posterior pole without optic nerve edema. Flame-shaped hemorrhages and cotton wool spots were also noted **(Fig. 14)**	Fundus	Deep, yellow, choroidal lesions under the posterior pole without optic nerve edema. Flame-shaped hemorrhages and cotton wool spots were also noted **(Fig. 14)**

(AC: anterior chamber; BCVA: best-corrected visual acuity; IOP: intraocular pressure; KP: keratic precipitates; OD: right eye; OS: left eye)

Work-up: Given the previous diagnosis of disseminated *Cryptococcal* infection, no additional laboratory studies were ordered.

Follow-up: After treatment of intravenous amphotericin B, the cryptococcal choroiditis resolved. The flame-shaped hemorrhages and cotton wool spots on examination were compatible with HIV microangiopathy, which improved with the start of cART.

Case 4

Personal data: A 22-year-old female presented with blurred vision in both eyes.

History of present illness: She was HIV positive and had concurrently developed a headache, weight loss, and vomiting. She was admitted for a systemic work-up and referred to the ophthalmology clinic for examination.

Physical examination: Her vision was 6/36 in the right eye and 6/60 in the left eye. Deep, yellow, multifocal choroidal lesions were noted without papilledema bilaterally **(Fig. 15)**.

Slit lamp examination: Slit lamp examination is shown in **Table 7**.

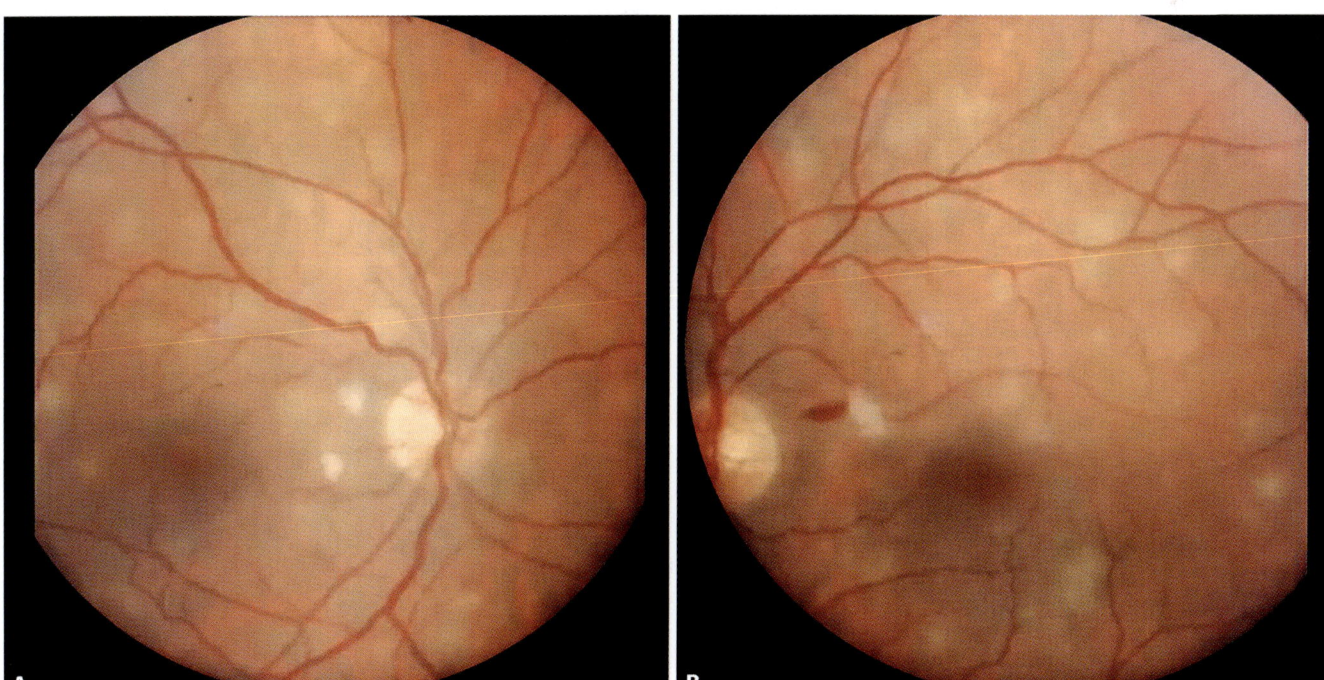

Fig. 14: Color fundus photos of both eyes showing yellow, multifocal choroidal lesions secondary to *Cryptococcus neoformans*. *Source:* Uveitis Webinar - Grand Round 12. International Uveitis Study Group (IUSG). 2025. https://youtu.be/1P4dx4IHwUc.[4]

TABLE 7: Slit lamp examination of the patient with choroiditis.

OD	*Parameter*	*OS*
6/36	BCVA	6/60
15	IOP	16
Normal	Exernal	Normal
Normal	Lids/lashes	Normal
White and quiet	Conjunctiva/sclera	White and quiet
Clear	Cornea	Clear
Normal	Iris	Normal
No cell or flare	AC	No cell or flare
Pigment deposits	Lens	Clear
Clear	Anterior vitreous	Clear
Deep, yellow, multifocal choroidal lesions, no papilledema	Fundus	Deep, yellow, multifocal choroidal lesions, no papilledema

(AC: anterior chamber; BCVA: best-corrected visual acuity; IOP: intraocular pressure; KP: keratic precipitates; OD: right eye; OS: left eye)

Work-up: On fluorescein angiography, the lesions blocked early and stained in the later frames **(Fig. 15)**. Indocyanine green imaging showed blockage in the areas of the lesions. Laboratory testing revealed a CD4+ count of 5 cells/mm and a viral load of over 500,000 copies. The CSF fluid obtained from the lumbar puncture was positive for *Cryptococcus* on both direct examination and on culture.

Follow-up: The patient was treated with intravenous amphotericin B leading to clinical improvement both systemically and on repeated ophthalmic examination, she had 6/6 vision in the right eye and 6/9 in the left eye. There was complete resolution of the choroidal lesions with pigmentary changes in the posterior pole of both eyes.

Discussion

Choroiditis due to *Cryptococcus* spp. presents with a classic yellow, bilateral, and symmetric lesions with minimal inflammation. When this is seen on examination, clinical suspicion for this entity should be high.[23] Infection

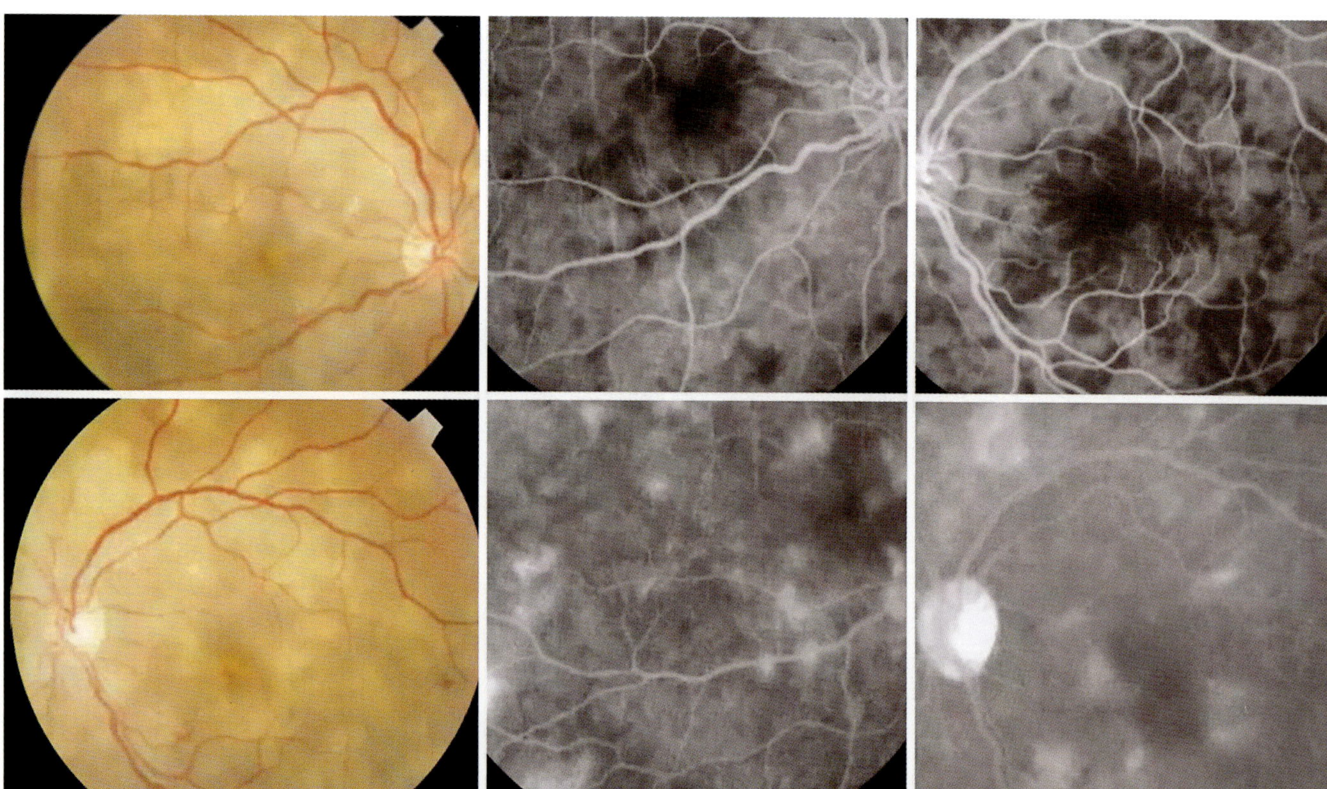

Fig. 15: Color fundus photos of both eyes (left) showing yellow, multifocal choroidal lesions secondary to *Cryptococcus neoformans*. On fluorescein angiography, the lesions block early (middle and right upper) and show staining in the later frames (middle and right lower). *Source:* Uveitis Webinar - Grand Round 12. International Uveitis Study Group (IUSG). 2025. https://youtu.be/1P4dx4IHwUc.[4]

often does not elicit any changes in visual acuity until there is optic nerve involvement.[24] The presentation of cryptococcal choroiditis without papilledema is very rare. Several cases of cryptococcal choroiditis have been presented recently, which have increased from prior and are reminiscent of the AIDS pandemic in the 1990s. Back then, CMV retinitis, acute retinal necrosis, toxoplasmosis, and syphilis were also more prevalent. This is likely due to increasing drug use and other socioeconomic factors contributing to increase in untreated HIV in our region.

When diagnosing infectious diseases in HIV, an important consideration is whether the affected area is retinal or choroidal in nature. This will help you narrow your differential, with retinal lesions more commonly resulting from CMV, HSV, or syphilis. Cryptococcal infection and lesions often arising secondary to tuberculosis and fungi are located in the choroid.

PARADOXICAL REACTION TO TUBERCULOSIS

Case Presentation

Personal Data

A 33-year-old female with a 10-year history of HIV and compliance with cART presented for examination. Her most recent laboratory studies showed a CD4+ count of 1,225 cells per cubic millimeter and an undetectable viral load.

History of Present Illness

While visiting family, the patient was admitted to a regional hospital with a 1-month history of headaches and vomiting. On admission, she reported a 1-month history of complete vision loss in the right eye and a 5-month history of vision loss in the left eye. A prior work-up included a CT scan of the head which showed diffuse nodular parenchyma, meningeal thickening, and bilateral intraocular dependent layering with retinal hypodensities. A lumbar puncture showed a slightly elevated opening pressure of 22 cmH_2O, a lymphocyte count of 6, normal protein levels, and low glucose levels. Cryptococcal antigen antibody testing was negative. She was transferred to our hospital for continued care and for ophthalmic evaluation.

Physical Examination

The vision in both eyes was no light perception. There was 4+ flare in the anterior chamber of both eyes and no fundus view bilaterally.

TABLE 8: Slit lamp examination of the patient having paradoxical reaction to tuberculosis.

OD	Parameter	OS
NLP	BCVA	NLP
Clear	Cornea	Clear
4+ flare, deep	AC	4+ flare, very shallow
Partially broken posterior synechiae	Iris/pupil	360° posterior synechiae
2+ PSC	Lens	Dense cataract
5 mm Hg	IOP	0 mm Hg
Yellow reflex, no fundal view	Fundus	No view

(AC: anterior chamber; BCVA: best-corrected visual acuity; IOP: intraocular pressure; NLP: no light perception; PSC: posterior subcapsular cataract; OD: right eye; OS: left eye)

Slit Lamp Examination

Slit lamp examination is shown in **Table 8**.

Initial Treatment

She was suspected to have meningitis and was started on empiric intravenous ceftriaxone and dexamethasone with subsequent placement of indwelling catheters. She was also started on prednisolone acetate and atropine eyedrops for the anterior chamber inflammation. A QFT-TB Gold test was also ordered.

Follow-up

The patient was admitted to the neurology service and was not seen again until 6 weeks later with improved vision of hand motions in the left eye. She was treated by neurology for presumed tuberculous meningitis based on the CT results from the outside hospital. With the antituberculosis treatment and prednisone, a view to the fundus was now visible in the left eye. It showed choroidal lesions in the posterior pole **(Fig. 16)**. Given improvement with treatment, it was presumed that tuberculosis was also the cause of her ophthalmic findings.

The patient returned 3 weeks later with worsening vision despite continued antituberculosis treatment, oral corticosteroids, and the restart of cART. The fundus examination showed more vitreous haze and an increase in the number and size of the choroidal lesions. Her case was presented at the hospital grand rounds to determine the cause of the worsening ophthalmic examination. Since the patient was a poor historian, possible causes included the patient not taking the antituberculosis medications as prescribed or discontinuing the use of the corticosteroids. Alternative explanations included a missed alternative diagnosis or the development of fungal endophthalmitis given the presence of multiple indwelling catheters. Finally, a paradoxical response to antituberculosis treatment was considered. The consensus was to continue the current treatment course. Three days later, the patient's vision again declined to light perception and a diagnostic vitrectomy was performed. Intraoperatively, a dense, white vitritis was seen, which appeared similar to cases of endophthalmitis. Once the vitreous was removed, subretinal lesions in the anterior choroid and ciliary body were noted with large choroidal granulomas in the posterior pole. Additionally, an exudative retinal detachment was noted without the presence of retinal tears. Vitreous samples were sent for bacterial and fungal cultures, auramine staining, cellular analysis, potassium hydroxide preparation, GeneXpert panels, and PCR testing for herpes viruses. All of the results were negative. Post-operatively, multiple choroidal granulomas were noted on examination to be smaller **(Fig. 17)**. The etiology of the transient worsening was presumed to be a paradoxical reaction to the anti-tuberculosis therapy. Three weeks later, the patient returned with a worsening retinal detachment. A choroidal biopsy was considered, but ultimately deferred.

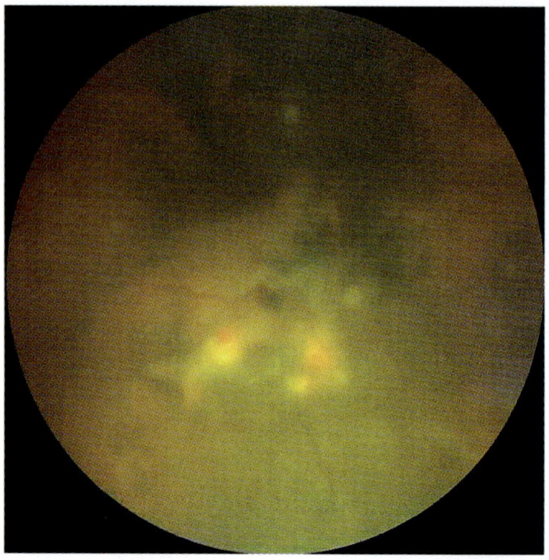

Fig. 16: A color fundus photo of the left eye showing vitreous opacities and choroiditis affecting the macula and optic nerve.
Source: Uveitis Webinar - Grand Round 12. International Uveitis Study Group (IUSG). 2025. https://youtu.be/1P4dx4lHwUc.[4]

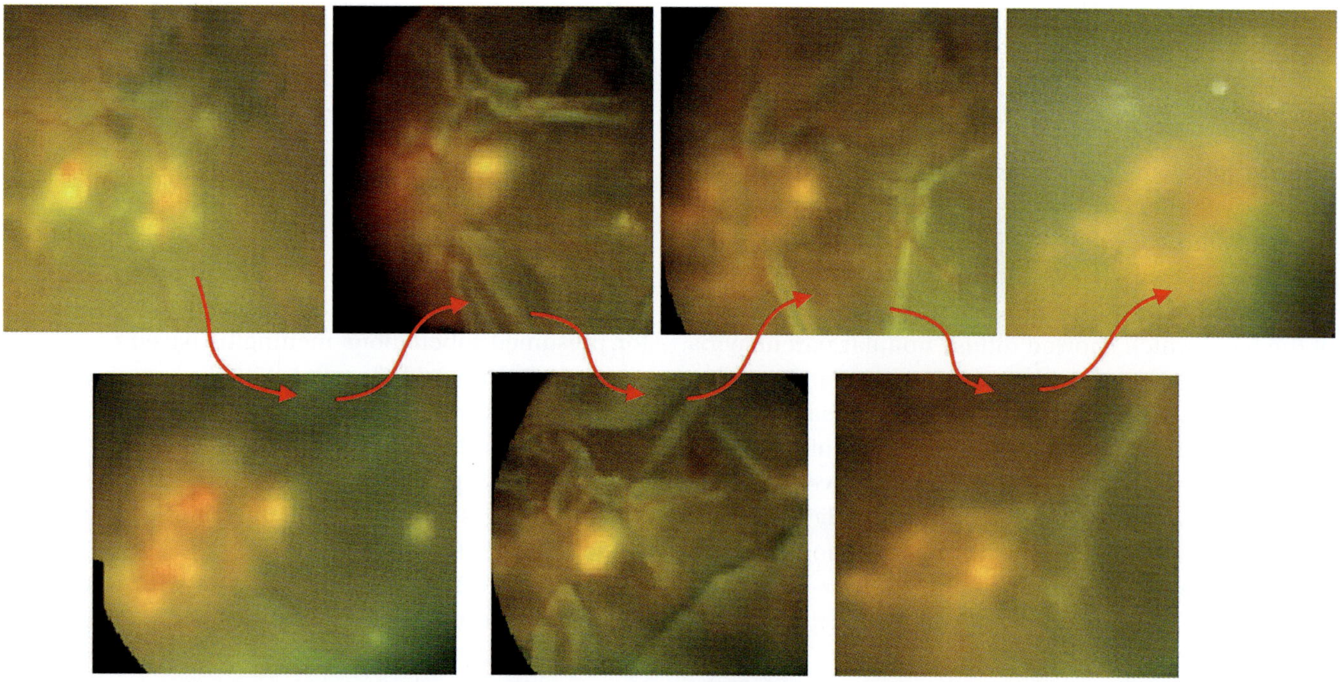

Fig. 17: A montage of color fundus photos of the left eye showing the initial presence of choroidal lesions in the posterior pole with transient worsening followed by resolution of the exudative detachment with smaller lesion sizes.
Source: Uveitis Webinar - Grand Round 12. International Uveitis Study Group (IUSG). 2025. https://youtu.be/1P4dx4lHwUc.[4]

Follow-up

Both the exudative detachment and the choroidal lesions slowly resolved with flattening of the retina after 5 months.

Discussion

The difficulty of this case was that the paradoxical worsening after initiation of antituberculosis treatment has been reported to occur in 2–4 weeks after initiation, and in our case, the worsening clinical picture occurred after day 40. In addition, the patient was not on the primary ophthalmology service, but rather was admitted to neurology. In cases such as these, it is important to review the medical records to construct a complete image of what has happened during the hospital admission. Developing your own differential diagnosis is important to identify any additional work-up that is needed. This case involved an acutely ill patient requiring multiple interventions, including indwelling catheters, that were of concern as a source for fungal endophthalmitis. In addition, there also existed a language barrier between patient and caregivers with the additional limitations posed by the patient's inability to recall medication usage and doses. Nonetheless, the decision to continue both the corticosteroids and antituberculosis medications was made given there were no other conditions that remained in the differential diagnosis after the vitrectomy. Pathologic examination of the fellow, pre-phthisical eye was also a consideration. Due to the disparate time frame of vision loss between the eyes, we were not sure if the same pathology occurred in the fellow eye. She previously may have developed CMV retinitis with a subsequent retinal detachment leading to the vision loss; however, the patient declined enucleation.

PEARLS FROM THE EXPERTS ON FREQUENTLY ASKED QUESTIONS

1. Is there any additional treatment recommended for large granulomas that develop secondary to tuberculosis?

Answer: You can treat with antituberculosis therapy alone, but given the size and nature of the infection, the time to resolution can be significant. You can consider comanagement with intravitreal anti-VEGF or moxifloxacin injections in these situations. Given the high VEGF titers, intravitreal injections are given every 10–14 days, as opposed to the monthly timing used in patients with wet macular degeneration or diabetic macular edema. It is important to note that atypical mycobacteria may present similarly to tuberculosis, but not clinically improve when treated with standard antituberculosis regimens.

2. In patients with HIV, can systemic corticosteroids be administered safely?

Answer: While CD4+ counts can have a wide range in patients with HIV, systemic corticosteroids are not contraindicated provided tuberculosis and the presence of other undiagnosed infectious diseases have been ruled out. Since the treatment of HIV requires multidisciplinary care, consultation with an infectious disease specialist is advised. As with any treatment, a discussion of the systemic risk and vision saving benefit ratio is needed.

3. Would a vitreous tap for culture and sensitivity be helpful in the diagnosis in these patients?

Answer: Yes, a vitreous tap or, as described in the last case, a vitrectomy was required for diagnostic certainty. Alternative tests besides a culture with sensitivities can include next-generation DNA sequencing, flow cytometry, cellular analysis, or an interleukin (IL)-6:10 ratio. IL-10 levels are more elevated in lymphoma and IL-6 in inflammatory or infectious causes. The ability to obtain fluid from the eye for testing can provide clarity if neuroimaging shows granulomas and both tuberculosis and central nervous system lymphoma remain in the differential diagnosis.

4. What are possible explanations for the series of patients with cryptococcal choroiditis in Brazil?

Answer: It is possible that there is an environmental factor to be considered, as sporotrichosis is also seen in immunosuppressed patients in Rio de Janeiro. The resurgence of HIV alone cannot explain the trend as cryptococcal choroiditis is also seen locally in immunocompetent patients, but with robust intraocular inflammation.

5. When should you suspect sarcoidosis versus tuberculosis in a patient with HIV?

Answer: Depending on the CD4+ cell count, autoimmune disorders can still occur. The clinical manifestations of sarcoidosis are similar in patients with or without HIV. However, immunologic tests, such as the quantiFERON gold assay, rely on normal CD4+ cell counts. False negatives can occur when the CD4+ count drops to ≤100 cells. As in the publication by Agrawal et al., some ocular immunologists consider sarcoidosis and tuberculosis as different ends of the same disease spectrum.[25]

FINAL WRAP-UP

New cases of HIV and AIDS are diagnosed worldwide on a daily basis. Testing is warranted in the setting of ocular opportunistic infections. The risk of death is very high in patients with low CD4+ cell counts. Prompt, multidisciplinary management for the treatment of systemic infections and the start of cART is lifesaving. Continued monitoring is necessary for the development of immune recovery uveitis and cystoid macular edema in patients with a history of CMV retinitis.

REFERENCES

1. WHO South Africa HIV Country Profile 2024. [online] Available from https://cfs.hivci.org/index.html [Last accessed February, 2026].
2. UNAIDS DATA 2023. Geneva: Joint United Nations Programme on HIV/AIDS; 2023. Available from https://www.genevaenvironmentnetwork.org/environment-geneva/organizations/joint-united-nations-programme-on-hiv-aids/ [Last accessed February, 2026].
3. Meyer D, Smit DP. Eyelid and Orbital Involvement in HIV Infection – An African Perspective. Ocul Immunol Inflamm. 2020;28(7):1022-30.
4. Smit DP, Esterhuizen TM, Meyer D. The prevalence of intraocular tuberculosis in HIV-positive and HIV-negative patients in South Africa using a revised classification system. Ocul Immunol Inflamm. 2018:26(6):830-7.
5. Odendaal LN, Andreae C, Sanderson-November M, Zaharie D, Smit DP. The prevalence of human papillomavirus in ocular Surface squamous neoplasia in HIV positive and negative patients in a South African population. Infection. 2024;52(4):1547-52.
6. Laaks D, Smit DP, Meyer D. Cryptococcal IRIS in the anterior segment of the eye. AIDS. 2013;27(3):489-90.
7. Radhakrishnan N, Smit DP, Prajna NV, Rathinam SR. Corneal Involvement in HIV-infected Individuals. Ocul Immunol Inflamm. 2021;29(6):1177-82.
8. Du Toit SH, Smit DP. Mooren's ulcer of the cornea after immune reconstitution. AIDS. 2014;28:139-40.
9. Rosberger DF, Heinemann M, Friedberg DN, Holland GN. Uveitis associated with human immunodeficiency virus infection. Am J Ophthalmol. 1998;125:301-5.
10. Rothova A, Schneider M, de Groot-Mijnes JD. Human immunodeficiency virus-induced uveitis: intraocular and plasma human immunodeficiency virus-1 RNA loads. Ophthalmology. 2008;115:2062-4.
11. Kunavisarut P, Sirirungsi W, Pathanapitoon K, Rothova A. Clinical manifestations of human immunodeficiency virus-induced uveitis. Ophthalmology. 2012;119:1455-9.
12. Smit DP, Meyer D. HIV-induced uveitis: would you recognize it if it looked straight at you? AIDS. 2017;31(12):1777-9.
13. Smit DP, Esterhuizen TM, Meyer D. The role of Quantiferon TB Gold and tuberculin skin test as diagnostic tests for intraocular tuberculosis in HIV-positive and HIV-neagtive patients in South Africa. Ocul Immunol Inflamm. 2018:16(6):853-8.
14. Smit DP, Meyer D, Esterhuizen TM, De Groot-Mijnes JDF. Polymerase chain reaction and Goldmann-Witmer coefficient testing in the diagnosis of infectious uveítis in HIV-positive and HIV-negative patients in South Africa. Ocul Imunol Inflamm. 2019;27(2):189-96.
15. Smit DP, Esterhuizen TM, Meyer D, de Boer JH, De Groot-Mijnes JDF. The etiology of intraocular inflammation in HIV positiveand HIv negative adults in a tertiary hospital in Cape Town, South Africa. Ocul Immunol Inflam. 2019;27(2):203-10.
16. Mathew D, Smit DP. Clinical and laboratory characteristics of ocular syphilis and neurosyphilis among individuals with and without HIV infection. Br J Ophthalmol. 2021;105(1):70-4.
17. Odendaal LN, Smit DP. A triple case series of uveitis caused by HIV, syphilis and tuberculosis coinfection. AIDS. 2022;36(1):155-6.
18. Kempen JH, Jabs DA, Dunn JP, West SK, Tonascia J. Retinal detachment risk in cytomegalovirus retinitis related to the acquired immunodeficiency syndrome. Arch Ophthalmol. 2001;119(1):33-40.
19. Kempen JH, Jabs DA, Wilson LA, Dunn JP, West SK, Tonascia JA. Risk of vision loss in patients with cytomegalovirus retinitis and the acquired immunodeficiency syndrome. Arch Ophthalmol. 2003;121(4):466-76.
20. Kempen JH, Jabs DA, Wilson LA, Dunn JP, West SK. Incidence of cytomegalovirus (CMV) retinitis in second eyes of patients with the acquired immune deficiency syndrome and unilateral CMV retinitis. Am J Ophthalmol. 2005;139(6):1028-34.
21. Kempen JH, Jabs DA, Wilson LA, Dunn JP, West SK, Tonascia J. Mortality risk for patients with cytomegalovirus retinitis and acquired immune deficiency syndrome. Clin Infect Dis. 2003;37(10):1365-73.
22. Kuo IC, Kempen JH, Dunn JP, Vogelsang G, Jabs DA. Clinical characteristics and outcomes of cytomegalovirus retinitis in persons without human immunodeficiency virus infection. Am J Ophthalmol. 2004;138(3):338-46.
23. Andreola C, Riberiro MP, deCarli CR, Gouvea AL, Curi AL. Multifocal choroiditis in disseminated *Cryptococcus neoformans* infection. Am J Ophthalmol. 2006;142(2):346-8.
24. Paiva A, Biancardi AL, Curi AL. Clinical-laboratory outcome of *Cryptococcus* sp. multifocal choroiditis in Acquired immunodeficiency Syndrome patients. Ocul Immunol Inflamm. 2024;32(10):2421-7.
25. Agrawal R, Kee AR, Ang L, Tun Hang Y, Gupta V, Kon OM, et al. Tuberculosis or sarcoidosis: Opposite ends of the same disease spectrum? Tuberculosis (Edinb). 2016;98:21-6.

CHAPTER 13

Juvenile Idiopathic Arthritis-associated Uveitis

Meghan Berkenstock, Alessandra Pagliara, Claudia Fabiani, Sara Abdel Jalil, Radgonde Amer, Panayiotis Maghsoudlou, Athimalaipet V Ramanan, Sara Prischak, Vishali Gupta, Alejandra de-la-Torre, Reema Bansal, John H Kempen

INTRODUCTION

Uveitis associated with juvenile idiopathic arthritis (JIA) is one of the leading causes of ocular morbidity in childhood. It can result in severe complications such as cataract, glaucoma, and irreversible vision loss if not treated promptly. Its asymptomatic course in the early stages, particularly in the oligoarthritis subtype, highlights the importance of regular ophthalmologic screening. Moreover, studying uveitis in these patients enhances our understanding of the relationship between systemic inflammation and ocular autoimmunity, allowing for improved management strategies and better patient outcomes.

THEMATIC LECTURE: JUVENILE IDIOPATHIC ARTHRITIS

JIA is the most commonly associated systemic condition with chronic ocular inflammation in children. It is clinically defined as arthritis lasting at least 6 weeks in children under 16 years of age. There are seven subtypes based on the number of joints involved at presentation, laboratory values, and associated systemic symptoms: Systemic onset (formerly known as Still's disease), oligoarthritis, polyarticular involvement with or without a positive serologic rheumatoid factor (RF), psoriatic, enthesitis-related, and undifferentiated (meets either none of the other categorical classifications or more than two classifications).[1] The subtypes with the lowest number of patients that develop uveitis are polyarticular involvement with RF positivity or systemic onset, with a frequency of 4–6%. Polyarticular involvement with RF positivity has a disease course akin to seropositive rheumatoid arthritis in adults. Polyarticular disease, by definition, has five or more joints affected at presentation, and those without a positive RF value develop uveitis in 5–25% of cases. The most commonly affected subtype is pauciarticular, with less than five joints inflamed at diagnosis. Persistent pauciarticular disease refers to four or less joints involved both at presentation and throughout the clinical course. Alternatively, extended pauciarticular disease involves more than 4 joints after 6 months. The highest risk for the development of uveitis is in patients who are younger than the age and in patients with negative RF and positive antinuclear antibodies (ANAs) on serologic testing. There is a female predominance, and 20–30% of those with pauciarticular disease will develop uveitis. Psoriatic and enthesitis-related JIA subtypes have up to 11% of cases that develop uveitis, with the latter predominantly affecting older boys, most of whom are human leukocyte antigen B27 (HLA-B27) positive.

The average age of uveitis onset in patients with JIA is at 6 years old and within 5–7 years after the disease onset. The timing of joint and ocular inflammation can be disparate, making screening slit lamp exams essential for detecting the development of uveitis. Only on an ophthalmic can inflammation be detected in eyes lacking erythema and in patients who may endorse minimal symptoms. Without early diagnosis and treatment, ocular complications can develop, including posterior synechiae, cataracts, band keratopathy, glaucoma, macular edema, and, in end-stage disease, phthisis bulbi. On examination, fine cells are seen with varying degrees of flare and are graded using the Standardization of Uveitis Nomenclature scales.[2] A standardized screening algorithm has been proposed, most recently by the American College of Rheumatology and the Arthritis Foundation in 2019.[3] An ophthalmic exam should be performed for screening every 3 months in high-risk patients with RF-negative oligoarthritis, psoriatic, or undifferentiated JIA and who are ANA positive with joint disease onset at <7 years old and with a disease duration of ≤4 years. Screening can be spaced out to every 6–12 months in patients with RF-negative oligoarthritis, psoriatic, or undifferentiated JIA who are ANA-negative, with joint disease onset at ≥7 years and a disease duration of >4 years, given a low or moderate risk. Screening exams can also be extended to 6–12 months from disease onset in other low-risk groups, including systemic-onset, RF-positive polyarticular, and enthesitis-related disease.

In addition to screening, early prescription of immunosuppressive therapies in patients with JIA has been shown to reduce the incidence of ocular complications. In a paper by Thorne et al., the risk of cataract development was independently associated with the use of prednisolone acetate 1% drops.[4] The dose-dependent increase in the rate of cataract formation rose with the use of more than three drops per day. Eyes receiving less than or equal to two drops per day had a risk of cataract formation of 0 per eye-year. If quiescence of anterior chamber inflammation can only be achieved using 3 or more drops per day, the start of systemic immunosuppression should be considered. In addition to cataract formation, elevation of intraocular pressures (IOPs) occurs in a dose- and route of administration-dependent manner, as reported in the Systemic Immunosuppressive Therapy for Eye Diseases Research Study (SITE).[5] Eyes receiving two to three drops daily of prednisolone acetate 1% had a two to threefold increased incidence of IOP elevation with escalation to a ninefold incidence with use four times daily. Similarly, the use of periocular corticosteroid injections had a seven- to eightfold risk of IOP elevation. In contrast, immunosuppressive therapy and a daily dose of prednisone ≤7.5 mg were not associated with a higher risk of elevated IOPs, even after adjusting for topical corticosteroid use. In addition to the use of periocular or topical corticosteroids, other risk factors for IOP elevation included poor vision at presentation, need for ocular surgeries, and longer duration of disease. The estimated incidence of any observed IOP elevation to ≥21 mm Hg was 33.4%, and to ≥30 mm Hg was 14.8%, respectively. Moreover, 16% of patients in the SITE study had an IOP ≥21 mm Hg at presentation. This is a reminder that the cumulative incidence of eyes with IOP elevation continued to rise throughout follow-up. While the rate of the rise tended to decrease over the study period, the cumulative incidence never returned to baseline, highlighting the continued need to monitor IOPs throughout the disease course.

Given the development of ocular complications with local corticosteroid use, most patients with JIA require initiation of non-corticosteroid immunosuppressive medications. The use of systemic corticosteroids is contraindicated over prolonged time periods, given the risk of developing side effects, including iatrogenic short stature due to premature closure of the epiphyses in young patients. Based on numerous papers over the last 40 years, a step-wise approach has been developed that strats with antimetabolite agents, including methotrexate, mycophenolate mofetil, or azathioprine.[6-9] In patients presenting with ocular complications or inflammation that is not completely controlled with anti-metabolite therapy, escalation to tumor necrosis factor alpha inhibitors (TNF-inhibitors) should be considered.[10] Several studies have shown the efficacy and safety of adalimumab for the treatment of JIA-associated uveitis. The SYCAMORE Study was a multicenter, double-blind, randomized, placebo-controlled trial that assessed the efficacy and safety of adalimumab in children ≥2 years old with active JIA-associated uveitis.[11] Those on a stable dose of methotrexate were randomly assigned in a 2:1 ratio to receive either adalimumab or placebo. The number of treatment failures was highly statistically significant, with only 27% in the adalimumab group versus 60% in the placebo group. The use of adalimumab also showed a sparing effect on the use of corticosteroid drops. These results were mirrored by the ADJUVITE Study, which was also a double-blind, randomized, placebo-controlled trial of 31 patients with ocular inflammation refractory to corticosteroids and methotrexate who were randomized to receive adalimumab or placebo.[12] After 60 days, 56% in the treatment group versus 20% in the control group had decreased inflammation measured by laser flare photometry.

While the prior studies showed the clinical efficacy of adalimumab, the ADJUST trial assessed whether discontinuing adalimumab after quiescence led to the recurrence of active uveitis.[13] With a multicenter, double-masked, randomized, placebo-controlled design, it assessed patients ≥2 years of age with controlled arthritis and uveitis for at least 1 year on adalimumab. Patients received adalimumab or placebo every other week until the 48-week visit or treatment failure. Only 14% in the adalimumab group and 68% in the placebo group had treatment failure, with a median time in the placebo group of 119 days [interquartile range (IQR 84–243)]. The median time to re-establishing sustained control of inflammation in the placebo group after restarting adalimumab was 105 days (IQR 63–196). Discontinuing adalimumab led to higher rates of recurrence of uveitis, arthritis, or both in patients with previously controlled JIA-associated uveitis, and all patients with treatment failure regained control by week 48.

In cases of adalimumab failure, studies support the use of other TNF inhibitors for the treatment of JIA-associated uveitis. A prospective, multicenter study conducted in patients with JIA-associated uveitis refractory to anti-metabolite or cyclosporine immunosuppressive therapy and who were systemically corticosteroid-dependent demonstrated a higher remission rate with the addition of adalimumab (60.0%) than with infliximab (20.3%).[14] However, the adalimumab group was larger (90 versus 32 subjects), and there was no randomization with prescription of adalimumab favored due to ease of administration with subcutaneous injections. Similarly, retention rates for patients on infliximab were lower. Nonetheless, it showed that quiescence could be achieved than infliximab. Similarly, one retrospective, single-center study assessed the efficacy of golimumab, in which 50% of children with JIA uveitis refractory to adalimumab achieved quiescence over 30 months.[15] Finally, one randomized, placebo-controlled, double-masked clinical trial conducted on children with active JIA-associated uveitis showed that etanercept did not provide a significant efficacy above placebo.[16] The difference in efficacy may lie in the unique mechanism of action as a soluble TNF-receptor. Other agents in the class are monoclonal antibodies that prevent TNF-alpha from binding cell surface receptors. While etanercept has shown efficacy in alleviating joint inflammation, cases of new-onset uveitis with use have been reported. Further evidence is needed on the effectiveness of other TNF inhibitors in treating JIA-associated uveitis.

When TNF inhibitors are contraindicated, or patients with active uveitis have failed methotrexate and two TNF inhibitors, the use of tocilizumab is recommended. Tocilizumab is a humanized monoclonal antibody that competitively inhibits interleukin-6 (IL-6) from binding its soluble and membrane-bound receptors. It is also available in subcutaneous and intravenous (IV) administrations. A retrospective study of 17 patients with treatment-resistant, active uveitis resulted in inactivity in 10 patients after a mean of 5.7 months.[17] Another multicenter study with 25 patients with active uveitis and macular edema showed that after 6 months of treatment, 79.2% of patients demonstrated less anterior chamber inflammation, corticosteroid-sparing success, and reduced macular edema.[18]

In addition to achieving clinical remission, an understanding the optimal timing for managing complications is needed. Given the concern for amblyopia in young children, cataracts should be removed after ≥3 months of quiescence without macular edema.[19] A pars plana vitrectomy and posterior capsulotomy should be performed during cataract surgery in children who are unable to undergo yttrium aluminum garnet (YAG)-laser capsulotomy for posterior capsular opacification. Before surgery, maximizing immunosuppressive dosing and prophylactic pretreatment with a short course of oral or topical corticosteroids is advised. Postoperative continuation of immunosuppressive medications is essential with close follow-up and escalation of immunosuppression for inflammation.[19] This is of the utmost importance as children mount a strong inflammatory response postoperatively, resulting in the formation of posterior capsular opacification, macular edema, and pupillary membranes. The decision to implant an intraocular lens (IOL) should be made on a case-by-case basis. Several considerations include the patient's age, risk for amblyopia, preoperative adherence to immunosuppressive therapy, and the ability to follow post-operative instructions. If the patient is left aphakic, will a contact lens be worn reliably, or are there contraindications due to disease severity, such as the presence of band keratopathy? If an IOL is inserted, placement in the ciliary sulcus, as opposed to in the lens capsule, can limit synechiae formation between the anterior capsule and the iris. However, there is always a risk of the IOLs dropping over time, irrespective of location, due to zonular laxity. In addition to surgical planning, the most effective way to reduce complications and the need for surgical intervention is to prevent structural damage from uncontrolled disease.

In summary, JIA-associated uveitis is a chronic condition requiring long-term follow-up. Corticosteroid drop and periocular injections have a dose- and route-of-administration-dependent increase in IOP. Patients frequently require early initiation of non-corticosteroid immunosuppressive therapy for control of inflammation and prevention of complications. Larger prospective, multicenter studies are needed to assess the efficacy of TNF-inhibitors other than adalimumab and third-line agents.

CLASSIC JUVENILE IDIOPATHIC ARTHRITIS-ASSOCIATED UVEITIS: A CASE-BASED APPROACH

Case 1

Personal Data

A 3-year-old female, previously diagnosed with oligoarticular JIA with ANA positivity. She presented at age 2 with joint symptoms affecting the proximal interphalangeal, elbow, and knee joints. Her family history was positive for rheumatoid arthritis and psoriasis in her maternal grandfather and mother, respectively.

History of Present Illness

She presented 4 months after diagnosis for a follow-up ophthalmic screening exam. Treatments included prednisone tablets, which were discontinued due to difficult administration, ibuprofen, and corticosteroid joint injections. Subcutaneous methotrexate injections (up to 7.5 mg/week) were also trialed and then discontinued due to nausea. She was then started on etanercept (0.8 mg/kg/week) and systemic corticosteroids, resulting in decreased joint pain. Previous ophthalmologic screening exams were negative.

Physical Examination

Visual acuity was 20/32 in both eyes. The anterior chambers had 2+ flare and 2+ cells in the right eye and 2+ flare and 3+ cells in the left eye. The posterior chamber examination was unremarkable **(Table 1)**.

TABLE 1: Physical examination of a patient having a classic juvenile idiopathic arthritis-associated uveitis Case 1.

OD	***Parameter***	***OS***
20/32	BCVA	20/32
14 mm Hg	IOP	14 mm Hg
Quiet	Conjunctiva	Quiet
Fine KPs	Cornea	Fine KPs
2+ cells, 2+ flare	Anterior chamber	3+ cells, 2+ flare
No synechiae	Iris	No synechiae
Clear	Lens	Clear
Unremarkable	Vitreous	Unremarkable
Normal, no macular edema	Fundus	Normal, no macular edema

(BCVA: best corrected visual acuity, IOP: intraocular pressure; KPs: keratic precipitates)

Uveitis Workup

Based on the prior history of JIA, no additional testing was ordered.

Initial Treatment

Etanercept was switched to adalimumab 20 mg administered subcutaneously every 14 days, in conjunction with a topical cycloplegic and corticosteroid drops. Tropicamide drops 10 mg/mL were administered three times daily for 2 weeks, then twice daily for 1 month, and finally once daily. Topical dexamethasone drops 1.5 mg/mL were administered four times daily for 1 week, then three times daily for 1 week, then two times daily for the next 2 weeks, and finally once daily for 2 weeks. Follow-up visits were scheduled every 2 weeks during this time, as well as 1 month after the corticosteroid taper.

Clinical Course

At the 1-week follow-up, there was 1+ cell and 1+ flare in both eyes. By week 3, the exam showed no cells or flare. At the final follow-up, there was a mild increase in uveitis activity to 1+ cell and 1 + flare, so topical corticosteroids and cycloplegics were reintroduced for two weeks, leading to quiescence.

Case 2

Personal Data

A 13-year-old male presented with blurred vision, redness, and pain in the left eye over the past 5 days. His last eye exam was 10 months before presentation and was within normal limits.

History of Present Illness

He was previously diagnosed with enthesitis-related arthritis with HLA-B27 positivity at 6 years old. There was a positive family history of HLA-B27+ ankylosing spondylitis in his father, father's twin brother, and paternal cousin. Treatment at presentation included methotrexate 15 mg/week administered subcutaneously, with the recent addition of etanercept 37.5 mg subcutaneously every 7 days.

He had discontinued adalimumab 2 months prior due to a loss of efficacy.

Physical Examination

Visual acuity was 20/20 in the right eye and 20/50 in the left eye. The anterior chamber was quiet on the right, but 4+ cell and fibrin formation were present in the left eye with posterior synechiae formation and conjunctival injection **(Table 2) (Fig. 1)**.

Ancillary Testing

Anterior segment optical coherence tomography (OCT) showed cellular reaction and fibrous membrane formation over the anterior lens capsule **(Fig. 2)**.

Uveitis Workup

Based on the prior history of JIA, no additional testing was ordered.

TABLE 2: Physical examination of a patient having classic juvenile idiopathic arthritis-associated uveitis Case 2.

OD	***Parameter***	***OS***
20/20	BCVA	20/50
14 mm Hg	IOP	14 mm Hg
Quiet	Conjunctiva	Perilimbal injection
Clear	Cornea	Fine KPs on the endothelium
Deep and quiet	Anterior chamber	4+ cells, 4+ flare with fibrin formation
No synechiae	Iris	Posterior synechiae
Clear	Lens	Clear
Unremarkable	Vitreous	Unremarkable
Normal, no macular edema	Fundus	Normal, no macular edema

(BCVA: Best corrected visual acuity, IOP: Intraocular pressure, KPs: keratic precipitates)

Initial Treatment

Etanercept was discontinued, and golimumab 50 mg was started subcutaneously monthly, with continued subcutaneous methotrexate at 15 mg/week. A concurrent prednisone taper was initiated, starting at 40 mg and tapered in decrements over 2 months. Topical therapy included hourly dexamethasone 1.5 mg/mL drops for 3 days while awake, followed by a taper of one drop per week down to two times per day. Dosing was then decreased to daily for 5 days before cessation. During this time, the patient also received 2.5% phenylephrine and tropicamide 1% drops twice daily. At 5 weeks postpresentation, the left eye was quiet with improved vision to 20/20.

Follow-up

Regular follow-up was scheduled every 2 months. After 1 year, he had no recurrence of inflammation and was

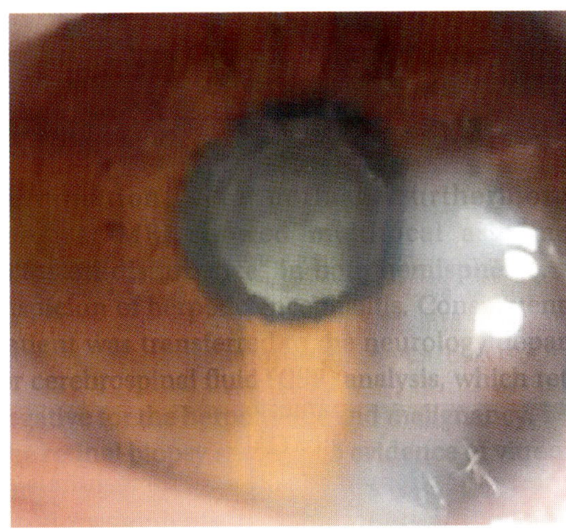

Fig. 1: Slit lamp photo of the left eye 1 day after presentation showing formation of a fibrin plaque over the lens capsule and posterior synechiae.
Source: Uveitis Webinar - Grand Round 13. International Uveitis Study Group (IUSG). 2025. https://www.youtube.com/watch?v=68KYOCmrTyl.

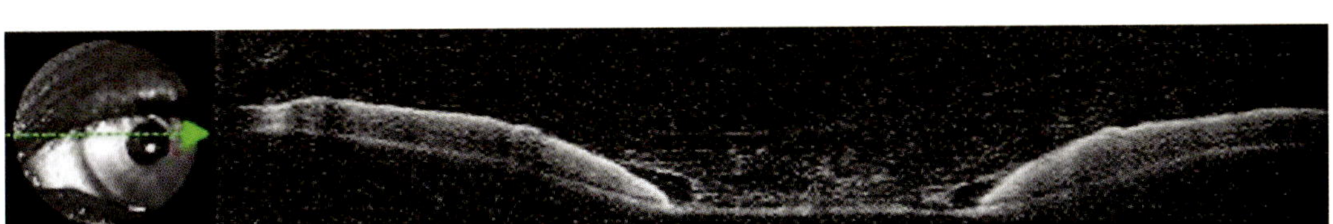

Fig. 2: An anterior segment OCT of the left eye at presentation showing fibrin deposition over the lens capsule and cells in the anterior chamber.
Source: Uveitis Webinar - Grand Round 13. International Uveitis Study Group (IUSG). 2025. https://www.youtube.com/watch?v=68KYOCmrTyl.

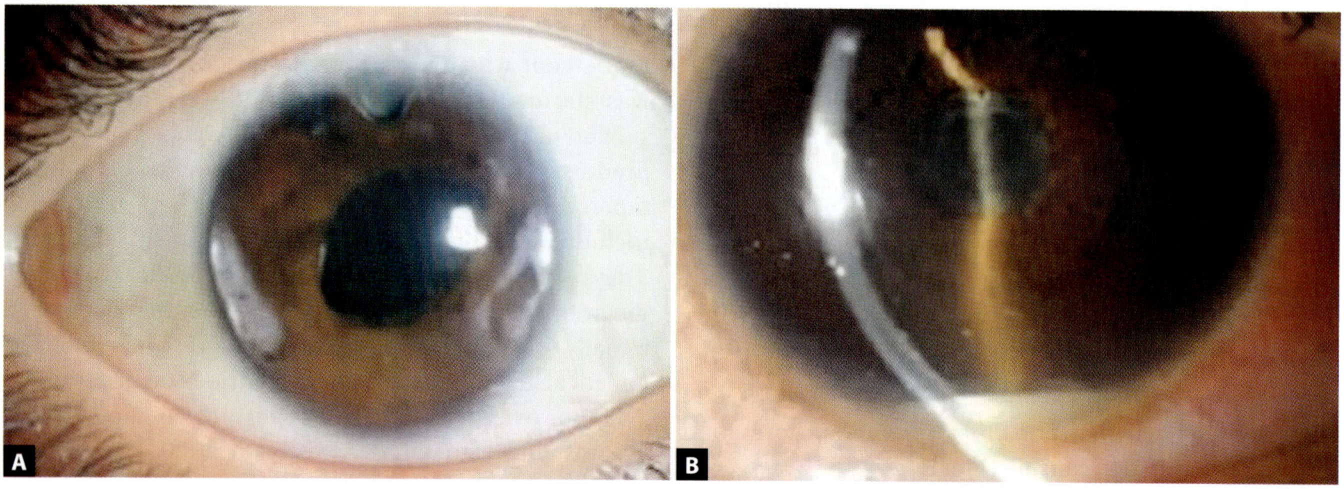

Figs. 3A and B: Slit lamp photo of an inflamed eye without injection in a patient with JIA-associated anterior uveitis (A). Another slit lamp photo (B) shows the more common presentation of conjunctival injection and hypopyon formation in active HLA-B27 anterior uveitis. (HLA-B27: human leukocyte antigen B27; IUSG: International Uveitis Study Group; JIA: juvenile idiopathic arthritis)
Source: Uveitis Webinar - Grand Round 13. International Uveitis Study Group (IUSG). 2025. https://www.youtube.com/watch?v=68KYOCmrTyl.

still on the same dose of golimumab and methotrexate in addition to one drop of tropicamide 10 mg/mL nightly.

Discussion

Children account for 6% of all cases of uveitis, and of these, 50% are due to JIA-associated uveitis.[20-22] The onset of JIA-associated uveitis peaks between 6 months and 4 years of age, with 90% of cases presenting within 4 years of diagnosis and only 3–7% experiencing ocular symptoms before joint inflammation. The most common presentations are chronic anterior uveitis (CAU) and acute or recurrent anterior uveitis. CAU in the pediatric patient often presents asymptomatically with an insidious onset, emphasizing the importance of screening exams. It is bilateral in 70–85% of patients and presents with a normal or reduced IOP, with the latter occurring in an inflamed eye. The characteristic appearance on exam is a white eye that lacks external signs of inflammation **(Figs. 3A and B)**, yet cells and flare are visible in the anterior chamber.

Human leukocyte antigen B27 positivity is associated with enthesitis-related JIA, and the gene is present in 8–10% of the Caucasian population. Most cases of ankylosing spondylitis-associated uveitis or enthesitis-related uveitis present as acute, non-granulomatous anterior uveitis.[23] Episodes may be monophasic or recurrent, unilateral, alternating, or rarely bilateral. The inflammatory episode is often highly symptomatic with photophobia. Pain and blurred vision typically are preceded by characteristic prodromal symptoms within three days of onset. During a flare, ophthalmic exams show intense ciliary flush, significant anterior chamber inflammation with cells and fibrin formation over the pupil with or without a hypopyon **(Figs. 3A and B)**. Synechiae formation and low IOP are also common. The posterior segment is usually unaffected, but macular or optic disc edema may be present in severe, untreated, or chronic cases.[24] Given the potential for these posterior pole complications, further examination with OCT scans through the macula and/or fluorescein angiography is recommended.[25]

Regarding topical treatment, initial dosage and choice of drug potency depend on the severity of uveitis, but it is typically dosed initially every 1 hour while awake to three drops per day **(Table 3)**. Tapering follows a typical pattern, reducing by one drop every 5–10 days. Prolonged use should be minimized in children to minimize the risk of cataract and glaucoma. Cycloplegic eye drops are commonly used to prevent posterior synechiae formation and reduce the pain of ciliary muscle spasm in cases of active uveitis. Unilateral cycloplegia is avoided in young children to prevent amblyopia. Mydriatics are used to break synechiae **(Table 4)**.

Methotrexate is the first-line corticosteroid-sparing systemic treatment for managing JIA-associated uveitis, followed by adalimumab and other monoclonal TNF-inhibitors, such as infliximab and golimumab. These biologics are increasingly used for both as monotherapy and in combination therapy **(Tables 5 and 6)** and have significantly enhanced the visual prognosis for these young patients.[26,27] A multidisciplinary approach, including a

TABLE 3: A list of commonly used corticosteroid eye drops for the treatment of anterior uveitis with dosing recommendations.

Drug name	***Potency***	***Key features***	***Initial frequency***
Prednisolone acetate 1%	++++	First-line treatment for severe active uveitis of cells 3–4+, with a higher risk of cataract and glaucoma	Every 1–2 hours, not available in all countries
Dexamethasone: 2 mg/mL, 1.5 mg/mL, 1 mg/mL	+++	First-line treatment for active uveitis with cells 2+, at medium risk for cataract or glaucoma	Every 1–2 hours to every 2–3 hours
Loteprednol etabonate 0.5%	++	Preferred for long-term use, with fewer side effects	Every 4–6 hours
Fluorometholone 0.1%	++	Lower risk of increased IOP	Every 4–6 hours
Rimexolone 1%	++	Lower risk of increased IOP	Every 4–6 hours

Source: Uveitis Webinar - Grand Round 13. International Uveitis Study Group (IUSG). 2025. https://www.youtube.com/watch?v=68KYOCmrTyI.

TABLE 4: A list of commonly used dilating or cycloplegic eye drops for the treatment of anterior uveitis with dosing recommendations.

Drug name	***Duration***	***Recommended use***	***Dosing***
Atropine 1% (0.5% in less severe cases)	7–14 days	The best choice for children with uveitis and a higher risk of synechiae development. It also has a higher risk for the development of anticholinergic side effects systemically	1 drop, one to two times daily
Cyclopentolate 1%	12–24 hours	These agents should be used in less severe cases	1 drop, two to three times daily
Homatropine 1%	24–48 hours	This is an alternative for mild cases	1 drop, two to three times daily
Tropicamide 1%	4–6 hours	It is generally insufficient for the treatment and prevention of synechiae. It is useful for diagnostic exams and as night-time dilation treatment	1 drop, one to four times daily
Phenylephrine 2.5%*	3–6 hours	A pure mydriatic is used in combination with atropine or cyclopentolate to enhance pupillary dilation	1 drop, two to three times daily

*Phenylephrine 10% causes a higher risk of systemic side effects and should only be used in patients with resistant synechiae with cardiac monitoring.
Source: Uveitis Webinar - Grand Round 13. International Uveitis Study Group (IUSG). 2025. https://www.youtube.com/watch?v=68KYOCmrTyI.

TABLE 5: A list of commonly used nonbiologic systemic immunosuppressive agents for the treatment of chronic JIA-associated anterior uveitis with dosing recommendations.

Drug	***Mechanism***	***Pediatric dosage***	***Side effects***	***Monitoring tests***	***Monitoring frequency***
Methotrexate (On-label for JIA and JIA-associated uveitis in Europe)	Dihydrofolate reductase inhibitor	10–15 mg/m^2/week (oral or SC)	Nausea, stomatitis, hepatotoxicity, myelosuppression	CBC, liver enzymes, creatinine	Every 4–8 weeks
Mycophenolate mofetil (off-label)	Purine synthesis inhibitor	600–1200 mg/m^2/day divided into two doses	Diarrhea, leukopenia, opportunistic infections	CBC, liver enzymes, creatinine	Every 4–8 weeks
Azathioprine (off-label)	Purine antagonist, lymphocyte proliferation inhibitor	1–3 mg/kg/day	Myelosuppression, hepatotoxicity, pancreatitis	CBC, liver enzymes, amylase, lipase	Every 4–8 weeks
Cyclosporine (off-label)	Calcineurin inhibitor, reduced lymphocyte activation	2–5 mg/kg/day in two doses	Hypertension, nephrotoxicity, and gingival hyperplasia	Blood pressure, creatinine, liver enzymes	Every 4–8 weeks
Tacrolimus (off-label)	Calcineurin inhibitor	0.05–0.2 mg/kg/day in two doses	Nephrotoxicity, hypertension	Blood pressure, creatinine	Every 4–8 weeks

(CBC: complete blood count; SC: subcutaneous)
Source: Uveitis Webinar - Grand Round 13. International Uveitis Study Group (IUSG). 2025. https://www.youtube.com/watch?v=68KYOCmrTyI.

TABLE 6: A list of commonly used biologic systemic immunosuppressive agents for the treatment of chronic JIA-associated anterior uveitis with dosing recommendations.

Drug	Mechanism	Dosage	Side effects	Monitoring tests	Monitoring frequency
Adalimumab (first choice agent), on label for JIA and JIA-associated uveitis in Europe	Monoclonal TNFα inhibitor	SQ: 20 mg/kg every 2 weeks (≤30 kg) 40 mg every 2 weeks (>40 kg)	Increased infection risk, injection site reactions, headache	Quanti-FERON gold, CBC, liver enzyme test	Before treatment, then every 3–6 months (Quanti-FERON gold every year)
Infliximab (off-label)	Monoclonal TNFα inhibitor	IV: 5–10 mg/kg every 4–8 weeks (Induction: week 0, 2, and 4)	Increased infection risk, injection site infusion reactions, headache	Quanti-FERON gold, CBC, liver enzyme test	Before treatment, then every 3–6 months (Quanti-FERON gold every year)
Golimumab (on-label)	Monoclonal TNFα inhibitor	SC: 30 mg/m^2/monthly (<40 kg) 50 mg/m^2/monthly (>40 kg)	Increased infection risk, injection site reactions	Quanti-FERON gold, CBC, liver enzyme test	Before treatment, then every 3–6 months (Quanti-FERON gold every year)
Tocilizumab (on-label)	IL-6 inhibitor	8–10 mg/kg every 4 weeks (IV or SC)	Increased infection risk, neutropenia, hyperlipidemia	Quanti-FERON gold, CBC, liver enzyme test, lipid profile	Every 4–8 weeks (Quanti-FERON gold every year)

(CBC: complete blood count; IL-6: interleukin-6; SQ: subcutaneous; IV: intravenous)
Source: Uveitis Webinar - Grand Round 13. International Uveitis Study Group (IUSG). 2025. https://www.youtube.com/watch?v=68KYOCmrTyl.

pediatric rheumatologist, is essential for the effective management of JIA-associated uveitis.

SEVERE JUVENILE IDIOPATHIC ARTHRITIS-ASSOCIATED UVEITIS WITH STRUCTURAL DAMAGE

Case Presentation

Personal Data

A 5-year-old girl whose mother noticed right eye redness and difficulty focusing.

History of Present Illness

She had recurrent episodes of redness of the right eye over the last few months, which were treated with a topical antibiotic ointment by the family doctor. A review of systems was negative for arthralgias, skin rash, fever, abdominal pain, diarrhea, or shortness of breath. The family history was positive for the patient's mother being diagnosed with rheumatoid arthritis at age 22 and treated with etanercept for 2 years. She was currently in remission. A brother also was diagnosed with Celiac disease.

Physical Examination

On presentation to the emergency room, the vision in the right eye was counting fingers, and 0.3 in the left eye. Band keratopathy and cataract formation were present in the right eye **(Table 7) (Fig. 4)**.

TABLE 7: Physical examination of a patient having severe JIA-associated uveitis with structural damage.

OD	Parameter	OS
CF	BCVA	0.3
24 mm Hg	IOP	16 mm Hg
Quiet	Conjunctiva	Quiet
Band keratopathy, white KP	Cornea	White KP
1+ cell, 3+ flare	Anterior chamber	1+ cell, 3+ flare
Posterior synechiae with atrophy	Iris	No synechiae
2+ cortical	Lens	Clear
No view due to cataract	Vitreous	Unremarkable
No view due to cataract	Fundus	Normal

(BCVA: best corrected visual acuity, IOP: intraocular pressure, CF: counting fingers, KP: keratic precipitates)

- *Ancillary testing:* A B-scan showed an attached retina with macular edema in the right eye **(Fig. 5)**. Testing for Celiac disease was negative. Rheumatology was consulted, and no systemic inflammation or joint inflammation was found.

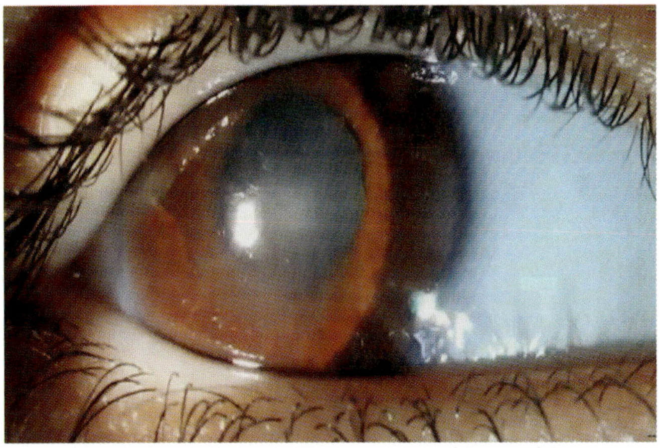

Fig. 4: Slit lamp photo of the right eye showing formation of band keratopathy without conjunctival injection.
Source: Uveitis Webinar - Grand Round 13. International Uveitis Study Group (IUSG). 2025. https://www.youtube.com/watch?v=68KYOCmrTyl.

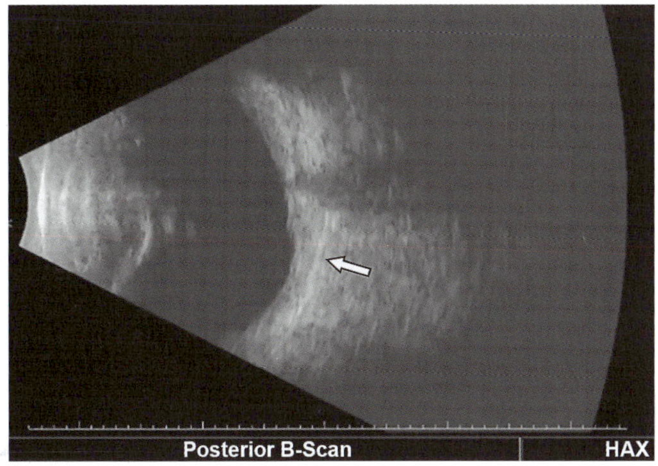

Fig. 5: A B-scan image of the right eye with the arrow highlighting the presence of macular edema.
Source: Uveitis Webinar - Grand Round 13. International Uveitis Study Group (IUSG). 2025. https://www.youtube.com/watch?v=68KYOCmrTyl.

Uveitis Workup

The patient was evaluated by a glaucoma specialist, and gonioscopy showed an open angle without anterior synechiae or neovascularization. Serologic testing revealed a positive ANA and a negative RF. Additional testing was negative for hepatitis B, hepatitis C, and anti-double-stranded DNA antibodies. The Manatoux test was also negative.

Anatomic Diagnosis

The differential diagnosis included JIA-associated uveitis, tubulointerstitial nephritis and uveitis syndrome, and sarcoidosis.

Initial Treatment

She was started on topical prednisolone acetate 1% three times a day in both eyes; timolol-dorzolamide drops twice a day in the right eye, and oral corticosteroids at 2 mg/kg/day. Two weeks later, subcutaneous methotrexate 5 mg/week was initiated.

Follow-up

Three weeks later, the patient returned to the emergency department with periorbital pain around the right eye for several hours. The IOP in the right eye was 40 mmHg, and she was given one drop of timolol-dorzolamide, brimonidine, pilocarpine, and latanoprost, resulting in a change to decrease in the IOP to 17 mmHg after 1 hour. She was discharged with plans to continue methotrexate 5 mg/week and taper the oral corticosteroids from 30 mg/day for 1 week to 20 mg/day until seen again in the clinic. She was also to continue timolol-dorzolamide two times a day, along with the addition of brimonidine three times a day, pilocarpine three times a day, and latanoprost once daily in the right eye.

The patient returned to the uveitis clinic 1 week later. Dense cataract formation led to anterior chamber angle narrowing and elevation of IOP to 46 mmHg in the right eye **(Figs. 6A and B)**, and she underwent urgent cataract removal and anterior vitrectomy without IOL placement the next day.

Two weeks postoperatively, her exam had improved. There was a decrease from 1+ to 0.5+ cells, and the IOP had fallen to 18 mmHg. The vision in the aphakic right eye was hand motion, and OCT imaging of the optic nerve showed diffuse nerve fiber thinning. An OCT scan through the macula showed cystoid macular edema **(Fig. 7)**. The patient was started on adalimumab 20 mg every 2 weeks, nepafenac drops three times a day in the right eye, and she was continued on the oral corticosteroid taper at 12 mg/day with methotrexate 5 mg/week.

At her final follow-up 3 years later, her best corrected visual acuity was 0.3 in the right eye with a contact lens and 1.00 in the left eye with glasses. The anterior chamber was quiet bilaterally with aphakia in the right eye. IOP was controlled at 18 mmHg and 14 mmHg in the right and left eyes, respectively. There were no signs of macular edema. Her treatment regimen consisted of 20 mg adalimumab every 2 weeks, 7.5 mg methotrexate injected

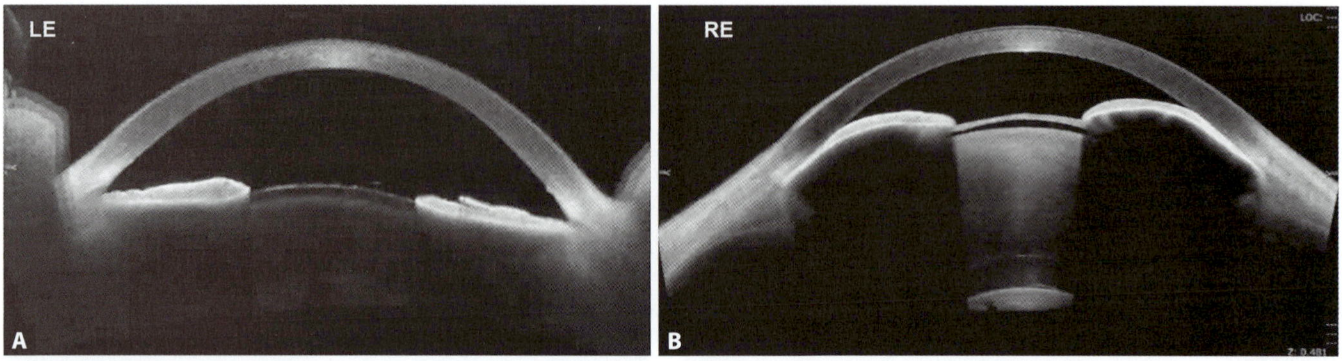

Figs. 6A and B: An anterior segment optical coherence tomography (OCT) showing an open angle in the left eye (LE) and angle closure in the right eye (RE).
Source: Uveitis Webinar - Grand Round 13. International Uveitis Study Group (IUSG). 2025. https://www.youtube.com/watch?v=68KYOCmrTyl.

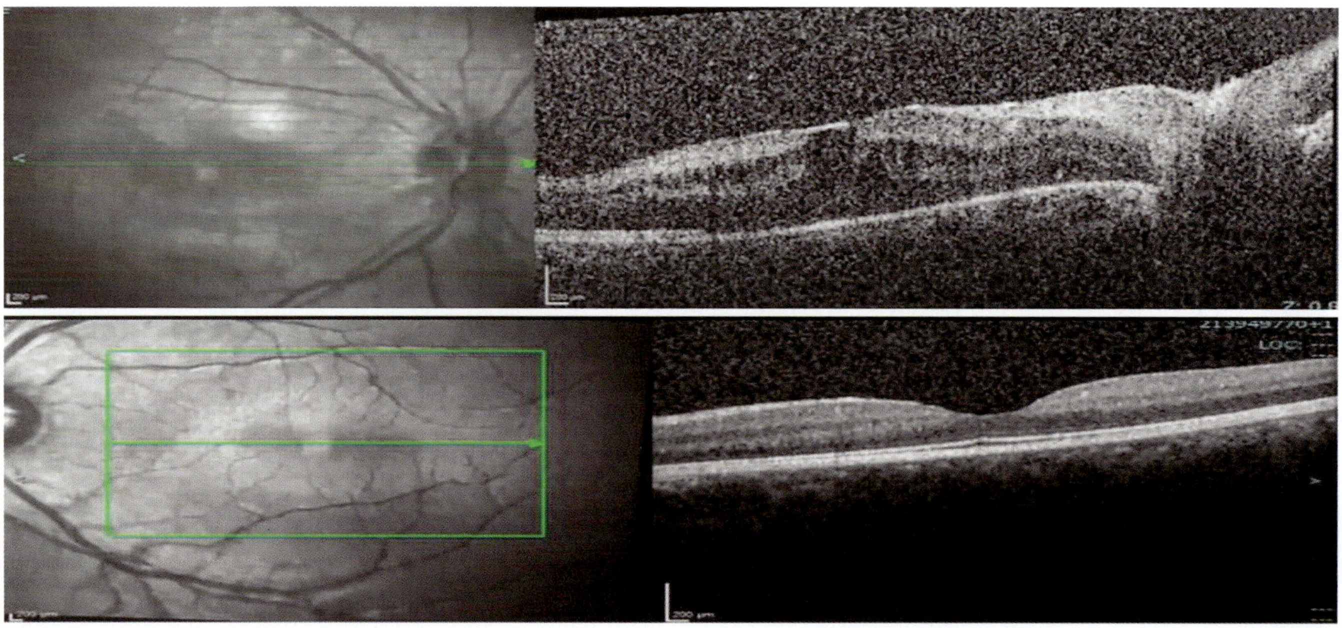

Fig. 7: A posterior segment of OCT with scans through the macula showing cystoid macular edema in the right eye (superior) and a preserved foveal contour in the left eye (inferior).
Source: Uveitis Webinar - Grand Round 13. International Uveitis Study Group (IUSG). 2025. https://www.youtube.com/watch?v=68KYOCmrTyl.

subcutaneously weekly, and both timolol-dorzolamide and brimonidine drops twice daily.

Discussion

Ocular complications of uveitis in this case included band keratopathy, posterior synechiae, a shallow anterior chamber, cataract, iris atrophy, glaucoma, and macular edema. Looking at the prevalence of these complications, numerous studies have documented ocular complications occurring in 30–67% of cases. The most common complications are posterior synechiae, cataract, and band keratopathy. Risk factors for ocular complications include the duration of uveitis, a short duration between diagnosis of arthritis and uveitis, ANA positivity, and the presence of ≥1+ anterior chamber flare at presentation. These are the same risk factors associated with poor vision or ≤20/50, at presentation.[28] Predictors of complications at the final visit include the presence of complications on the first visit (Odds ratio = 80.2) and having uveitis before the diagnosis of arthritis (Odds ratio: 20.8).[29]

Cataract is the most common complication causing reversible vision loss. It occurs in approximately one-third of patients, and in children, it is known to lead to amblyopia. Several studies have confirmed this increased incidence in patients with uveitis, with one paper from Scandinavia reporting cataract development in all patients who were diagnosed with uveitis before joint involvement.[30] Another study reported that the presence of posterior synechiae at the time of diagnosis of uveitis resulted in a significantly shorter interval to cataract extraction compared to those without synechiae development (3.5 vs. 6.6 years).[31] When methotrexate was started during the first year after the diagnosis of uveitis, the development of cataract was postponed by 3.5 years. This study also demonstrated that, among children who initially presented with uveitis rather than joint disease, the interval to cataract extraction was significantly shorter. It was concluded that the presence of posterior synechiae may be an indication for prompt treatment with methotrexate to delay the time until cataract extraction is needed (3.5 versus 6.6 years).

Since the introduction of immunosuppressive medications, the treatment goal has been a zero tolerance of inflammation. This improved outcomes of cataract surgery in patients with JIA-associated uveitis. It is recommended that the anterior chamber be free of inflammation for at least 3 months, and that patients receive perioperative corticosteroids before surgery. However, the surgical treatment of JIA-associated cataract remains challenging, with a major point of controversy surrounding whether to implant an IOL. Risks with IOL implantation include increased inflammation and the formation of membranes over the IOL. This leads to cocooning of the IOL, displacement, pupillary distortion, and cyclitic membrane formation. Such complications can eventually result in chronic hypotony and phthisis bulbi. The surgical approach needs to be considered on a patient-specific basis.

One might consider IOL implantation in patients with JIA-associated uveitis who are given adequate immunosuppression and have well-controlled inflammation. Others may choose to perform a combined lensectomy-vitrectomy without IOL implantation with postoperative contact lens use. In 2010, a study showing the long-term ocular complications in pseudophakic versus aphakic eyes found no difference in complication rates between the two groups and better corrected vision in the IOL group.[32] Another study comparing lensectomy with primary versus secondary IOL implantation showed secondary implantation with a delay of 1 year had a lower rate of inflammation-related complications, including secondary glaucoma and retrolental membrane formation.[33] In 2021, a comparison of biologic and antimetabolite immunosuppressive therapies showed similar ages at diagnosis; however, patients receiving biologic therapy were older at the time of surgery.[34] It was concluded that immunotherapy with biologic immunosuppressive agents improved visual outcomes after cataract surgery in JIA-associated uveitis patients, but did not significantly reduce post-operative ocular complications.

A second complication that occurs with JIA-associated uveitis is macular edema. This complication is present in approximately 3% of eyes at presentation. A study examining retinal changes on OCT in patients with JIA-associated uveitis reported an incidence of maculopathy of 84%, compared with 12% reported in the literature.[35] Manifestations included perifoveolar thickening, macular edema, foveal detachment, and atrophic changes. A study from the Netherlands in 2015 concluded that macular edema was a later complication, occurring in 26.5% of patients, with a mean of 11.6 years after diagnosis.[36] Another study showed that uveitis as the first manifestation of JIA was an independent risk factor for macular edema and that increased macular thickness was negatively correlated with the best corrected vision.[37] This was confirmed in a later study from Germany, which showed that macular edema is a late complication, occurring approximately 5.3 years after a diagnosis of uveitis. Patients with macular edema were generally older and had experienced more ocular complications. Flare was also noted to increase in the 6 months leading up to the diagnosis of macular edema. Fortunately, clinical outcomes are improving for patients with JIA-associated uveitis in the era of biologic therapy. In patients diagnosed after 2010, there has been a decrease in cataract surgery, secondary glaucoma, legal blindness, and visual impairment due to early referrals for tertiary ophthalmic care and the early initiation of immunosuppressive therapies.[38]

Though similar, is there a need for different treatments in patients with idiopathic CAU versus JIA-associated uveitis? A study of the prospective, nationwide pediatric rheumatologic database (NPRD) in Germany stratified patients into groups of those diagnosed with uveitis alone, arthritis before uveitis, or uveitis before arthritis. The phenotype of those with uveitis was similar between all three groups: (1) anteriorly located, (2) bilateral, and (3) insidious in onset. Visual acuity was worse in eyes with uveitis only or those who had uveitis diagnosed before arthritis. The better vision in patients presenting with arthritis first was deemed the result of the referral to ophthalmology for screening exams. Similarly, complication rates were also highest in patients with uveitis only or who developed uveitis first. There were no differences in the groups with regard to the use of systemic corticosteroids, antimetabolites, or biologic therapies. However, a minimal difference was observed across subgroups in the frequency of quiescence.[39] Thus, the study concluded that these are analogous diseases that require immunosuppression.

This case highlights several important concepts, including the risk of visual impairment, the necessity for early diagnosis and initiation of treatment, and the need for universal vision screening in childhood.

TABLE 8: Physical examination of a patient having juvenile idiopathic arthritis-associated uveitis.

OD	*Parameter*	*OS*
6/6	BCVA	6/36
14 mm Hg	IOP	12 mm Hg
White and quiet	Conjunctiva	White and quiet
Clear	Cornea	Band keratopathy
Quiet	Anterior chamber	3+ cells
No synechiae	Iris	360° of synechiae
Clear	Lens	Clear
Unremarkable	Vitreous	Unremarkable
Normal	Fundus	Cystoid macular edema

(BCVA: best corrected visual acuity, IOP: intraocular pressure)

A CHALLENGING CASE OF JUVENILE IDIOPATHIC ARTHRITIS-ASSOCIATED UVEITIS

Case Presentation

Personal Data

A 2-year-old boy presented with stiff and aching joints, worse in the morning and predominantly in the ankles.

History of Present Illness

He was diagnosed with oligoarthritic JIA and initially managed with non-steroidal anti-inflammatory medications. After a few months with poor response, he was admitted for intra-articular corticosteroid injections and concurrently started on prednisone at 15 mg for one week, then 10 mg for 1 week, then it was discontinued. He was also started on oral methotrexate 15 mg/m^2/weekly. Throughout treatment, ophthalmic screenings were negative.

Physical Examination

On presentation to our clinic, he had severe left-sided anterior chamber inflammation with 360 posterior synechiae formation, cystoid macular edema, band keratopathy, and an associated reduction in visual acuity resulting in amblyopia **(Table 8)**.

Ancillary Testing

Optical coherence tomography imaging showed cystoid macular edema of the left eye.

Uveitis Workup

Based on the history of JIA, no additional testing was ordered.

Anatomic Diagnosis

The patient was diagnosed with CAU associated with oligoarthritic JIA and amblyopia.

Initial Treatment

He was admitted to the hospital for IV methylprednisolone 1 g daily for 3 days, a sub-Tenon injection of triamcinolone performed in the left eye, and the patient was enrolled into the SYCAMORE (Safety and Cost-effectiveness of Adalimumab in Combination with Methotrexate for the Treatment of Juvenile Idiopathic Arthritis associated Uveitis) trial with randomization to adalimumab 20 mg every 2 weeks. He was additionally started on methotrexate 10mg weekly and prednisolone acetate 1% hourly, reducing by 1 drop per week decrements according to clinical response **(Fig. 8)**.

Follow-up

The patient was followed from 2008 to 2012. While the cystoid macular edema resolved, an epiretinal membrane formed in the left eye. He underwent patching for treatment of amblyopia in addition to the use of atropine drops. His eyes remained quiet with amblyopia improving to 6/9.5. He requested to stop adalimumab at that time; however, three months later, he presented with bilateral, 2+ anterior chamber cells, and adalimumab was restarted.

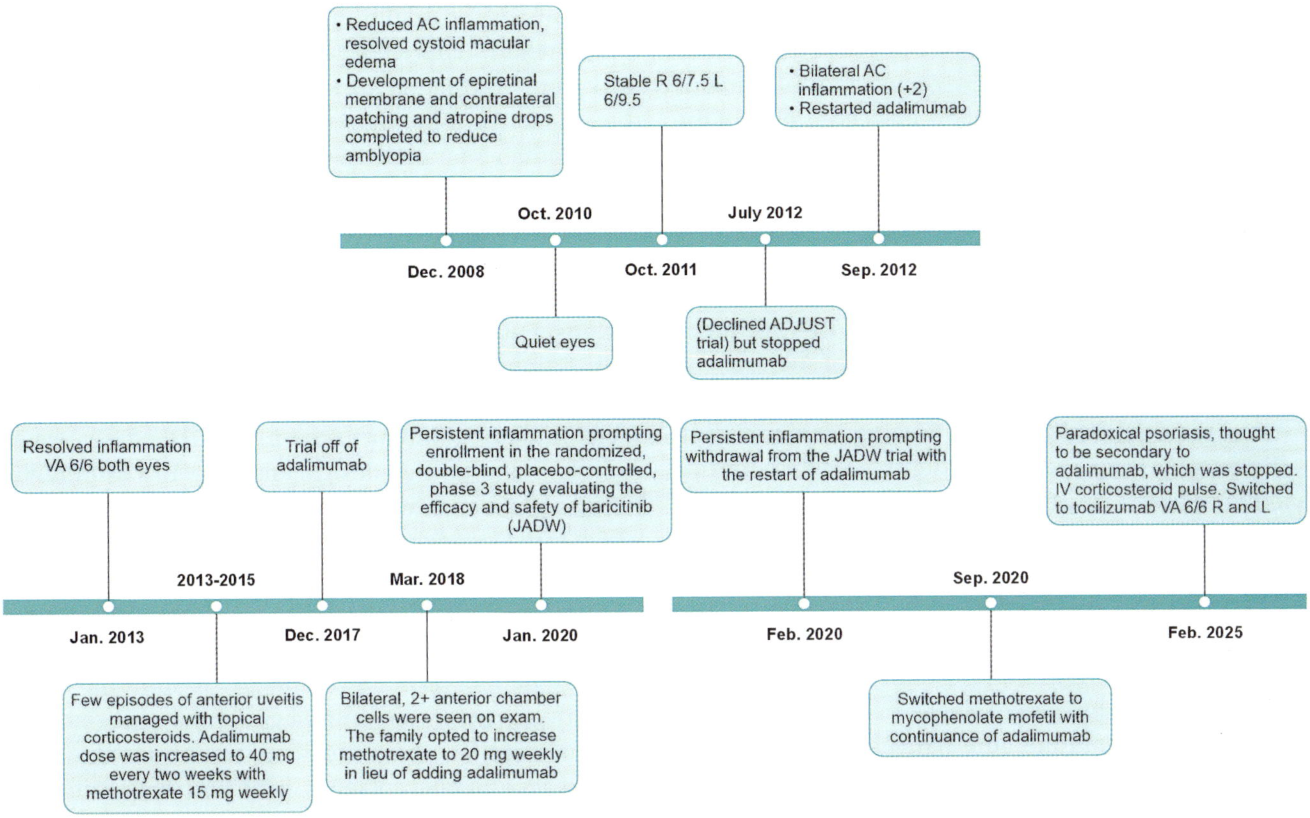

Fig. 8: A timeline of the clinical activity and treatments. (VA: visual acuity; AC: anterior chamber; IV: intravenous.)
Source: Uveitis Webinar - Grand Round 13. International Uveitis Study Group (IUSG). 2025. https://www.youtube.com/watch?v=68KYOCmrTyl.

Over the next 5 years, he developed several flares of anterior uveitis, which were managed with topical corticosteroids and dosing of adalimumab was increased to 40 mg every 2 weeks with 15 mg methotrexate weekly.

He again tried discontinuing adalimumab in December of 2017, but had a relapse of uveitis 3 months later. He was recruited for the JADW trial, which assessed the efficacy of baricitinib 4 mg daily in biologic and antimetabolite treatment-resistant JIA-uveitis. Persistent inflammation resulted in withdrawal from the trial a month later with resumption of adalimumab. Seven months later, methotrexate was changed to mycophenolate mofetil in September 2020. Most recently, he experienced paradoxical psoriasis due to adalimumab. He was treated with an IV corticosteroid pulse and switched to tocilizumab. The patient continues to have 6/6 visual acuity in both eyes with controlled IOPs.

Discussion

In the SYCAMORE trial, our key goal was to include JIA-associated uveitis patients because the regulatory bodies, such as the United States Food and Drug Administration and the European Medicines Agency, did not recognize that CAU without arthritis is the same disease.[11] Through multiple publications, it has been shown that adalimumab decreases ocular inflammation and allows for a significant drop in topical corticosteroid use to less than two drops per day. The ultimate goal is achieving no anterior chamber cells on examination without the use of topical corticosteroid drops, which is possible with adalimumab use.

One trial not mentioned in the earlier discussion is the APTITUDE trial.[39] When adalimumab became the standard of care in methotrexate refractory patients, a head-to-head trial comparing the efficacy of adalimumab to tocilizumab became difficult. We recruited children who had already failed methotrexate and a TNF-inhibitor and started subcutaneous tocilizumab, as many children do not want to come into the hospital for IV infusions. In children with arthritis, we had already shown that subcutaneous and IV administrations of tocilizumab were equally effective. This was an open-label, single-arm, phase 2 trial using a stop-and-go, two-stage design. The first 10 children received open-label access to tocilizumab with a pre-specified requirement of two to three patients meeting clinical endpoints to allow for recruitment of the full complement of 21 patients. Of the 22 patients that were recruited, one child dropped out for logistical reasons. In the remaining 21 patients, seven had a 2-step decrease in anterior chamber cell count by week 12. Considering these patients had previously failed both methotrexate and one anti-TNFα, treatment with an anti-IL-6 agent was successful in 1/3 of patients. Another 20% of subjects had one-step improvement by week 12, which is a limitation of using the Standardization of Uveitis Nomenclature grading scale. If you recruit patients with 1+ anterior chamber cells, it is very hard to achieve no cells compared to achieving a 2-step decrease in patients with 3+ or 4+ cells at enrollment.

There are two reasons why it is a struggle to stop adalimumab. One possibility is that we are missing the immunological window of opportunity. If biologics are initiated too late, the patient needs to stay on the drug for longer periods of time. Alternatively, uveitis may be more proinflammatory than arthritis, and patients may need long-term treatment. The key variables to mention are the need to have inactive uveitis for 1 year, where most enrollees had inactive uveitis for two full years. The data show that even 2 full years of inactive disease is not enough to stop the drug. The reason for this may be a combination of both reasons previously mentioned.

A newer class of medications that show promise in the treatment of JIA-associated uveitis is Janus kinase (JAK) inhibitors. They are upstream modifiers that affect hematopoiesis and Th17 cell differentiation. Clinical efficacy has been demonstrated in the treatment of inflammatory bowel disease, given the alteration of the IL-12 and IL-23 axes. The pleotropic effects of cytokines have also led to clinical trials to determine efficacy in alopecia, atopic dermatitis, and hidradenitis suppurativa. In the JUVE-BRIGHT trial, which is currently under review, 20 patients with chronic uveitis refractory to methotrexate and adalimumab received open-label baricitinib in this active-controlled, phase 3 study.[40] A reference arm to comparative efficacy was comprised of another 10 patients randomized to adalimumab or baricitinib. The primary endpoint was a two-step decrease in anterior chamber cells per the Standardization of Uveitis Nomenclature (SUN) criteria by week 24. In the cohort, 19 patients refractory to both adalimumab and methotrexate, compared with 5 patients in the adalimumab arm who had only failed methotrexate. There was a 30% response to baricitinib in patients refractory to adalimumab. When assessing the efficacy of a biologic medication in naive patients, adalimumab is far more effective than a JAK inhibitor.

The take-home message is that adalimumab remains the first-choice agent after methotrexate. In patients who have continued inflammation despite treatment with adalimumab, tocilizumab or baricitinib are third-line options. Future directions include assessing the efficacy of IL-17 inhibitors. We have completed the first phase of the TURTLE trial, which examined IL-17 inhibition with secukinumab.[41] Similar to the APTITUDE study, we are using the stop-and-go design, enrolling 10 TNF-inhibitor refractory patients into the high-dose secukinumab arm, which is the same dose used to treat psoriasis rather than psoriatic arthritis. If clinical endpoints are met for three or more patients, there will be a 1:1 randomization of secukinumab versus adalimumab. As uveitis specialists, we have patients who are refractory to multiple agents. Local therapy with intravitreal corticosteroids remains a treatment option, and we plan on starting a trial to assess the efficacy and safety of intravitreal fluocinolone implants (0.19 mg) in children with non-infectious posterior and panuveitis.

PEARLS FROM THE EXPERTS ON FREQUENTLY ASKED QUESTIONS

1. How often do you see a family history of autoimmune disease in patients with JIA-uveitis?

Answer: While this is not common, it is not unexpected. Data show an increased risk of the same or different autoimmune disorders in immediate family members.

2. In patients refractory to adalimumab, should drug and antibody levels be measured?

Answer: Yes, checking both drug and antibody levels is important to understand the cause of the lack of response to adalimumab. There appears to be a biphasic pattern to a lack of clinical response, either at 3–6 months or 18–24 months. High anti-adalimumab antibodies and low drug levels in a patient not on methotrexate warrant a trial of mycophenolate as an alternative. Conversely, escalating to weekly dosing of adalimumab is another option. If you have normal drug levels and no antibody formation without efficacy, a switch of immunosuppressive therapies should be considered.

3. Is there concern in other countries about the ingredients of certain topical therapies? What risks and benefits are there?

Answer: Band keratopathy is composed of calcium phosphate, and instillation of topical corticosteroids containing phosphate may worsen the condition. Other eye drops contain borate, which has been linked to sterility in patients treated with systemic, borate-containing medications. However, the amount present in eye drops is low, and it is questionable whether there is enough of the compound in the formulation to cause sterility. It is worth considering alternatives when present, such as prednisolone acetate versus prednisolone phosphate.

4. What do you think about adalimumab as monotherapy and the first line before methotrexate? Is there a group of patients who can receive adalimumab alone?

Answer: There are studies looking at the efficacy of adalimumab alone versus adalimumab plus methotrexate. As a sole agent, adalimumab is effective. One problem is that methotrexate intolerance has a high prevalence in the West. If a patient has developed ocular complications at presentation, adalimumab should be initiated. One of the primary limitations of adalimumab as monotherapy is cost, which is now less problematic with the release of biosimilars.

5. Is CAU in pediatric patients without associated joint symptoms considered to be part of the JIA spectrum of disease?

Answer: The incidence and prevalence of JIA-associated uveitis are variable for two reasons. First, the early initiation of immunosuppression to treat CAU in a child may prevent the manifestation of joint symptoms and disease. Conversely, early and aggressive use of immunosuppression in patients with joint symptoms lowers the risk for developing uveitis. Recent studies have shown that JIA-associated uveitis is declining as the use of immunosuppressive therapy in these groups increases.[42]

6. Is there a standardized perioperative corticosteroid regimen that is recommended for pediatric patients with a history of uveitis undergoing cataract surgery?

Answer: Due to the risk of IOP rises in children with intravitreal and periocular corticosteroid injections, systemic and topical corticosteroids are preferred pre- and postoperative treatment options. Alternative strategies include the administration of IV methylprednisolone at the time of surgery followed by a short oral corticosteroid taper. Systemic administration has more flexible dosing, and when used over several days, causes limited long-term side effects.

7. How effective are IL-6 inhibitors in treating macular edema?

Answer: A primary cytokine in the development of macular edema is IL-6, with aqueous humor levels that correlate with macular thickness. While access to medication may be limited by cost or insurance approval, use of tocilizumab can be a consideration in patients with both JIA-associated uveitis and macular edema.

8. What is the stepwise treatment approach in patients who are refractory to TNF-inhibitors? Is there a role for anti-CD20 medications?

Answer: The decision of which third-line agent to prescribe should be made on a patient-specific basis. Cost, insurance coverage, and preference for the route of administration are all considerations. Oral formulations in the JAK-inhibitor class do not require injections, and subcutaneous tocilizumab is more convenient than IV infusions. The current literature is not robust enough to determine the effectiveness of anti-CD20 medications.

FINAL WRAP-UP

Juvenile idiopathic arthritis-associated uveitis classically presents as silent, CAU. It may only become symptomatic when ocular complications are present, or vision is compromised. Ophthalmologic screening is essential to prevent complications such as band keratopathy, posterior synechiae, cataract, glaucoma, and macular edema. Risk factors include age at JIA onset of <6–7 years of age, female sex, oligoarthritis subtype, ANA+, and uveitis within the first year of diagnosis. Early initiation of immunosuppression can mitigate the development of ocular complications, and it is escalated in a stepwise approach. First-line agents include antimetabolites followed by adalimumab and other TNF-inhibitors in refractory cases. In patients with a TNF-inhibitor contraindication or in those with continued inflammation, clinical trials have shown some efficacy with the use of tocilizumab and baricitinib.

REFERENCES

1. Long AM, Marston BM. Juvenile Idiopathic Arthritis. Pediatrics in Review. 2023;44(10):565-77.
2. Jabs DA, Nussenblatt RB, Rosenbaum JT; Standardization of Uveitis Nomenclature (SUN) Working Group. Standardization of uveitis nomenclature for reporting clinical data. Results of the First International Workshop. Am J Ophthalmol. 2005;140(3):509-16.

3. Angeles-Han ST, Ringold S, Beukelman T, Lovell D, Cuello CA, Becker ML, et al. 2019 American College of Rheumatology/Arthritis Foundation Guideline for the Screening, Monitoring, and Treatment of Juvenile Idiopathic Arthritis-Associated Uveitis. Arthritis Rheumatol. 2019;71(6):864-77.
4. Thorne JE, Woreta FA, Dunn JP, Jabs DA. Risk of cataract development among children with juvenile idiopathic arthritis-related uveitis treated with topical corticosteroids. Ophthalmology. 2010;117(7):1436-41.
5. Kothari S, Foster CS, Pistilli M, Liesegang TL, Daniel E, Sen HN, et al. The Risk of Intraocular Pressure Elevation in Pediatric Noninfectious Uveitis. Ophthalmology 2015;122(10):1987-2001.
6. Jabs DA. Immunosuppression for the Uveitides. Ophthalmology. 2018;125(2):193-202.
7. Goebel JC, Roesel M, Heinz C, Michels H, Ganser G, Heiligenhaus A. Azathioprine as a Treatment Option for Uveitis in Patients with Juvenile Idiopathic Arthritis. Br J Ophthalmol. 2011;95(2):209-13.
8. Sobrin L, Christen W, Foster CS. Mycophenolate Mofetil after Methotrexate Failure or Intolerance in the Treatment of Scleritis and Uveitis. Ophthalmology. 2008;115(8):1416-21.
9. Simonini G, Paudyal P, Jones GT, Cimaz R, Macfarlane GJ. Current Evidence of Methotrexate Efficacy in Childhood Chronic Uveitis: A Systematic Review and Meta-Analysis Approach. Rheumatology (Oxford). 2013;52(5):825-31.
10. Levy-Clarke G, Jabs DA, Read RW, Rosenbaum JT, Vitale A, Van Gelder RN. Expert panel recommendations for the use of anti-tumor necrosis factor biologic agents in patients with ocular inflammatory disorders. Ophthalmology. 2014;121(3):785-96.e3.
11. Ramanan AV, Dick AD, Jones AP, McKay A, Williamson PR, Compeyrot-Lacassagne S, et al. Adalimumab plus Methotrexate for Uveitis in Juvenile Idiopathic Arthritis. N Engl J Med. 2017;376(17):1637-46.
12. Quartier P, Baptiste A, Despert V, Allain-Launay E, Koné-Paut I, Belot A, et al. ADJUVITE: a double-blind, randomised, placebo-controlled trial of adalimumab in early onset, chronic, juvenile idiopathic arthritis-associated anterior uveitis. Ann Rheum Dis. 2018;77(7):1003-11.
13. Acharya NR, Ramanan AV, Coyne AB, Dudum KL, Rubio EM, Woods SM, et al. Stopping of adalimumab in juvenile idiopathic arthritis-associated uveitis (ADJUST): a multicentre, double-masked, randomised controlled trial. Lancet 2025;405(10475):303-13.
14. Cecchin V, Zannin ME, Ferrari D, Pontikaki I, Miserocchi E, Paroli MP, et al. Longterm Safety and Efficacy of Adalimumab and Infliximab for Uveitis Associated with Juvenile Idiopathic Arthritis. J Rheumatol. 2018;45(8):1167-72.
15. Lanz S, Seidel G, Skrabl-Baumgartner A. Golimumab in juvenile idiopathic arthritis-associated uveitis unresponsive to Adalimumab. Pediatr Rheumatol Online J. 2021;19(1):132.
16. Smith JA, Thompson DJS, Whitcup SM, Suhler E, Clarke G, Smith S, et al. A Randomized, Placebo-Controlled, Double-Masked Clinical Trial of Etanercept for the Treatment of Uveitis Associated with Juvenile Idiopathic Arthritis. Arthritis Rheum. 2005;53(1):18-23.
17. Tappeiner C, Mesquida M, Adán A, Anton J, Ramanan AV, Carreno E, et al. Evidence for Tocilizumab as a Treatment Option in Refractory Uveitis Associated with Juvenile Idiopathic Arthritis. J. Rheumatol. 2016;43(12):2183-8.
18. Iannone C, Marelli L, Costi S, Pellico MS, Franca LL, Caprali R, et al. Tocilizumab in Juvenile Idiopathic Arthritis Associated Uveitis, a Narrative Review. Children (Basel). 2023;10(3):434.
19. Phatak S, Lowder C, Pavesio C. Controversies in intracoular lens implantation in pediatric uveítis. J Ophthalmic Inflamm Infect. 2016;6(1):12.
20. Smith JA, Mackensen F, Sen HN, Leigh JF, Watkins AS, et al. Epidemiology and course of disease in childhood uveitis. Ophthalmology. 2009;116 (8):1544-51.
21. Shin Y, Kang J, Lee J, Lee CS, Lee SC, Ahn JG. Epidemiology of pediatric uveitis and associated systemic disease. Ped Rheumatol Online J. 2021;19(1):48.
22. Paivonsalo-Hietanen T, Tuominen J, Saari KM. Uveitis in children: population-based study in FInland. Acta Ophthalmol Scand. 2000;78(1):84-8.
23. Robinson PC, Claushuis TAM, Cortes A, Martin TM, Evans DM, Leo P, et al. Genetic dissection of acute anterior uveitis releavels similaritis and differences in associations observed with ankylosing spondylitis. Arthritis and Rheumatism. 2015;67(1):140-51.
24. Paroli MP, Fabiani C, Spinucci G, Abicca I, Sapta A, Spadea L. Severe macular edema in patient with juvenile idiopathic arthritis-related uveitis. Case Rep Ophthalmol Med. 2013;2013:803989.
25. Pichi F, Neri P, Hay S, Parrulli S, Zicarelli F, Invernizzi A. An en face swept source optical coherence tomography study of the vitreous in eyes with anterior uveitis. Acta Ophthalmol. 2022;100(3):e820-6.
26. Tarsia M, Vitale A, Gaggiano C, Sota J, Maselli A, Bellantonio C, et al. Effectiveness and Safety of Biosimilars in Pediatric Non-infectious Uveitis: Real-Life Data from the International AIDA Network Uveitis Registry. Ophthalmol Ther. 2024;13(3):761-74.
27. Vitale A, Casa FD, Guerriero S, Ragab G, Mauro A, Caggiano V, et al. Efficacy and Safety of Adalimumab in Pediatric Non-infectious Non-anterior Uveitis: Real-life Experience From the International AIDA Network Uveitis Registry. Ophthalmol Ther. 2023;12(4):1957-71.
28. Rypdal V, Glerup M, Songstad NT, Bertelsen G, Christoffersen T, Arnstad ED, et al. Uveitis in Juvenile Idiopathic Arthritis: 18-Year Outcome in the Population-based Nordic Cohort Study. Ophthalmology. 2021;128(4):598-608.
29. Sijssens KM, Rothova A, Van De Vijver DAMC, Stilma JS, De Boer JH. Risk factors for the development of cataract

requiring surgery in uveitis associated with juvenile idiopathic arthritis. Am J Ophthalmol. 2007;144(4):574-9.
30. Sijssens KM, Los LI, Rothova A, Schellekens Pa WJF, van de Does P, Stilma JS, et al. Long-term ocular complications in aphakic versus pseudophakic eyes of children with juvenile idiopathic arthritis-associated uveitis. Br J Ophthalmol. 2010;94(9):1145-9.
31. Magli A, Forte R, Rombetto L, Alessio M. Cataract Management in Juvenile Idiopathic Arthritis: Simultaneous versus Secondary Intraocular Lens Implantation. Ocul Immunol Inflamm. 2014;22(2):133-7.
32. Bolletta E, Coassin M, Iannetta D, Mastrofilippo V, Aldigeri R, Invernizzi A, et al. Cataract Surgery with Intraocular Lens Implantation in Juvenile Idiopathic Arthritis-Associated Uveitis: Outcomes in the Era of Biological Therapy. J Clin Med 2021;10(11):2437.
33. Ducos de Lahitte G, Terrada C, Tran THC, Cassoux N, LeHoang P, Kodjikian L, et al. Maculopathy in uveitis of juvenile idiopathic arthritis: an optical coherence tomography study. Br J Ophthalmol. 2008;92(1):64-9.
34. de Boer J, Steijaert A, van den Bor R, Stellato R, Ossewaarde-van Norel J. Development of macular edema and impact on visual acuity in uveitis associated with juvenile idiopathic arthritis. Ocul Immunol Inflamm. 2015;23(1):67-73.
35. Tappeiner C, Bae HS, Rothaus K, Walscheid K, Heiligenhaus A. Occurrence and Risk Factors for Macular Edema in Patients with Juvenile Idiopathic Arthritis-Associated Uveitis. J Clin Med. 2021;10(19):4513.
36. Wennink RAW, Kalinina Ayuso V, Pameijer EM, Dekkers CC, Bozkir I, de Boer JH. Improved clinical outcomes in patients with juvenile idiopathic arthritis associated uveitis in the last decade. Acta Ophthalmol. 2022;100(7):781-7.
37. Heiligenhaus A, Klotsche J, Niewerth M, Horneff G, Ganser G, Haas J-P, et al. Similarities in clinical course and outcome between juvenile idiopathic arthritis (JIA)-associated and ANA-positive idiopathic anterior uveitis: data from a population-based nationwide study in Germany. Arthritis Res Ther. 2020;22(1):81.
38. Horton S, Jones AP, Guly CM, Hardwick B, Beresford MW, Lee RW, et al. Adalimumab in Juvenile Idiopathic Arthritis–Associated Uveitis: 5-Year Follow-up of the Bristol Participants of the SYCAMORE Trial. Am J Ophthalmol. 2019;207:170-4.
39. Ramanan AV, Dick AD, Guly C, McKay A, Jones AP, Hardwick B, et al. Tocilizumab in patients with anti-TNF refractory juvenile idiopathic arthritis-associated uveitis (APTITUDE): a multicentre, single-arm, phase 2 trial. Lancet Rheumatol. 2020;2(3):e135-41.
40. Ramanan AV, Guly CM, Keller SY, Schlichting DE, de Bono S, Liao R, et al. Clinical effectiveness and safety of baricitinib for the treatment of juvenile idiopathic arthritis-associated uveitis or chronic anterior antinuclear antibody-positive uveitis: study protocol for an open-label, adalimumab active-controlled phase 3 clinical trial (JUVE-BRIGHT). Trials. 2021;22(1):689.
41. A Randomized Controlled Trial of SecUkinumab VeRsus Adalimumab for the Treatment of JuveniLe Idiopathic Arthritis (JIA) AssociatEd Uveitis using a Bayesian Design – TURTLE. https://www.turtle-trial.org/. Accessed March 16, 2026.
42. Marshall RM, Thorne JE, Berkenstock MK. Prevalence and Incidence of Juvenile Idiopathic Arthritis-Associated Uveitis and Medication Trends in the TriNetX Database. Br J Ophthalmol. 2025;110(1):46-51.

CHAPTER 14

Ocular Complications of Behçet's Disease

Ilknur Tugal-Tutkun, Merve Inanç Tekin, Pinar Ozdal, Wijden Nabi, Moncef Khairallah, Shruthika Bhimewar, Kalpana Babu Murthy, Ramesh Jois, Maggie Feng, Vishali Gupta, John H Kempen, Reema Bansal, Alejandra de-la-Torre, Meghan Berkenstock

INTRODUCTION

Behçet disease (BD) is a systemic vascular inflammatory disorder first described in 1937 and is defined by the triad of recurrent aphthous and genital ulcers with ocular inflammation. Ocular involvement occurs in 50–70% of patients with the predominant features of uveitis and occlusive retinal vasculitis. Given the high risk of visual impairment and progression to legal blindness without treatment, systemic immunosuppressive therapy is required. Understanding the ocular manifestations and therapeutic options in Behçet disease can promote an early diagnosis, treatment, and prevention of both ocular and systemic complications.

THEMATIC LECTURE: AN OVERVIEW OF BEHÇET UVEITIS

Behçet disease was first described as a triple symptom complex of recurrent oral and genital ulcers and uveitis. It is now known that the disease involves several other organ systems characterized by recurrent episodes of inflammation.[1] The disease has the highest prevalence in countries along the ancient "Silk Road," ranging from the Mediterranean basin to Asia. These populations also have the highest prevalences of human leukocyte antigen (HLA)-B51 positivity, with the greatest number occurring in Turkey. The HLA-B51 gene was introduced into modern humans in Eurasia during the Neanderthal period. Genome-wide association studies have confirmed shared genetic factors in the endemic regions.[2] While HLA-B51 has the strongest association with Behçet disease, other weaker associations and non-HLA gene associations have also been identified. An important finding was the epistatic interaction between HLA-B51 and ERAP1, specifically in the Hap10 haplotype.[3] This increases the odds of developing Behçet disease by 11-fold. Hap10 has low enzymatic activity, and this may alter the peptidome affinity for HLA-B51, which results in an altered immune response. It is now thought that environmental factors trigger the disease in genetically susceptible individuals, and this results in a hyperactivated innate immune system and polarized adaptive immunity with organ or tissue specificity. Heterogeneous presentations and phenotypic clusters have been identified.[4-8]

Patients with Behçet disease–associated uveitis stand out as a separate cluster, and uveitis may be the initial or only manifestation of the disease. There is no specific diagnostic test, and HLA-B51 is not a diagnostic criterion in all clinical criteria sets. Ocular lesions have been vaguely defined, even in the Standardization of Uveitis Nomenclature (SUN) classification criteria.[9] Fulfillment of International Study Group for Behçet Disease (ISG) criteria, which was released in 1990, is still required in the recently published criteria set.[10]

Behçet disease–associated uveitis is a distinct uveitic syndrome classically defined as non-granulomatous panuveitis and retinal vasculitis. The natural course is characterized by recurrent, symptomatic, acute inflammatory episodes. Between the inflammatory episodes, there is spontaneous resolution of symptoms, but persistent optic disc and retinal capillary leakage. Patients with Behçet disease are typically young adults, as the onset of disease is rare in children and after 50 years of age, with a more severe disease course and predominance in males.

Signs of inflammation include non-granulomatous, acute anterior segment inflammation, and absent or mild

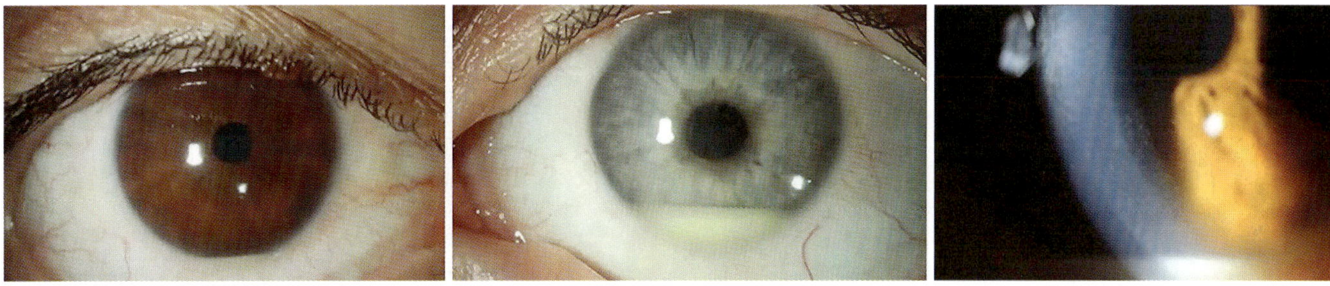

Fig. 1: Slit lamp photos showing several examples of hypopyon without ciliary flush as a common manifestation of Behçet disease-associated uveitis.
Source: Uveitis Webinar - Grand Round 14. International Uveitis Study Group (IUSG). 2025. https://youtu.be/-E8PbG9PkxE?si=XcEXr31C7XMY23RX.

Fig. 2: A color fundus photo of a right eye showing dense vitreous haze limiting the view to the posterior pole in a flare of Behçet disease-associated uveitis.
Source: Uveitis Webinar - Grand Round 14. International Uveitis Study Group (IUSG). 2025. https://youtu.be/-E8PbG9PkxE?si=XcEXr31C7XMY23RX.

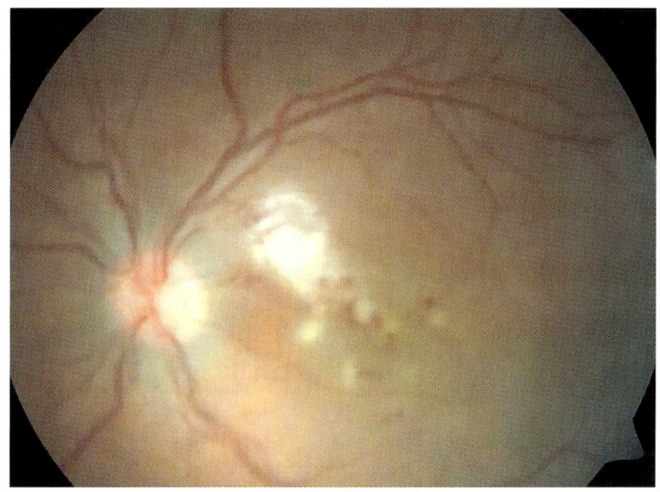

Fig. 3: A color fundus photo of a left eye showing retinal infiltrates extending into the macula with associated capillary hemorrhages.
Source: Uveitis Webinar - Grand Round 14. International Uveitis Study Group (IUSG). 2025. https://youtu.be/-E8PbG9PkxE?si=XcEXr31C7XMY23RX.

ciliary injection that is disproportionate to the high-grade cells. Additionally, a smooth-layered shifting hypopyon and a rapid response to topical corticosteroid treatment support the diagnosis of Behçet disease-associated uveitis **(Fig. 1)**. Granulomatous keratic precipitates (KPs), iris nodules, and a chronic course of anterior uveitis should exclude Behçet disease from the differential diagnosis. Isolated, recurrent anterior uveitis is seen in around 10% of patients. These are mostly women with only mucocutaneous manifestations, but the majority of Behçet disease-associated uveitis patients have significant posterior segment inflammation.

Diffuse vitritis is a constant feature of posterior segment inflammation with the grade of vitreous haze varying based on the episode severity. In severe attacks, the fundus may not even be visualized **(Fig. 2)**. Retinal infiltrates of any size, location, or number are the most commonly seen inflammatory lesions in the fundus **(Fig. 3)**. Fluorescein angiography characteristically shows profuse and predominately capillary leakage. Optical coherence tomography (OCT) scans through the retinal lesions show hyperreflective thickening with variable amounts of subretinal fluid. Occlusive retinal periphlebitis rarely involves the central retina vein, but commonly affects the peripheral or distal branches. Clinically, this is observed as diffuse sheathing of the retinal vessels that phenotypically resembles frosted branch angiitis. This accompanied by extensive hemorrhages in the involved areas leads to the description of Behçet disease-associated uveitis retinal findings as a hemorrhagic, occlusive retinal vasculitis **(Fig. 4)**. The optic disc is invariably inflamed during flares, but isolated inflammation of the optic disc

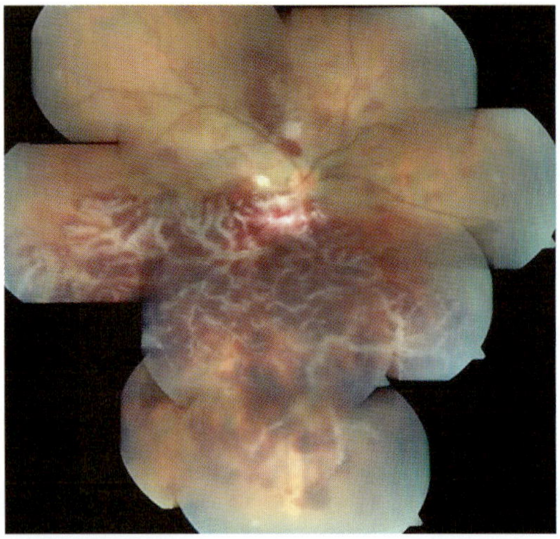

Fig. 4: A montage color fundus photo of a right eye showing occlusive retinal periphlebitis with diffuse sheathing of retinal vessels and retinal hemorrhages.
Source: Uveitis Webinar - Grand Round 14. International Uveitis Study Group (IUSG). 2025. https://youtu.be/-E8PbG9PkxE?si=XcEXr31C7XMY23RX.

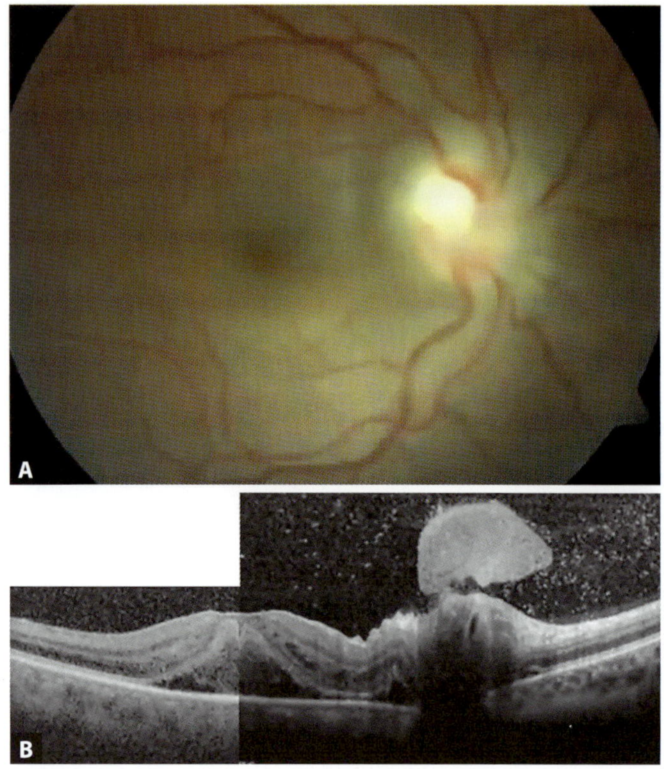

Figs. 5A and B: A color fundus photo (A) showing vitritis and blurred disc margins and (B) an optical coherence tomography (OCT) of the optic nerve (inferior) showing vitreous debris overlying the optic nerve head and subretinal fluid with extension into the macula.
Source: Uveitis Webinar - Grand Round 14. International Uveitis Study Group (IUSG). 2025. https://youtu.be/-E8PbG9PkxE?si=XcEXr31C7XMY23RX.

presents similarly to neuroretinitis with a macular star, which were formerly called disc infiltrates. With the use of OCT, a cloud of hyperreflective infiltrate in the vitreous can be seen overlying the optic disc **(Figs. 5A and B)**. In cases of isolated optic nerve involvement, infectious causes of neuroretinitis still need to be ruled out. A clinically distinguishing feature is the rapid resolution of the infiltrates and retinal exudates with Behçet disease–associated uveitis compared to infectious cases of neuroretinitis.

The frequency and the severity of uveitis flares determine the long-term visual outcome. The severity of a flare is variable and can be asymmetric in cases of bilateral involvement. A scoring system was devised to assess the severity of a flare called the Behcet Disease Ocular Attack Score 24 (BOS24).[11,12] Using a semiquantitative system, anterior chamber cells and vitreous haze are graded based on SUN criteria.[13] Active retinal and optic nerve lesions are also scored. The sum of these scores during each flare is significantly associated with the long-term visual outcome.

In the convalescent phase of the disease, the gradual resolution of flare signs and symptoms takes several days to a couple of weeks, as anterior chamber cells are rapidly cleared. The resolution of vitreous haze is more gradual with the appearance of inferior, pearl-like precipitates on the surface of the retina or the posterior hyaloid. The presence of these precipitates is a very helpful diagnostic clue, as they are not seen in any other non-infectious entity **(Figs. 6A and B)**. Uncommonly, a similar finding can be seen in infectious retinitis, such as toxoplasmosis or syphilis. The resolution of retinal infiltrates occurs within several days without visible chorioretinal scarring. However, the development of retinal atrophy and nerve fiber layer defects can be seen most clearly on OCT imaging **(Figs. 7A and B)**.

The use of multimodal imaging is essential in helping narrow down the cause of the retinal infiltrates given a broad differential diagnosis.[14-16] Images also can document sequelae after a flare. OCT findings are similar to those seen in neuroretinitis from *Bartonella* spp. or in post-fever viral retinitis. However, fluorescein angiography in Behçet disease–associated uveitis will show diffuse capillary leakage, as opposed to other infectious entities. After resolution of the inflammation, focal atrophy of the retina gives a pseudo-foveal appearance with elevation of the outer plexiform layer with a corresponding retinal nerve fiber layer defect and a scotoma on visual field testing.

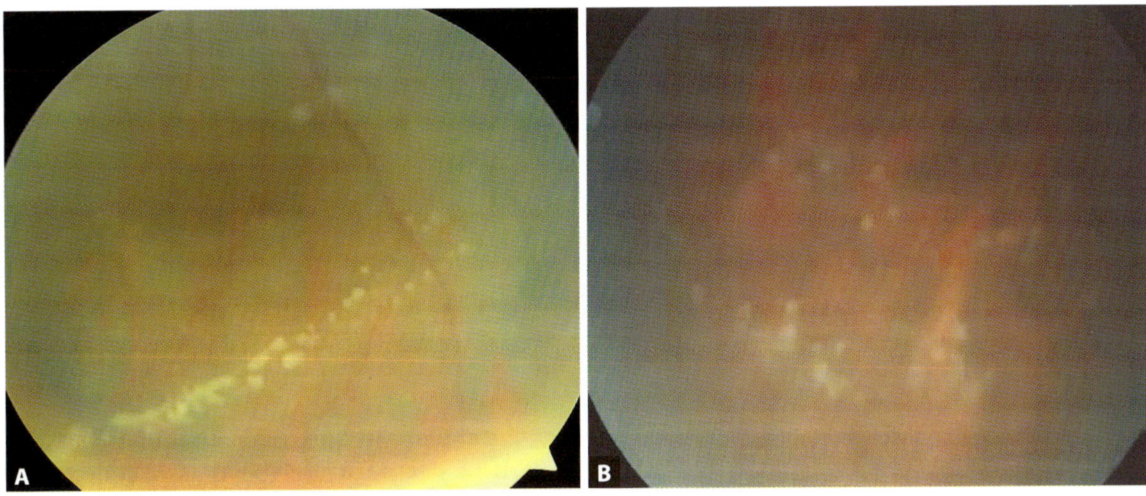

Figs. 6A and B: Color fundus photos of the peripheral retina showing inferior pearl-like precipitates during the resolution of a Behçet disease-associated uveitis flare.
Source: Uveitis Webinar - Grand Round 14. International Uveitis Study Group (IUSG). 2025. https://youtu.be/-E8PbG9PkxE?si=XcEXr31C7XMY23RX.

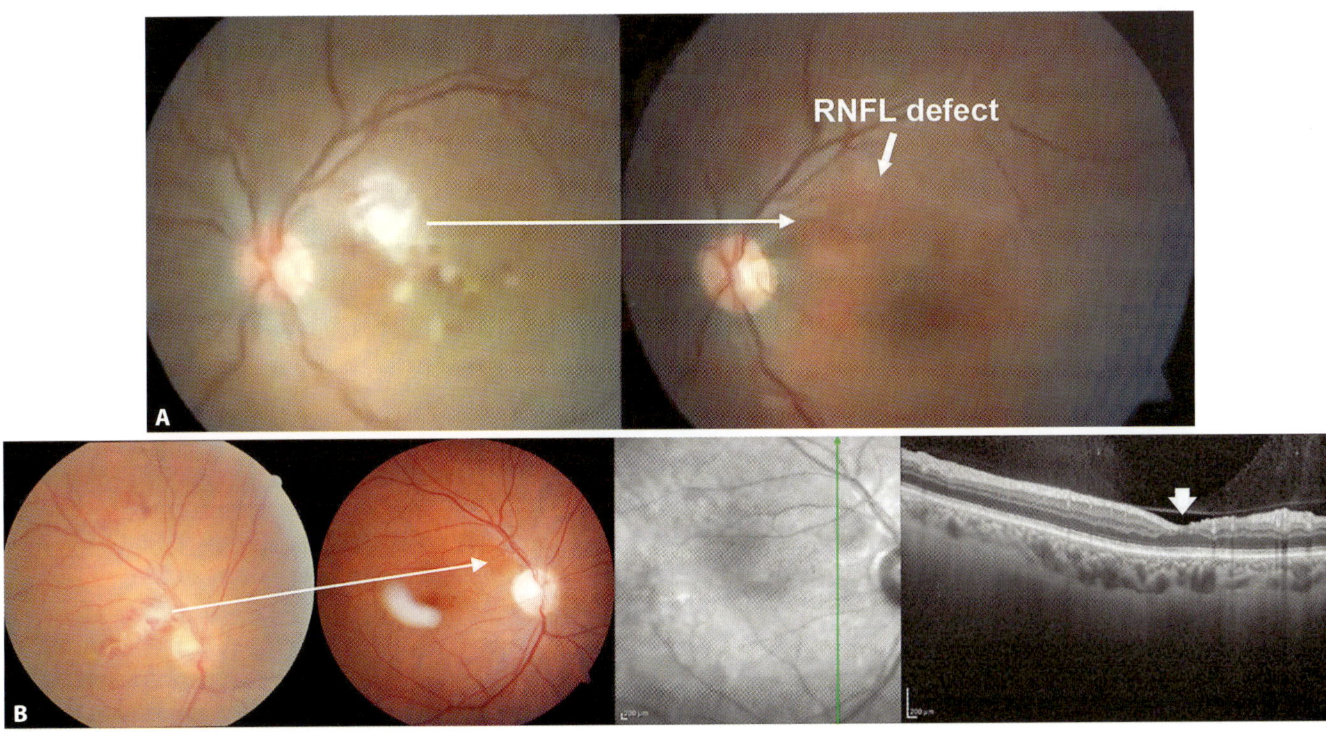

Figs. 7A and B: Color fundus photos and an optical coherence tomography (OCT) scan through the macula during a flare (left top and bottom) show retinal infiltrates, hemorrhages, and retinal edema. With clinical resolution, the retinal infiltrates disappear within days without visible chorioretinal scarring (right top and middle). The resulting inner retinal atrophy (arrow shows a nerve fiber layer defect) is seen best on OCT imaging (bottom right). (RNFL: retinal nerve fiber layer)
Source: Uveitis Webinar - Grand Round 14. International Uveitis Study Group (IUSG). 2025. https://youtu.be/-E8PbG9PkxE?si=XcEXr31C7XMY23RX.

After retinal vascular occlusions, there will be resolution of perivascular sheathing and fading of retinal hemorrhages. With milder episodes, only gliotic, thin sheathing of the retinal veins can be seen. However, after severe episodes, ghost vessels form and patches of extensive retinal non-perfusion result. Diffuse leakage in non-occluded areas can be seen **(Fig. 8)**. The development of shunt vessels, rarely neovascularization elsewhere, can occur in Behçet disease-associated uveitis. The ischemic retina becomes atrophic with window defects on fluorescein angiography. Areas of nonperfusion do not need laser photocoagulation in most cases, as aggressive anti-inflammatory treatment will induce clinical regression of the vascular inflammation.

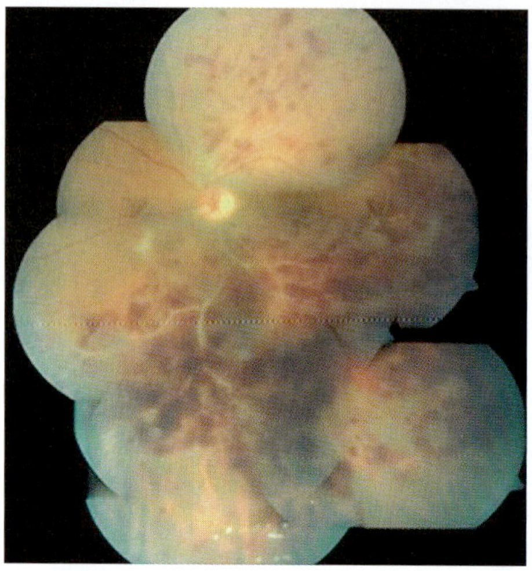

Fig. 8: A color fundus photo of a left eye showing extensive areas of hemorrhagic, occlusive retinal vasculitis inferiorly. This resulted in a large area of non-perfusion on fluorescein angiography inferiorly with small vessel leakage superiorly in areas without occlusion.
Source: Uveitis Webinar - Grand Round 14. International Uveitis Study Group (IUSG). 2025. https://youtu.be/-E8PbG9PkxE?si=XcEXr31C7XMY23RX.

Clinical remission is defined by the absence of any inflammation in the eye. The fundus may look completely normal on dilated fundoscopy, but complete remission can only be determined if there is angiographic quiescence. Subclinical inflammation may only be detected with the use of fluorescein angiography. As seen in **Figures 9 and 10**, diffuse leakage can be seen despite the absence of any inflammatory signs on examination. Even in eyes with advanced damage, fluorescein will differentiate between burnt-out disease versus persistent subclinical inflammation and small vessel leakage, which will need to be treated.

Optic disc staining and retinal capillary leakage in a fern-like pattern are the most frequent fluorescein angiography findings in Behçet disease-associated uveitis, both in active episodes and during clinical remission periods in patients with inadequately controlled disease **(Fig. 11)**. This finding is not specific to Behçet disease-associated uveitis. A similar fluorescein angiographic picture is seen in intermediate uveitis, idiopathic cases, or any inflammatory etiology affecting the posterior pole.

Multimodal imaging is very helpful in cases without systemic involvement. As seen in **Figure 12**, a 25-year-old male without systemic symptoms presented with bilateral vitritis and recurrent visual blurring with spontaneous improvement. The fluorescein angiography showed bilateral disc staining and peripheral leakage. Focal retinal atrophy was seen on OCT scans with elevation of the outer

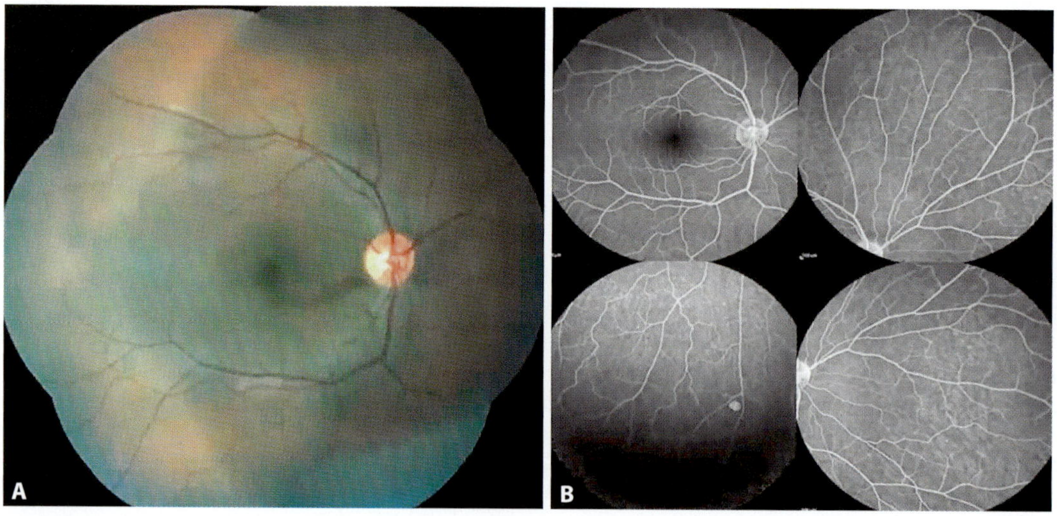

Figs. 9A and B: A color fundus photo of a right eye (left) showing no retinal lesions or vascular sheathing. A late phase fluorescein angiogram (right) showing remission without vascular leakage or occlusions. This is the gold standard for monitoring Behçet disease-associated uveitis.
Source: Uveitis Webinar - Grand Round 14. International Uveitis Study Group (IUSG). 2025. https://youtu.be/-E8PbG9PkxE?si=XcEXr31C7XMY23RX.

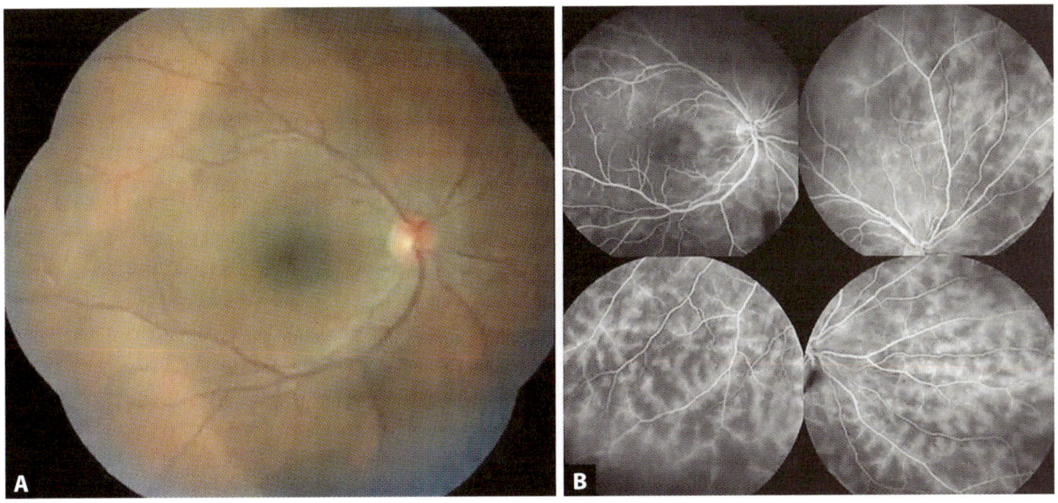

Figs. 10A and B: A color fundus photo showing no retinal lesions or vascular sheathing (A). However, late phase fluorescein angiography (B) shows active small vessel leakage.
Source: Uveitis Webinar - Grand Round 14. International Uveitis Study Group (IUSG). 2025. https://youtu.be/-E8PbG9PkxE?si=XcEXr31C7XMY23RX.

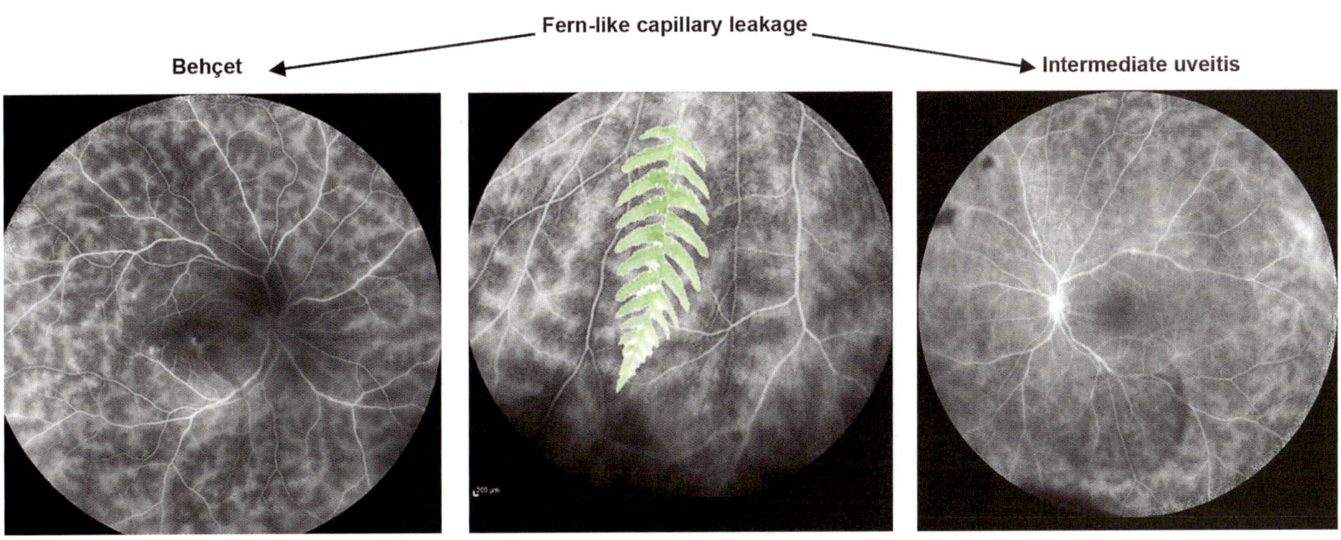

Fig. 11: A late phase fluorescein angiogram of a right eye in a patient with Behçet disease-associated uveitis (left). The fern-like capillary leakage pattern is similar to the late phase angiogram in a patient with intermediate uveitis (right).
Source: Uveitis Webinar - Grand Round 14. International Uveitis Study Group (IUSG). 2025. https://youtu.be/-E8PbG9PkxE?si=XcEXr31C7XMY23RX.

plexiform layer. These findings, as previously mentioned, are indicative of prior retinal infiltrates at the location of the retinal atrophy and strongly suggests a diagnosis of Behçet disease-associated uveitis.

An algorithm for the clinical diagnosis of Behcet disease-associated uveitis in adults was published by Tugal-Tutkun et al. in 2021.[17] A Classification and Regression Tree (CART) uses the presence or absence of clinical findings to aid in making the diagnosis. The probability of Behçet disease as the associated systemic cause, with or without extraocular manifestations, increases with the presence of several criteria. These include diffuse vitritis, the absence of granulomatous anterior uveitis or choroiditis, superficial retinal infiltrates or their sequelae, regressed or active occlusive retinal periphlebitis, and diffuse capillary leakage on fluorescein angiography.

A single, severe flare can cause irreversible damage and visual loss, which requires the immediate start

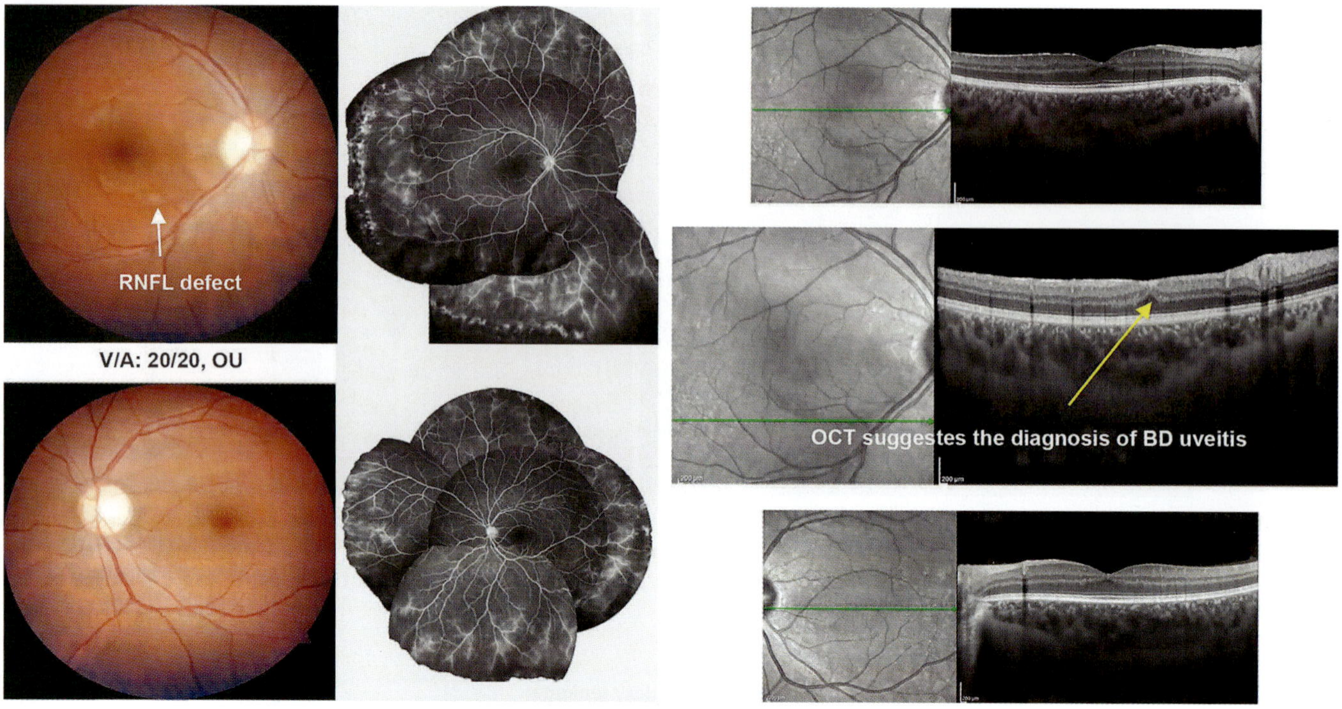

Fig. 12: Color fundus photos of both eyes (left) show a small nerve fiber layer defect in the inferior macula of the right eye (white arrow). Centrally, fluorescein angiography late frames show peripheral leakage in both eyes. Optical coherence tomography (OCT) scans of the macula retina (right upper and lower) are unremarkable, but the central scan shows an area of atrophy with outer plexiform layer giving the appearance of a pseudo-foveal contour (right center). (RNFL: retinal nerve fiber layer; VA: visual acuity)
Source: Uveitis Webinar - Grand Round 14. International Uveitis Study Group (IUSG). 2025. https://youtu.be/-E8PbG9PkxE?si=XcEXr31C7XMY23RX.

of immunosuppressive agents. Recurrent attacks cause cumulative structural and functional damage, necessitating long-term immunomodulatory treatment to prevent recurrence. Persistent subclinical retinal inflammation can result in neovascularization of the disc, optic atrophy, chorioretinal atrophy, cystoid macular edema, and low vision **(Figs. 13A and B)**. Therefore, fluorescein angiographic monitoring of subclinical retinal inflammation is essential, especially during remission periods, with adjustment of immunosuppressive treatment according to disease activity.[18]

Improved visual outcomes have been reported with the reduction of capillary leakage.[19,20] Laser flare photometry measures anterior chamber flare as a non-nvasive, surrogate marker of fluorescein angiography leakage during remission periods.[21] Elevation of anterior chamber flare has been associated with a higher risk of recurrent attacks.[22] Again, the long-term goal is preservation of vision through angiographic remission.

Corticosteroids are widely used for the treatment of acute inflammation, starting with intravenous methylprednisolone in combination with a corticosteroid-sparing agent. Local depot corticosteroids should be used as an adjunct treatment only in severe, unilateral attacks or for the treatment of persistent macular edema. Both azathioprine and cyclosporine have proven efficacy as corticosteroid-sparing agents.[23] However, visual loss may not be prevented in resistant cases with disease-modifying antirheumatic drugs (DMARDs) alone. Interferon-alpha is a biologic that has shown clinical efficacy, but has limited regional availability. The major advantage is the induction of a durable, drug-free remission; however, side effect tolerability limits use.[24-30]

There are only a few randomized, controlled trials on Behçet disease-associated uveitis treatment. In a small pilot study from China, the efficacy of interferon-alpha was compared to cyclosporine A.[31] Interferon-alpha showed less time to resolution and reduction of flare severity at 12 months. In another trial, the efficacy of adalimumab, interferon-alpha, and cyclosporine A were compared head-to-head.[32] The adalimumab group had the lowest annual relapse rate. Finally, a randomized, controlled trial from the United Kingdom compared interferon-alpha to infliximab, and both were found to be equally effective

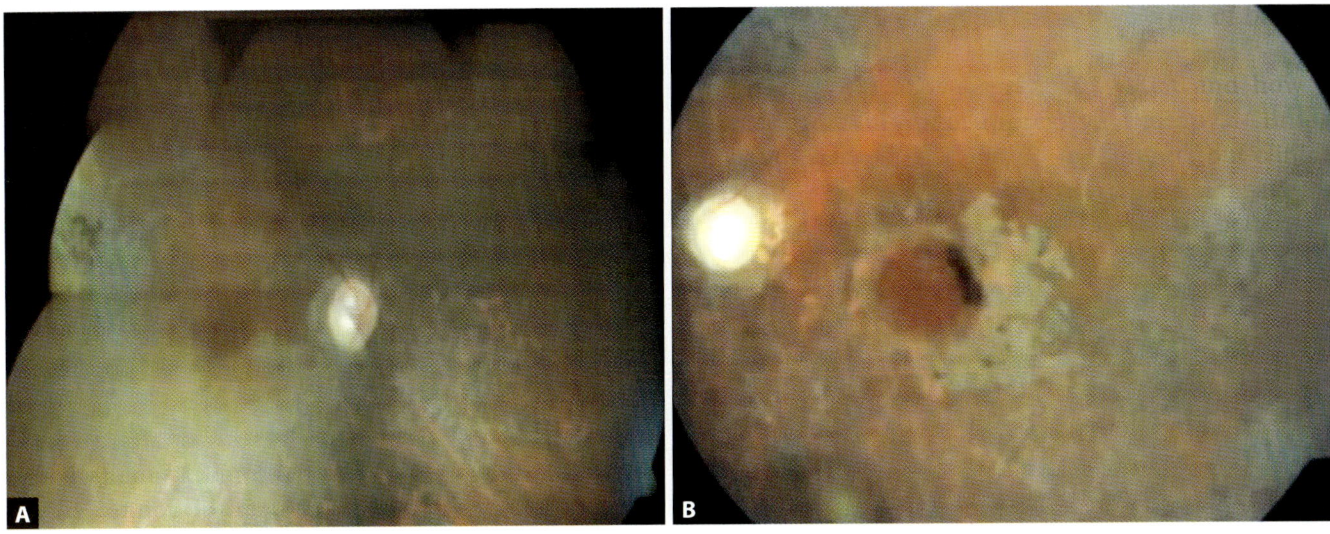

Figs. 13A and B: Color fundus photos of a right eye showing optic disc pallor, chorioretinal atrophy with scarring, and sclerotic vessels (left). The fundus photo of the left eye shows a macular hole, perifoveal atrophy, optic nerve pallor, and sclerotic peripheral vessels (right). *Source:* Uveitis Webinar - Grand Round 14. International Uveitis Study Group (IUSG). 2025. https://youtu.be/-E8PbG9PkxE?si=XcEXr31C7XMY23RX.

in the reduction of the Behçet Disease Activity Index at 12 weeks and secondary outcomes, including organ involvement, at 24 weeks.[33] Unfortunately, few patients in the trial had ocular involvement. Efficacy could not be proven in placebo-controlled trials with daclizumab, secukinumab, or gevokizumab in Behçet disease-associated uveitis.[34-36]

Anti-tumor necrosis factor (TNF) agents are effective and widely used for the treatment of active inflammation in Behçet disease and to prevent flares as corticosteroid-sparing immunosuppressive agents. In case of inadequate response, dose escalation or shortening of the dosing interval can be considered. If non-response continues at the maximum dose and the shortest interval, an alternative TNF-inhibitor can be initiated. In patients who fail anti-TNF inhibitors, tocilizumab, an interleukin-6 (IL-6) inhibitor, is an alternative along with anti-IL-1 agents. There are recent small case series that show a beneficial effect of Janus kinase (JAK) inhibitors for the treatment of Behçet disease-associated uveitis. Biologic agents should be combined with a conventional DMARD agent to limit antibody formation to the monoclonal antibodies.

Better outcomes have been reported when TNF agents are administered as first-line treatments in Behçet disease–associated uveitis, as recommended by the American Uveitis Society expert panel.[37] Earlier treatment with TNF agents provided higher rates of drug-free remission.[38] Both infliximab and adalimumab are effective, but head-to-head trials comparing the efficacy or safety of these agents for the treatment of Behçet disease-associated uveitis are lacking.[39] Infliximab infusions are preferred for the treatment of severe inflammation due to the rapid and potent anti-inflammatory effect.[40] The dose can also be titrated based on the severity of inflammation and the patient's body weight. Higher doses are used in Behçet disease patients both at initiation and during monthly maintenance infusions. Although adalimumab has been approved for the treatment of non-infectious intermediate, posterior, and panuveitis, including Behçet disease, it seems to be safer and more effective for long-term disease control.[41,42] However, the approved standard dose is usually inadequate with the majority of patients requiring weekly injections. The TNF retention rates and adverse event profiles for adalimumab and infliximab are shown in **Table 1**.[43-46]

In severe cases, combination therapy with multiple immunosuppressive agents may be required. As seen in **Figure 14**, a patient presented with inflammatory neovascularization of the optic disc and diffuse peripheral leakage on fluorescein angiography. Infliximab infusions were started at 4,000 mg (67 kg body weight) concurrently with azathioprine 100 mg daily after a pulse of 1 g of methylprednisolone for 3 days. Combination therapy facilitates a more rapid taper and discontinuation of oral corticosteroids. After 4 months of treatment, there was marked improvement on fluorescein angiography with

TABLE 1: Antitumor necrosis factor retention rates and adverse event profiles in patients with Behçet disease-associated uveitis.

Study	*No. of patients*	*Drug*	*Retention rate*	*Discontinued due to inefficacy*	*Discontinued due to adverse events*	*Discontinued due to clinical remission*
Fabiani Italy, 2018	54	ADA	77% @ 1 year 64% @ 4 years	9% primary inefficacy 13% secondary failure	7%	0
Fabiani Italy, 2019	40	IFX	89% @ 1 year 47% @ 10 years	5% primary inefficacy 15% secondary failure	10%	5%
Atienza-Matteo Spain, 2019	74 103	ADA IFX	95% @ 1 year 85% @ 1 years	15% 17%	5% 9%	8% 19%
Takeuchi Japan, 2023	140	IFX	76% @ 10 year	4%	14%	6%

(ADA: adalimumab; IFX: infliximab)

Source: Uveitis Webinar - Grand Round 14. International Uveitis Study Group (IUSG). 2025. https://youtu.be/-E8PbG9PkxE?si= XcEXr31C7XMY23RX.

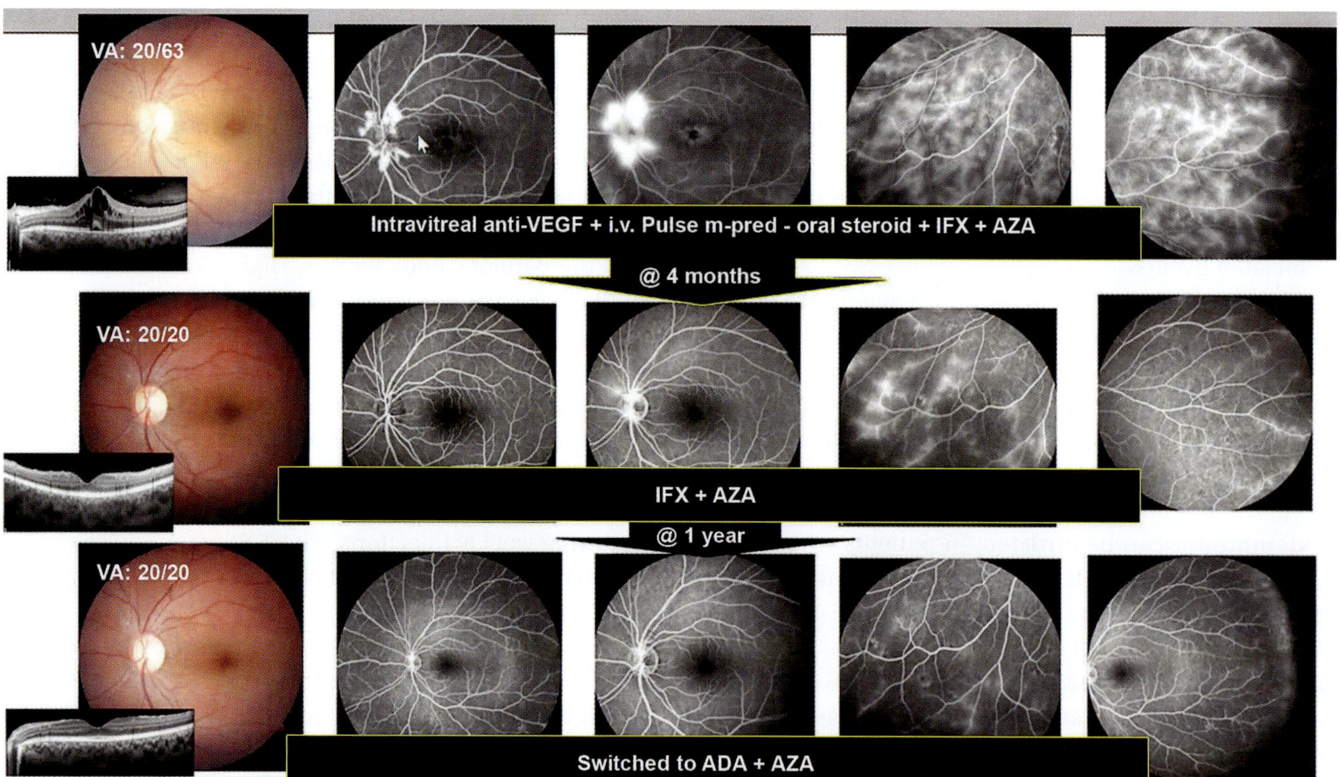

Fig. 14: Color fundus photos of a left eye (left column) showing optic disc neovascularization, which is visible on early (inner left column) and late fluorescein angiograms (middle column) along with peripheral fern-like leakage (right columns). The optic nerve leakage resolved over the following year (bottom row) with the start of infliximab (IFX) then later adalimumab (ADA) and azathioprine (AZA). There was almost complete angiographic resolution of peripheral leakage as well. (M-pred: methylprednisolone; VEGF: vascular endothelial growth factor; VA: visual acuity)

Source: Uveitis Webinar - Grand Round 14. International Uveitis Study Group (IUSG). 2025. https://youtu.be/-E8PbG9PkxE?si= XcEXr31C7XMY23RX.

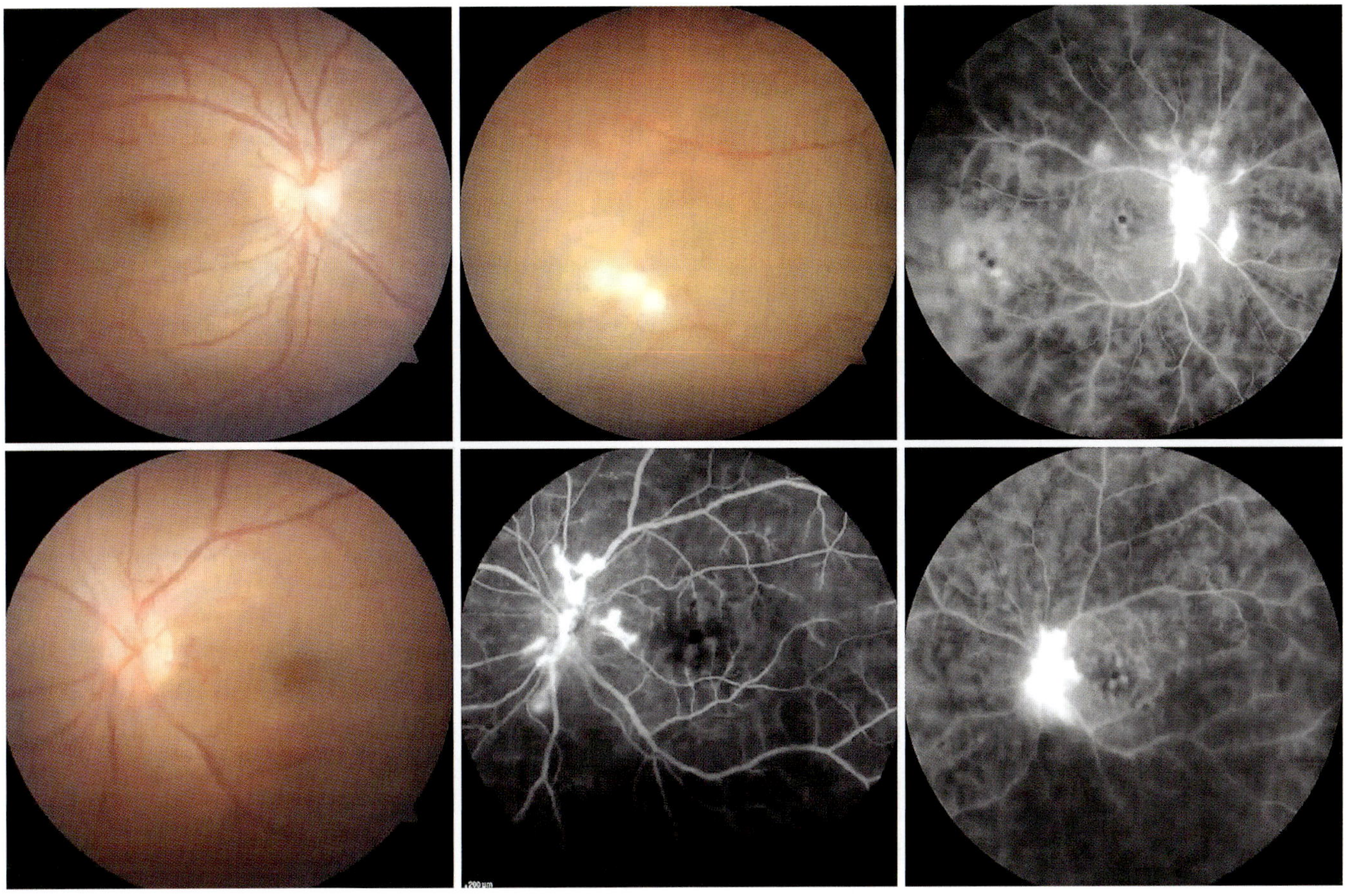

Fig. 15: Color fundus photos of both eyes eye (left column) showing hazy media. Retinal infiltrates are seen in the upper central fundus photo in addition to diffuse vascular and optic nerve leakage on fluorescein angiography (inferior middle and right column).
Source: Uveitis Webinar - Grand Round 14. International Uveitis Study Group (IUSG). 2025. https://youtu.be/-E8PbG9PkxE?si=XcEXr31C7XMY23RX.

almost complete angiographic remission at 1 year. The patient was ultimately switched to adalimumab 40 mg every other week for maintenance of the remission.

In another example, a patient was referred for recurrent flares on treatment with adalimumab 40 mg every 2 weeks in combination with azathioprine 100 mg daily and prednisone 10 mg daily. On fluorescein angiography, diffuse leakage can be seen with inflammatory neovascularization of the disc in both eyes **(Fig. 15)**. On fundus examination, retinal infiltrates and cystoid macular edema were also present in the right eye. Given the severity of the inflammation, the patient was switched to infliximab 4,000 mg (72 kg body weight) in lieu of escalation to weekly injections of adalimumab for disease control.

Cystoid macular edema is the most common complication involving the posterior pole in patients with Behçet disease–associated uveitis. In a multicentered retrospective study by Barroso-Garcia et al., three TNF-inhibitors (adalimumab, infliximab, and certolizumab pegol) were compared head-to-head with no significant difference in the reduction of macular thickness.[47] Of note, 7 of the 10 patients in the certolizumab group were previously treated with adalimumab, infliximab, or both. In another study by Barroso-Garcia et al., a comparison of infliximab, adalimumab, or tocilizumab for treatment of macular edema in patients with Behçet disease–associated uveitis found no significant difference between the agents.[48] Similarly, subjects in the tocilizumab group had previously been treated with infliximab or adalimumab without clinical resolution of the macular edema. Given the available evidence, tocilizumab should be considered a second-line agent for patients who fail TNF treatment. In a meta-analysis by Arida et al., tocilizumab induced remission of uveitis in all TNF naive patients, though the number of patients was small ($N = 5$).[49] The same effect was found in 24 of 28 subjects previously treated with a TNF agent.

A multicenter study by Khitri et al. reported tocilizumab showed corticosteroid-sparing reduction in inflammation in more than 80% of patients with Behçet disease-associated uveitis.[50]

TNF inhibitors effectively treat all clinical manifestations of Behçet's disease. Only 3% of patients with Behçet disease treated for uveitis with infliximab or adalimumab develop new organ system involvement.[51-53] Therefore, tapering or discontinuation of a biologic immunosuppressant may be considered when complete ocular remission, including lack of leakage on a fluorescein angiogram, is achieved. It is important to achieve an absence of ocular inflammation as visual prognosis has improved with the use of biologic immunosuppressive agents due to the prevention of both disease and corticosteroid-related complications.[48,54,55] However, there continues to be an unmet need for patients with ocular inflammation that is refractory to all available biologic agents. Future research is needed to develop immunosuppressive agents with different mechanisms of action.[56] A novel approach to prevent or treat Behçet disease may lie in personalized medicine and include suppression of more selective inflammatory pathways, selective modulation of endoplasmic reticulum aminopeptidase-1 (ERAP) activity, immunopeptidome blockage, microRNA regulation, and modulation of microbiota.

DIAGNOSING AND TREATING BEHÇET UVEITIS

Case Presentation

Case 1

Personal data: A 34-year-old male patient with a history of Behçet disease was referred by the rheumatology department for ophthalmic examination given active genital and aphthous ulcers. He had a previous history of uveitis that was diagnosed 1.5 years prior.

History of present illness: The patient presented with blurred vision in both eyes on treatment with azathioprine 50 mg twice daily.

Physical examination: The best-corrected visual acuity was 20/20 in both eyes. Disc hyperemia was noted in the right eye and both eyes had 1+ vitreous cells. There was no retinitis or vasculitis on fundus examination in both eyes **(Table 2)**.

TABLE 2: Physical examination of a patient having Behçet disease–associated uveitis Case 1.

OD	Parameter	OS
20/20	BCVA	20/20
14 mm Hg	IOP	12 mm Hg
White and quiet	Conjunctiva	White and quiet
Fine KPs on the endothelium	Cornea	Fine KPs on the endothelium
0.5+ cells	Anterior chamber	0.5+ cells
No synechiae	Iris	No synechiae
Clear	Lens	Clear
1+ cell	Vitreous	1+ cell
Optic disc hyperemia	Fundus	Normal, no macular edema

(BCVA: best-corrected visual acuity, IOP: intraocular pressure; KPs: keratic precipitates; OD: right eye; OS: left eye)

Ancillary testing: Fluorescein angiography showed peripheral retinal leakage and disc hyperfluorescence in both eyes. While there was no angiographic macular edema, OCT imaging showed thinning of the inner retinal layers temporal to the optic nerve in the left eye **(Fig. 16)**.

Uveitis workup: A complete blood count (CBC) and a comprehensive metabolic panel (CMP) were normal. Syphilis and HIV testing were negative. A pathergy test was positive.

Initial treatment: Based on both the clinical and imaging findings, cyclosporine 100 mg twice daily and prednisolone 24 mg daily were added to the treatment regimen. The dose of prednisolone was tapered by 8 mg/week.

Follow-up: However, 3 months later, two new foci of retinitis were noted on dilated fundus examination of the right eye **(Fig. 17)**. A repeat fluorescein angiogram showed continued late peripheral leakage and disc hyperfluorescence. The immunosuppressive therapy was changed to adalimumab 40 mg subcutaneously every other week, but the patient did not agree with this plan. Alternatively, the dose of azathioprine was increased to 50 mg three times daily with reinstitution of prednisolone 32 mg daily.

The patient was lost to follow-up for 6 months, during which time he tapered the prednisolone on his own and developed symptoms of a flare. He restarted the prednisolone again at 48 mg/day. His vision changed in the right eye to 20/40 and remained 20/20 in the left eye. On slit lamp examination, he had 1+ anterior chamber cells and 2+ vitreous cells in both eyes. The immunosuppressive regimen was again changed to adalimumab 40 mg every other week and azathioprine 50 mg three times daily.

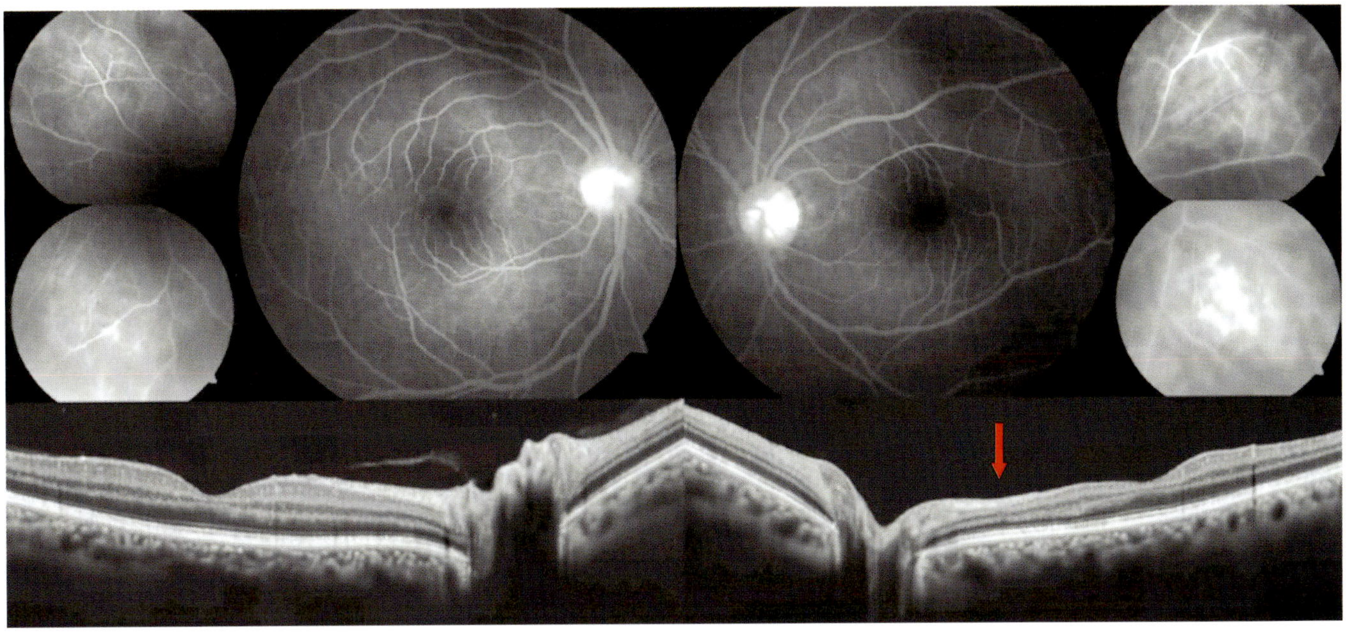

Fig. 16: Fluorescein angiography of both eyes (upper images) showing late optic disc and peripheral leakage. Optical coherence tomography (OCT) scans of the macula in both eyes (lower images) show no cystoid macular edema. An orange arrow (bottom right) depicts thinning of the inner retinal layers temporal to the left disc.
Source: Uveitis Webinar - Grand Round 14. International Uveitis Study Group (IUSG). 2025. https://youtu.be/-E8PbG9PkxE?si=XcEXr31C7XMY23RX.

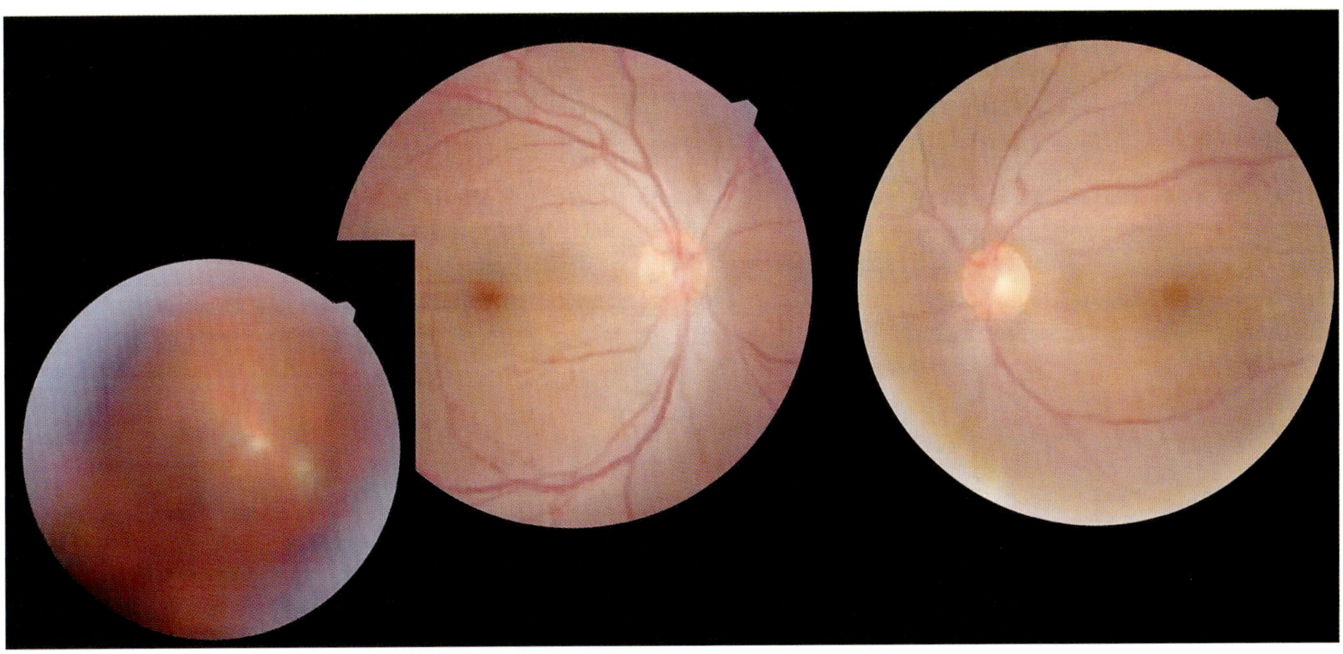

Fig. 17: A color fundus photo of both eyes showing two foci of retinitis in the periphery of the right eye.
Source: Uveitis Webinar - Grand Round 14. International Uveitis Study Group (IUSG). 2025. https://youtu.be/-E8PbG9PkxE?si=XcEXr31C7XMY23RX.

Three months later, there were no signs of inflammation on clinical examination or on fluorescein angiography activation. Given quiescence, the azathioprine dose was decreased to 50 mg twice daily. After 28 months of follow-up, the patient has remained without reactivation, and the azathioprine dose was again lowered to 50 mg daily.

Case 2

Personal data: A 31-year-old female patient presented with decreased vision in both eyes for 1 week. Systemically, she also had active oral ulcers, papulopustular skin lesions, and a history of deep vein thrombosis.

Physical examination: The best-corrected visual acuity was 20/400 in the right eye and 20/200 in the left eye. Focal areas of retinitis were noted in the right periphery and superonasal macula **(Table 3 and Fig. 18)**.

Ancillary testing: OCT images of the macula in the left eye showed nerve fiber layer loss and submacular fluid was present in both eyes **(Fig. 19)**. Fluorescein angiography showed intense leakage with a fern-like appearance and disc hyperfluorescence in both eyes on late frames **(Fig. 19)**.

Uveitis workup: On laboratory investigation, both CBC and CMP values were normal. Serological tests for HIV and syphilis were negative.

Initial treatment: The patient was given a 3-day course of intravenous methylprednisolone 1 g daily followed by 1 mg/kg of prednisolone tapered by 8 mg/week.

Follow-up: Two weeks after presentation, the best-corrected visual acuities improved to 20/100 in the right eye and 20/40 in the left eye. With clearing of the vitreous haze, a serous retinal detachment was visible and regressing on OCT images. The prednisone taper was continued, and interferon-alpha was added to the treatment regimen intravenously at 6 million units three times per week.

After 5 months of follow-up, the retinal edema had resolved completely. However, thinning of the inner retinal layers temporal to the optic disc were visible on OCT

TABLE 3: Physical examination of a patient having Behçet disease–associated uveitis Case 2.

OD	*Parameter*	*OS*
20/400	BCVA	20/200
18 mm Hg	IOP	15 mm Hg
Mild hyperemia	Conjunctiva	Mild hyperemia
Fine KPs on the endothelium	Cornea	Fine KPs on the endothelium
3+ cell	Anterior chamber	2+ cell
No synechiae	Iris	No synechiae
Clear	Lens	Clear
3+ cell, 2+ haze	Vitreous	2+ cell, 1+ haze
Focal area of retinitis superotemporal to the macula under the superior arcade and inferiorly in the periphery. Macular edema was present	Fundus	Macular edema was present

(BCVA: best-corrected visual acuity; IOP: intraocular pressure; KPs: keratic precipitates; OD: right eye; OS: left eye)

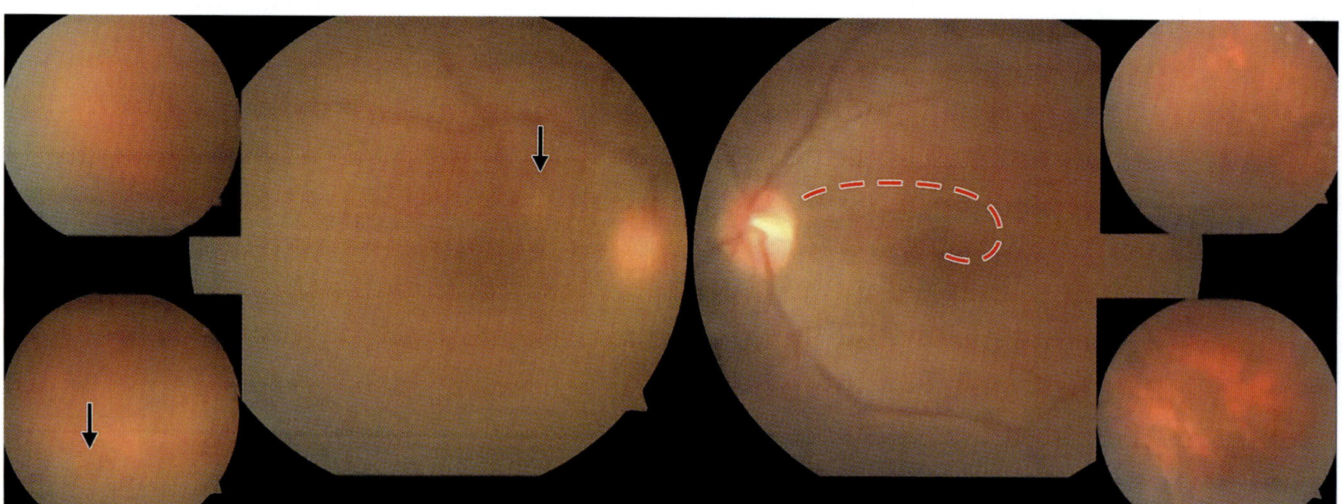

Fig. 18: Color fundus photos of both eyes show new foci of retinitis superonasal to the macula of the right eye (middle black arrow) and in the periphery (bottom left black arrow). Retinal nerve fiber layer loss was also noted in the left eye (red dotted line).
Source: Uveitis Webinar - Grand Round 14. International Uveitis Study Group (IUSG). 2025. https://youtu.be/-E8PbG9PkxE?si=XcEXr31C7XMY23RX.

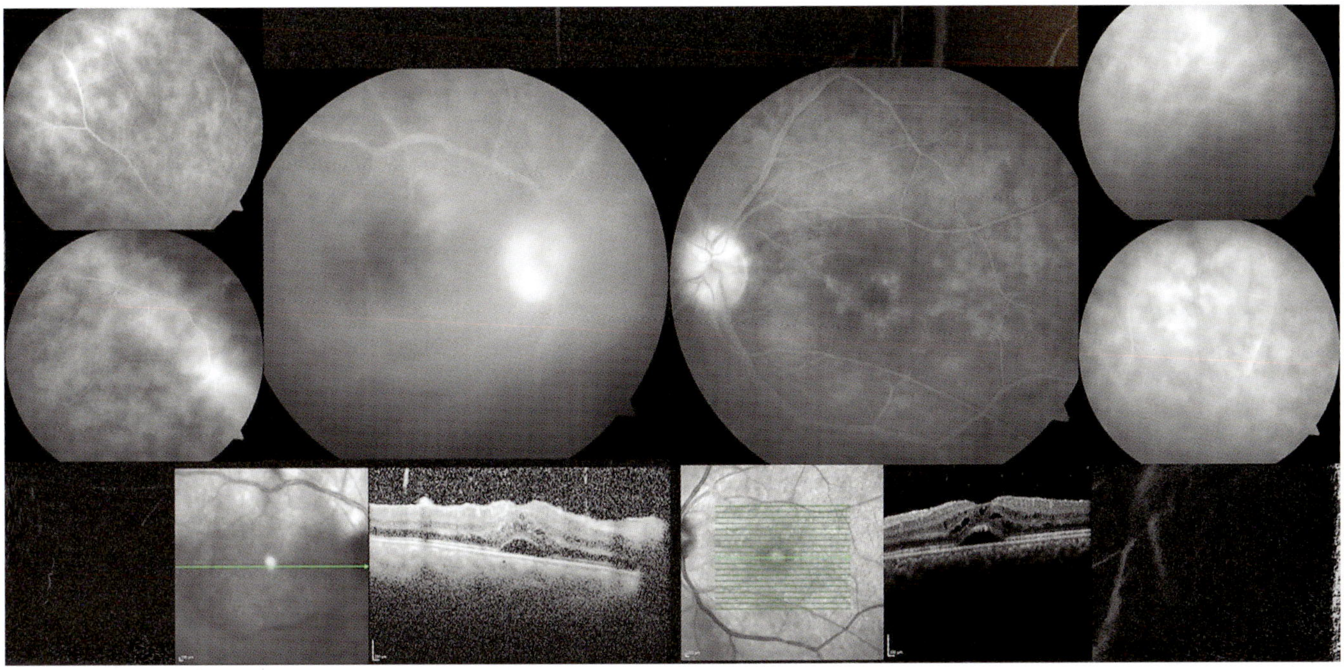

Fig. 19: Fluorescein angiography of both eyes showed late fern-like leakage and disc hyperfluorescence. Optical coherence tomography (OCT) scans (bottom) show intraretinal and subretinal fluid.
Source: Uveitis Webinar - Grand Round 14. International Uveitis Study Group (IUSG). 2025. https://youtu.be/-E8PbG9PkxE?si=XcEXr31C7XMY23RX.

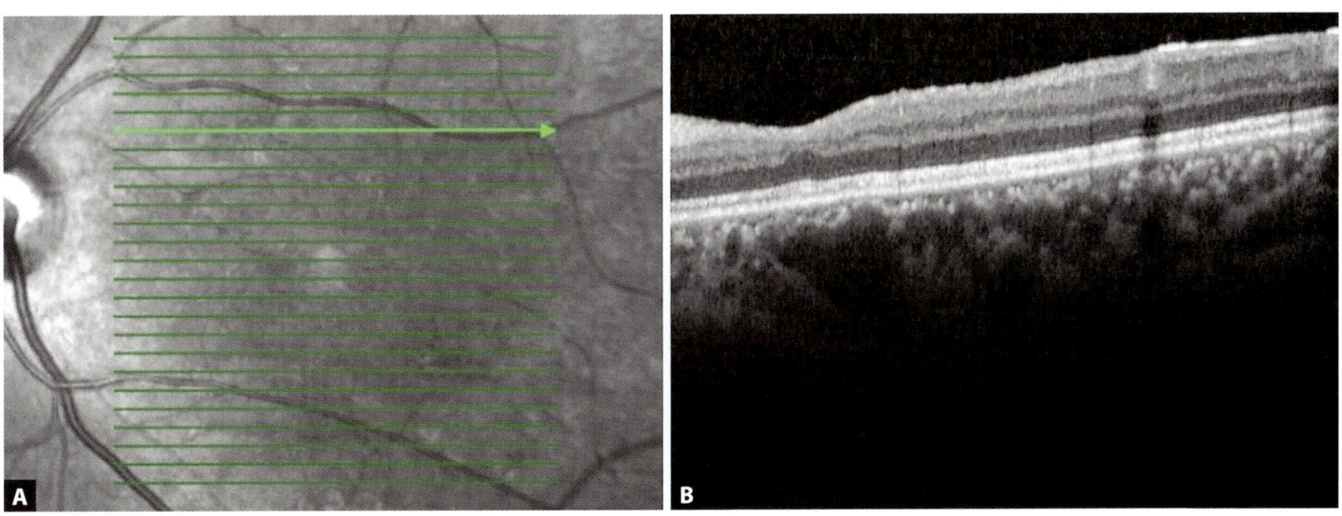

Figs. 20A and B: An optical coherence tomography (OCT) scan through the macula of the left eye showed no edema but thinning of the inner retinal layers temporal to the optic disc.
Source: Uveitis Webinar - Grand Round 14. International Uveitis Study Group (IUSG). 2025. https://youtu.be/-E8PbG9PkxE?si=XcEXr31C7XMY23RX.

imaging **(Figs. 20A and B)**. Interferon-alpha infusions were continued.

At the seventh month visit, there was a new focus of resolving retinitis, and the patient was experiencing excessive hair loss. Infliximab 5 mg/kg every 4 weeks was stared in lieu of interferon-alpha infusions, in addition to azathioprine 50 mg twice daily. Five months later (1 year after presentation), there was no clinical inflammation on examination. However, peripheral leakage was noted on fluorescein angiography. The dose of the infliximab was increased to 7 mg/kg every 4 weeks with continuance of azathioprine 50 mg three times daily **(Fig. 21)**.

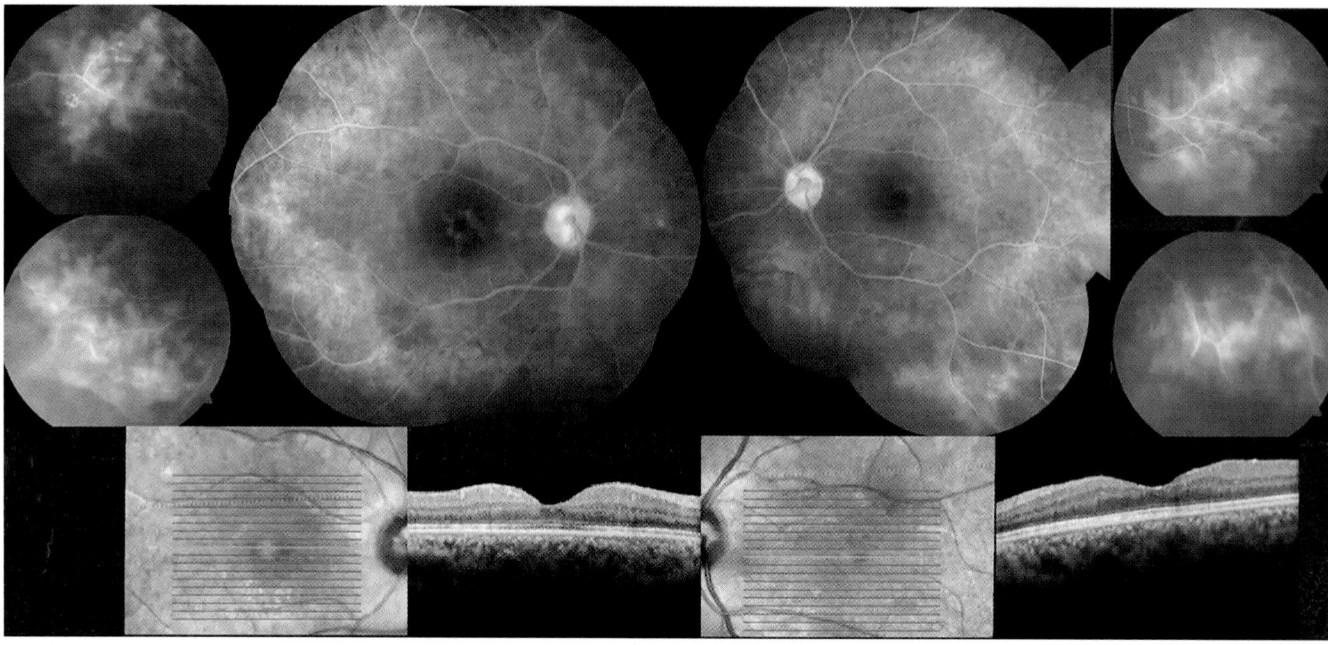

Fig. 21: Fluorescein angiography showed peripheral leakage in both eyes in late frames (superiorly) without macular edema on optical coherence tomography (OCT) scans of the macula (bottom).
Source: Uveitis Webinar - Grand Round 14. International Uveitis Study Group (IUSG). 2025. https://youtu.be/-E8PbG9PkxE?si=XcEXr31C7XMY23RX.

Twenty-four months after presentation, the best corrected visual acuities improved to 20/32 in both eyes with no clinical activity, but there was again late peripheral leakage on fluorescein angiography. Immunosuppressive therapy was changed to adalimumab 40 mg weekly and azathioprine 50 mg three times a day. No active inflammation was detected over the subsequent year, and the dose of adalimumab was decreased to 40 mg every other week. Most recently at 5 years after presentation, the best-correct visual acuity is 0.7 in the right eye and 0.8 in the left eye without clinical reactivation. She remains on adalimumab 40 mg every other week, and azathioprine was decreased to 50 mg twice daily.

Discussion

The two cases presented highlight the varying severities of inflammation in Behçet disease-associated uveitis. The first case was diagnosed by the rheumatologist due to systemic manifestations, but he also had some characteristic ocular findings compatible with Behçet disease-associated uveitis. In this relatively milder case, the preferred step ladder treatment approach started with conventional immunosuppressive therapies of azathioprine and cyclosporine in combination. However, the second patient presented to the ophthalmology clinic first and had the characteristic ocular findings. These included vitreous cells and haze, retinal infiltrates, vitreous precipitates, a focal nerve fiber layer defect, and leakage on fluorescein angiography which confirmed the diagnosis of Behçet disease-associated uveitis. While the patient also had extraocular manifestations of the disease, the diagnosis could be made by the typical ophthalmic findings alone. Given the poor presenting vision and severe intraocular inflammation, biologic treatment was started as the first-line therapy.

Several ocular findings are highly suggestive for Behçet disease-associated uveitis. The presence of retinal infiltrates, occlusive retinal vasculitis, diffuse retinal capillary leakage on fluorescein angiography, vitritis, and the absence of granulomatous anterior uveitis or choroiditis are characteristic. Additionally, localized retinal nerve fiber layer defects secondary to superficial retinal infiltrates and pearl-like vitreous precipitates occurring after the resolution of vitritis are also typical diagnostic findings.[17]

There are two main factors which determine the visual prognosis. First, and most importantly, early and appropriate treatment with conventional or biologic immunosuppressive therapies to treat persistent vascular leakage and prevent recurrent flares.[23,57-59] Adherence to treatment is the second most important factor for the visual prognosis. There is a clear association between treatment adherence and improvement of the best-corrected visual acuity with less uveitis flares.[60-62]

The severity of the clinical picture is important in determining the treatment choice. Fluorescein angiography should be a key determinant in clinical decision making, as vascular leakage can be seen in patients without clinical signs of retinal vasculitis or retinitis. Active leakage is a surrogate marker for uncontrolled disease necessitating an escalation in the current immunosuppressant dose or addition of another agent. Additionally, Behçet disease is a systemic disorder requiring oral, intravenous, or subcutaneous treatments. Behçet disease-associated uveitis cannot be treated with corticosteroid drops or ointments alone. Periocular or intravitreal corticosteroids can be used as adjuvant therapies to treat acute flares or refractory macular edema, especially in unilateral cases. Similarly, systemic corticosteroids should only be used in high doses and as bridging therapy for the treatment of severe posterior and panuveitis flares. The concurrent use of non-corticosteroid immunosuppressive therapies in a stepwise manner begins with DMARDs then biologics for the long-term treatment of the disease. Due to the side effect profile, corticosteroid monotherapy is contraindicated.

Any posterior segment involvement, even if mild or only angiographic, needs treatment with immunosuppressive therapies. A stepwise therapeutic approach should be followed, starting with DMARDs as first-line agents followed by biologics.[63-67] Depending on practice location, interferon-alpha may not be available, leaving infliximab and adalimumab as first-line biologics. Third-line treatment consist of other biologic medications, such as tocilizumab, IL-1 inhibitors, and JAK inhibitors. In patients presenting with severe, sight-threatening posterior segment involvement, biologic therapy should be prescribed first. Both infliximab and adalimumab provide the rapid and effective suppression of ocular inflammation. Infliximab has a more rapid and potent anti-inflammatory effect, but adalimumab has better long-term inflammation control and patient compliance. In patients having recurrences with infliximab or adalimumab, an increase in the dose or the frequency of dose administration should be implemented. Failure of one TNF inhibitor does not predict a poor response to a second. In cases where there is decreased clinical efficacy, check both serum drug and medication-specific antibodies levels. After failure of both infliximab and adalimumab, another class of biologic agent should be started.

There is no consensus about when and how to discontinue immunosuppressive therapy. Clinical quiescence for at least 2 years is required, but clinical inactivity should be confirmed with no leakage on fluorescein angiography. Treatments should be tapered to avoid an abrupt cessation. With a gradual taper, the treatment should be continued for an additional 1–3 years.

SEVERE BEHÇET DISEASE-ASSOCIATED UVEITIS WITH STRUCTURAL DAMAGE

Case Presentation

Personal Data

A 37-year-old male presented with blurred vision in both eyes.

History of Present Illness

He had a history of recurrent oral ulcers and pseudofolliculitis.

Physical Examination

The best-corrected visual acuity was 20/40 in the right eye and 20/32 in the left eye. Vitreous haze was present in both eyes. A focal, yellow retinal lesion was seen superior to the macula in the right eye. Fine macular retinal hemorrhages were noted in the left eye **(Table 4 and Fig. 22)**.

TABLE 4: Physical examination of a patient having severe Behçet disease-associated uveitis with structural damage.

OD	Parameter	OS
20/40	BCVA	20/32
18 mm Hg	IOP	19 mm Hg
White and quiet	Conjunctiva	White and quiet
Fine KPs	Cornea	Fine KPs
0.5+ cell	Anterior chamber	0.5+ cell
Normal	Iris	Normal
Clear	Lens	Clear
2+ cell, 2+ haze	Vitreous	2+ cell, 2+ haze
Focal, yellow, retinal lesion superior to the macula	Fundus	Fine macular retinal hemorrhages

(BCVA: best-corrected visual acuity; IOP: intraocular pressure; KPs: keratic precipitates; OD: right eye; OS: left eye)

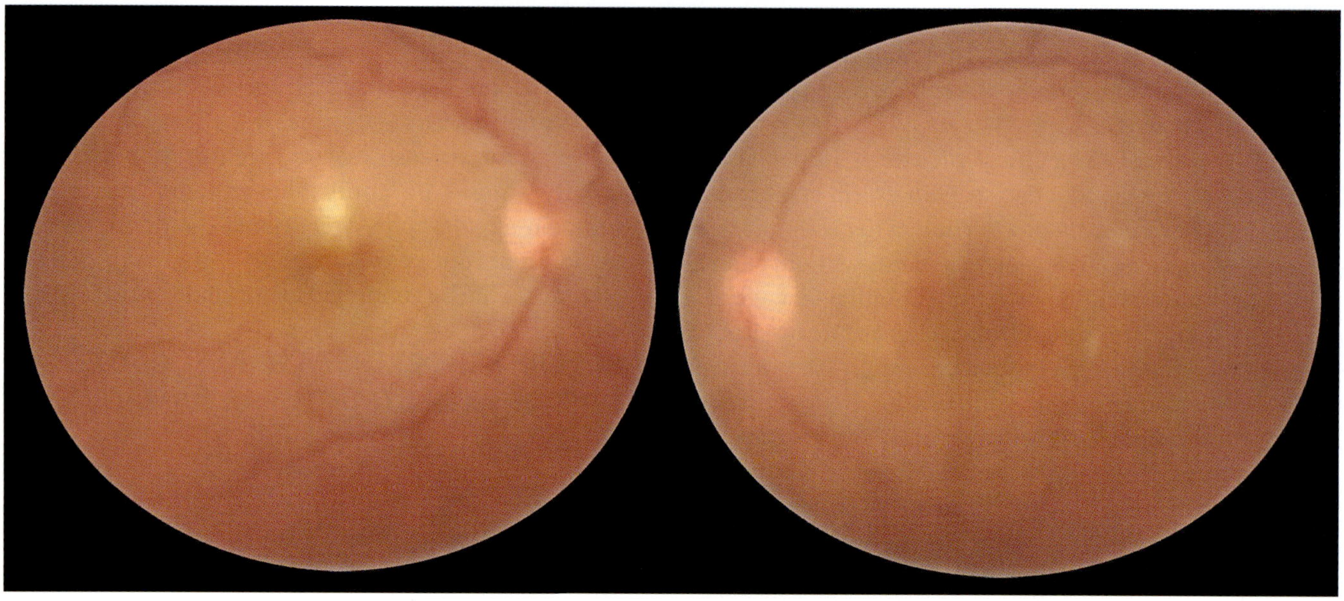

Fig. 22: Color fundus photos of both eyes showing vitreous haze. Superior to the macula, there is a yellow retinal lesion in the right eye. *Source:* Uveitis Webinar - Grand Round 14. International Uveitis Study Group (IUSG). 2025. https://youtu.be/-E8PbG9PkxE?si=XcEXr31C7XMY23RX.

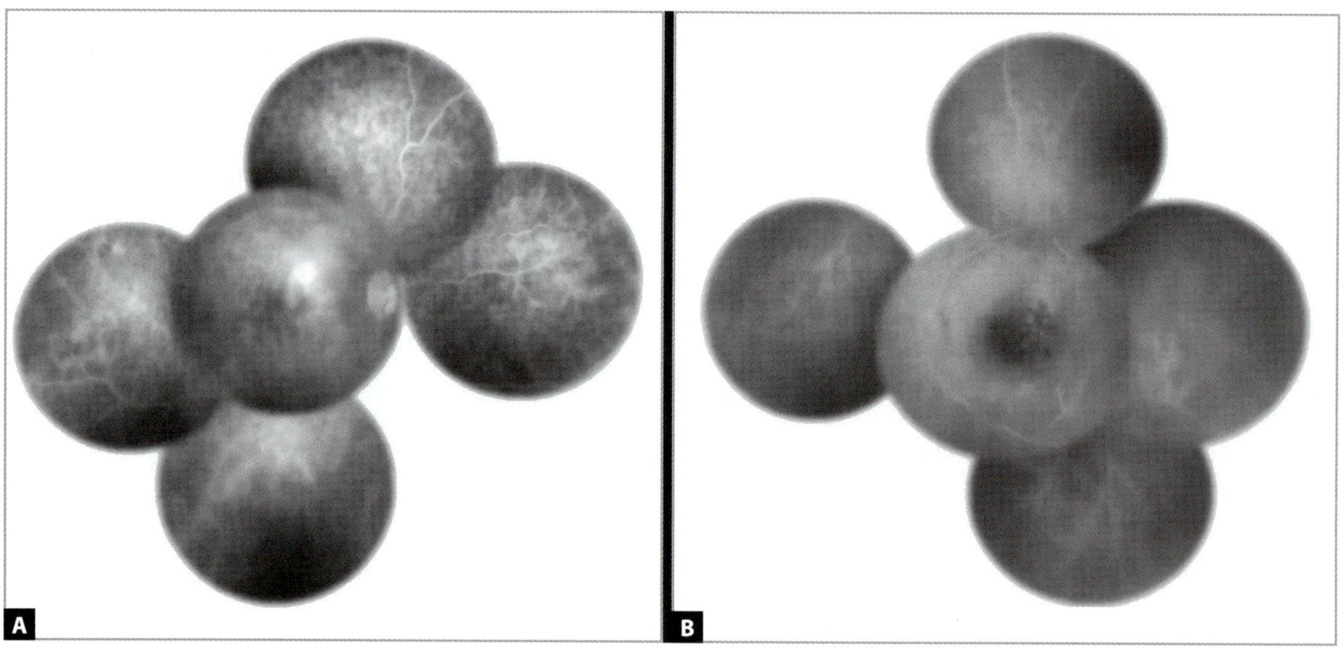

Figs. 23A and B: Late phase fluorescein angiography images showing diffuse vascular leakage and hyperfluorescence superior to the macula in the right eye (A), and punctate hyperfluorescence in the left eye (B).
Source: Uveitis Webinar - Grand Round 14. International Uveitis Study Group (IUSG). 2025. https://youtu.be/-E8PbG9PkxE?si=XcEXr31C7XMY23RX.

Ancillary Testing

Fluorescein angiography showed late staining of the retinal lesion in the right eye and diffuse retinal vasculitis in both eyes. Punctate macular hyperfluorescence was seen in the left eye **(Figs. 23A and B)**. OCT scans showed focal inner retinal thickening and hyperreflectivity corresponding to the retinal lesion associated with macular edema and subretinal fluid in the right eye. The scans of the left eye

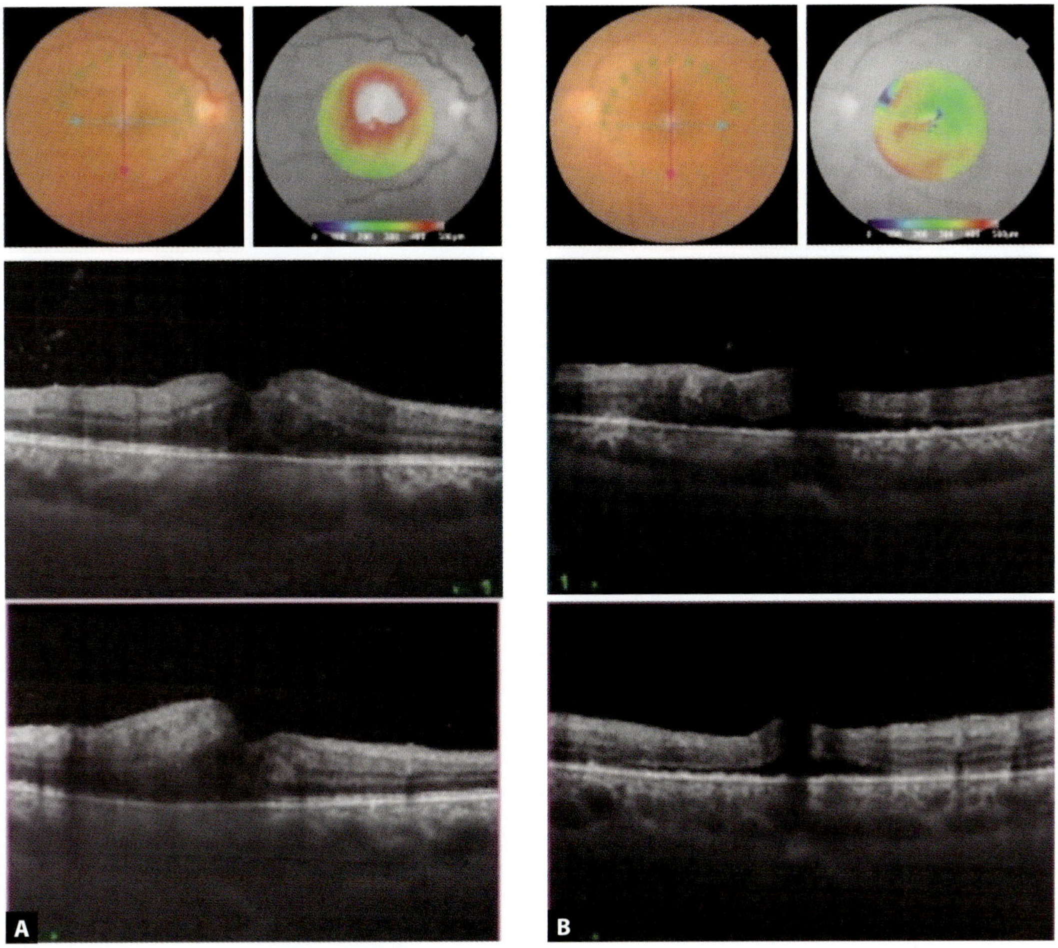

Figs. 24A and B: Optical coherence tomography (OCT) scans of the macula of the right eye (left) showing focal inner retinal thickening and hyperreflectivity corresponding to the retinal infiltrate associated with macular edema and a serous retinal detachment. OCT scans of the macula of the left eye (right) showing multifocal thickening of the RPE with a macular serous retinal detachment and an area of posterior shadowing due to vitreous condensations.
Source: Uveitis Webinar - Grand Round 14. International Uveitis Study Group (IUSG). 2025. https://youtu.be/-E8PbG9PkxE?si=XcEXr31C7XMY23RX.

showed focal thickening of the RPE with a serous retinal detachment. There was an area of posterior shadowing due to vitreous condensations **(Figs. 24A and B)**.

Uveitis Workup

The baseline CBC and CMP were normal. The Mantoux test was negative.

Initial Treatment

The diagnosis of Behçet disease-associated uveitis was made based on a score of five according to International Criteria for Diagnosis of Behçet Disease. The patient was given oral prednisone 1 mg/kg/day, started on azathioprine 2.5 mg/kg/day followed by gradual corticosteroid taper: 10 mg every 10 days until 40 mg then 5 mg every 10 days until 20 mg.

Follow-up

Four months later, the prednisone dose was decreased to 20 mg daily, and the patient developed recurrent inflammation. On examination, visual acuity was 20/100 in the right eye and 20/200 in the left eye. There were pearl-like inferior vitreous opacities with retinitis and macular hemorrhages in the right eye. The left eye exhibited vitreous haze and retinal hemorrhages. Ultra-wide field fluorescein angiography showed diffuse retinal vasculitis with a fern-like appearance **(Figs. 25A and B)**. Adalimumab was started initially at 80 mg once as a loading dose followed by 40 mg every other week.

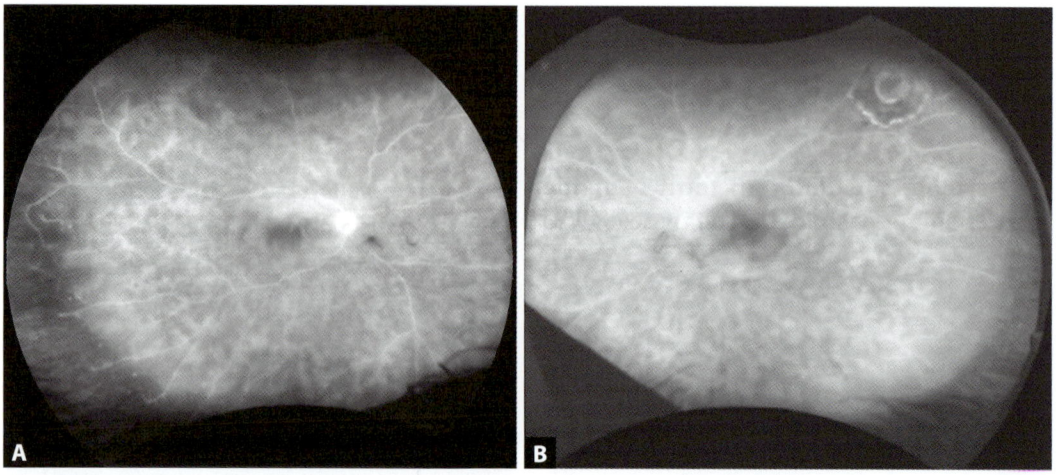

Figs. 25A and B: Late frames in the fluorescein angiography show diffuse vascular leakage in a fern-like pattern in the right eye (A) and the left eye (B).
Source: Uveitis Webinar - Grand Round 14. International Uveitis Study Group (IUSG). 2025. https://youtu.be/-E8PbG9PkxE?si=XcEXr31C7XMY23RX.

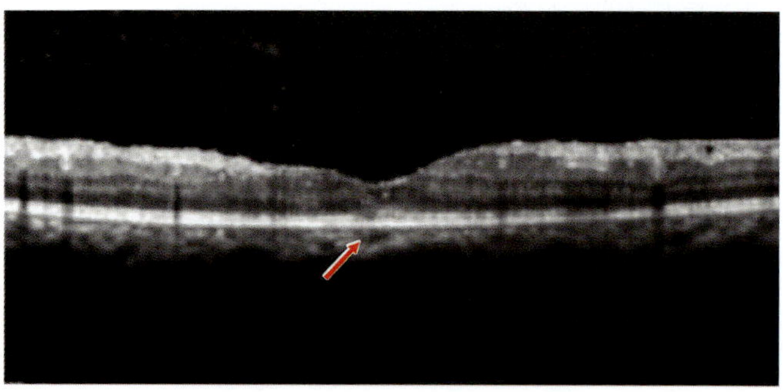

Fig. 26: An optical coherence tomography (OCT) scan through the macula of the right eye showing ellipsoid zone disruption (red arrow).
Source: Uveitis Webinar - Grand Round 14 International Uveitis Study Group (IUSG). 2025. https://youtu.be/-E8PbG9PkxE?si=XcEXr31C7XMY23RX.

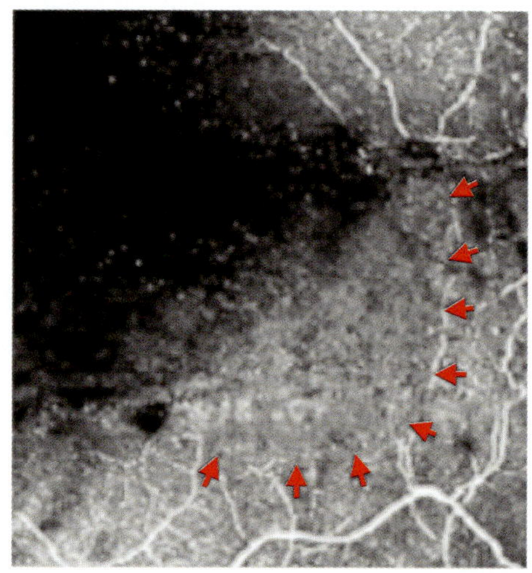

Fig. 27: An optical coherence tomography (OCTA) image of the left macula showing a large flow void temporal to the macula (red arrows) leading to enlargement of the foveal avascular zone.
Source: Uveitis Webinar - Grand Round 14. International Uveitis Study Group (IUSG). 2025. https://youtu.be/-E8PbG9PkxE?si=XcEXr31C7XMY23RX.

Three months later, the visual acuity of the right eye had improved to 20/40 with resolution of the inflammatory changes. Macular central thickness was 284 μm. There was an epiretinal membrane and a focal disruption of the ellipsoid zone on OCT. Enlargement with irregularity of the central avascular zone on OCT angiography (OCTA) was also noted **(Fig. 26)**. Visual acuity of the left eye remained unchanged at 20/200, and there was a mild subcapsular cataract. OCT showed a marked macular atrophy (central macular thickness was 198 μm) and a large area of ellipsoid zone disruption. OCTA showed a large flow deficit **(Fig. 27)**.

Discussion

Objective assessment and quantification of the severity of active Behçet disease-associated uveitis can be made using the SUN criteria, the BOS 24, and the fluorescein angiography scoring system.[13,68,69] The use of multimodal imaging including fluorescein angiography and spectral domain OCT (SD-OCT) is essential to evaluate extramacular and macular structural changes. Infiltrative and ischemic events involving the retinal layers of the macula can cause irreversible reductions in visual acuity that develop gradually with severe attacks, recurrent flares, or chronic, subclinical inflammation. The resulting retinal atrophy can be seen in areas of prior retinitis or occlusive

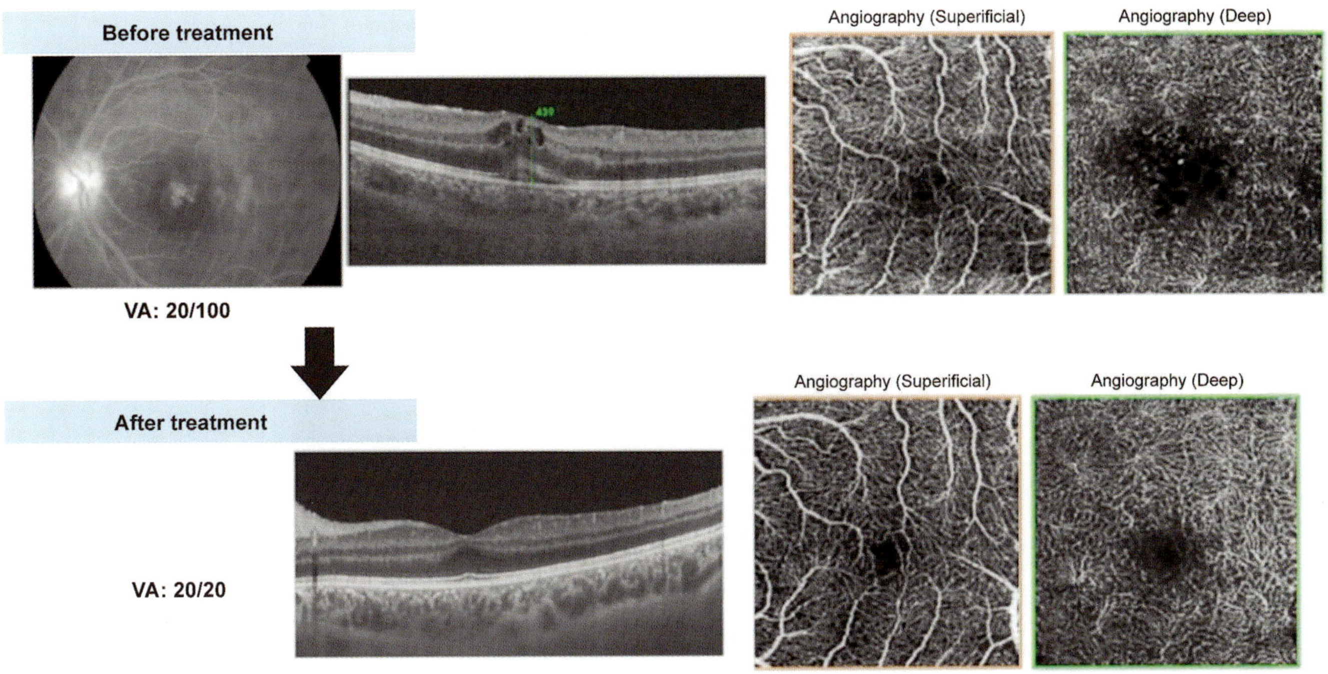

Fig. 28: Multimodal imaging of a left eye during a Behçet disease-associated uveitis flare and after resolution. Superiorly, the fluorescein angiogram shows disc and macular leakage in late frames (top left) and macular edema on optical coherence tomography (OCT) (top center). OCT angiography slabs show decreased flow in the superficial and deep plexi (top right). Resolution of the cystoid macular edema and increased flow are seen (inferior right). (VA: visual acuity)
Source: Uveitis Webinar - Grand Round 14. International Uveitis Study Group (IUSG). 2025. https://youtu.be/-E8PbG9PkxE?si=XcEXr31C7XMY23RX.

retinal vasculitis. A new clinical grading system has been proposed for staging the structural damage.[70] However, OCT remains the gold standard to evaluate the severity of structural damage in Behçet disease-associated uveitis.[71] Findings may include focal or diffuse areas of ellipsoid zone disruption, disorganization of the inner retinal layers, macular atrophy, epiretinal membranes, subfoveal fibrosis, microcystic degeneration, and retinal nerve fiber layer defects.

OCTA is also an important tool to evaluate structural damage in Behçet disease-associated uveitis.[72] Vascular changes with ischemia, mainly involving the deep capillary plexus, can be well visualized. Atrophy on SD-OCT and ischemia on OCTA scans are seen in tandem and are characteristic of the inflammation in Behçet disease-associated uveitis. For example, macular edema resolved in the first case and, there was an improvement of visual acuity to 20/20. The OCT and OCTA scans were normal after clinical resolution **(Fig. 28)**.

Conversely, in the second case despite treatment, the visual acuity improved to only 20/40, and there were persistent ellipsoid zone disruptions on OCT with the presence of areas of capillary non-perfusion on OCTA **(Fig. 29)**.

In conclusion, in Behçet disease-associated uveitis, it is important to make a distinction between active inflammatory changes with potentially reversible vision loss versus permanent tissue damage. It is important to keep in mind that early diagnosis, aggressive immunosuppressive treatment, and close follow-up are essential to prevent the development and progression of sight-threatening structural damage.

DOUBLE TROUBLE: DISSEMINATED TUBERCULOSIS IN BEHÇET'S DISEASE

Case Presentation

Personal Data

A 33-year-old female was referred for a second opinion for a sudden decrease in vision of both eyes in May 2021.

History of Present Illness

Her past medical history included a 7-year history of occlusive retinal vasculitis with panuveitis in both eyes.

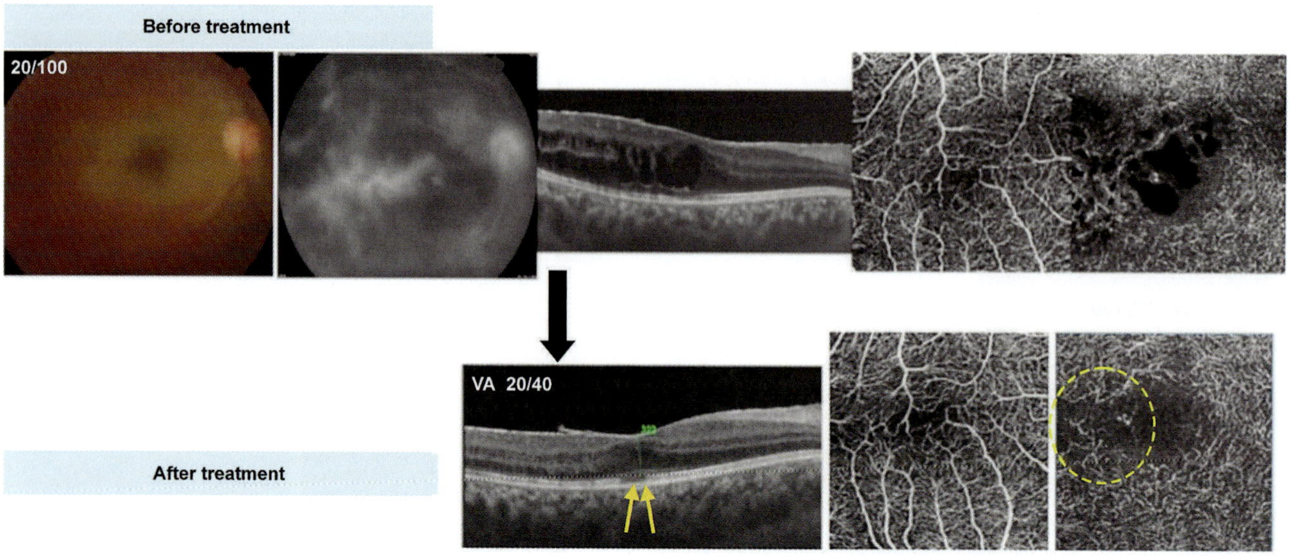

Fig. 29: Multimodal imaging of a right eye during a Behçet disease-associated uveitis flare and after treatment. Superiorly, the fluorescein angiogram shows disc and macular leakage in late frames (top left) and macular edema on optical coherence tomography (OCT) (top center). OCT angiography (OCTA) slabs show decreased flow in the deep capillary plexus (top right). Resolution of the cystoid macular edema with ellipsoid zone loss is seen on OCT, which corresponds to the nasal loss of capillary perfusion remains on OCTA (bottom left and right, respectively).

Source: Uveitis Webinar - Grand Round 14. International Uveitis Study Group (IUSG). 2025. https://youtu.be/-E8PbG9PkxE?si=XcEXr31C7XMY23RX.

Treatment included several tapers of oral corticosteroids and multiple sub-Tenon triamcinolone injections in both eyes. She developed increased intraocular pressures in both eyes, which was managed with topical antiglaucoma medications. She also underwent cataract removal with lens implantation in both eyes. A diagnosis of Behçet disease was made 4 years prior when she developed recurrent oral and genital ulcers and tested positive for the HLA-B51 antigen. She was referred to a rheumatologist at that time and started on azathioprine 100 mg/day. With multiple recurrences, she was advised to start infliximab infusions, but was lost to follow-up due to pregnancy. In January 2020, she developed panuveitis in both eyes with hypopyon formation after recovering from herpes zoster. As she was breastfeeding, she was restarted oral corticosteroids, azathioprine 2 mg/kg, and cyclosporine 3 mg/kg. Despite this, she continued to develop a flare on taper of oral corticosteroids to less than 20 mg/day.

Physical Examination

On presentation, her vision was 20/80 in the right eye and hand motion in the left eye. Both eyes showed optic disc pallor and sclerotic retinal vessels in all quadrants **(Table 5 and Fig. 30)**.

TABLE 5: Physical examination of a patient having disseminated tuberculosis in Behçet disease–associated uveitis.

OD	*Parameter*	*OS*
20/80	BCVA	HM
18 mm Hg	IOP	16 mm Hg
Normal	Conjunctiva	Normal
Fine KPs on the endothelium	Cornea	Fine KPs on the endothelium
0.5+ cell	Anterior chamber	0.5+ cell
Scattered posterior synechiae	Iris	Scattered posterior synechiae
Posterior chamber intraocular lens	Lens	Posterior chamber intraocular lens
2+ cell, 2+ haze	Vitreous	2+ cell, 2+ haze
Optic nerve pallor and 360° of sclerotic vessels	Fundus	Optic nerve pallor and 360° of sclerotic vessels

(BCVA: best-corrected visual acuity; HM: hand motion IOP: intraocular pressure; KPs: keratic precipitates; OD: right eye; OS: left eye)

Ancillary Testing

Fluorescein angiography showed fern-like leakage in all quadrants **(Fig. 31)**. A month later, when she presented

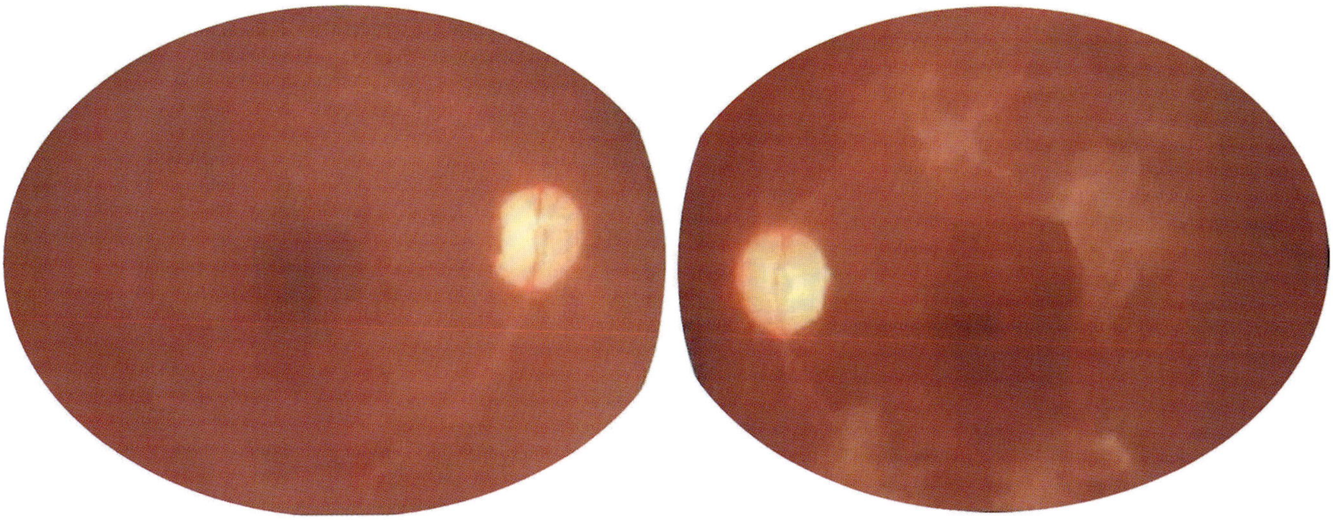

Fig. 30: Color fundus photos of both eyes showing optic disc pallor and sclerotic retinal vessels in all quadrants.
Source: Uveitis Webinar - Grand Round 14. International Uveitis Study Group (IUSG). 2025. https://youtu.be/-E8PbG9PkxE?si=XcEXr31C7XMY23RX.

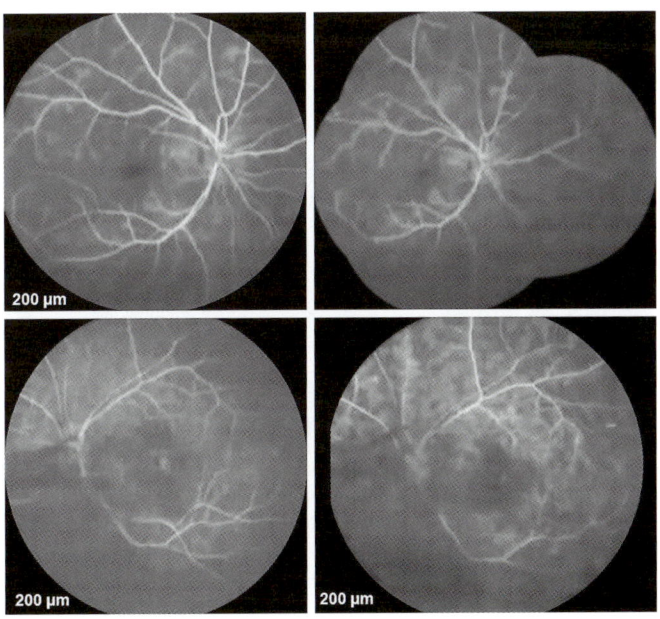

Fig. 31: Fluorescein angiogram images of the right eye (superior) and the left eye (inferior) showing late fern-like leakage. Early and late images showed blocking from vitritis in the left eye.
Source: Uveitis Webinar - Grand Round 14. International Uveitis Study Group (IUSG). 2025. https://youtu.be/-E8PbG9PkxE?si=XcEXr31C7XMY23RX.

to us for the second opinion, she had active panuveitis in both eyes and retinitis in the left eye. The vision in the right eye was 20/400 and light perception in the left eye. OCT scans of both eyes showed epiretinal membrane formation and foveal atrophy with retinal layer disorganization **(Figs. 32A and B)**.

Uveitis Workup

Since she had an extensive prior laboratory and radiographic work-up with rheumatology, no additional studies were ordered.

Initial Treatment

She was started on intravenous methylprednisolone 1 g/day for 3 days, followed by prednisone at 1 mg/kg, azathioprine 100 mg/day, and cyclosporine 100 mg/day. After obtaining negative serologic results for syphilis and tuberculosis, she was prescribed adalimumab 40 mg subcutaneously every 2 weeks. She was unable to start adalimumab due to financial constraints. Through a pharmaceutical patient assistance program, she was able to receive free samples of adalimumab.

Follow-up

In October 2021, cyclosporine was stopped, while azathioprine and adalimumab were continued. Prednisone was tapered to 15 mg/day. At that time, she had no clinical signs of inflammation. By December 2021, prednisone was tapered to 10 mg/day. She concurrently developed oral ulcers and a headache. An MRI of the brain did not reveal any abnormalities. In May 2022, prednisone was further tapered to 7.5 mg/day and a small patch of retinitis was noted in her right eye. Prednisone was increased to 20 mg and cyclosporine was added again at 50 mg/day. In July 2022, prednisone was tapered down to 12.5 mg/day while continuing azathioprine 100 mg/day and adalimumab

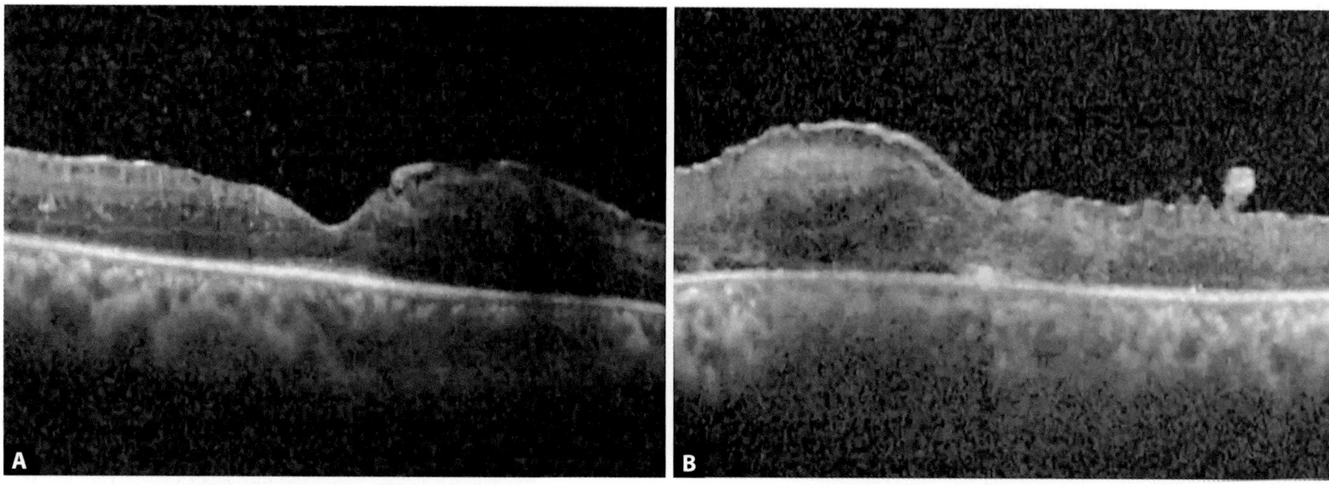

Figs. 32A and B: Optical coherence tomography (OCT) scans of the right (A) and left (B) eyes showing epiretinal membrane formation, retinal atrophy, and loss of retinal layer architecture.
Source: Uveitis Webinar - Grand Round 14. International Uveitis Study Group (IUSG). 2025. https://youtu.be/-E8PbG9PkxE?si=XcEXr31C7XMY23RX.

40 mg every other week. Despite improvement in the vitritis and retinitis, she developed new oral and genital ulcers. Colchicine 1 mg/day was added, and the cyclosporine dose was increased to 100 mg/day. By March 2023, she was on a regimen of alternate day dosing of 7.5 and 10 mg of prednisone, azathioprine 100 mg/day, adalimumab every 2 weeks, colchicine 0.5 mg/day, and cyclosporine 100 mg/day. As she did not have any flares in ocular or systemic inflammation, cyclosporine was discontinued and prednisone was tapered to 7.5 mg/day.

In July 2023, she developed 3 weeks of fever, night sweats, and a cough. Her mother had died of miliary tuberculosis 5 months prior, which was previously not disclosed. A high-resolution CT scan of the thorax showed multiple centrilobular pulmonary nodules prompting the stop of adalimumab. Oral corticosteroids were tapered to 5 mg/day with continuation of the azathioprine and colchicine. Genexpert testing of the sputum came back positive for Mycobacterium tuberculosis (MTB), which was sensitive to both rifampicin and isoniazid. The patient was started on four drug anti-tubercular therapy (ATT). A month later, she was diagnosed with a proximal deep vein thrombosis of the right leg, and coumadin 1 mg/day was started, preventing further increases in prednisone dosing.

In September 2023, the sputum culture for acid fast bacilli was negative, while new retinitis patches were noted in the right eye with a corresponding drop in vision to counting fingers at 3 meters. Given she was now monocular, cyclosporine 100 mg/day was added, prednisone was increased to 10 mg daily, and azathioprine 100 mg/day

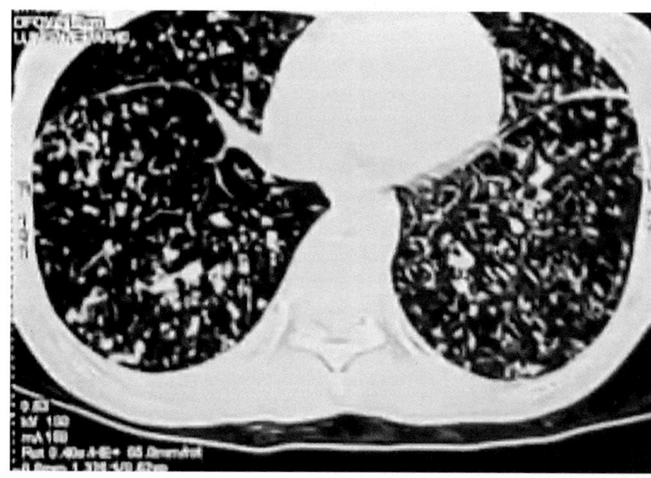

Fig. 33: A high-resolution CT scan of the lungs showing multifocal nodules consistent with Mycobacterium tuberculosis infection.
Source: Uveitis Webinar - Grand Round 14. International Uveitis Study Group (IUSG). 2025. https://youtu.be/-E8PbG9PkxE?si=XcEXr31C7XMY23RX.

was continued. A month later, regression of the pulmonary nodules on a repeat CT scan was seen. With the intensive phase of ATT over, adalimumab 40 mg every other week was restarted in collaboration with pulmonology. Concurrently, cyclosporine was discontinued, and ATT was continued **(Fig. 33)**.

In November 2023, her sputum culture for acid fast bacilli was again negative and she was maintained on oral corticosteroids at 7.5 mg/day, azathioprine 100 mg/day, adalimumab 40 mg every other week, and ATT. But a month later, in December 2023, she developed a fever

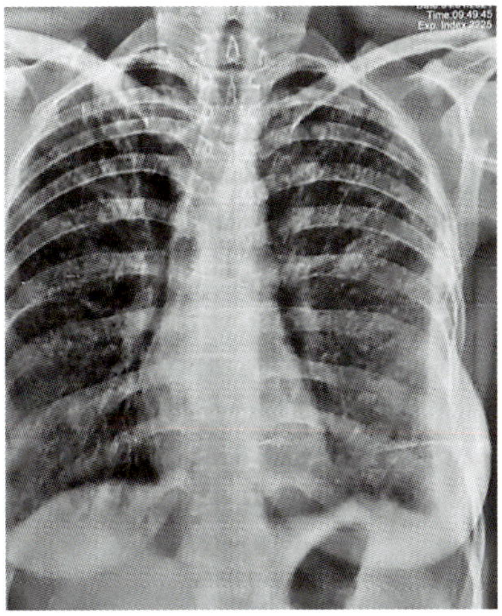

Fig. 34: A posteroanterior view chest X-ray showing increased miliary nodules in both lungs, a patch of consolidation, and a left pleural effusion.
Source: Uveitis Webinar - Grand Round 14. International Uveitis Study Group (IUSG). 2025. https://youtu.be/-E8PbG9PkxE?si=XcEXr31C7XMY23RX.

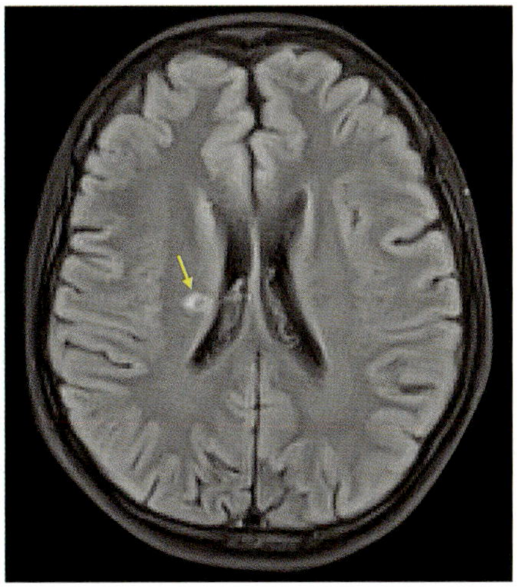

Fig. 35: A T1-weighted MRI image of the brain showing a tuberculoma with surrounding edema near the right lateral ventricle (yellow arrow).
Source: Uveitis Webinar - Grand Round 14. International Uveitis Study Group (IUSG). 2025. https://youtu.be/-E8PbG9PkxE?si=XcEXr31C7XMY23RX.

and a headache. She was readmitted at the tuberculosis sanatorium, where adalimumab was discontinued. A chest X-ray showed increased miliary nodules with patches of consolidation in both lungs and a left pleural effusion. In January 2024, a repeat CT scan of the chest showed extensive miliary nodules with continued consolidation and a left pleural effusion. A pleural paracentesis was performed, but did not yield fluid for culture. A cartridge-based nucleic acid amplification test and line probe assay of the bronchoalveolar lavage were sent to test for MTB. No drug resistance was found. Azathioprine and prednisone were continued at the same doses **(Fig. 34)**.

A month later, an MRI of the brain showed a ring enhancing lesion with surrounding edema, suggestive of tuberculoma. Azathioprine and prednisone were stopped, and only ATT was continued. This time, it was decided that ATT without immunosuppressive agents would be continued for 2 years. While her chest X-ray continued to show pulmonary lesions in follow-up, repeat MRIs of the brain in August 2024 and December 2024 showed a stable tuberculoma. In February 2025, 1 year after her last eye examination, her right eye vision was 20/80 and light perception in the left eye. There was no evidence of vitritis or retinitis. Based on multidisciplinary discussion, ATT was continued without the restart of immunosuppressive medications. But a month later, the visual acuity remained stable despite the development of vitritis without retinitis. Given the inflammation was in her better seeing eye, azathioprine 50 mg/day and cyclosporine 100 mg/day were started **(Fig. 35)**.

Discussion

This was a very challenging case since the diagnosis of Behçet disease was made late in the disease course leading to a delay in the initiation of systemic immunosuppression. At the time of the referral, bilateral optic atrophy and structural damage were already present. The patient was also functionally monocular. There were many therapeutic challenges. The ocular inflammation was refractory and required oral corticosteroids in high doses for almost 10 years. She had also failed the combination of azathioprine and cyclosporine, leaving little choice to start a biologic therapy. Cost was also a major limiting factor, as biologic drugs were not covered by her insurance and treatment was self-funded by the patient. Fortunately, through a patient assistance program, she was able to start adalimumab injections. This highlights a socioeconomic barrier to care, where biologic medications are not covered by many insurances in India.

Another consideration that complicated her care was the endemic nature of MTB in India. The patient also lived in an overcrowded environment while on a combination of corticosteroids and TNF agents for many years. She also had a primary contact who died of miliary TB, which she did not initially disclose. However, the immunosuppressive medications were able to be discontinued, and she was sensitive to ATT. Her ocular disease was complicated by recurrent vitritis then retinitis in the better seeing eye. Despite improvement of the MTB infection and the reinstitution of adalimumab, she unfortunately developed recurrent, disseminated MTB with both pulmonary and central nervous system involvement necessitating a stop of the immunosuppressive agents. She developed vitritis after approximately 14 months of ATT. Whether the underlying infection triggered the immunologic reactions in the disease course is debatable. She is starting to again develop recurrences leading to uncertainty on future options for systemic immunomodulation.

Discussion

From a rheumatologic perspective, there are a few things to highlight about Behçet disease–associated uveitis. Assessing if there is systemic versus isolated ocular involvement helps decide the choice of therapy. There are certain manifestations of systemic involvement that would require the prescription of other medications, which may not be the first choice for ocular disease. For example, in cases of Behçet disease with vascular involvement and ocular inflammation, cyclophosphamide may be the preferred immunosuppressant. It is important to understand that oral and genital ulcers might precede or follow ocular findings making the diagnosis of Behçet disease very difficult. In addition, there are no specific laboratory, histopathologic, or genetic findings to confirm the diagnosis.

The clinical utility of HLA-B51 testing is limited by the frequency within different ethnic populations. There is low endemicity for Behçet disease in India, rendering it an uncommon disease seen in rheumatology practice. Studies have shown that the prevalence of HLA-B51 in those without Behçet disease ranges from 3.8% to 15.6% depending on region of India. The strength of association also varies among clinical phenotypes with isolated ocular involvement having a lower positivity rate for HLA-B51 compared to cases with vascular or neurologic involvement. Given these limitations, there is a reliance on the ophthalmologist to assess if the retinitis or panuveitis are compatible with Behçet's disease.

Initial treatment consists of a combination of azathioprine and cyclosporine. For a woman who weighed barely 45 kg, she was on 100 mg of azathioprine and 150 mg of cyclosporine. Additionally, this is an endemic area for tuberculosis. However, all of the MTB screening tests were done before initiation of TNF therapy, and infliximab would have been a good choice. The dose for Behçet disease with ophthalmic involvement versus treating other organ systems has a large variation. For example, in rheumatoid arthritis, infliximab is dosed at 3 mg/kg; however, in Behçet disease, it is dosed at approximately 5–10 mg/kg. India does not have a state-supported or insurance-based coverage of biologic therapies, leaving access relegated to paying capacity. Luckily for this patient, she obtained pharmaceutical company funding for her treatment. Even after obtaining the adalimumab, she was not given the loading dose. She remained on a dose of 40 mg every other week due to the cost of treatment. The severity of her inflammation required triple therapy, where DMARDs were not stopped despite the addition of a biologic.

Intermittent flares despite the continuance of azathioprine, cyclosporine, and adalimumab left few other options available. Even after the start of ATT and the resumption of immunosuppression therapies, she developed miliary tuberculosis with a tuberculoma in the brain. Interferon-alpha is not available in India; however, it would have been a good choice in the setting of endemic tuberculosis. Apart from adalimumab, golimumab is also available. Unfortunately, the data on the efficacy of golimumab in the treatment of Behçet disease are limited. Tocilizumab is a good option with a lower incidence of tuberculosis. Again, cost is a limiting factor for both intravenous and subcutaneous administrations. The only other option with known efficacy is cyclophosphamide, which is the only affordable treatment available yet contraindicated with a disseminated MTB infection.

The British Association of Dermatologists and the British Society for Rheumatology recently developed guidelines for managing Behçet disease.[73] One of the biggest problems in highly endemic countries is screening for tuberculosis in all patients. Screening is multifold and includes a clinical history, examination, and latent MTB screening with a Mantoux test, QuantiFERON, or another gamma interferon assay. A chest X-ray or helical chest CT is ordered as needed. If any of these results are positive, two-drug ATT is started: isoniazid and rifampicin. Contact tracing becomes very important. The patient never disclosed that her mother had died of pulmonary tuberculosis.

Infections, including tuberculosis, are still rare with the use of biologics in India. One of the biggest hurdles, even if biologic medications are not cost prohibitive, is the increased risk of infection with higher doses. Several trials have shown that the rate of infection exponentially rises with a higher dose. Using an infliximab dose of 5 mg/kg with escalation to 7–10 mg/kg can lead to the development of disseminated infections. Anecdotally, we treated another patient with Behçet disease with a previous history of genitourinary tuberculosis. The patient developed pulmonary tuberculosis when stated on infliximab at 5 mg/kg despite many years of inactive disease. The unmet need in highly endemic countries is a drug that has a lower incidence of tuberculosis infection. Progress can be made on generating more data on the incidence of active tubercular infection with the use of tocilizumab.

Another class of immunosuppressants to consider are JAK inhibitors, although there have been case reports of the development of tuberculosis while on therapy. Still, the incidence of tuberculosis is far less compared to the TNF agents. This patient's repeated episodes of tuberculosis indicated a poor prognosis. Fortunately, she responded to the conventional ATT drug regimen due to lack of infection with a multidrug-resistant organism. Now, there is cautious waiting to slowly restart the azathioprine for the treatment of Behçet disease with the later addition of cyclosporine. Maximizing the dose of both drugs requires continuing ATT. Another future strategy will be the addition of tocilizumab if there are continued flares of Behçet disease.

PEARLS FROM THE EXPERTS ON FREQUENTLY ASKED QUESTIONS

1. What are your views regarding the strategy of tapering TNF agents by increasing the gap between injections and/or infusions? What is the concern for the development of antidrug antibodies, which would then decrease the efficacy of the medication over time?

Answer: There is no clear evidence on a preferred course for treatment in this circumstance. When any TNF treatment is interrupted, patients are prone to developing antidrug antibodies leading to decreased clinical efficacy. This occurs more frequently with infliximab given the murine component of the antibody. If it is not possible to discontinue the biologic agent, the infusion or injection intervals can be extended to assess for breakthrough activation clinically or on the fluorescein angiogram. If another disease-modifying drug is added, such as azathioprine, the chances of antibody formation are much less. When tapering is required and both a DMARD and biologic agent are prescribed, the biologic dose should be lowered first then the DMARD.

2. Is wide field angiography needed to evaluate for retinal vasculitis and to monitor patients with Behçet disease-associated uveitis?

Answer: Yes, using wide field or ultra-wide field fluorescein angiography with peripheral sweeps helps visualize the entire retina for non-perfusion or leakage. Even in clinically inactive patients, focal, mild leakage in the far periphery may be visualized and may be secondary to other causes, including vitreous traction at the ora serrata.

3. When starting a biologic medication, is there a need for tuberculosis screening? Where does anterior chamber aspiration for MTB PCR fall into management strategies?

Answer: Screening with an interferon-gamma release assay is useful as high-dose corticosteroids need to be started right away in clinically active disease. Rapid results of the assay, compared to the Mantoux test, which is read 48–72 hours later, allows for the start of intravenous methylprednisolone 1 g for 3 days with isoniazid. If there is latent MTB, chest imaging is required (chest X-ray or CT chest).

4. Is it difficult to distinguish between MTB and Behçet disease-associated uveitis?

Answer: Normally, there is no confusion between the diagnosis of MTB and Behçet disease at presentation. Anecdotally, we have only had two patients with retinitis-like lesions on presentation with MTB-associated uveitis. Here, we discussed a patient with Behçet disease who developed recurrent ocular inflammation after developing MTB secondary to immunosuppression use. This is a complicated case with the development of a disseminated infection in the setting of rheumatologic disease with both etiologies capable of causing ocular inflammation. Even in this complex case, PCR is not routinely performed. Rheumatologists do order gamma interferon release assays or Mantoux tests to assess for latent MTB infection. If either is positive, ATT is started with later addition of biologic immunosuppression.

A patient with occlusive retinal vasculitis, compared to Behçet disease-associated vasculitis, is not truly occlusive at first. The initial phase of inflammation begins with capillary leakage then later with later large vessel occlusions. Another point of differentiation is that MTB-related ocular inflammation involves the retinal pigment epithelium. If hypoautofluorescent areas are noted on wide field autofluorescence imaging prior to indocyanine green angiography, it is less likely

Behçet disease-associated uveitis and more likely MTB as the cause of the ocular inflammation. Another disease in the differential diagnosis for Behçet disease is Crohns disease in terms of both the systemic and ocular manifestations.

5. How is autoimmune disease differentiated from tuberculosis? When there is a flare, is the inflammation secondary to the autoimmune disease or tuberculosis?

Answer: There is an interesting interaction between MTB and Behçet disease with overlapping genetic disease susceptibility. There are studies on the incidence and prevalence of MTB in patients with Behçet disease. For example, there is a study from Turkey, comparing the incidence of active MTB infection in patients on TNF treatment by a rheumatologist. The incidence was 8% in those with Behçet disease versus less than 1% in all other diagnoses, including rheumatoid arthritis and the spondyloarthropathies. Heat shock protein 65, a mycobacterial protein that leads to leukocyte activation, shows molecular mimicry with heat shock protein 60 in humans. It has been hypothesized that molecular mimicry in MTB infection may be related to the onset and recurrence of Behçet disease.

6. What is the importance of HLA-B52? Are there other genes that have been associated with Behçet disease?

Answer: Only HLA-B51 has been associated with the development of Behçet disease in Turkey. In Japan, HLA-A26 is associated with the development of ocular disease. While there are some other genes that have been implicated, they are weaker disease associations. The mechanism of HLA genes causing Behçet disease is complex and not fully understood. Alleles confer susceptibility or protection from developing Behçet disease, and the interaction of the genetic effects varies both individually and by region.

7. In addition to genetic testing, does pathergy testing play a role in the diagnosis of Behçet disease?

Answer: Yes, if the pathergy test is positive, it is very helpful. However, in most cases, it is negative. Research is being conducted on how to improve the reliability and sensitivity of the pathergy test by employing the pneumococcal vaccine to be placed at the injection site.

8. Is the rate of isolated anterior uveitis, which is estimated to account for 10% of Behçet disease-associated cases, underestimated secondary to overestimation of vitritis and posterior pole involvement?

Answer: That figure comes from a past study where fluorescein angiography was not routinely performed and did not include sweeping images of the peripheral retina. If fluorescein angiogram was performed on every patient presenting with any grade of anterior chamber inflammation, the true percentage of posterior segment involvement would likely be higher.

9. Does alteration of gut microflora have any role in the treatment? Are there data on the development of autoinflammatory disease due to gut flora and gene susceptibility in patients with Behçet disease?

Answer: Yes, alterations of gut microbiota have been reported by several investigators. Giacomo Emmi has tried to modulate microbiota through diet modification and butyrate supplements. While the microbiota were altered, the clinical expression of the disease was not changed. More research is needed in this area. If asked by patients about what they should eat, we recommend probiotics. There are also anecdotal stories from patients that certain foods increase the risk of oral ulcers, such as the consumption of walnuts. Again, data are lacking on the impact of specific foods on clinical disease. The problem lies in understanding which microbiota need to be replaced.

FINAL WRAP-UP

Behçet disease is a multiorgan inflammatory condition requiring aggressive prescription of corticosteroids for initial control of inflammation with transition to DMARDs and biologics for long-term management. Screening for and continued assessment for risk factors associated with MTB infection are needed with the use of biologic therapies. More research is needed to identify new immunosuppressive agents that are both effective to treat the inflammation in Behçet disease with a lower risk of disseminated MTB infection. Additional studies are also needed to identify how changes in the gut flora can alter the severity of Behçet disease.

REFERENCES

1. Tugal-Tutkun I. Behçet's Disease. Int Ophthalmol Clin. 2010;50(2):1-19.
2. Abi-Rached L, Jobin MJ, Kulkarni S, McWhinnie A, Dalva K, Gragert L, et al. The shaping of modern human immune systems by multiregional admixture with archaic humans. Science. 2011;334(6052):89-94.
3. Kirino Y, Bertsias G, Ishigatsubo Y, Mizuki N, Tugal-Tutkun I, Seyahi E, et al. Genome-wide association analysis identifies new susceptibility loci for Behçet's disease and epistasis between HLA-B*51 and ERAP1. Nat Genet. 2013;45(2):202-7.

4. Kuiper JJ, Prinz JC, Stratikos E, Kuśnierczyk P, Arakawa A, Springer S, et al. EULAR study group on 'MHC-I-opathy': identifying disease-overarching mechanisms across disciplines and borders. Ann Rheum Dis. 2023;82(7): 887-96.
5. Mattioli I, Bettiol A, Saruhan-Direskeneli G, Direskeneli H, Emmi G. Pathogenesis of Behçet's Syndrome: Genetic, Environmental and Immunological Factors. Front Med (Lausanne). 2021;8:713052.
6. Tunc R, Keyman E, Melikoglu M, Fresko I, Yazici H. Target organ associations in Turkish patients with Behçet's disease: a cross sectional study by exploratory factor analysis. J Rheumatol. 2002;29(11):2393-6.
7. Soejima Y, Ohno S, Kirino Y, Takeno M, Kurosawa M, Takeuchi M, et al. Changes in the proportion of clinical clusters contribute to the phenotypic evolution of Behçet's disease in Japan. Arthritis Res Ther. 2021;23(1):49.
8. Li C, Li L, Wu X, Shi J, Liu J, Zhou J, Wang L, Tian X, Zeng X, Zheng W. Clinical manifestations of Behcet's disease in a large cohort of Chinese patients: gender- and age-related differences. Clin Rheumatol. 2020;39(11):3449-54.
9. Standardization of Uveitis Nomenclature (SUN) Working Group. Development of classification criteria for uveitis of Behçet's disease. Am J Ophthalmol. 2021;228:201-10.
10. International Study Group for Behcet's Disease. Criteria for diagnosis of Behcet's disease. Lancet. 1990;335(8697): 1078-80.
11. Kaburaki T, Namba K, Sonoda KH, Kezuka T, Keino H, Fukuhara T, et al. Ocular Behçet Disease Research Group of Japan. Behçet's disease ocular attack score 24: evaluation of ocular disease activity before and after initiation of infliximab. Jpn J Ophthalmol. 2014;58(2):120-30.
12. Tanaka R, Murata H, Takamoto M, Ohtomo K, Okinaga K, Yoshida A, et al. Behçet's disease ocular attack score 24 and visual outcome in patients with Behçet's disease. Br J Ophthalmol. 2016;100(7):990-94.
13. Jabs DA, Nussenblatt RB, Rosenbaum JT; Standardization of Uveitis Nomenclature (SUN) Working Group. Standardization of uveitis nomenclature for reporting clinical data: Results of the first international workshop. Am J Ophthalmol. 2005;140(3):509-16.
14. Oray M, Onal S, Bayraktar S, Izgi B, Tugal-Tutkun I. Nonglaucomatous localized retinal nerve fiber layer defects in Behçet uveitis. Am J Ophthalmol. 2015;159(3): 475-81.e1.
15. Tugal-Tutkun I, Ozdal PC, Oray M, Onal S. Review for Diagnostics of the Year: Multimodal Imaging in Behçet Uveitis. Ocul Immunol Inflamm. 2017;25(1):7-19.
16. Kido A, Uji A, Morooka S, Kuroda Y, Arichika S, Akagi T, et al. Outer Plexiform Layer Elevations as a Marker for Prior Ocular Attacks in Patients With Behcet's Disease. Invest Ophthalmol Vis Sci. 2018;59(7):2828-32.
17. Tugal-Tutkun I, Onal S, Stanford M, Akman M, Twisk JWR, Boers M, et al. An algorithm for the diagnosis of Behcet disease uveitis in adults. Ocul Immunol Inflamm. 2021;29(6):1154-63.
18. Tugal-Tutkun I, Herbort C, Khairallah M, the Angiographic Scoring for Uveitis Working Group (ASUWOG). Scoring of dual fluorescein and ICG inflammatory angiographic signs for the grading of posterior segment inflammation (dual fluorescein and ICG angiographic scoring system for uveitis). Int Ophthalmol. 2010;30(5):539-52.
19. Keino H, Okada AA, Watanabe T, Nakayama M, Nakamura T. Efficacy of Infliximab for Early Remission Induction in Refractory Uveoretinitis Associated with Behçet Disease: A 2-year Follow-up Study. Ocul Immunol Inflamm. 2017;25(1):46-51.
20. Shirahama S, Kaburaki T, Matsuda J, Tanaka R, Nakahara H, Komae K, et al. The Relationship between Fluorescein Angiography Leakage after Infliximab Therapy and Relapse of Ocular Inflammatory Attacks in Ocular Behçet's Disease Patients. Ocul Immunol Inflamm. 2020;28(8):1166-70.
21. Tugal-Tutkun I, Cingü K, Kir N, Yeniad B, Urgancioglu M, Gül A. Use of laser flare-cell photometry to quantify intraocular inflammation in patients with Behcet uveitis. Graefes Arch Clin Exp Ophthalmol. 2008;246(8):1169-77.
22. Guner MK, Guner ME, Oray M, Tugal-Tutkun I. Correlation between widefield fundus fluorescein angiography leakage score and anterior chamber flare in Behçet uveitis. Ocul Immunol Inflamm. 2024;32(1):123-30.
23. Tugal-Tutkun I, Onal S, Altan-Yaycioglu R, Altunbas HH, Urgancioglu M. Uveitis in Behçet disease: an analysis of 880 patients. Am J Ophthalmol. 2004;138(3):373-80.
24. Tugal-Tutkun I, Güney-Tefekli E, Urgancioglu M. Results of interferon-alfa therapy in patients with Behçet uveitis. Graefes Arch Clin Exp Ophthalmol. 2006;244(12):1692-5.
25. Kötter I, Zierhut M, Eckstein AK, Vonthein R, Ness T, Günaydin I, et al. Human recombinant interferon alfa-2a for the treatment of Behcet's disease with sight threatening posterior or panuveitis. Br J Ophthalmol. 2003;87(4):423-31.
26. Gueudry J, Wechsler B, Terrada C, Gendron G, Cassoux N, Fardeau C, et al. Long-term efficacy and safety of low-dose interferon alpha2a therapy in severe uveitis associated with Behcet disease. Am J Ophthalmol. 2008;146(6):837-44.e1.
27. Sobaci G, Erdem U, Durukan AH, Erdurman C, Bayer A, Köksal S, et al. Safety and effectiveness of interferon alpha-2ᵃ in treatment of patients with Behcet's uveitis refractory to conventional treatments. Ophthalmology. 2010;117(7):1430-5.
28. Deuter CM, Zierhut M, Möhle A, Vonthein R, Stöbiger N, Kötter I. Long-term remission after cessation of interferon-alpha treatment in patients with severe uveitis due to Behcet's disease. Arthritis Rheum. 2010;62(9):2796-805.
29. Onal S, Kazokoglu H, Koc A, Akman M, Bavbek T, Direskeneli H, et al. Long-term efficacy and safety of low-dose and dose-escalating interferón alfa-2a therapy in refractory Behcet uveítis. Arch Ophthalmol. 2011;129(3):288-94.
30. Diwo E, Guedry J, Saadoun D, Weschler B, LeHoang P, Bodaghi B. Long-term efficacy of interferon in severe uveitis

associated with Behcet disease. Ocul Immunol Inflamm. 2017;25(1):76-84.

31. Qian Y, Qu Y, Gao F, Pei M, Liang A, Xiao J, et al. Comparison of the Safety and Efficacy of Interferon Alpha-2a and Cyclosporine-A When Combined With Glucocorticoid in the Treatment of Refractory Behçet's Uveitis: A Randomized Controlled Prospective Study. Front Pharmacol. 2021;12:699903.
32. Zhong Z, Deng D, Gao Y, Bu Q, Dai L, Feng X, et al. immunomodulatory agents for prevention of uveitis relapse in patients with severe Behçet's disease already on corticosteroid therapy: a randomised, open-label, head-to-head trial. Lancet Rheumatol. 2024;6(11):e780-e790.
33. Moots RJ, Fortune F, Jackson R, Thornburn T, Morgan AW, Carr DF, et al. Predicting response to infliximab and interferon-α in Behçet's syndrome: An exploratory analysis from the BIO-BEHÇET'S randomized controlled trial. Rheumatol Immunol Res. 2025;6(2):70-79. doi: 10.1515/rir-2025-0010. eCollection 2025 Jun.
34. Buggage RR, Levy-Clarke G, Sen HN, Ursea R, Srivastava SK, Suhler EB, et al. A double-masked, randomized study to investigate the safety and efficacy of daclizumab to treat the ocular complications related to Behçet's disease. Ocul Immunol Inflamm. 2007;15(2):63-70.
35. Dick AD, Tugal-Tutkun I, Foster S, Zierhut M, Melissa Liew SH, Bezlyak V, et al. Secukinumab in the treatment of noninfectious uveitis: results of three randomized, controlled clinical trials. Ophthalmology. 2013;120(4):777-87.
36. Tugal-Tutkun I, Pavesio C, De Cordoue A, Bernard-Poenaru O, Gül A. Use of Gevokizumab in Patients with Behçet's Disease Uveitis: An International, Randomized, Double-Masked, Placebo-Controlled Study and Open-Label Extension Study. Ocul Immunol Inflamm. 2018;26(7):1023-33.
37. Levy-Clarke G, Jabs DA, Read RW, Rosenbaum JT, Vitale A, Van Gelder RN. Expert panel recommendations for the use of anti-tumor necrosis factor biologic agents in patients with ocular inflammatory disorders. Ophthalmology. 2014;121(3):785-96.e3.
38. Yang S, Huang Z, Hu Y, Zhang J, Liu X, Li H, et al. The Efficacy of Adalimumab as an Initial Treatment in Patients with Behcet's Retinal Vasculitis. Front Pharmacol. 2021;12:609148.
39. Sfikakis PP, Markomichelakis N, Alpsoy E, Assaad-Khalil S, Bodaghi B, Gul A, et al. Anti-TNF therapy in the management of Behçet's disease. Arthritis Rheumatol. 2017;69(2):392-401.
40. Markomichelakis N, Delicha E, Masselos S, Fragiadaki K, Kaklamanis P, Sfikakis PP, et al. A single infliximab infusion vs corticosteroids for acute panuveitis attacks in Behçet's disease: a comparative 4-week study. Rheumatology (Oxford). 2011;50(3):593-7.
41. Jaffe GJ, Dick AD, Brézin AP, Nguyen QD, Thorne JE, Kestelyn P, et al. Adalimumab in patients with active noninfectious uveitis. N Engl J Med. 2016;375(10):932-43.
42. Nguyen QD, Merrill PT, Jaffe GJ, Dick AD, Kurup SK, Sheppard J, et al. Adalimumab for prevention of uveitis flare in patients with inactive non-infectious uveitis controlled by corticosteroids (VISUAL II): a multicentre, double-masked, randomised, placebo-controlled phase 3 trial. Lancet. 2016;388(10050):1183-92.
43. Fabiani C, Sota J, Vitale A, Rigante D, Emmi G, Vannozzi L, et al. Cumulative retention rate of adalimumab in patients with Behcet's disease-related uveitis: a four-year follow-up study. Br J Ophthalmol. 2018;102(5):637-41.
44. Fabiani C, Sota J, Vitale A, Emmi G, Vannozzi L, Bacherini D, et al. Ten-Year Retention Rate of Infliximab in Patients with Behcet's Disease-Related Uveitis. Ocul Immunol Inflamm. 2019;27(1):34-9.
45. Atienza-Mateo B, Martín-Varillas JL, Calvo-Río V, Demetrio-Pablo R, Beltrán E, Sánchez-Bursón J, et al. Comparative Study of Infliximab Versus Adalimumab in Refractory Uveitis due to Behcet's Disease: National Multicenter Study of 177 Cases. Arthritis Rheumatol. 2019;71(12):2081-89.
46. Takeuchi M, Usui Y, Namba K, Keino H, Takeuchi M, Takase H, et al. Ten-year follow-up of infliximab treatment for uveitis in Behçet disease patients: A multicenter retrospective study. Front Med (Lausanne). 2023;10:1095423.
47. Barroso-Garcia N, Martín-Varillas JL, Ferraz-Amaro I, Sánchez-Bilbao L, Martín-Gutiérrez A, Adán A, et al. Comparative study of adalimumab, infliximab and certolizumab pegol in the treatment of cystoid macular edema due to Behçet's disease. J Clin Med. 2024;13(2):1234.
48. Barroso-Garcia N, Atienza-Mateo b, Ferraz-Amaro I, Prieto-Peña D, Beltrán E, Adán A, et al. Anti-TNF vs tocilizumab in refractory uveitic cystoid macular edema due to Behçet's disease. Multicenter study of 49 patients. Semin Arthritis Rheum. 2023;58:152153.
49. Arida A, Saadoun D, Sfikakis PP. IL-6 Blockade for Behçet's disease: review on 31 anti-RNF naïve and 45 anti-TNF experienced patients. Clin Exp Rheumatol. 2022;40(8):1575-83.
50. Khitri MY, Bartoli A, Maalouf G, Deroux A, Salvarani C, Emmi G, et al. Tocilizumab in Behçet's disease: a multicenter study of 30 patients. J Rheumatol. 2023;50(7):916-23.
51. Ozguler Y, Ozdede A, Hatemi G. Recent Insights into the Management of Behçet Syndrome. J Inflamm Res. 2021;14: 3429-41.
52. Tukek NB, Esatoglu SN, Hatemi G, Calıskan EB, Ozyazgan Y, Ucar D, et al. Emergence of new manifestations during infliximab treatment in Behcet's syndrome. Rheumatology (Oxford). 2022;61(9):3746-53.
53. Esatoglu SN, Sonmez O, Ucar D, Kaymaz E, Ozguler Y, Ugurlu S, et al. De novo manifestations during adalimumab treatment in Behçet's syndrome. Rheumatology (Oxford). 2025;64(4): 2034-40.

54. Ohno S, Umebayashi I, Matsukawa M, Goto T, Yano T. Safety and efficacy of infliximab in the treatment of refractory uveoretinitis in Behçet's disease: a large-scale, long-term postmarketing surveillance in Japan. Arthritis Res Ther. 2019;21(1):2.
55. Sener H, Evereklioglu C, Horozoglu F, Gunay Sener AB. Efficacy and safety of adalimumab in patients with Behçet uveitis: a systematic review and meta-analysis. Ocul Immunol Inflamm. 2024;32(1):89-97.
56. Tugal-Tutkun I, Özdal PÇ. Behçet's disease uveitis: is there a need for new emerging drugs? Expert Opin Emerg Drugs. 2020;25(4):531-47.
57. Taylor SR, Singh J, Menezo V, Wakefield D, McCluskey P, Lightman S. Behcet disease: visual prognosis and factors influencing the development of visual loss. Am J Ophthalmol. 2011;152(6):1059-66.
58. Cingu AK, Onal S, Urgancioglu M, Tugal-Tutkun I. Comparison of presenting features and three-year disease course in Turkish patients with Behcet uveitis who presented in the early 1990s and the early 2000s. Ocul Immunol Inflamm. 2012;20(6):423-8.
59. Keino H, Okada AA, Watanabe T, Nakayama M, Nakamura T. Efficacy of Infliximab for Early Remission Induction in Refractory Uveoretinitis Associated with Behcet Disease: A 2-year Follow-up Study. Ocul Immunol Inflamm. 2017;25(1):46-51.
60. Khabbazi A, Karkon Shayan F, Ghojazadeh M, Kavandi H, Hajialiloo M, Esalat Manesh K, et al. Adherence to treatment in patients with Behcet's disease. Int J Rheum Dis. 2018;21(12):2158-66.
61. Zayed HS, Medhat BM, Seif EM. Evaluation of treatment adherence in patients with Behcet's disease: its relation to disease manifestations, patients' beliefs about medications, and quality of life. Clin Rheumatol. 2019;38(3):761-8.
62. Oklar M, Zorlutuna Kaymak N, Tanyildiz B, Tezcan ME, Şimşek Ş. Treatment Adherence Effect on the Visual Acuity of Behcet's Uveitis Patients. Ocul Immunol Inflamm. 2024;32(8):1698-706.
63. Hatemi G, Christensen R, Bang D, Bodaghi B, Celik AF, Fortune F, et al. 2018 update of the EULAR recommendations for the management of Behcet's syndrome. Ann Rheum Dis. 2018;77(6):808-18.
64. Calvo-Río V, Blanco R, Beltrán E, Sánchez-Bursón J, Mesquida M, Adán A, et al. Anti-TNF-alpha therapy in patients with refractory uveitis due to Behcet's disease: a 1-year follow-up study of 124 patients. Rheumatology (Oxford). 2014;53(12):2223-31.
65. Horiguchi N, Kamoi K, Horie S, Kurozumi-Karube H, Takase H, Ohno-Matsui K. A 10-year follow-up of infliximav monotherapy for refractory uveítis in Behcet síndrome. Sci Rep. 2020;10(1):22227.
66. Hu Y, Huang Z, Yang S, Chen X, Su W, Liang D. Effectiveness and Safety of Anti-Tumor Necrosis Factor-Alpha Agents Treatment in Behcets' Disease-Associated Uveitis: A Systematic Review and Meta-Analysis. Front Pharmacol. 2020;11:941.
67. Vallet H, Seve P, Biard L, Baptiste Fraison J, Bielefeld P, Perard L, et al.; French Uveitis Network. Infliximab Versus Adalimumab in the Treatment of Refractory Inflammatory Uveitis: A Multicenter Study From the French Uveitis Network. Arthritis Rheumatol. 2016;68(6):1522-30.
68. Kaburaki T, Namba K, Sonoda KH, Kezuka T, Keino H, Fukuhara T, et al. Behçet's disease ocular attack score 24: evaluation of ocular disease activity before and after initiation of infliximab. Jpn J Ophthalmol. 2014;58(2):120-30.
69. Keorochana N, Homchampa N, Vongkulsiri S, Choontanom R. Fluorescein angiographic findings and Behcet's disease ocular attack score 24 (BOS24) as prognostic factors for visual outcome in patients with ocular Behcet's disease. Int J Retina Vitreous. 2021;7(1):48.
70. Ozyazgan Y, Ucar D, Oto BB, Esatoglu SN, Ozguler Y, Hatemi G, et al. A proposal of a new tool for the assessment of damage in Behçet syndrome uveitis: Cerrahpasa Ocular Damage Grading System. Ocul Immunol Inflamm. 2024;232-8.
71. Oray M, Onal S, Bayraktar S, Izgi B, Tugal-Tutkun I. Nonglaucomatous localized retinal nerve fiber layer defects in Behçet uveitis. Am J Ophthalmol. 2015;159(3):475-481.e1.
72. Khairallah M, Abroug N, Khochtali S, Anis Mahmoud, Bechir Jelliti, Gabriel Coscas, et al. Optical coherence tomography angiography in patients with Behçet uveitis. Retina. 2017;37(9):1678-86.
73. Murphy R, Moots RJ, Brogan P, Çelik AF, Clement-Jones M, Coulson I, et al.; British Association of Dermatologists and British Society for Rheumatology living guideline for managing people with Behçets 2024. Br J Dermatol. 2024;191(5):e8-e25.

CHAPTER

15 Non-Infectious Posterior Uveitis (NIPU)

Janet Davis, Lawrence Chan, Anita Agarwal, Alessandro Feo, Shahin Faghihi, David Sarraf, Russel Dinh, Sapna Gangaputra, Maggie Feng, Vishali Gupta, Marc de Smet, John H Kempen, Reema Bansal, Alejandra de-la-Torre, Meghan Berkenstock

INTRODUCTION

"White Dot Syndrome" is a non-specific term used by many to describe a group of inflammatory disorders of the eye characterized by multiple white lesions at the level of the outer retina, retinal pigment epithelium, and/or choroid. Although their precise etiology remains unclear, immune-mediated mechanisms are believed to play a central role. Advances in multimodal imaging (MMI) and immunopathological understanding have improved diagnostic accuracy and management. Tailored therapy helps control inflammation, prevent structural damage, and preserve visual function. A nuanced approach based on disease phenotype, lesion location, and patient profile enhances outcomes and minimizes treatment-related risks.

THEMATIC LECTURE: WHITE DOT SYNDROMES: IMPROVED DEFINITIONS AND DIAGNOSTIC TOOLS

This work was inspired by the exceptionally successful *Inflammatio* conference held in November 2024 in Singapore. We would like to retire the term White Dot Syndromes (WDS) and transition to discussing non-infectious posterior uveitides. These following case studies show the expanded range of inflammatory diseases that we need to consider when we talk about this class of ocular inflammation. Here are three cases that look like a non-infectious posterior uveitis **(Fig. 1)**. The fundus autofluorescence image superiorly is due to use of the heparinase inhibitor, fondaparinux. Similar to pentosan polysulfate sodium, the class effect of this drug causes retinal pigment epithelial changes that resemble acute posterior multifocal placoid pigment epitheliopathy (APMPPE). What differentiates the clinical appearance is that fondaparinux changes are more symmetric, but still result in the same convalescent appearance with hyperreflectivity and hypertrophy of the retinal pigment epithelium creating hyperautofluorescent scars. The color fundus photo in the middle shows chorioretinal scarring in a patient with chronic variable immunodeficiency resulting from multiple prior infections. As opposed to multifocal choroiditis, the lesions are very atrophic and progress in an unusual manner over time. The last image shows early and late fluorescein angiogram images showing a case of late onset CEP250 retinal degeneration with inflammatory features.

The timeline of the Standardization of Uveitis Nomenclature (SUN) II is important to discuss as it defined research criteria for diagnosing of the WDS.[1] The project was conceived in 2012, which is when the use of MMI started. Data were collected between 2012 and 2016, which included fundus photographs. Data were curated in 2017, and machine learning occurred in 2018. The manuscript was written in 2019 with approval at the end of the year and final publication occurred in 2021. It was a long process for an extremely well-done project. The basis of the *Inflammatio* meeting was to reach a consensus vote on the basic imaging set required to make the diagnosis of a WDS. This is part of a larger MMI in Uveitis (MUV) project, which will look at the minimal imaging set required for infectious uveitides as well. The initial MUV project took about a year and a half and it is still not complete. Manuscripts resulting from the Delphi process will be published in the *American Journal of Ophthalmology*.

The WDS encompass six specific entities with defined diagnostic criteria, as specified in SUN II. The first diagnosis we will discuss is APMPPE, which is defined as

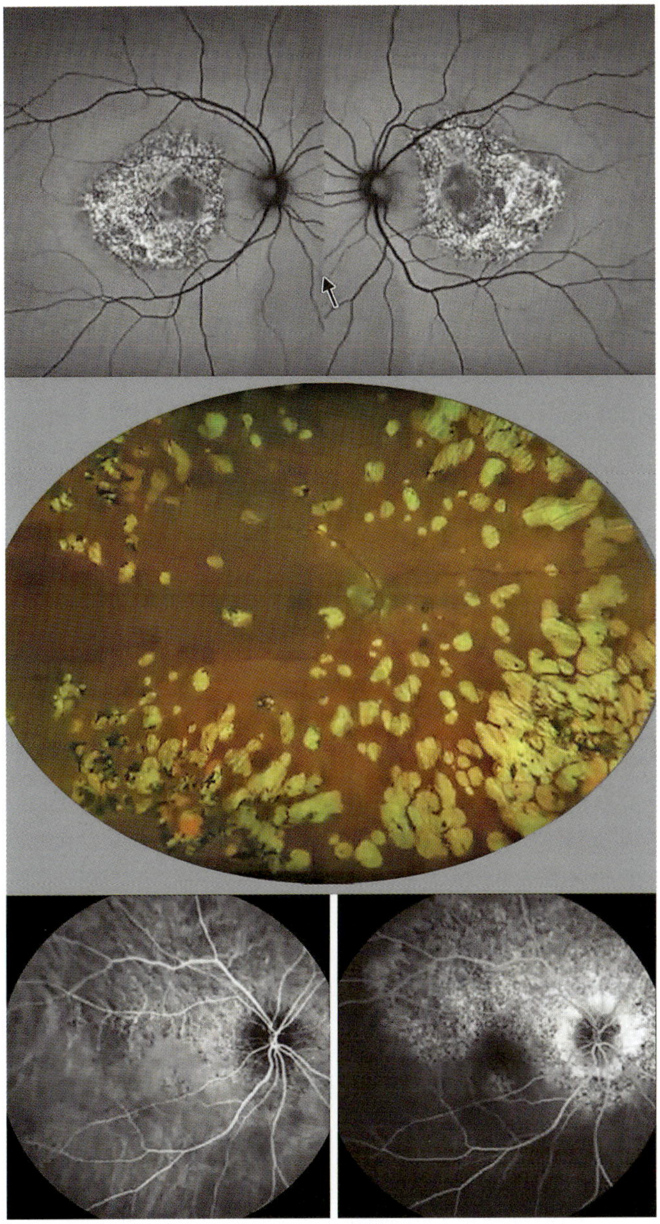

Fig. 1: Fundus autofluorescence images (superiorly) in a patient using a heparinase inhibitor, fondaparinux. The color fundus photo (middle) shows atrophic scars in a patient with chronic variable immune deficiency. The early and late fluorescein angiography images (bottom) show window defects and staining in a case of late-onset CEP250 retinal degeneration.
Source: Uveitis Webinar - Grand Round 15. International Uveitis Study Group (IUSG). 2025. https://youtu.be/zWjjQGAAxh4?si=KrNaSnT3l5p4Mzkt.

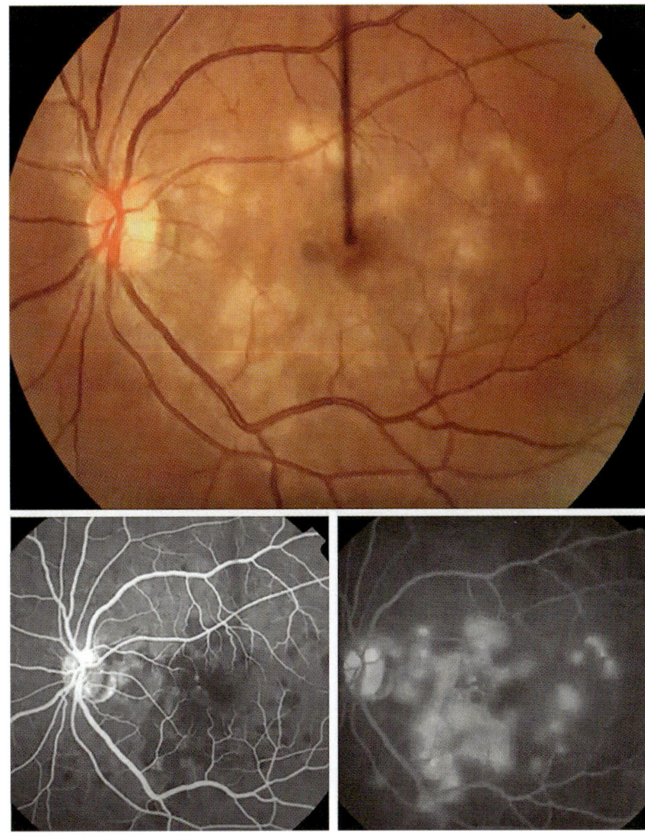

Fig. 2: A color fundus photo of a left eye showing macular, yellow, plaque-like lesions (top). An early-phase fluorescein angiogram (bottom left) shows blocking of the lesions and late staining (bottom right) in acute posterior multifocal placoid pigment epitheliopathy.
Source: Uveitis Webinar - Grand Round 15. International Uveitis Study Group (IUSG). 2025. https://youtu.be/zWjjQGAAxh4?si=KrNaSnT3l5p4Mzkt.

paucifocal or multifocal, plaque-like lesions on fundus photography.[2] On fluorescein angiography, there is blocking of the lesions with late staining **(Fig. 2)**. The imaging findings in the convalescent phase of the disease were not addressed in SUN II. Similarly, the appearance of lesions on indocyanine green (ICG) was not discussed. An important part of the diagnostic criteria, which is consistent across all WDS, is the exclusion of alternative etiologies, such as syphilis or sarcoidosis.

The next disease that was studied was birdshot chorioretinopathy. The SUN II criteria had pauci-imaging requirements for this entity, as images with the appearance of birdshot lesions were accepted.[3] However, this diagnosis can be challenging for clinicians who are not uveitis specialists. Imaging was not required if fundus photos had birdshot appearing lesions with minimal vitritis or if HLA-A29 testing was positive in the clinical setting of multifocal choroiditis. An ICG was not required, except in rare cases where spots were not visible, which differs from many clinical practices, where it is commonly performed

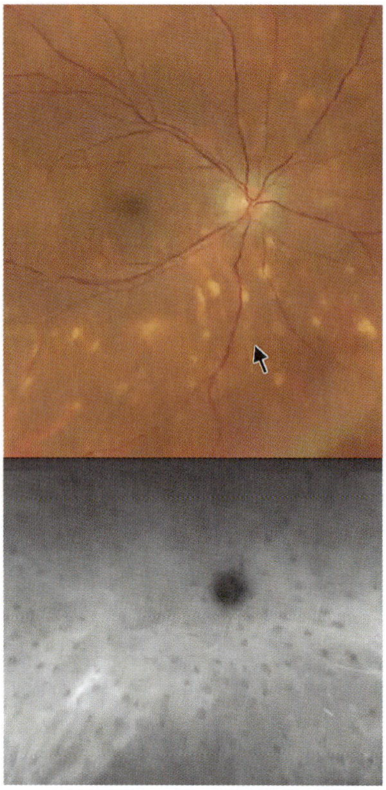

Fig. 3: A color fundus photo of a right eye showing peripapillary, yellow, ovoid lesions characteristic of birdshot chorioretinitis (top). An indocyanine green image showing multiple hypocyanescent spots in late frames (bottom).
Source: Uveitis Webinar - Grand Round 15. International Uveitis Study Group (IUSG). 2025. https://youtu.be/zWjjQGAAxh4?si=KrNaSnT3l5p4Mzkt.

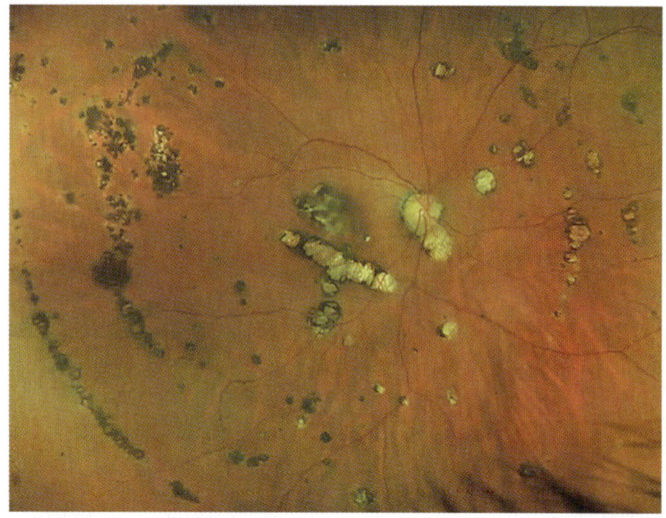

Fig. 4: A color fundus photo of a right eye showing multifocal punched-out lesions involving the peripheral retina with pigmentation at the borders in a patient with multifocal choroiditis and panuveitis.
Source: Uveitis Webinar - Grand Round 15. International Uveitis Study Group (IUSG). 2025. https://youtu.be/zWjjQGAAxh4?si=KrNaSnT3l5p4Mzkt.

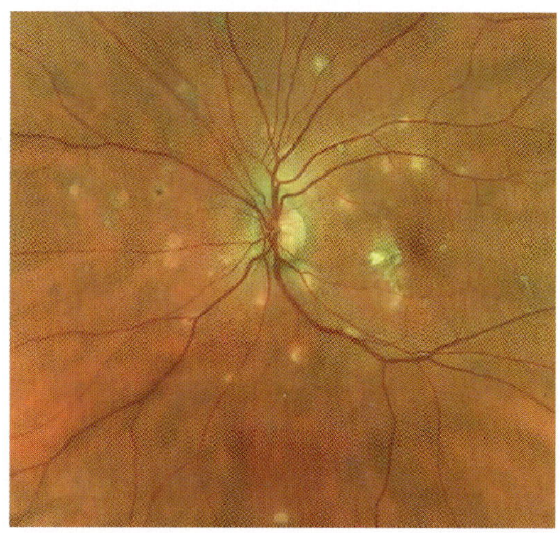

Fig. 5: A color fundus photo of a left eye showing small, yellow lesions involving the posterior pole in punctate inner choroidopathy.
Source: Uveitis Webinar - Grand Round 15. International Uveitis Study Group (IUSG). 2025. https://youtu.be/zWjjQGAAxh4?si=KrNaSnT3l5p4Mzkt.

(Fig. 3). Intraocular lymphoma needed to also be excluded for this diagnosis per SUN II criteria.

The diagnostic criteria for multifocal choroiditis with panuveitis (MFC) in SUN II required lesions that were active or punched-out, oval or round, and >125 µm **(Fig. 4)**.[4] There could be activity with a few cells and lesions had to involve the peripheral retina. Involvement of the posterior pole was not required.

The fourth condition studied was punctate inner choroidopathy (PIC). Many uveitis specialists feel this is not a unique disease, but rather a phenotype on the spectrum of disease with MFC. Criteria for diagnosis included involvement of the posterior pole and small lesions measuring <250 µm **(Fig. 5)**.[5] In addition, minimal vitreous cells were allowed on examination.

For the diagnosis of multiple evanescent white dot syndrome (MEWDS), the SUN II criteria listed foveal granularity with gray-white spots in a wreath-like pattern on fluorescein angiography.[6] Additional required imaging included outer retinal hyperreflectivity on OCT **(Fig. 6)**.

Serpiginous choroidopathy is called serpiginous choroiditis in SUN II. Shape is important as it is an ameboid or serpentine multifocal choroiditis that has minimal vitritis.[7] Early hypofluorescence is replaced by

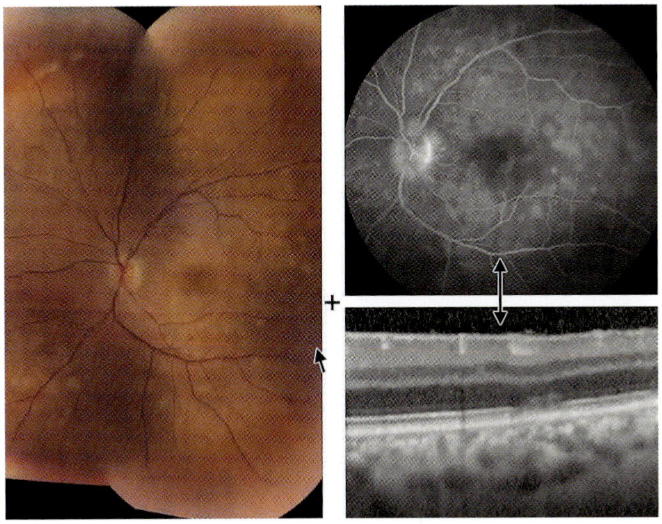

Fig. 6: A color fundus photo of a left eye showing subtle gray-white spots (left) and a fluorescein angiogram in late frames (superior right) highlighting the wreath-like lesions with staining. Outer retinal hyperreflectivity is also seen on the optical coherence tomography (OCT) scan of the retina in multifocal evanescent white dot syndrome (inferior right).
Source: Uveitis Webinar - Grand Round 15. International Uveitis Study Group (IUSG). 2025. https://youtu.be/zWjjQGAAxh4?si=KrNaSnT3l5p4Mzkt.

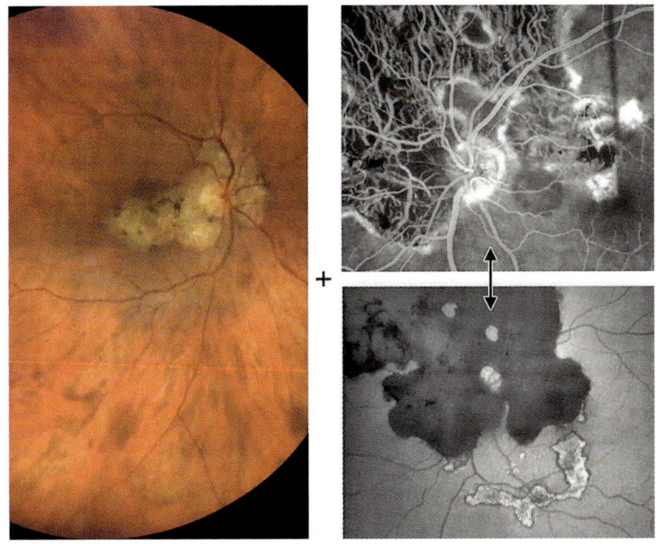

Fig. 7: A color fundus photo of a right eye showing a serpiginoid-shaped lesion adjacent to the optic nerve (left). A fluorescein angiogram with staining at the lesion border (superior right) in active disease. A hyperautofluorescent border seen inferiorly extending from a hypoautofluorescent lesion suggesting disease activity (inferior right).
Source: Uveitis Webinar - Grand Round 15. International Uveitis Study Group (IUSG). 2025. https://youtu.be/zWjjQGAAxh4?si=KrNaSnT3l5p4Mzkt.

staining at the borders on the fluorescein angiogram and hyperautofluorescence can be seen at the lesion border in active disease **(Fig. 7)**.

Retrospectively, how did the SUN II criteria compare to clinical diagnostic practices? A study conducted at the University of Colorado found there was a high percentage of patients who met the SUN II criteria for diagnosis.[8] There were also very few cases of each of these diseases with more cases of birdshot chorioretinitis and MFC. Another study from Korea also assessed the clinical utility of the SUN II criteria.[9] They assessed 100 eyes of 75 patients who were considered to have multifocal choroiditis. Of these, 29 eyes were diagnosed as multifocal choroiditis-PIC, 15 eyes were diagnosed as multifocal choroiditis, and 56 eyes could not be diagnosed as either by the SUN II criteria. Many categories overlap with PIC and MFC in terms of what the clinicians in the study diagnosed, including myopic fundus changes. SUN II criteria allowed cases that overlap to be segregated out by lesion size and location. This is an artificial construct that relates more to pattern recognition than a consideration of the pathogenesis and appearance on MMI.

How did the SUN II criteria perform prospectively? There were concerns about the ability to diagnose new cases using old criteria and old imaging techniques. There has also been an explosion in the use of MMI to diagnose, detect activity, monitor the treatment, and identify complications of the non-infectious uveitides. The new field of photo-pathology is very relevant to these investigations, especially with a focus on the outer retinal choriocapillaris complex.

Figure 8 shows the classic fundus appearance of APMPPE, as it is defined in SUN II. When MMI is used, there is a different appearance due to the analysis of individual retina layers. The OCT and OCT angiography (OCTA) can show flow voids and avascular areas through assessing both the deep and superficial retinal plexi. Areas of hypoperfusion can be visualized and intensity scans can be shown in enface images.

Optical coherence tomography angiography scans of the choriocapillaris layer show that there is clearly choriocapillaris closure, which is defined better than in the ICG **(Fig. 9)**. This is the gold standard for diagnosing APMPPE, based on choriocapillaris hypoperfusion, which is likely the pathophysiology of the disorder.

Inspired by this, a group of 12 uveitis experts conducted a systematic review of the literature.[10] Concentration was placed in the years after SUN II (2018–2024) to review

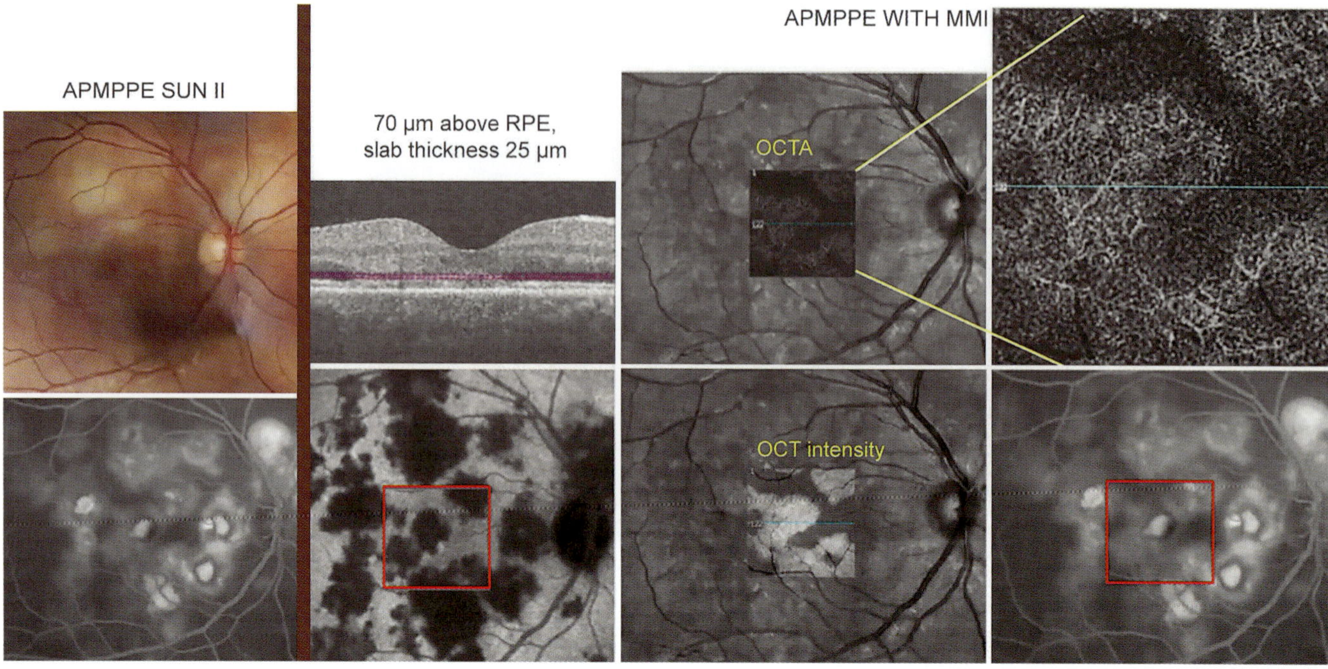

Fig. 8: Multimodal imaging of acute posterior multifocal placoid pigment epitheliopathy (APMPPE) is shown with color fundus photos showing the characteristic large yellow lesions (left top) and late staining on fluorescein angiography (left bottom). Newer modalities of optical coherence tomography (OCT) (center top) show hyperreflectivity of the outer retina. Fundus autofluorescence (center bottom) shows hypoautofluorescence in the area of the lesions. The modality of OCT angiography (right) shows both the intensity of (right bottom) and the location of hypoperfusion in the deep capillary plexus (right top).
Source: Uveitis Webinar - Grand Round 15. International Uveitis Study Group (IUSG). 2025. https://youtu.be/zWjjQGAAxh4?si=KrNaSnT3l5p4Mzkt.

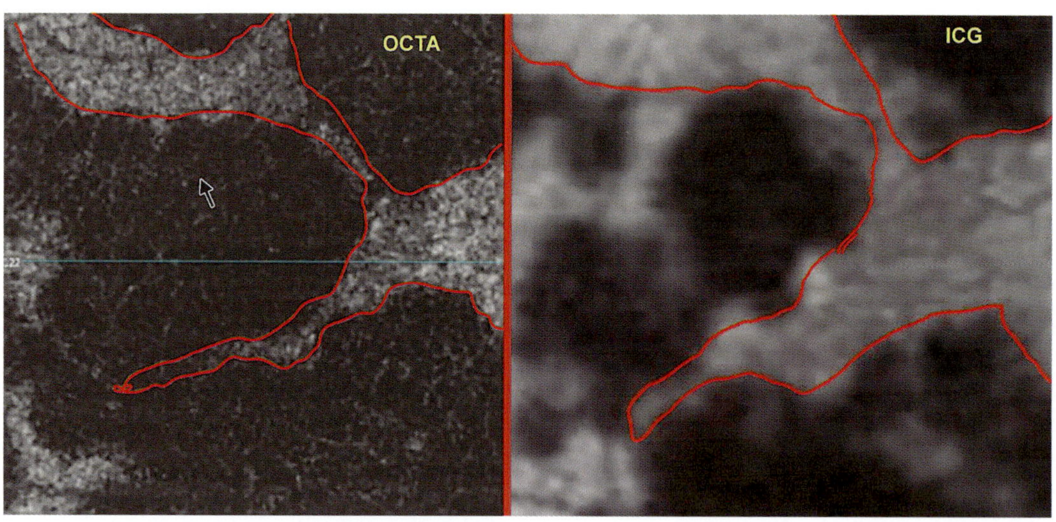

Fig. 9: An optical coherence tomography angiography (OCTA) enface image of the choriocapillaris (left) showing a larger area of flow restriction than captured on indocyanine green (ICG) (right).
Source: Uveitis Webinar - Grand Round 15. International Uveitis Study Group (IUSG). 2025. https://youtu.be/zWjjQGAAxh4?si=KrNaSnT3l5p4Mzkt.

images, diagnoses, and cases to assess what had changed since the initial review of this topic and the formation of the SUN II criteria. Professional research library software was used to perform the extensive literature review. Given the number of papers generated in the search, a closer review was conducted for the manuscripts published between

Flowchart 1: Illustrating the literature search with exclusion criteria for the multimodal imaging in uveitis systematic review on literature discussing multimodal imaging in non-infectious posterior uveitides.

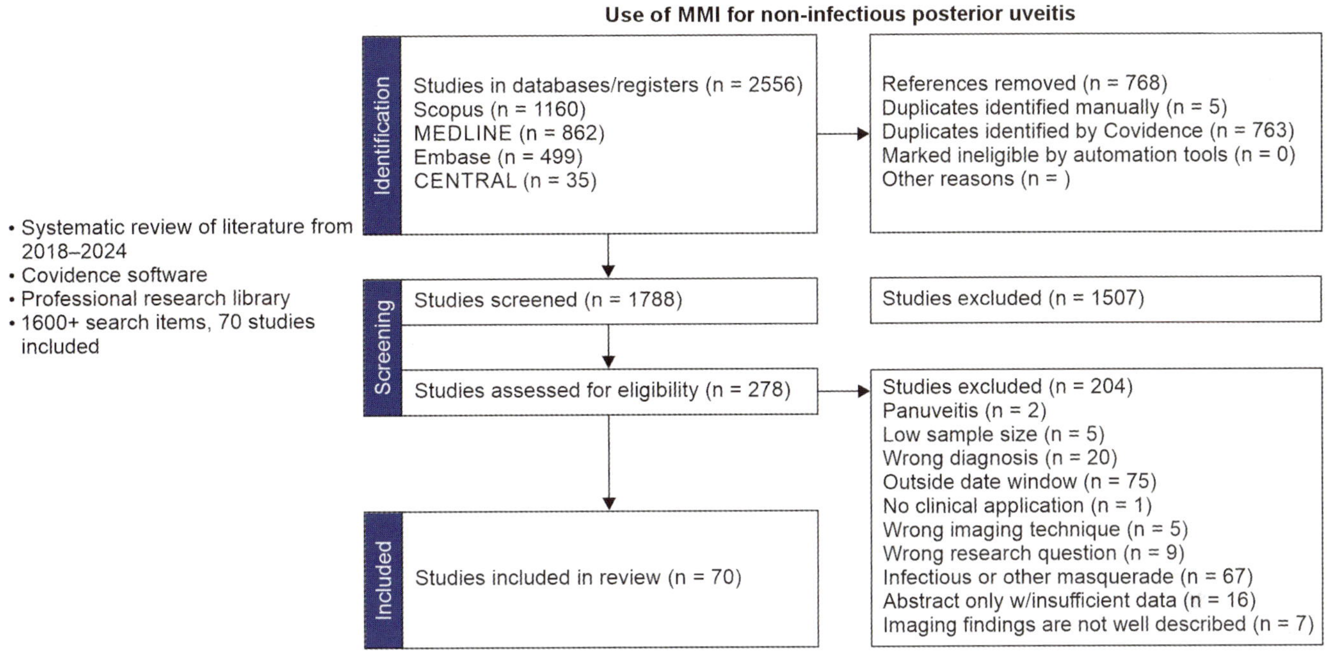

Source: Uveitis Webinar - Grand Round 15. International Uveitis Study Group (IUSG). 2025. https://youtu.be/zWjjQGAAxh4?si=KrNaSnT3l5p4Mzkt.

2012 and 2017, as fundamental findings from these papers informed later studies. From over 1,600 manuscripts, a final total of 70 papers were included in the review from 2018 to 2024 with very important papers published back to 2012, particularly in 2016 and 2015 **(Flowchart 1)**.

The findings of the systematic review were complicated. **Figure 10** shows the number of imaging tests performed, as shown by the numbers of patients not the number of eyes. For APMPPE, the number of imaging modalities were low. From 2018 to 2024, there were 109 examinations in only 14 papers, and seven manuscripts on MMI. In the papers published prior to 2018, there were 17 papers that discussed imaging features leaving any clinical utility statements developed for OCT from two papers, two papers on OCTA, and two papers on MMI. In comparison, birdshot chorioretinitis had more reported patient examinations and papers on the topic. There was more interest from 2018 to 2024 in terms of publications with more clinical utility statements. Two papers specifically discussed the use of MMI in diagnosing birdshot chorioretinitis.

The findings for MFC were similar, but there were more papers that not only described multifocal choroiditis, but also segregated out PIC **(Fig. 11)**. There was a very large number of patients due to the higher number of imaging studies for this disorder and the heterogeneity in this classification. Many of the diseases called multifocal choroiditis may turn out to be a different condition. However, there is no evidence that multifocal choroiditis is different from multifocal PIC other than by lesion size and location. Both of these characteristics are artificial and can certainly change over time. In other words, PIC can later look like multifocal choroiditis, and they likely represent the same disease process.

The papers on MMI for both MEWDS and serpiginous choroiditis are shown in **Figure 12**. Serpiginous choroiditis is a rare disorder with a paucity of papers published on the topic with the majority published between 2018 and 2024.

Understanding the number of papers on each condition can be better conceptualized using a heat map **(Fig. 13)**. The dark colors represent most of the patients studied with the majority having MFC, MEWDS, and in multifocal choroiditis-PIC rather than APMPPE or birdshot choroiditis.

Based on the number of publications, most of the clinical utility statements focused on the diagnosis of MFC and multifocal choroiditis-PIC as opposed to the diagnosis, activity, and monitoring in MEWDS **(Fig. 14)**.

A particular research interest within the MUV study group was determining the minimum amount of MMI **(Fig. 15)**.[11] This color-coded graph shows which imaging

APMPPE	*Color*	*FAF*	*OCT*	*FA*	*ICGA*	*OCTA*	*MMI*	*Total*
Tests performed 2018–2024	36	30	19	4	3	17	—	109
Imaging statements 2018–2024 (papers)	4	2	4	1	1	2	—	14 (5)
Supporting statements pre-2018 (papers)	5	1	5	2	2	2		17 (6)
Clinical utility statements 2018–2024	1		2			2	2	7
Birdshot chorioretinitis	*Color*	*FAF*	*OCT*	*FA*	*ICGA*	*OCTA*	*MMI*	*Total*
Tests performed 2018–2024	50	54	228	235	29	85	—	681
Imaging statements 2018–2024 (papers)	3	2	6	9	5	3	—	28 (12)
Supporting statements pre-2018 (papers)	3	0	2	4	4	2		15 (6)
Clinical utility statements 2018–2024	1	2	8	5	4	4	2	26

Fig. 10: A table showing the publications that discussed the use of multimodal imaging in acute posterior multifocal placoid pigment epitheliopathy and birdshot chorioretinitis from prior to 2018 compared to 2018-2024. The number of studies that specifically mention the utility of an imaging modality for diagnosing either condition is listed in the clinical utility statements row at the bottom of each table.
Source: Uveitis Webinar - Grand Round 15. International Uveitis Study Group (IUSG). 2025. https://youtu.be/zWjjQGAAxh4?si=KrNaSnT3l5p4Mzkt.

Multifocal choroiditis	*Color*	*FAF*	*OCT*	*FA*	*ICGA*	*OCTA*	*MMI*	*Total*
Tests performed 2018–2024	461	428	479	440	351	88	—	2247
Imaging statements 2018–2024 (papers)	10	12	12	11	6	8	—	59 (18)
Supporting statements pre-2018 (papers)	4	4	5	6	2	2		23 (7)
Clinical utility statements 2018–2024	4	5	9	3	2	5	8	36
Multifocal choroiditis — PIC	*Color*	*FAF*	*OCT*	*FA*	*ICGA*	*OCTA*	*MMI*	*Total*
Tests performed 2018–2024	265	243	319	279	266	236	—	1608
Imaging statements 2018–2024 (papers)	7	5	10	6	5	6	—	39 (14)
Supporting statements pre-2018 (papers)	2	3	6	1	3	0		15 (9)
Clinical utility statements 2018–2024	1	3	7	4	0	7	5	27

Fig. 11: A table showing the publications that discussed the use of multimodal imaging in multifocal choroiditis and multifocal choroiditis-punctate inner choroidopathy from prior to 2018 compared to 2018–2024. The number of studies that specifically mentioned the utility of an imaging modality for diagnosing either condition are listed in the clinical utility statements row at the bottom of each table.
Source: Uveitis Webinar - Grand Round 15. International Uveitis Study Group (IUSG). 2025. https://youtu.be/zWjjQGAAxh4?si=KrNaSnT3l5p4Mzkt.

MEWDS	Color	FAF	OCT	FA	ICGA	OCTA	MMI	Total
Tests performed 2018–2024	270	320	420	317	260	39	—	1626
Imaging Statements 2018–2024 (papers)	12	9	16	11	14	1	—	63 (17)
Supporting statements pre-2018 (papers)	5	4	7	3	4	1		24 (8)
Clinical utility statements 2018–2024	4	3	11	2	4	3	9	36

Serpiginous choroiditis	Color	FAF	OCT	FA	ICGA	OCTA	MMI	Total
Tests performed 2018–2024	36	47	55	41	42	45	—	266
Imaging statements 2018–2024 (papers)	3	4	4	4	4	6	—	25 (7)
Supporting statements pre-2018 (papers)	1	1	1	0	0	0		3 (1)
Clinical utility statements 2018–2024	0	4	2	1	3	6	3	19

Fig. 12: A table showing the publications that discussed the use of multimodal imaging in multiple evanescent white dot syndrome and serpiginous choroiditis from prior to 2018 compared to 2018–2024. The number of studies that specifically mentioned the utility of an imaging modality for diagnosing either condition is listed in the clinical utility statements row at the bottom of each table.
Source: Uveitis Webinar - Grand Round 15. International Uveitis Study Group (IUSG). 2025. https://youtu.be/zWjjQGAAxh4?si=KrNaSnT3l5p4Mzkt.

	Color	FAF	OCT	FA	ICG	OCTA	
APMPPE	36	30	19	4	3	17	Patients
	4	4	5	2	2	4	Studies
Birdshot	50	54	228	235	29	85	Patients
	4	3	10	8	4	4	Studies
MFC	461	428	479	440	351	88	Patients
	15	13	15	13	9	6	Studies
MEWDS	270	320	420	317	260	39	Patients
	12	14	16	13	13	6	Studies
Serpiginous	36	47	55	41	42	45	Patients
	5	5	7	4	5	5	Studies
MFC-PIC	265	243	319	279	266	236	Patients
	10	9	13	10	9	11	Studies

Quartile	1	2	3	4

Fig. 13: A heat map showing the number of patients diagnosed with each white dot syndrome and the imaging modality studied.
Source: Uveitis Webinar - Grand Round 15. International Uveitis Study Group (IUSG). 2025. https://youtu.be/zWjjQGAAxh4?si=KrNaSnT3l5p4Mzkt.

	Diagnosis	Activity	Monitoring	Complications
APMPPE	13	5	9	9
Birdshot	24	19	24	9
MFC	49	29	23	23
MEWDS	52	45	53	6
Serpiginous	11	11	8	8
MFC-PIC	34	28	23	23
Quartile	1	2	3	4

Fig. 14: A heat map showing the number of publications that discuss the diagnosis, activity, monitoring, and complications in each white dot syndrome.
Source: Uveitis Webinar - Grand Round 15. International Uveitis Study Group (IUSG). 2025. https://youtu.be/zWjjQGAAxh4?si=KrNaSnT3l5p4Mzkt.

Disease	Diagnosis classification pathogenesis	Activity monitoring treatment	Complications
APMPPE	Color * OCT FA OCTA or ICG	Color OCT OCTA	Color OCT OCTA
Birdshot	Color * FA ICG	Color OCT FA ICG	Color OCT FA ICG
MFC	Color * OCT	Color OCT	Color OCTA
MEWDS	Color * OCT * AF	Color OCT	Color OCT AF FA ICG
Serpiginous	Color * AF *	Color AF	Color OCT

Fig. 15: A color-coded graph showing the imaging modalities needed to assess the diagnosis, activity, and complication development in the WDS. An asterisk represents an imaging modality that was recommended for the indication listed in the column header by the SUN II criteria.
Source: Uveitis Webinar - Grand Round 15. International Uveitis Study Group (IUSG). 2025. https://youtu.be/zWjjQGAAxh4?si=KrNaSnT3l5p4Mzkt.

modalities are needed to assess the diagnosis, activity, and complication development in the WDS. An asterisk means that the modality was recommended for the indication listed in the column header by the SUN II criteria. For diagnosis, classification, and pathogenesis there are many imaging studies that are important. For activity and monitoring, the need for imaging remains robust. Particular to birdshot chorioretinitis, almost all modalities are needed for detecting complications. Serpiginous has the least imaging need associated with any of these disorders. This figure represents the studies a clinical practice could accomplish without sophisticated equipment to provide the standard of care for patients. OCTA has the most applications for evaluating APMPPE.

Validation of the minimum imaging set was based on the ability to diagnose and detect activity. It was assessed with projected images with real-time anonymous voting. This was attempted at the *Inflammatio* meeting with statistical confirmation. Color fundus photos were a surrogate marker for the clinical examination. Masquerade diagnoses that phenotypically mimicked the WDS were also shown. The results showed that autofluorescence improves sensitivity and specificity compared to color fundus photos alone **(Fig. 16)**. Autofluorescence was useful in MEWDS, whereas ICG improved the sensitivity and specificity for diagnosis and monitoring in birdshot chorioretinopathy. This is interesting as it was not even mentioned in the SUN II criteria. OCT improved diagnosis and activity monitoring compared with OCTA, thereby increasing sensitivity for the development of complications in multifocal choroiditis-PIC.

We found a gap in our knowledge of APMPPE that warrants consideration. While APMPPE is usually self-resolving, there are exceptions. MEWDS is self-resolving, and so quickly, that few papers have assessed a timeline of changes on imaging. Nonetheless, there is continual resolution. APMPPE remains interesting throughout the disease course due to the characteristic pattern of retinal pigment epithelial hypertrophy. Heparinase inhibitors prevent extracellular matrix breakdown, and their use can lead to the development of a phenotypically similar syndrome. The improvement of APMPPE is perhaps linked to heparinase assisting in tissue remodeling **(Fig. 17)**. The resulting retinal pigment epithelium scarring has sight-threatening implications.

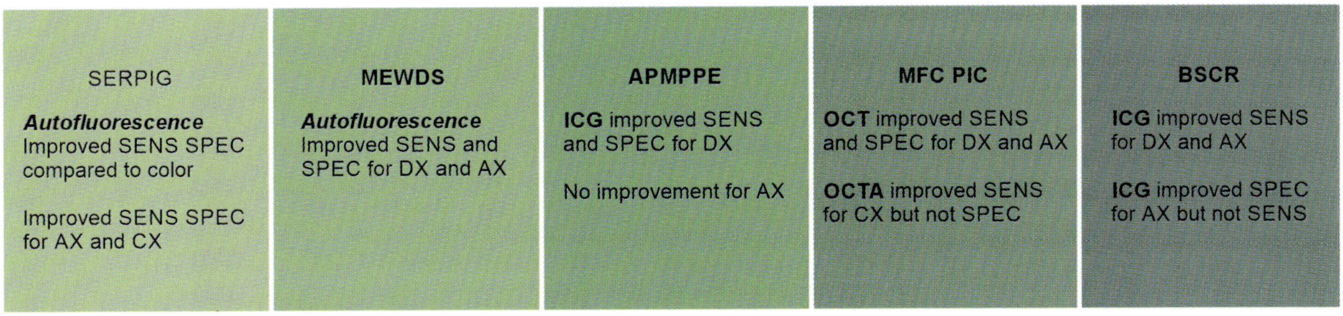

Fig. 16: A schematic showing the findings validated for a minimum imaging set from the *Inflammatio* meeting. (AX: activity; CX: complications; DX: diagnosis; ICG: indocyanine green angiography; OCTA: OCT angiography; SENS: sensitivity; SPEC: specificity)
Source: Uveitis Webinar - Grand Round 15. International Uveitis Study Group (IUSG). 2025. https://youtu.be/zWjjQGAAxh4?si=KrNaSnT3l5p4Mzkt.

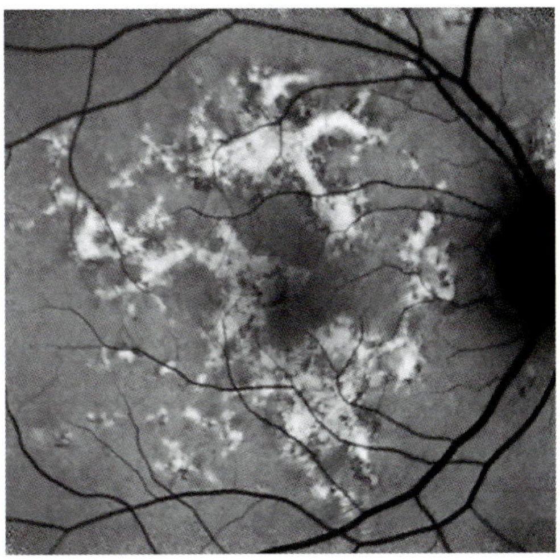

Fig. 17: A fundus autofluorescence photo of a right eye showing hyperautofluorescence with surrounding hypoautofluorescence in areas of retinal pigment epithelial hypertrophy in a patient with acute posterior multifocal placoid pigment epitheliopathy.
Source: Uveitis Webinar - Grand Round 15. International Uveitis Study Group (IUSG). 2025. https://youtu.be/zWjjQGAAxh4?si=KrNaSnT3l5p4Mzkt.

The next steps are to validate the clinical utility of MMI. How many images do you need to provide comprehensive and financially responsible care? Not all six imaging modalities are needed for every patient. There is a lot of work that needs to be done.

CLASSIC MULTIPLE EVANESCENT WHITE DOT SYNDROME

Case Presentation

Personal Data

A 46-year-old female presented with temporal flashes and a dark spot in her right eye for several days.

TABLE 1: Physical examination of a patient having classic multiple evanescent white dot syndrome.

OD	*Parameter*	*OS*
20/50	BCVA	20/20
12 mm Hg	IOP	14 mm Hg
Quiet	Conjunctiva	Quiet
Clear	Cornea	Clear
Deep and quiet	Anterior chamber	Deep and quiet
No synechiae	Iris	No synechiae
Clear	Lens	Clear
Trace cells	Vitreous	Clear
Multiple gray-white lesions surrounding the optic nerve and extending to the equator superiorly and inferiorly	Fundus	Normal

(BCVA: best corrected visual acuity; IOP: intraocular pressure; KPs: keratic precipitates)

History of Present Illness

About 2 weeks prior, she had an upper respiratory tract infection with sneezing and headaches. Her past ocular, medical, and surgical histories were unremarkable and she was not taking any systemic medications.

Physical Examination

The best corrected vision in the right eye was 20/50, and in the left eye, 20/20. Fundus examination showed multiple, gray-white lesions scattered across a posterior pole that extended to the equator superiorly and inferiorly in the right eye **(Table 1 and Fig. 18)**.

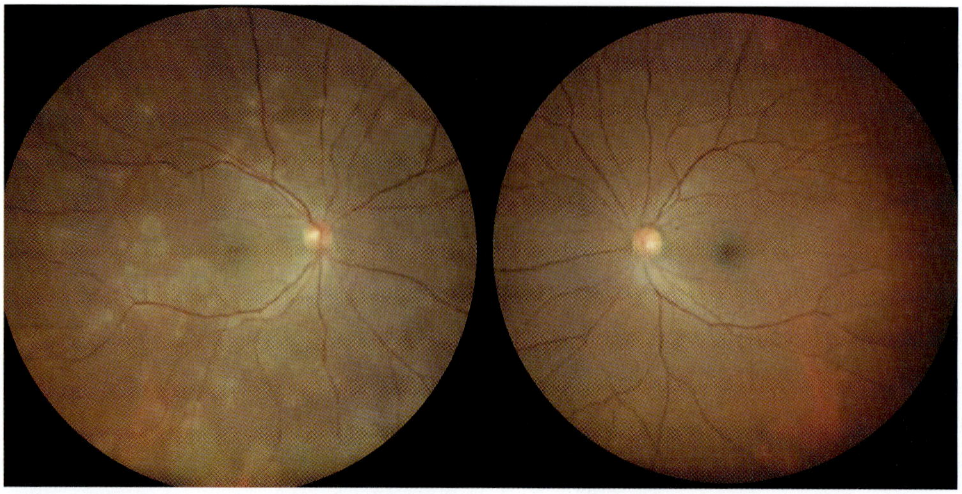

Fig. 18: Color fundus photos of both eyes showing multiple, grey lesions in the posterior pole and surrounding the arcades in the right eye and a normal fundus appearance in the left eye.
Source: Uveitis Webinar - Grand Round 15. International Uveitis Study Group (IUSG). 2025. https://youtu.be/zWjjQGAAxh4?si=KrNaSnT3l5p4Mzkt.

Ancillary testing: Fundus autofluorescence showed hyperautofluorescence in the area of the lesions **(Fig. 19)** and on fluorescein angiography, a few areas of punctate hyperfluorescence with late staining in a wreath-like pattern were seen **(Fig. 20)**. Optical coherence tomography (OCT) scans showed disruption of the outer retina with patchy loss of the ellipsoid zone. Vertical flare lines were seen extending from the ellipsoid zone through the outer nuclear layer **(Fig. 21)**.

Uveitis work-up: The differential diagnosis included MEWDS, multifocal choroiditis, PIC, acute idiopathic blind spot enlargement (AIBSE), syphilitic retinopathy, and APMPPE if this was a bilateral presentation. Syphilis serologies and quantiFERON testing were negative. Given the imaging findings, the final diagnosis was MEWDS.

Initial treatment: The plan was to observe with close clinical follow-up.

Follow-up: 1 month later, resolution of the lesions was noted on clinical examination, with a reduction in hyperautofluorescence **(Fig. 22)**. On OCT imaging, there was a restoration of the ellipsoid zone **(Fig. 23)**.

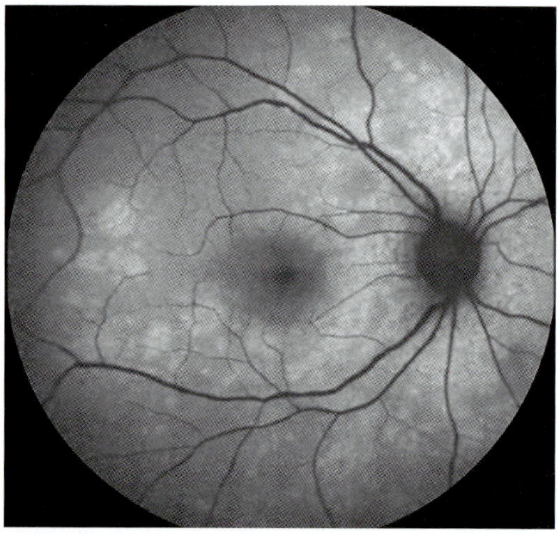

Fig. 19: An autofluorescence image of the right eye showing hyperautofluorescence in the area of the retinal lesions.
Source: Uveitis Webinar - Grand Round 15. International Uveitis Study Group (IUSG). 2025. https://youtu.be/zWjjQGAAxh4?si=KrNaSnT3l5p4Mzkt.

Discussion

Multiple evanescent white dot syndrome is an idiopathic condition that affects the outer retina and the retinal pigment epithelium. It primarily affects young myopic women and can present after a self-limited viral prodrome that resolves within weeks without or with very minimal sequelae. The acute presentation includes blurry vision, photopsias, scotomas, floaters, and rarely dyschromatopsia in one eye. Given the spontaneous recovery, the visual prognosis is good and observation with serial MMI is recommended. Syphilis serologies should be assessed since they can manifest with variable phenotypic presentations.

Figure 24 shows the orange granular dots, called Jampol dots, within the macula.[12] If the characteristic MEWDS lesions have already disappeared due to the evanescent

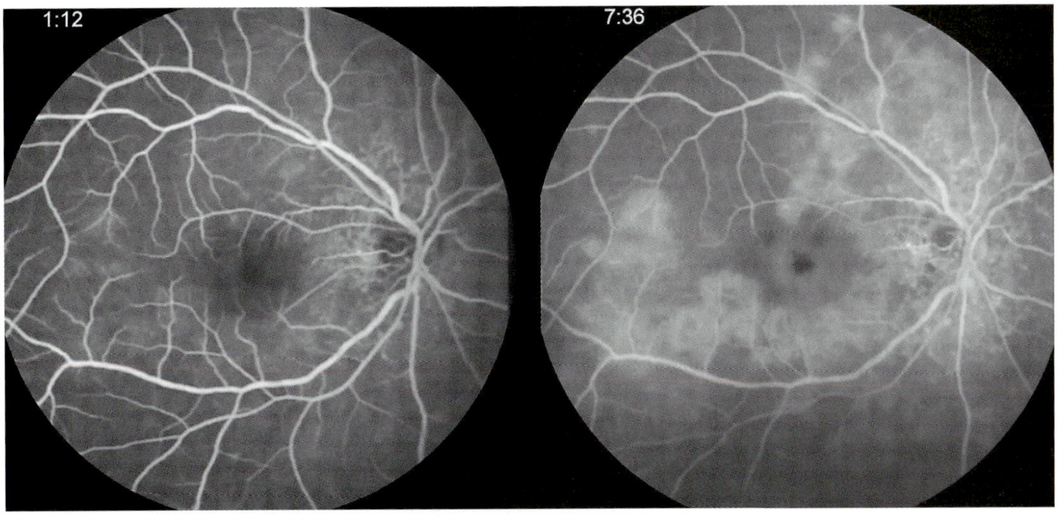

Fig. 20: A fluorescein angiogram showing early punctate hyperfluorescence (left) and late staining of the retinal lesions in a wreath-like pattern of the right eye (right).
Source: Uveitis Webinar - Grand Round 15. International Uveitis Study Group (IUSG). 2025. https://youtu.be/zWjjQGAAxh4?si=KrNaSnT3l5p4Mzkt.

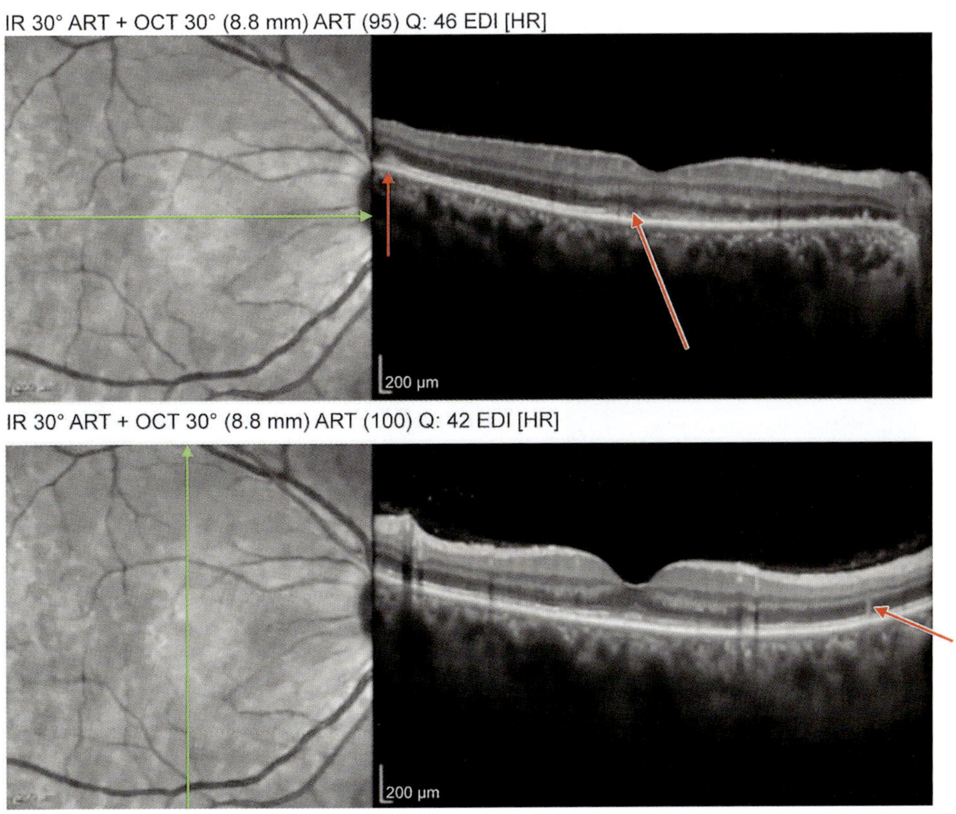

Fig. 21: An OCT of the macula in the right eye showing disruption of the outer retina with patchy loss of the ellipsoid zone (top, red arrow).
Source: Uveitis Webinar - Grand Round 15. International Uveitis Study Group (IUSG). 2025. https://youtu.be/zWjjQGAAxh4?si=KrNaSnT3l5p4Mzkt.

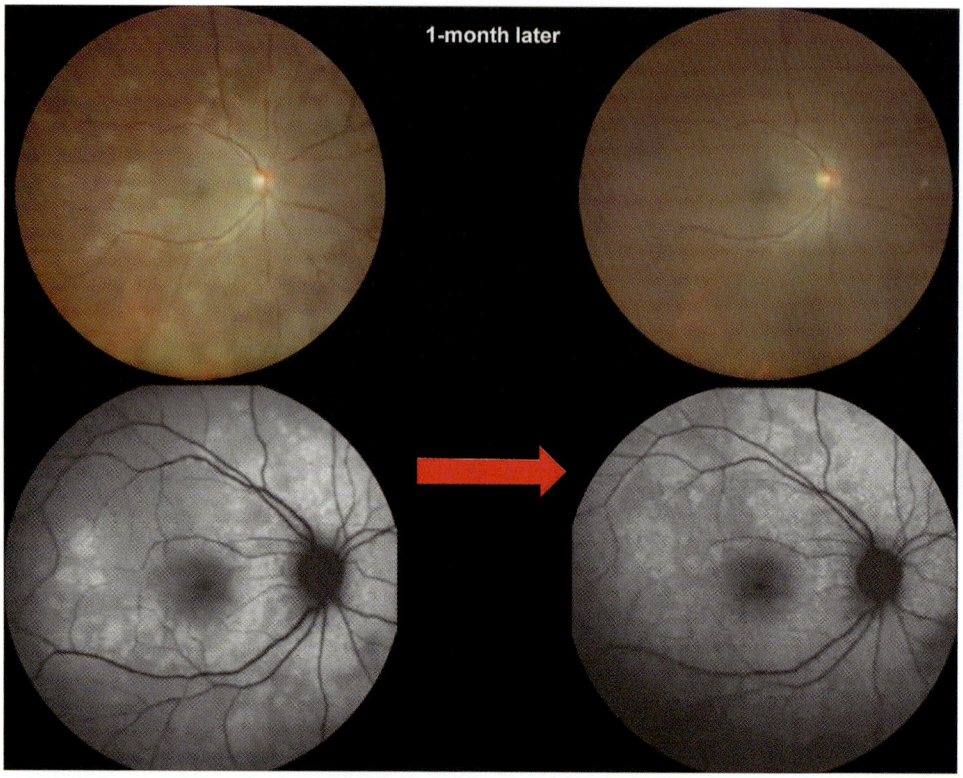

Fig. 22: Color fundus (top) and autofluorescence (bottom) images at presentation (left) and after 1-month (right) showing clinical resolution of the retinal lesions and fading of the hyperautofluorescence.
Source: Uveitis Webinar - Grand Round 15. International Uveitis Study Group (IUSG). 2025. https://youtu.be/zWjjQGAAxh4?si=KrNaSnT3l5p4Mzkt.

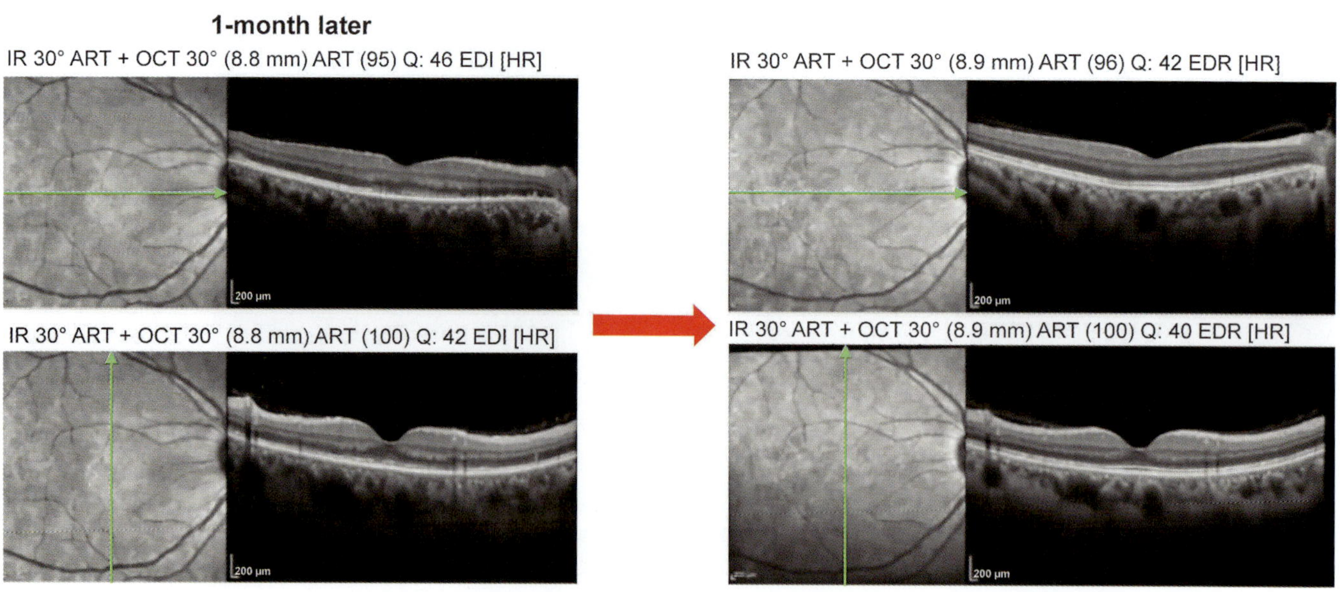

Fig. 23: optical coherence tomography (OCT) images of the right eye at baseline (left) after 1 month (right) showing restoration of the ellipsoid zone.
Source: Uveitis Webinar - Grand Round 15. International Uveitis Study Group (IUSG). 2025. https://youtu.be/zWjjQGAAxh4?si=KrNaSnT3l5p4Mzkt.

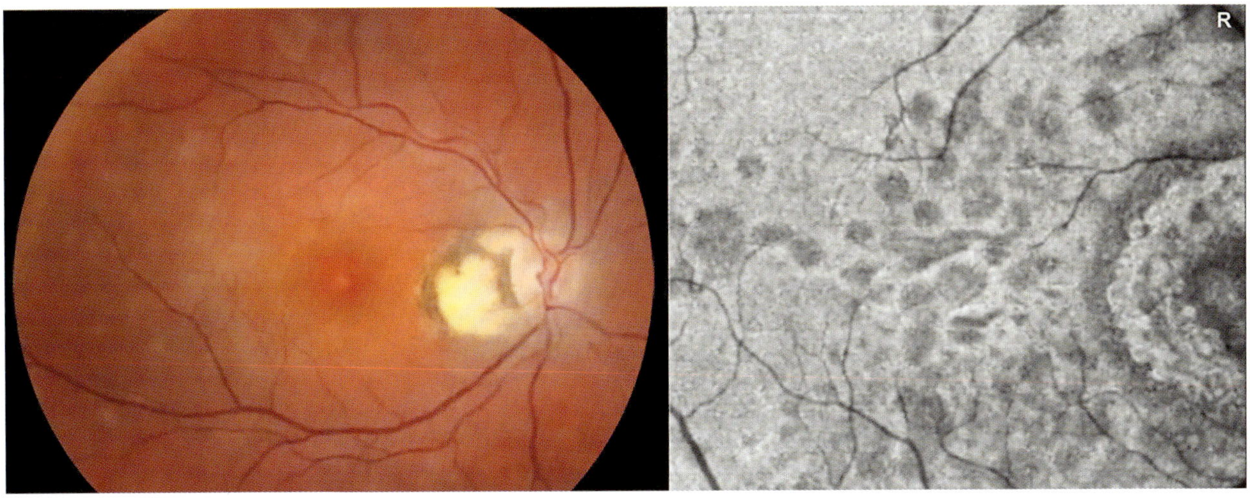

Fig. 24: A color fundus photo of the right eye (left) showing orange dots within the macula called Jampol dots, which can be seen on fundus autofluorescence (right) as hypoautofluorescent lesions.
Source: Uveitis Webinar - Grand Round 15. International Uveitis Study Group (IUSG). 2025. https://youtu.be/zWjjQGAAxh4?si=KrNaSnT3l5p4Mzkt.

nature of the disease, the only findings that can assist in the diagnosis are these orange foveolar dots. The lesions are at the level of the photoreceptors, and correspond to the location of most gray-white lesions.

Atypical features of MEWDS can overlap with PIC and acute zonal occult outer retinopathy (AZOOR). Additionally, the concept of secondary MEWDS has been discussed in recent years. Secondary MEWDS has been brought up by Dr. Lee Jampol and his colleagues.[13] Most patients who have MEWDS fall into the category previously described. However, older or highly myopic patients who were recently vaccinated or with a pre-existing retinal condition, such as choroidal neovascularization, pseudoxanthoma elasticum, Best disease, or prior retinal surgery are now being considered as secondary MEWDS.

This is a case of a patient with a retinal detachment status post vitrectomy with a laser barricade of a peripheral tear. Prior to presentation, his best corrected vision was 20/20 which dropped to 20/100. He had photopsias and an enlarged blind spot with temporal field loss. In myopic patients, assessment for a retinal detachment is essential; however, he had gray-white lesions that were more subtle than seen in the previous example **(Fig. 25)**. On autofluorescence images, areas of hyperautofluorescence corresponding to the lesions are widespread to the equator. The hypoautofluorescent lesions are from his prior laser scars **(Fig. 25)**.

Optical coherence tomography scans show diffuse and widespread loss of the ellipsoid zone and areas of patchy loss or clumping of the outer retina. The outer nuclear layer is preserved, which is a feature of MEWDS, leading to the subsequent visual and anatomic recovery **(Fig. 26)**.

Additional testing with a fluorescein angiogram and an ICG were performed. The early phases of the ICG were normal, but dark spots appeared in the late frames **(Fig. 27)**. Although the lesions are not in the choroid, they are the result of overlying opacification of retinal pigment epithelial cells blocking the dye and leading to the appearance of dots and spots. Again, MEWDS lesions do not occur in the choroid, but may affect the adjacent choriocapillaris. Thus, it is not a disease similar to PIC or birdshot chorioretinopathy. The fluorescein angiogram showed very clearly the hyperfluorescence of the MEWDS lesions are made of multiple small dots. The lesions show hyperfluorescence early in the angiogram with either staining or prominence with fading in the late phase **(Fig. 28)**.

The patient's symptoms improved without any treatment for about 3 weeks, but then he returned with worsening visual field loss with central involvement. The vision decreased from 20/40 to counting fingers. He was prescribed 40 mg of prednisone as OCT images showed photoreceptor disorganization. While the normal architecture of the outer retina had returned, a portion of the nasal macula had not improved **(Fig. 29)**. He subsequently underwent injection with a dexamethasone implant and mycophenolate mofetil 2 g/day was started along with a 6-week taper off of prednisone.

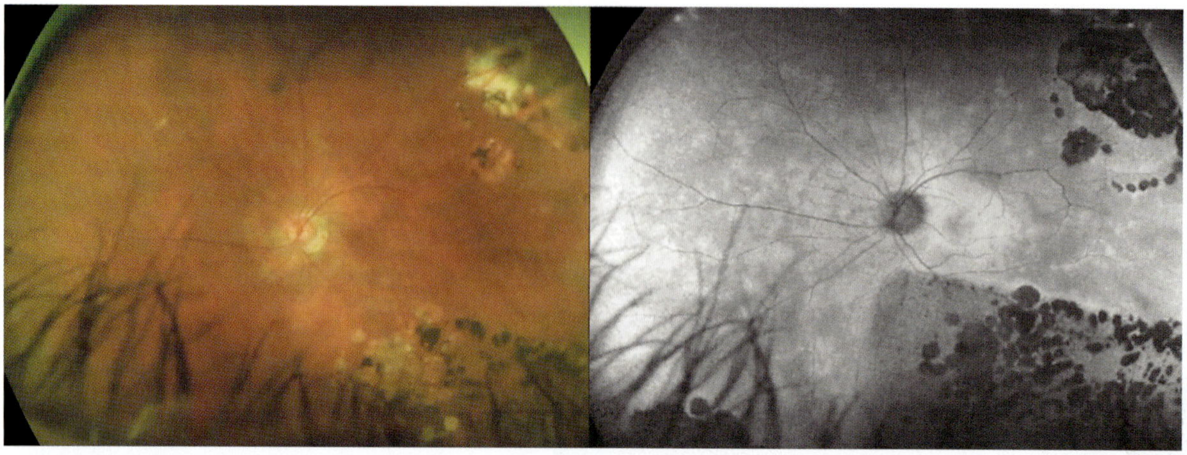

Fig. 25: A color fundus photo of a left eye showing prior laser barricade scars and faint, widespread gray-white lesions (left). These lesions are highlighted as hyperautofluorescent areas on fundus autofluorescence imaging (right). The prior laser scars are seen as hypoautofluorescent areas.
Source: Uveitis Webinar - Grand Round 15. International Uveitis Study Group (IUSG). 2025. https://youtu.be/zWjjQGAAxh4?si=KrNaSnT3l5p4Mzkt.

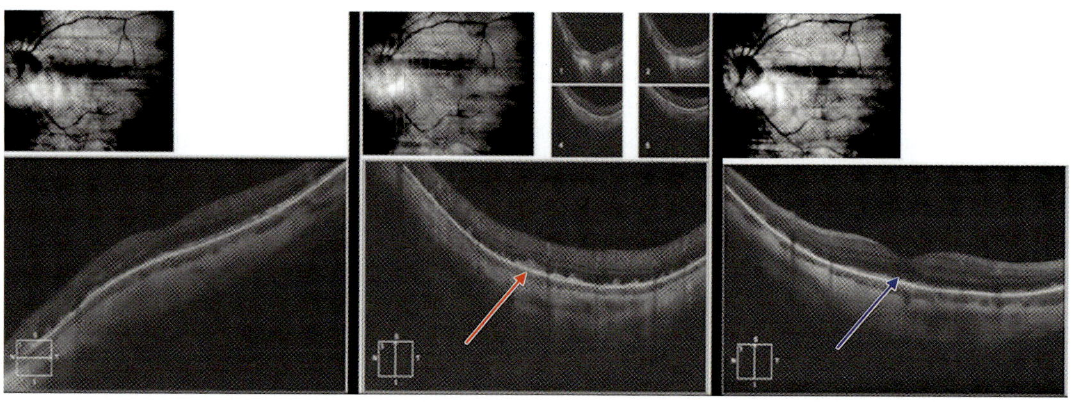

Fig. 26: Optical coherence tomography (OCT) scans of the macula showing clumping (red arrow) and patchy loss of the ellipsoid zone and outer retina (blue arrow).
Source: Uveitis Webinar - Grand Round 15. International Uveitis Study Group (IUSG). 2025. https://youtu.be/zWjjQGAAxh4?si=KrNaSnT3l5p4Mzkt.

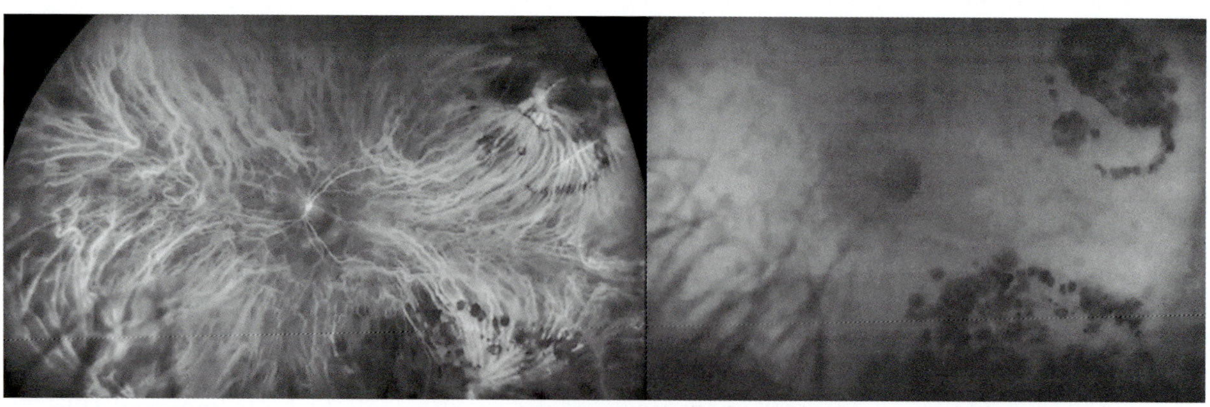

Fig. 27: Early (left) and late (right) indocyanine green angiography images showing the lack of hypocyanescent spots in early frames. Seen only in late frames, the hypocyanescence is due to blockage from opacification of the overlying retinal pigment epithelial cells.
Source: Uveitis Webinar - Grand Round 15. International Uveitis Study Group (IUSG). 2025. https://youtu.be/zWjjQGAAxh4?si=KrNaSnT3l5p4Mzkt.

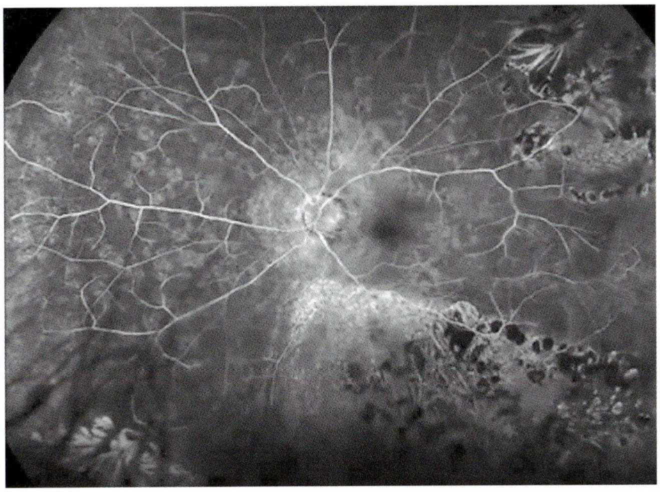

Fig. 28: A late frame image of a fluorescein angiogram showing staining of the multiple evanescent white dot syndrome (MEWDS) lesions in a wreath-like pattern, most noticeably nasal to the optic disc.
Source: Uveitis Webinar - Grand Round 15. International Uveitis Study Group (IUSG). 2025. https://youtu.be/zWjjQGAAxh4?si=KrNaSnT3l5p4Mzkt.

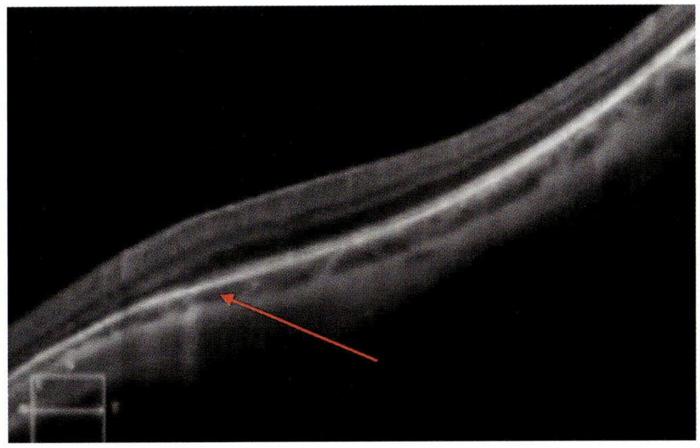

Fig. 29: An optical coherence tomography (OCT) scan of the macula of the left eye showing continued disruption of the photoreceptor layer (red arrow).
Source: Uveitis Webinar - Grand Round 15. International Uveitis Study Group (IUSG). 2025. https://youtu.be/zWjjQGAAxh4?si=KrNaSnT3l5p4Mzkt.

Over the next 6–8 weeks, the hyperautofluorescence decreased on imaging, but did not completely resolve around the disc, as would be expected with MEWDS. In addition, he developed PIC-like lesions over the following several months, which can be seen on repeated autofluorescent imaging **(Fig. 30)**. Over time, his vision improved to 20/25 on a repeated prednisone taper that lasted 5 months with concurrent use of mycophenolate. Eventually, all his symptoms stabilized. He was still left with a nasal macular photoreceptor loss causing an enlarged blind spot, although his central vision improved.

Two years later, there are still residual hyperautofluorescent lesions that are reminiscent of AZOOR. The photoreceptors in AZOOR can recover if they are caught early and treated with corticosteroids and possibly valacyclovir. AZOOR can result in residual field loss and residual hyperautofluorescent lesions that were present in this patient. This gentleman presented with exuberant MEWDS and ended up with a residual field defect. He also developed PIC-like lesions with atrophy nasal to the disc forming a complex picture of a WDS overlap with a disease course on the AZOOR spectrum. In summary, corticosteroids should only be used if there is an atypical course. Rarely, partial field defects and photopsias can persist for months even after the fundus examination findings resolve.

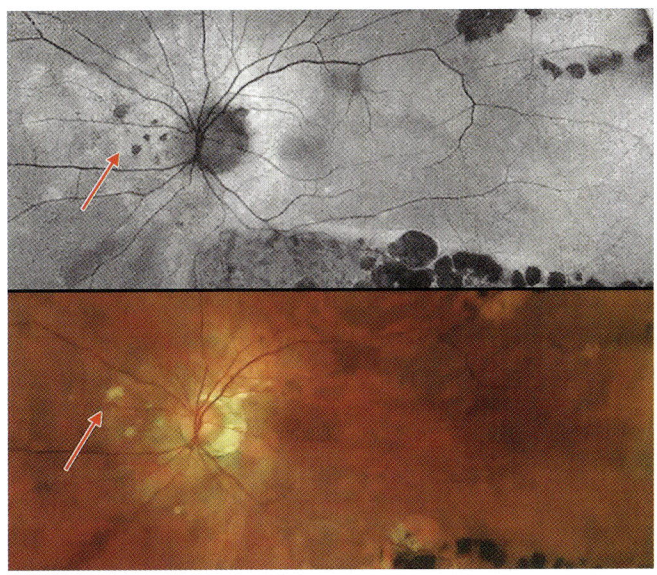

Fig. 30: An autofluorescence image (top) showing new areas of hypoautofluorescence in the areas of PIC-like lesions seen on color fundus photography (bottom) with red arrows.
Source: Uveitis Webinar - Grand Round 15. International Uveitis Study Group (IUSG). 2025. https://youtu.be/zWjjQGAAxh4?si=KrNaSnT3l5p4Mzkt.

ACUTE POSTERIOR MULTIFOCAL PLACOID PIGMENT EPITHELIOPATHY

Case Presentation

Personal Data

A 46-year-old male presented with blurred vision in the right eye in 2019.

History of Present Illness

He had no prior ocular history and denied flashes and floaters.

Physical Examination

Vision was 20/60 in the right eye and 20/20 in the left eye. Fundus examination showed multiple gray-white lesions surrounding the optic nerve and extending around the vascular arcades into the macula characteristic of APMPPE or persistent placoid maculopathy **(Table 2 and Fig. 31)**.

Ancillary testing: The creamy white lesions in the posterior pole corresponded to hyper and hypoautofluorescent changes on fundus autofluorescence images **(Fig. 32)**. OCT slices showed acute, oblique hyperreflectivity at the level of the outer retina and the Henle nerve fiber layer. This has been termed the angular sign of Henle fiber layer hyperreflectivity (ASHH) lesions, which correspond to an alteration of the proximal part of the photoreceptor cells in placoid lesions. This is thought to be secondary to anterograde spread of primary choroidal ischemia **(Fig. 33)**. Areas of hypocyanescence represent areas of choroidal hypoperfusion or ischemia on ICG testing in late frames **(Fig. 34)**.

Uveitis work-up: Serologic testing showed negative quantiFERON, TP-PA, Lyme ELISA, anti-nuclear antibodies, rheumatoid factor, beta-2 glycoprotein, cardiolipin, anticytoplasmic nuclear antibodies, direct Russel's viper venom time, and anti-cyclic citrullinated peptide results. Normal values were obtained with ESR and CRP testing. Systemic evaluation showed no joint swelling or central nervous system inflammation.

Initial treatment: The plan was to observe with close clinical follow-up.

Follow-up: 4 years later, despite an improvement in vision in the right eye to 20/40, he developed neovascular

TABLE 2: Physical examination of a patient having acute posterior multifocal placoid pigment epitheliopathy.

OD	***Parameter***	***OS***
20/60	BCVA	20/20
15 mm Hg	IOP	12 mm Hg
Quiet	Conjunctiva	Quiet
Clear	Cornea	Clear
Deep and quiet	Anterior chamber	Deep and quiet
No synechiae	Iris	No synechiae
Clear	Lens	Clear
Trace cells	Vitreous	Clear
Multiple gray-white lesions surrounding the optic nerve and extending around the vascular arcades into the macula	Fundus	Multiple gray-white lesions surrounding the optic nerve and extending around the vascular arcades into the macula

(BCVA: best corrected visual acuity, IOP: intraocular pressure; KPs: keratic precipitates)

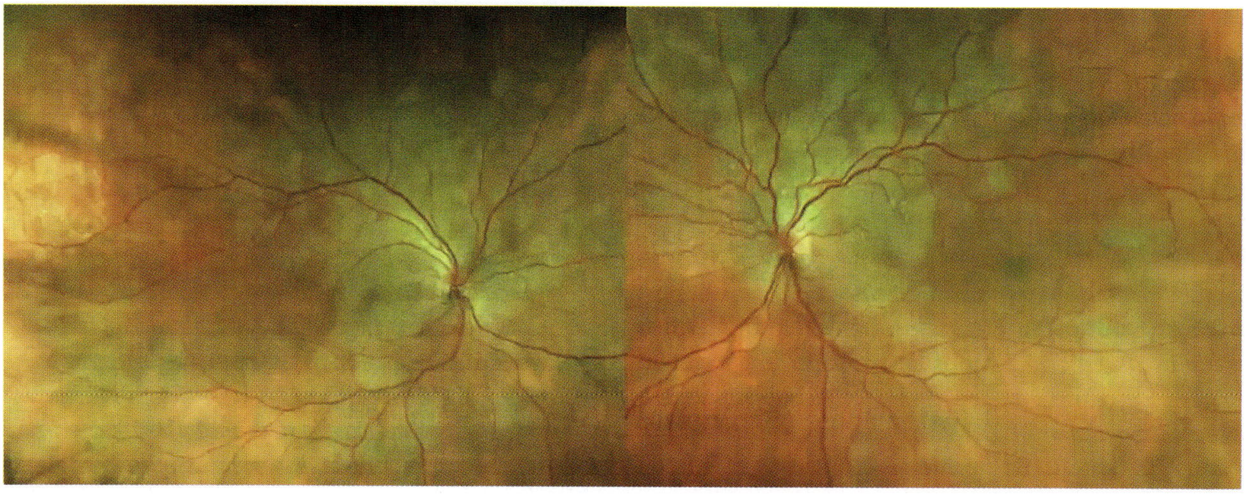

Fig. 31: Color fundus photos of both eyes showing gray-white placoid lesions surrounding the optic nerves and the vascular arcades with more macular involvement in the right eye.
Source: Uveitis Webinar - Grand Round 15. International Uveitis Study Group (IUSG). 2025. https://youtu.be/zWjjQGAAxh4?si=KrNaSnT3l5p4Mzkt.

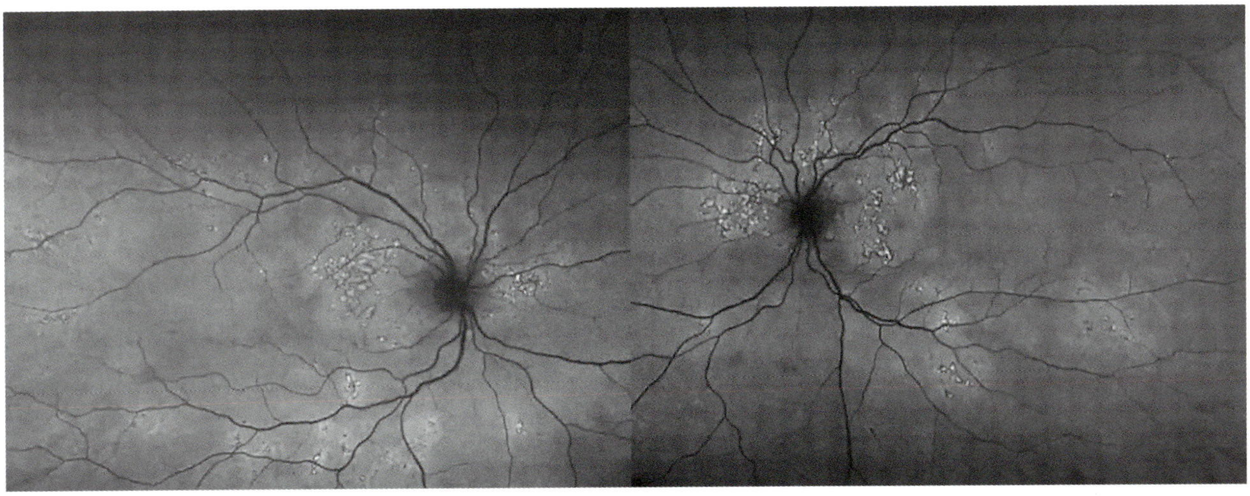

Fig. 32: Fundus autofluorescence images showing multifocal areas of hyperautofluorescence surrounding circumscribed hypoautofluorescent lesions.
Source: Uveitis Webinar - Grand Round 15. International Uveitis Study Group (IUSG). 2025. https://youtu.be/zWjjQGAAxh4?si=KrNaSnT3l5p4Mzkt.

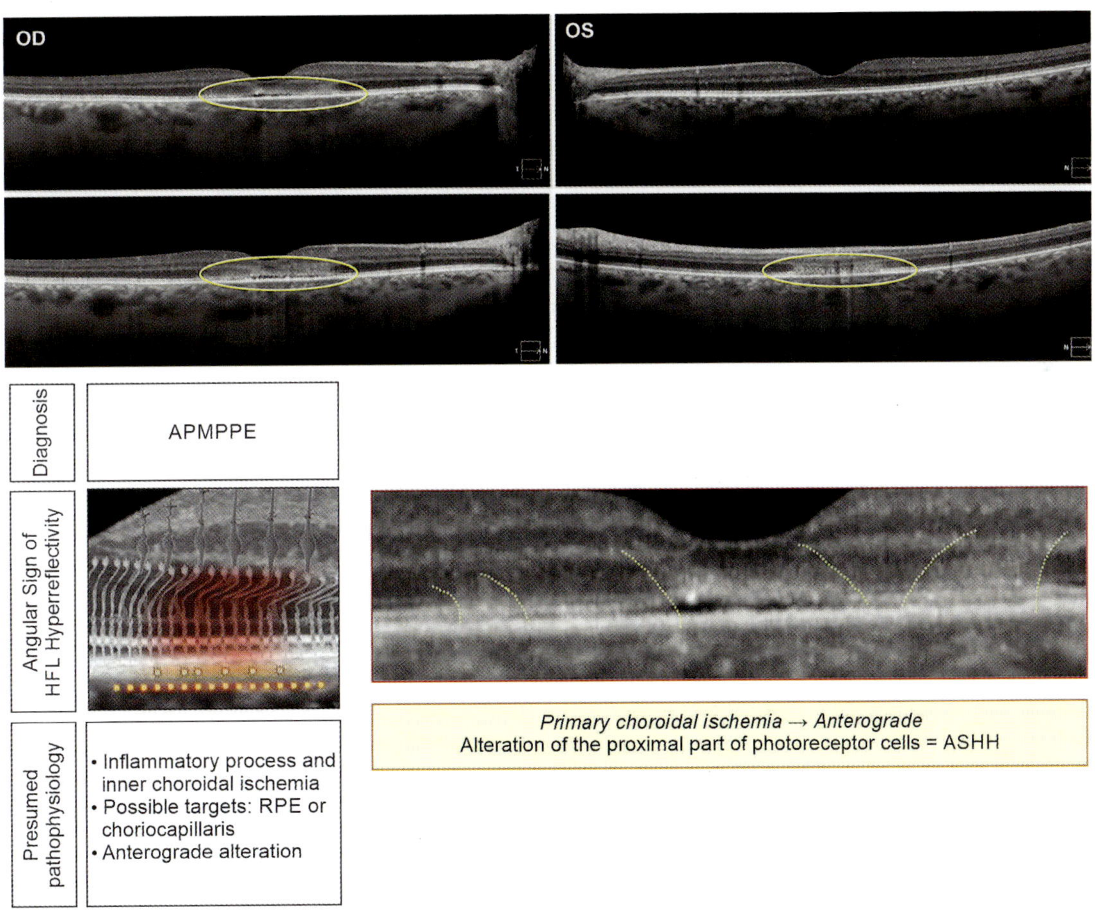

Fig. 33: Optical coherence tomography (OCT) images of the macula in both eyes showing acute hyperreflective lesions at the level of the outer retina (yellow circles, top). The pathophysiology of the lesions results from the anterograde effects of choroidal ischemia as seen in the bottom images.
Source: Uveitis Webinar - Grand Round 15. International Uveitis Study Group (IUSG). 2025. https://youtu.be/zWjjQGAAxh4?si=KrNaSnT3l5p4Mzkt.

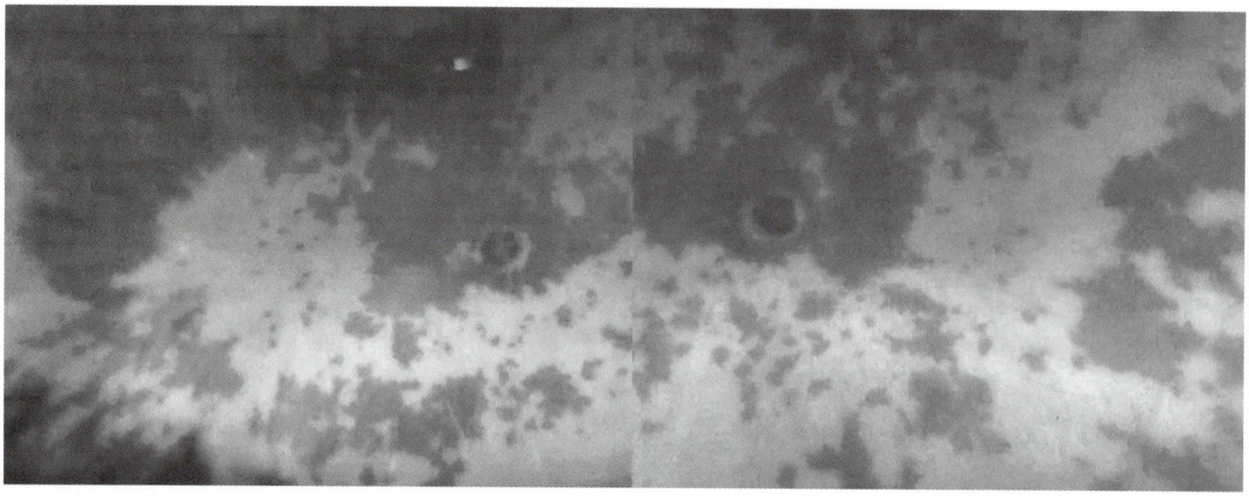

Fig. 34: An indocyanine green late frame image shows patchy areas of hypocyanescence representing choroidal ischemia or hypoperfusion.
Source: Uveitis Webinar - Grand Round 15. International Uveitis Study Group (IUSG). 2025. https://youtu.be/zWjjQGAAxh4?si=KrNaSnT3l5p4Mzkt.

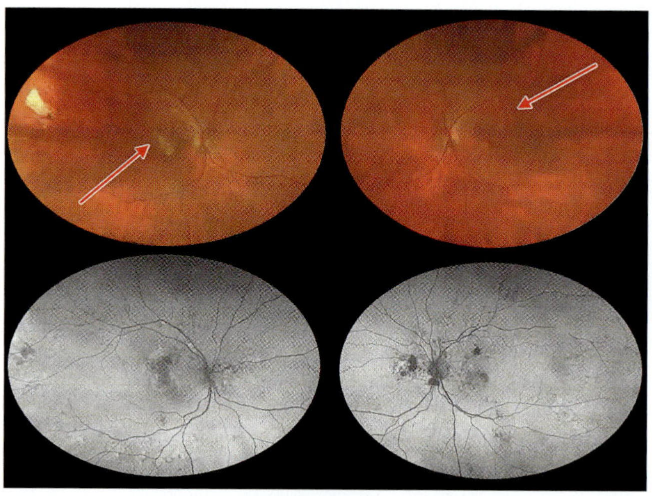

Fig. 35: Color fundus photos (top) and autofluorescence images of both eyes (bottom) showing new macular lesions in the right eye and retinal lesions in the left eye (red arrows) that correspond to areas of hypoautofluorescence (bottom).
Source: Uveitis Webinar - Grand Round 15. International Uveitis Study Group (IUSG). 2025. https://youtu.be/zWjjQGAAxh4?si=KrNaSnT3l5p4Mzkt.

complications. Given the MMI showing progressive choroidal ischemia, the diagnosis was felt to be persistent placoid maculopathy, not APMPPE. This guided clinical management to start azathioprine 50 mg/day. It was discontinued due to dyspepsia and replaced with mycophenolate mofetil 2 g/day for 1 year. He was switched to 10 mg of methotrexate weekly for the following year. His regimen was continued from October 2020 to April 2021. With the recurrence of the lesions in January 2023, he was restarted on mycophenolate 2 g/day. The immunosuppressive therapies were accompanied with repeated injections of aflibercept (23 in the right eye and 21 in the left eye).

On repeated color fundus photos, a dense area of white material was seen in the macula of the right eye with creamy lesions in the left eye **(Fig. 35)**. Again, the autofluorescence images showed hypo- and hyperautofluorescence of the lesions **(Fig. 35)**. OCT images showed the presence of a dense area of subretinal, hyperreflective material in the right eye and multiple areas of subretinal, hyperreflective material (SHRM) in the left eye **(Fig. 36)**.

Additional testing with enface OCTA imaging in the right eye showed the development of a dense, inactive type 2 neovascularization. Surrounding choroidal ischemia or hypoperfusion on the choriocapillaris slab is represented by hyporeflective areas **(Fig. 37)**.

Follow-up OCTA imaging showed a stable neovascular membrane after many aflibercept injections. The choriocapillaris slab again showed stable choroidal ischemia **(Fig. 38)**.

More interestingly, the left eye also developed a choroidal neovascular membrane as seen in an enface OCTA image segmented to the level of the choriocapillaris **(Fig. 39)**. Focusing specifically on the area highlighted by the yellow circle, there is no ischemia in July 2023. When followed a few months later in January 2024, this patient developed a new area of ischemia, which is visible

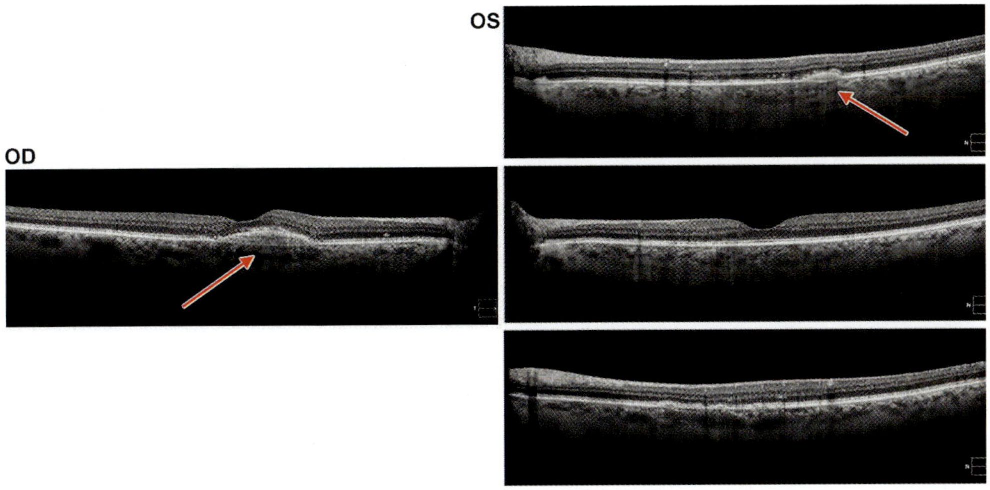

Fig. 36: Optical coherence tomography (OCT) images of both maculae showing a dense area of subretinal, hyperreflective material in the right eye on the left (red arrow) and multiple areas of subretinal, hyperreflective material in the left eye in the right images (red arrow).
Source: Uveitis Webinar - Grand Round 15. International Uveitis Study Group (IUSG). 2025. https://youtu.be/zWjjQGAAxh4?si=KrNaSnT3l5p4Mzkt.

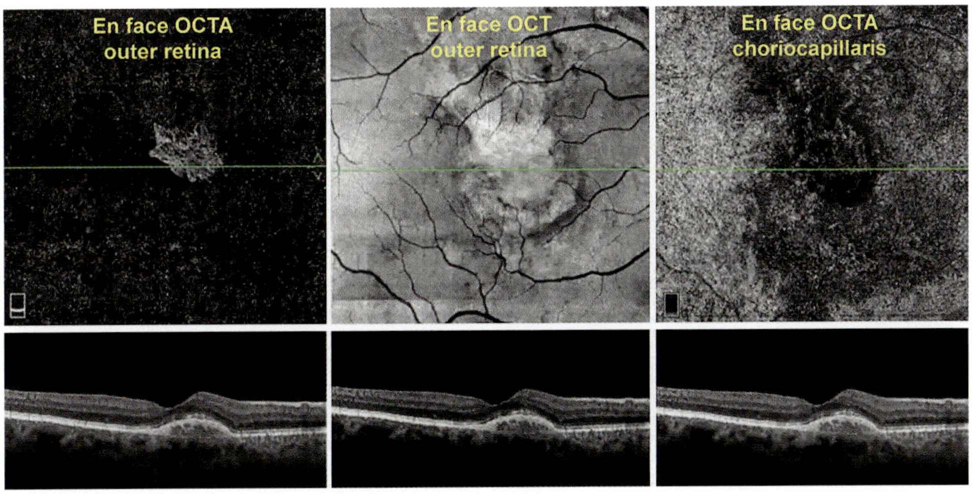

Fig. 37: Optical coherence tomography (OCT) and optical coherence tomography angiography (OCTA) images of the right macula showing a choroidal neovascular membrane on the outer retinal slab extending from the choriocapillaris with areas of hyporeflectivity representing hypoperfusion at the level of the choriocapillaris.
Source: Uveitis Webinar - Grand Round 15. International Uveitis Study Group (IUSG). 2025. https://youtu.be/zWjjQGAAxh4?si=KrNaSnT3l5p4Mzkt.

as a round area of hyporeflectivity **(Fig. 40)**. There is a corresponding enface scan with SHRM starting to develop at the same time.

Two months later, in march 2024, the same area of neovascular ischemia underwent the development of a type 2 choroidal neovascular membrane with both SHRM and subretinal fluid noted. This required treatment with repeated aflibercept injections. There are two take home messages from the evolution using MMI. First, primary choroidal ischemia represents the main pathogenesis of this type of placoid disorder. The ischemia drives both the development of the super acute ASHH lesions, which was the presentation in this case, but also the development of the neovascular complications such as a type two choroidal neovascular membrane. Therapy requires a dual approach with the use of both immunosuppressive therapy and anti-vascular endothelial growth factor (VEGF) intravitreal injections. This case also highlights the

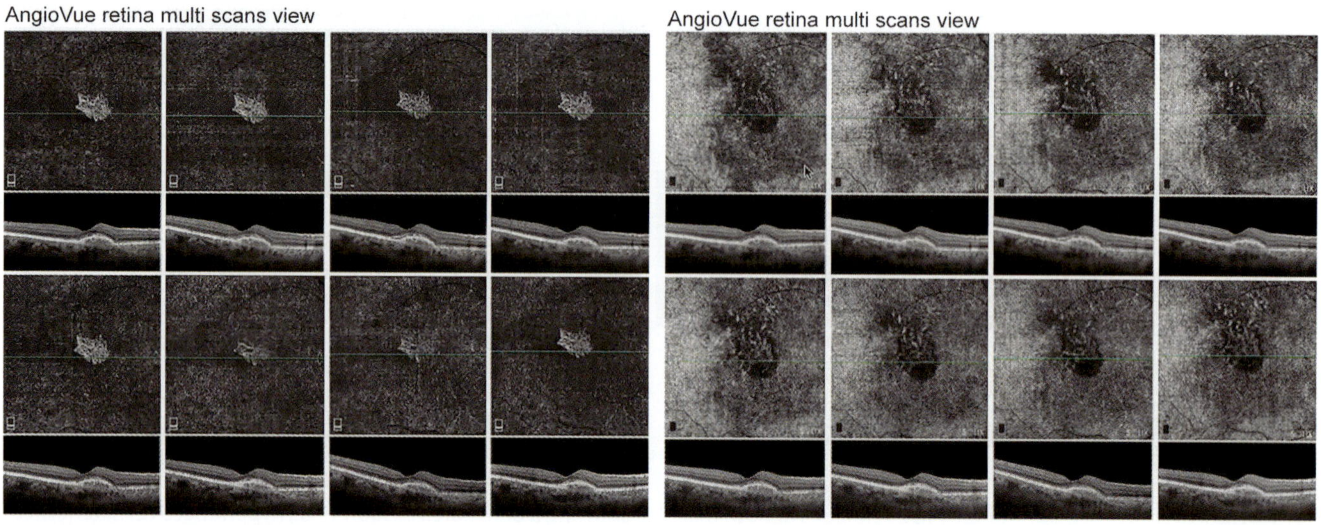

Fig. 38: Optical coherence tomography (OCT) and optical coherence tomography angiography (OCTA) images of the right macula showing a stable choroidal neovascular membrane on the outer retinal slab (left) and choriocapillary ischemia with stable areas of hyporeflectivity (right) over follow-up visits.
Source: Uveitis Webinar - Grand Round 15. International Uveitis Study Group (IUSG). 2025. https://youtu.be/zWjjQGAAxh4?si=KrNaSnT3l5p4Mzkt.

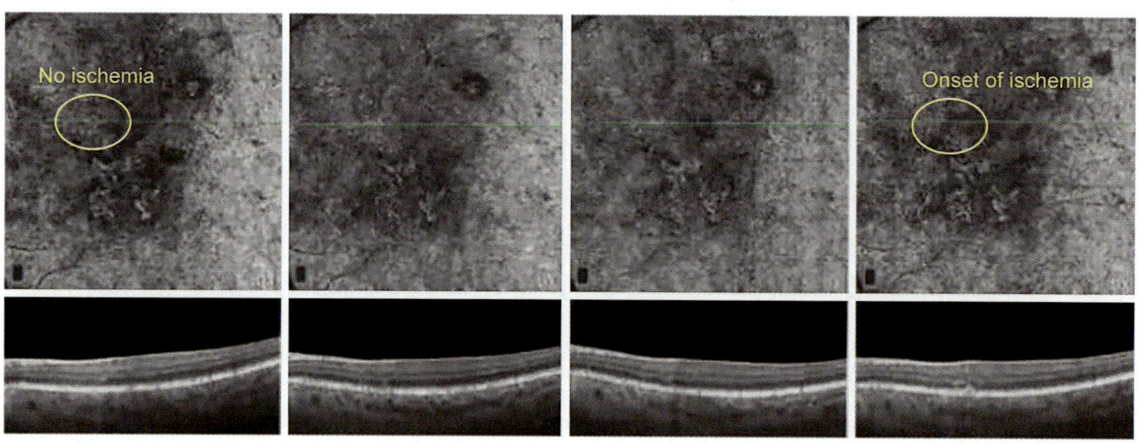

Fig. 39: Optical coherence tomography (OCT) and optical coherence tomography angiography (OCTA) images of the left macula showing no ischemia in the yellow circle (left) with increased choriocapillary ischemia seen with more hyporeflectivity in January 2024 (right yellow circle).
Source: Uveitis Webinar - Grand Round 15. International Uveitis Study Group (IUSG). 2025. https://youtu.be/zWjjQGAAxh4?si=KrNaSnT3l5p4Mzkt.

use of enface OCT and OCTA imaging to non-invasively visualize and monitor these patients to optimize both treatment approaches.

Case Presentation

Personal Data

A 57-year-old female with a history of multiple anti-VEGF injections presented with decreased vision in the left eye.

History of Present Illness

The patient denied flashes, floaters, or prior eye surgeries.

Physical Examination

The best corrected visual acuity on presentation was 20/50 in the right eye and 20/100 in the left eye. Dilated fundus examination showed tilted optic nerves with peripapillary atrophy. Yellow lesions extended from

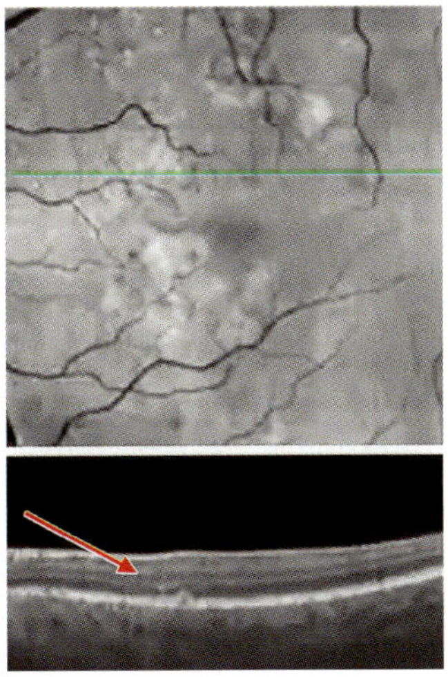

Fig. 40: Optical coherence tomography (OCT) and optical coherence tomography angiography (OCTA) image of the left macula showing the corresponding enface scan from January 2024 showing early subretinal, hyperreflective material (SHRM) formation (red arrow) with the choroidal ischemia.
Source: Uveitis Webinar - Grand Round 15. International Uveitis Study Group (IUSG). 2025. https://youtu.be/zWjjQGAAxh4?si=KrNaSnT3l5p4Mzkt.

TABLE 3: Physical examination of a patient having multiple anti-vascular endothelial growth factor (VEGF) injections presented with decreased vision in the left eye.

OD	***Parameter***	***OS***
20/50	BCVA	20/100
17 mm Hg	IOP	17 mm Hg
Quiet	Conjunctiva	Quiet
Clear	Cornea	Clear
Deep and quiet	Anterior chamber	Deep and quiet
No synechiae	Iris	No synechiae
1+ nuclear sclerosis	Lens	1+ nuclear sclerosis
Trace cells	Vitreous	Clear
Peripapillary atrophy with subretinal scarring with adjacent yellow lesions	Fundus	Peripapillary atrophy with subretinal scarring with adjacent yellow lesions

(BCVA: best corrected visual acuity, IOP: intraocular pressure; KPs: keratic precipitates)

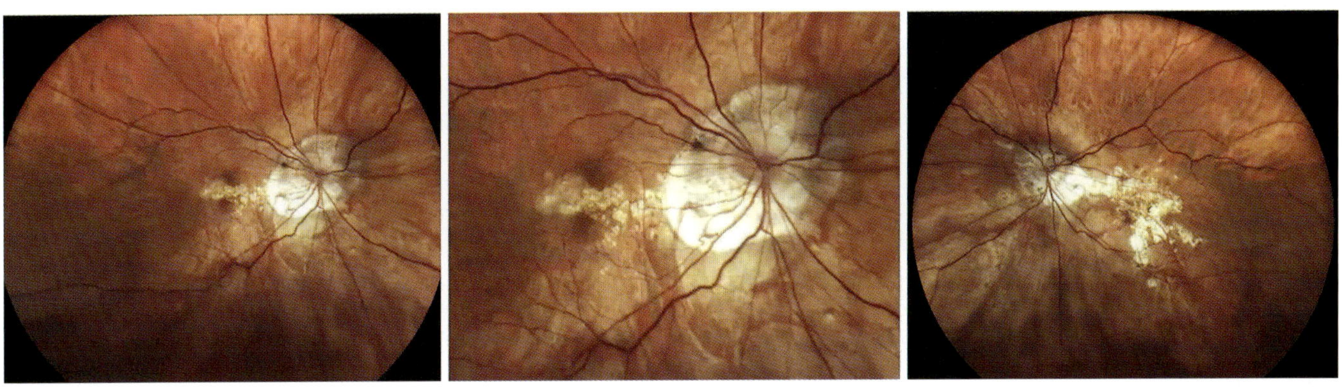

Fig. 41: Color fundus photos of both eyes showing tilted optic nerves, peripapillary atrophy, and yellow lesions extending from the peripapillary atrophy into the maculae.
Source: Uveitis Webinar - Grand Round 15. International Uveitis Study Group (IUSG). 2025. https://youtu.be/zWjjQGAAxh4?si=KrNaSnT3l5p4Mzkt.

the peripapillary atrophy into the macula in both eyes **(Fig. 41)**. The temporal portion of the lesion had a creamy, blurred border **(Table 3)**.

Ancillary testing: OCT scans of the macula show drusenoid subretinal deposits in both eyes and an epiretinal membrane in the left eye with inner retinal schisis **(Fig. 42)**. Fluorescein angiography showed early hyperfluorescence in the temporal area of the lesion in the right eye with a corresponding area of hypocyanescence on ICG testing **(Fig. 43)**. The left eye shows a serpiginoid pattern with late staining on fluorescein angiography with hypocyanescence of the same lesion on ICG **(Fig. 44)**. The highest diagnostic yield came from use of OCTA imaging. In the upper left area of the lesion on the choriocapillaris slab, ischemia, along with surrounding satellite islands of hypoperfusion **(Fig. 45)**. These findings were not related

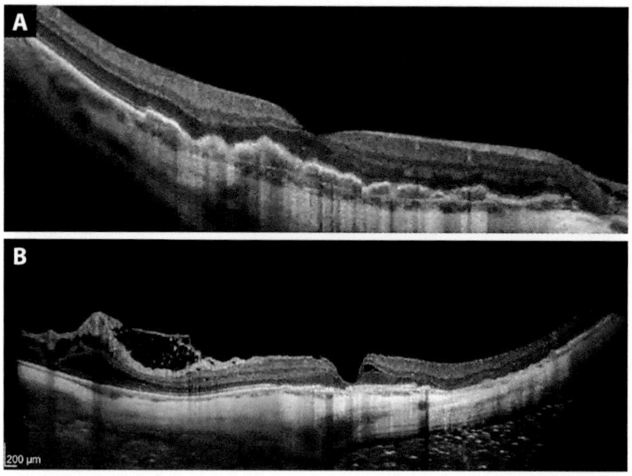

Figs. 42A and B: Optical coherence tomography (OCT) of the macula in the right eye showing drusenoid deposits under the macula (A) and an epiretinal membrane with retinoschisis in the left eye (B).
Source: Uveitis Webinar - Grand Round 15. International Uveitis Study Group (IUSG). 2025. https://youtu.be/zWjjQGAAxh4?si=KrNaSnT3l5p4Mzkt.

to shadowing since the enface OCT shows a bright outer retinal layer.

Uveitis work-up: Baseline testing with a complete blood count and comprehensive panel was normal. Syphilis testing was negative.

Initial treatment: All the information from the MMI confirmed the diagnosis of macular-involving serpiginous choroiditis. The patient was treated with 1.5 g of mycophenolate mofetil twice a day with a prednisone taper starting at 80 mg daily.

Follow-up: After several weeks, the visual acuity improved to 20/25 in the right eye. After 3 months, there was anatomical improvement in the right eye with decreased subretinal lesion thickness and reduced ischemia on OCTA, as seen in **Figure 46**. Color fundus photos also showed the evolution of the creamy, blurred edge of the temporal lesion to a clearer border with atrophy in the right eye **(Fig. 47)**.

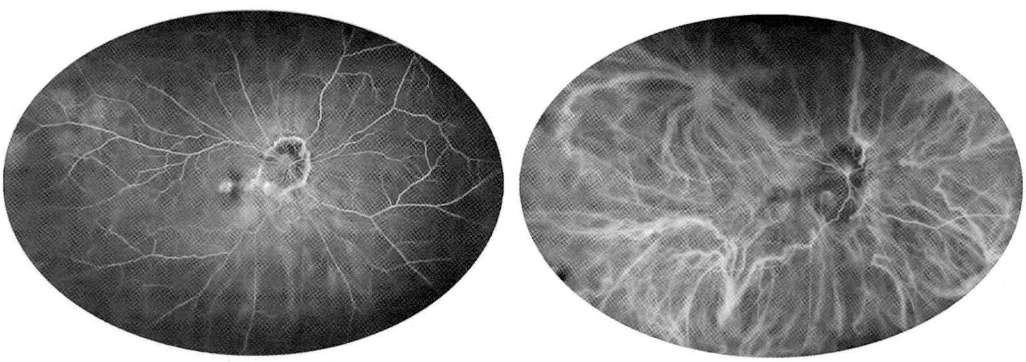

Fig. 43: Fluorescein angiography of the right eye showing early hyperfluorescence in the temporal area of the lesion (left). The corresponding area is hypocyanescent on indocyanine green testing (right).
Source: Uveitis Webinar - Grand Round 15. International Uveitis Study Group (IUSG). 2025. https://youtu.be/zWjjQGAAxh4?si=KrNaSnT3l5p4Mzkt.

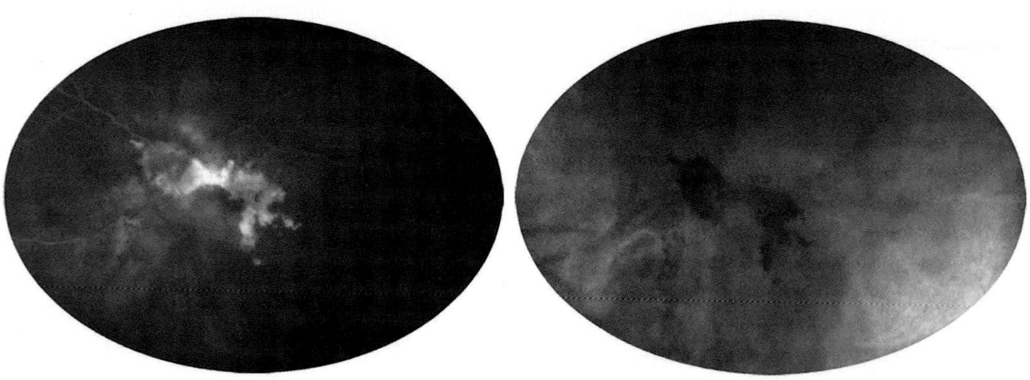

Fig. 44: Fluorescein angiography of the left eye showing a serpiginoid pattern with late staining (left) with hypocyanescence of the same lesion on indocyanine green (ICG) testing (right).
Source: Uveitis Webinar - Grand Round 15. International Uveitis Study Group (IUSG). 2025. https://youtu.be/zWjjQGAAxh4?si=KrNaSnT3l5p4Mzkt.

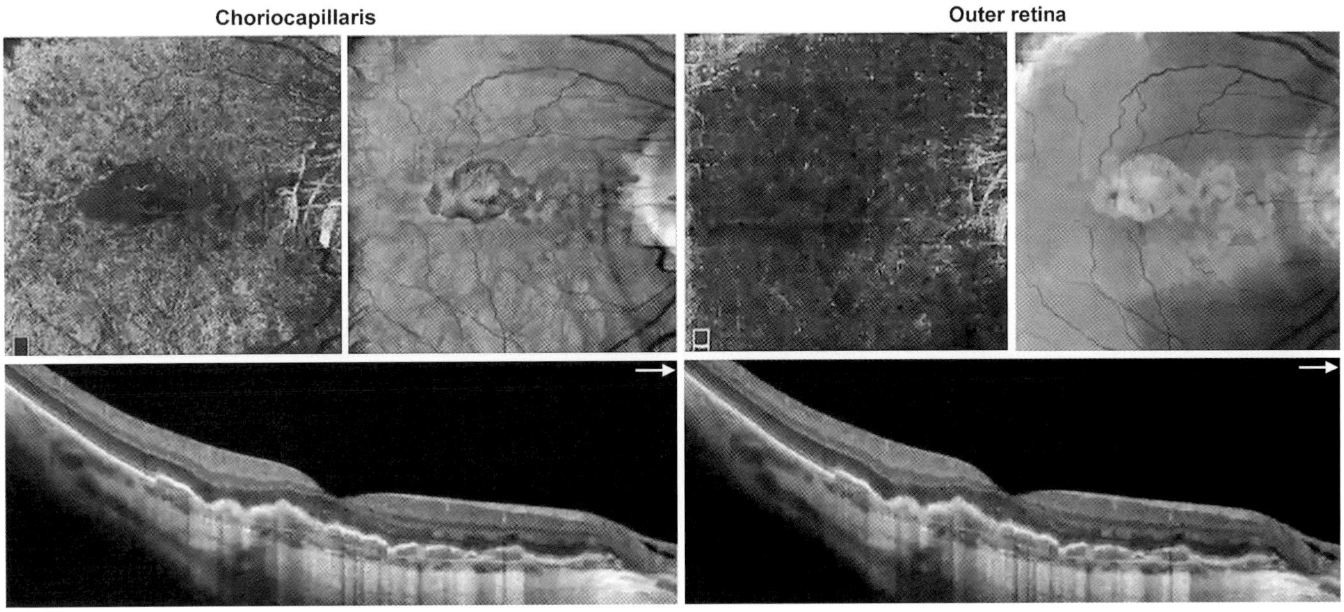

Fig. 45: An optical coherence tomography angiography (OCTA) segment image of the right eye showing in the upper left area of the lesion, on the choriocapillaris slab, ischemia is noted with surrounding satellite islands of hypoperfusion (left). These findings were not related to shadowing since the enface optical coherence tomography (OCT) image shows a bright outer retinal layer (right).
Source: Uveitis Webinar - Grand Round 15. International Uveitis Study Group (IUSG). 2025. https://youtu.be/zWjjQGAAxh4?si=KrNaSnT3l5p4Mzkt.

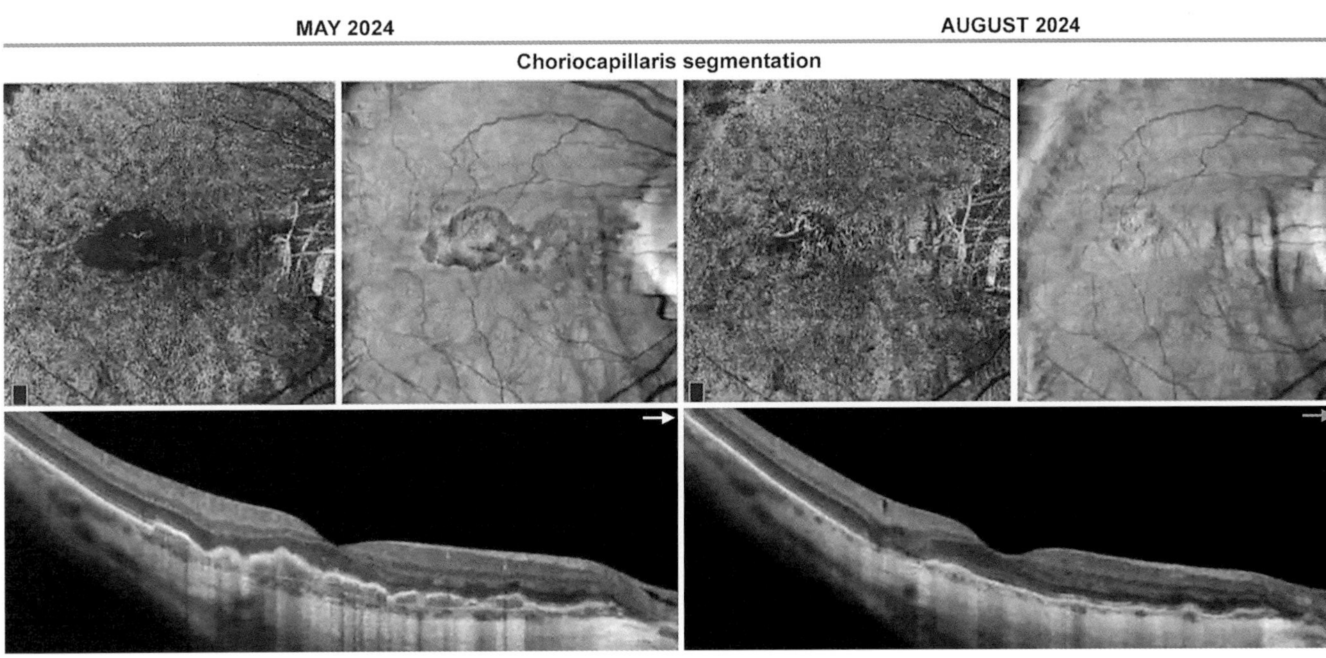

Fig. 46: An optical coherence tomography angiography (OCTA) segment image at the level of the choriocapillaris showing less hypoperfusion represented by less hyporeflective areas near the temporal lesion over 3 months of follow-up (top). The subretinal lesion thickness also decreased with improved vision (bottom).
Source: Uveitis Webinar - Grand Round 15. International Uveitis Study Group (IUSG). 2025. https://youtu.be/zWjjQGAAxh4?si=KrNaSnT3l5p4Mzkt.

Several articles have discussed the role of OCTA in monitoring the response to treatment in cases of persistent placoid maculopathy and APMPPE. In addition, overlaying the OCTA with the ICG to compare MMI modalities has been described. The second manuscript, by Cheng et al., presented a case series of eight patients with persistent

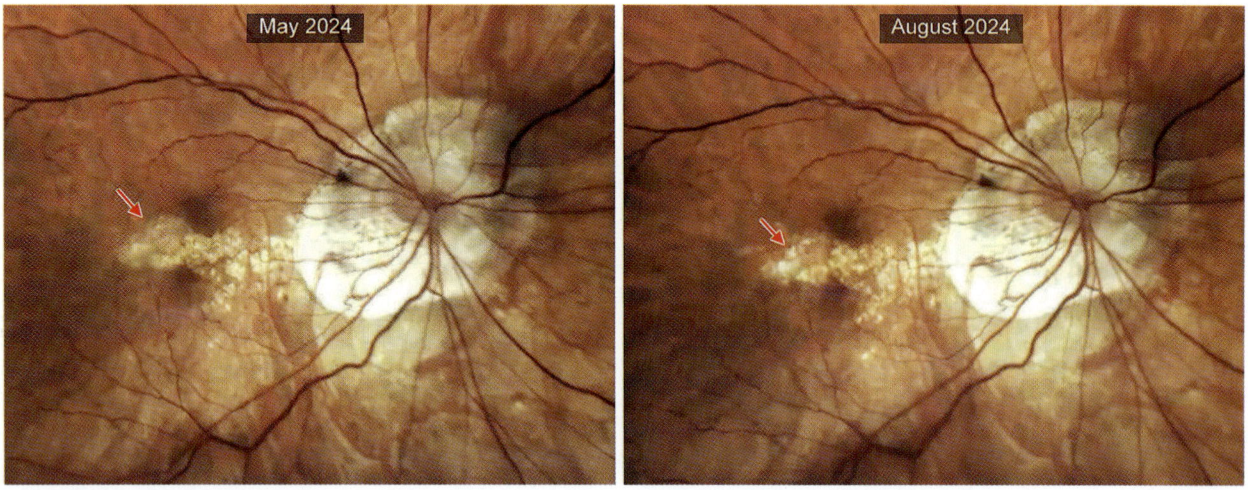

Fig. 47: Color fundus photos of the right eye show a clearer temporal border with atrophy after 3 months of treatment with mycophenolate mofetil and prednisone.
Source: Uveitis Webinar - Grand Round 15. International Uveitis Study Group (IUSG). 2025. https://youtu.be/zWjjQGAAxh4?si=KrNaSnT3l5p4Mzkt.

placoid maculopathy that showed ASHH lesions at clinical presentation evolving to drusen-like lesions, which were complicated with neovascularization requiring treatment with anti-VEGF intravitreal injections.

Discussion

The patient in the first case presented with classic APMPPE given the placoid lesions seen on color photographs and the presence of ischemia on both the ICGA and the OCTA images. Ischemia is the driving pathophysiology with this condition, as the choriocapillaris hypoperfusion seen on OCTA corresponds to ASHH lesions on cross-sectional OCT and to the development of neovascularization.[14-16] Areas of neovascularization can progress despite several years of anti-VEGF treatment, and in this particular case, the patient also developed progressive inner choroidal ischemia. Perhaps this was APMPPE that evolved to persistent placoid chorioretinitis, and for that aspect of the disease, we started mycophenolate mofetil at the maximum dose as immunomodulatory therapy. I have taken care of this patient for almost a decade, and it illustrates the difficulty of treating these conditions. The progression of the disease started as APMPPE that evolved into a persistent placoid maculopathy with secondary neovascularization with flares of active disease separated by years.

The second case is a little bit more complicated. Outer retinal and Henle fiber layer changes seen in the hyperacute phase were absent on presentation. Instead, retinal pigment epithelial changes typical of the subacute phase of APMPPE were seen on MMI. The inner choroidal ischemia was captured only by OCTA, which led to the diagnosis. This reiterates that inner choroidal ischemia is the driving pathogenic mechanism in placoid diseases like APMPPE and macular-involving serpiginous choroiditis. Both cases highlight the concept that lesions start with hyperacute changes in the outer retina and the Henle fiber layer (ASHH lesion) progressing to retinal pigment epithelial changes in the subacute phase. In older patients, these retinal pigment epithelial changes can masquerade as age-related macular degeneration.[17-18] It is important to use OCTA images to capture inner choroidal ischemia and identify any secondary complications, such as choroidal neovascularization.[19]

PUNCTATE INNER CHOROIDOPATHY

Case Presentation

Personal Data

An 18-year-old female presented with a smudge in the vision of the left eye for the past 6 months.

History of Present Illness

She had no pain, photophobia, flashes, or floaters. She was a high myope with contact lens use, and her past medical history included hypothyroidism, treated with levothyroxine, and migraine headaches.

Physical Examination

On examination, her best corrected visual acuity was 20/20 in the right eye and 20/200 in the left eye. Her anterior segment was normal, and her refraction was approximately -10 and -12 in the right and left eyes, respectively. The macula of the left eye had a hyperpigmented lesion in the fovea and a small hypopigmented punctate lesion in the infratemporal macula **(Table 4 and Fig. 48)**.

Ancillary testing: In the early arteriovenous phase of the fluorescein angiogram, there was mild hyperfluorescence in the fovea surrounded by hypofluorescence in the left eye. This area shows staining in the late phases with mild leakage **(Fig. 49)**. An OCT scan through the fovea of the left eye showed subretinal mixed hyperreflectivity with no significant intraretinal fluid **(Fig. 50)**.

TABLE 4: Physical examination of a patient having punctate inner choroidopathy.

OD	***Parameter***	***OS***
20/20	BCVA	20/200
14 mm Hg	IOP	13 mm Hg
Quiet	Conjunctiva	Quiet
Clear	Cornea	Clear
Deep and quiet	Anterior chamber	Deep and quiet
No synechiae	Iris	No synechiae
Clear	Lens	Clear
Clear	Vitreous	Clear
Normal	Fundus	Hyperpigmented lesion in the fovea and a small hypopigmented punctate lesion in the infratemporal macula

(BCVA: best corrected visual acuity; IOP: intraocular pressure)

Uveitis work-up: No laboratory studies were ordered at this time.

Initial treatment: In summary, an 18-year-old female with a history of high myopia presented with a chorioretinal lesion and a choroidal neovascular membrane in the left eye. The differential diagnosis included PIC and MFC, although she had no inflammation on examination. Other conditions that were considered were myopic maculopathy with choroidal neovascular membrane formation, tuberculosis, syphilis, and sarcoidosis. The patient was diagnosed with PIC based on the elevated pigmented lesion, likely a choroidal neovascular membrane complex, and the small hypopigmented lesion in the inferotemporal macula. For the macular neovascularization, the plan was to administer a series of three anti-VEGF injections. However, she only received one injection and was lost to follow-up for 5 years.

Follow-up: She presented again with metamorphopsia in her right eye. Two small hypopigmented lesions in the macula of the right eye and several more lesions in the left eye were seen on examination **(Fig. 51)**.

Repeat OCT testing through both maculas showed sparing of the fovea in the right eye and a subretinal lesion

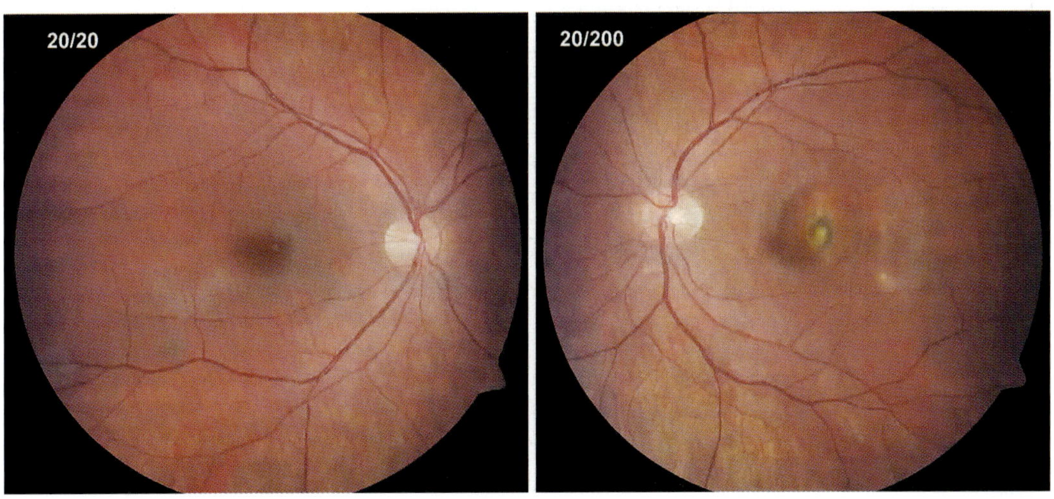

Fig. 48: Color fundus photos of both eyes showing a normal fundus in the right eye (left) and a hyperpigmented lesion in the fovea with a small hypopigmented punctate lesion in the infratemporal macula of the left eye (right).
Source: Uveitis Webinar - Grand Round 15. International Uveitis Study Group (IUSG). 2025. https://youtu.be/zWjjQGAAxh4?si=KrNaSnT3l5p4Mzkt.

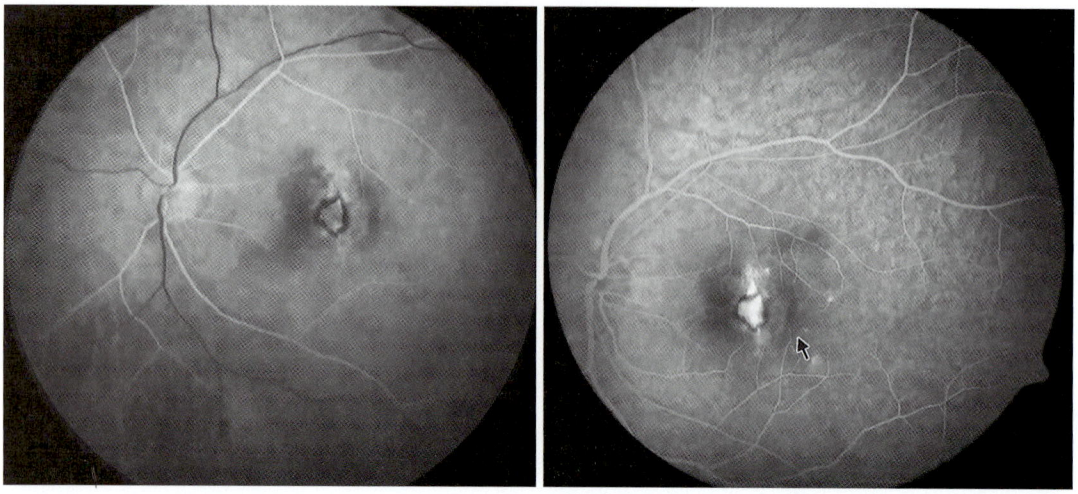

Fig. 49: Early (left) and late frame (right) fluorescein angiograms of the left eye. Mild hyperfluorescence in the fovea surrounded by hypofluorescence in the left eye occurs in the arteriovenous phase. This area shows staining in the late phases with mild leakage.
Source: Uveitis Webinar - Grand Round 15. International Uveitis Study Group (IUSG). 2025. https://youtu.be/zWjjQGAAxh4?si=KrNaSnT3l5p4Mzkt.

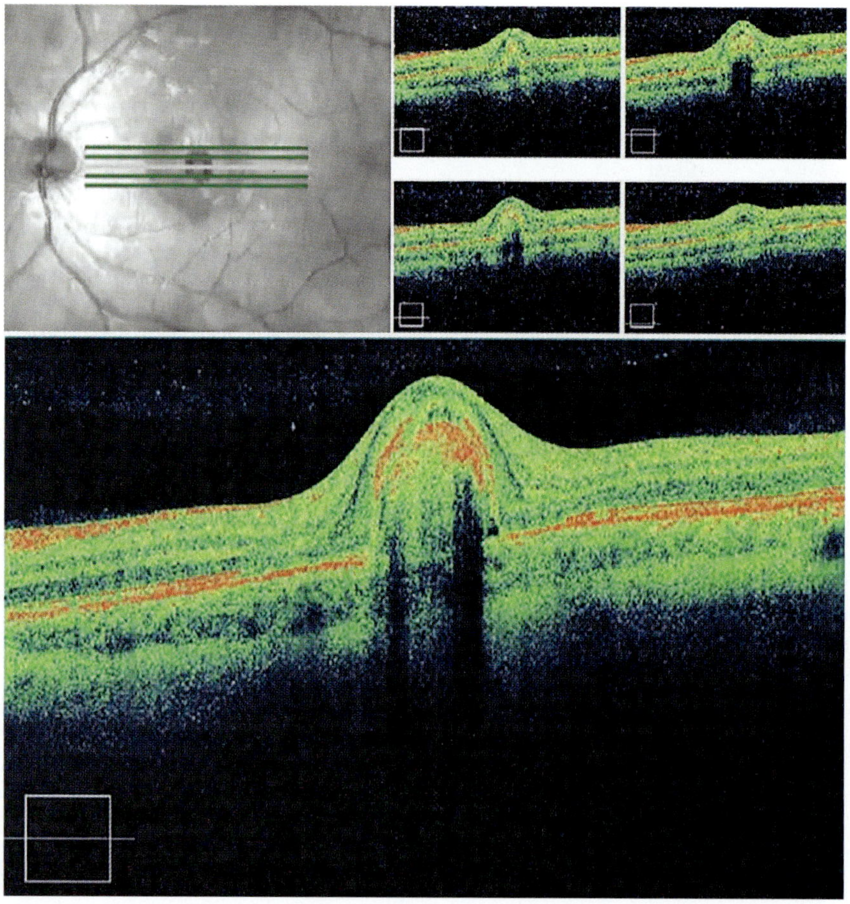

Fig. 50: An optical coherence tomography (OCT) scan through the fovea of the left eye showed subretinal mixed hyperreflectivity suggestive of the presence of a choroidal neovascular membrane.
Source: Uveitis Webinar - Grand Round 15. International Uveitis Study Group (IUSG). 2025. https://youtu.be/zWjjQGAAxh4?si=KrNaSnT3l5p4Mzkt.

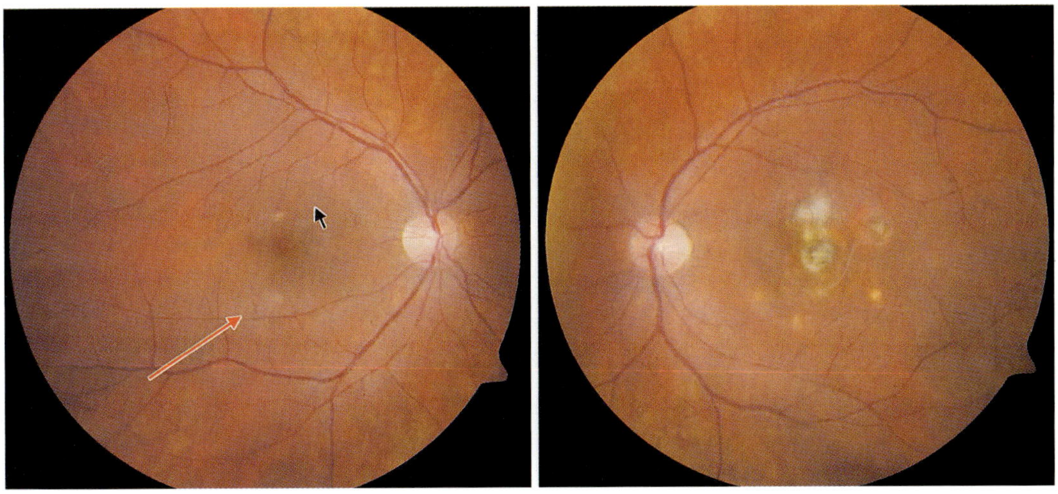

Fig. 51: Color fundus photos of both eyes show new punctate lesions in the macula of the right eye (red arrow, left) and new yellow lesions inferior to the macula in the left eye (right).
Source: Uveitis Webinar - Grand Round 15. International Uveitis Study Group (IUSG). 2025. https://youtu.be/zWjjQGAAxh4?si=KrNaSnT3l5p4Mzkt.

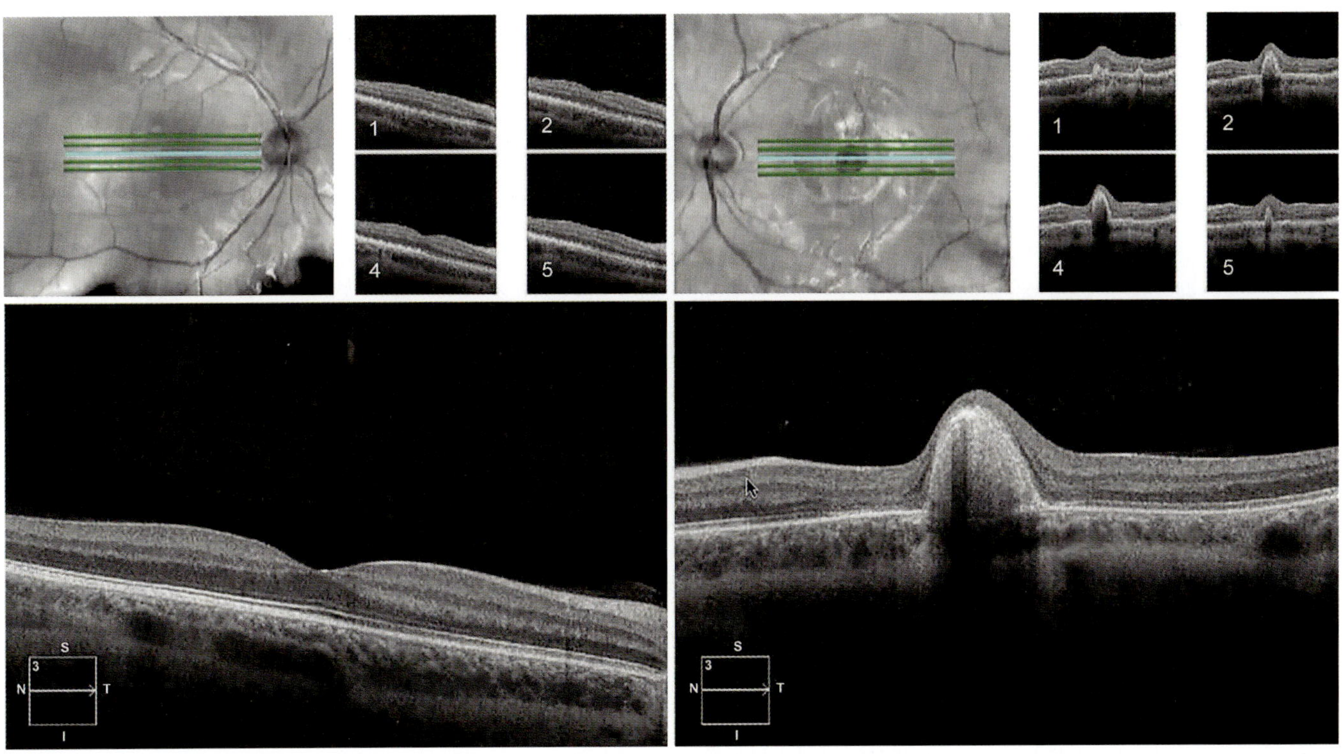

Fig. 52: An optical coherence tomography (OCT) scan through the fovea of the right eye with a preserved macular contour (left). The left eye scan showed a subretinal lesion without significant intraretinal fluid (right).
Source: Uveitis Webinar - Grand Round 15. International Uveitis Study Group (IUSG). 2025. https://youtu.be/zWjjQGAAxh4?si=KrNaSnT3l5p4Mzkt.

in the left eye **(Fig. 52)**. While her scan did not capture the new lesion in her right eye, we found a representative OCT image from a patient with a similar examination. On near infrared, there are numerous punctate lesions near a focal, hyperreflective, subretinal outer retinal lesion, and loss of the ellipsoid zone **(Fig. 53)**. The ellipsoid disruption extends further than the lesion itself and shows active disease.

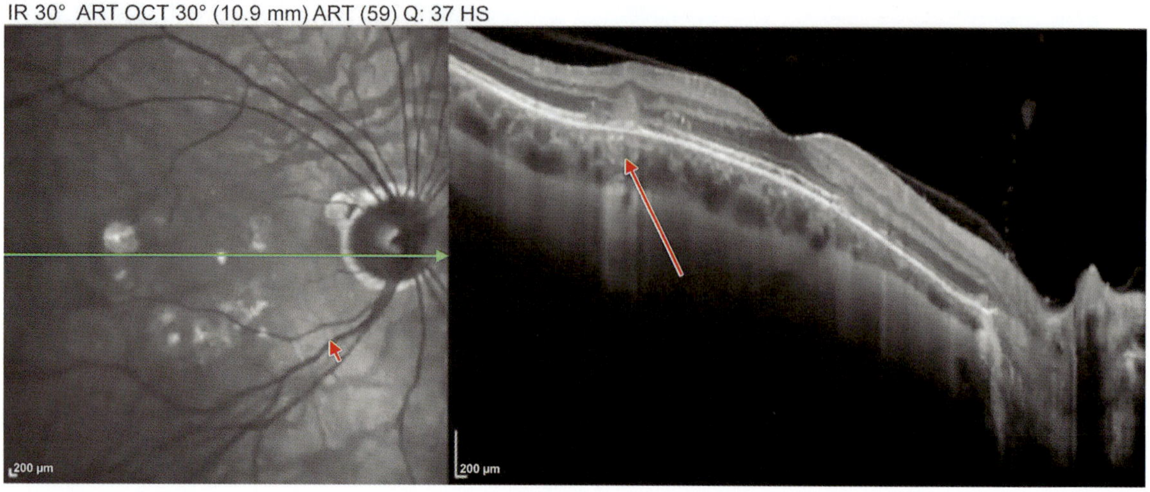

Fig. 53: An optical coherence tomography (OCT) scan through the perifovea of the right eye showed a focal, hyperreflective, outer retinal lesion with ellipsoid zone disruption representing an active lesion (red arrow).
Source: Uveitis Webinar - Grand Round 15. International Uveitis Study Group (IUSG). 2025. https://youtu.be/zWjjQGAAxh4?si=KrNaSnT3l5p4Mzkt.

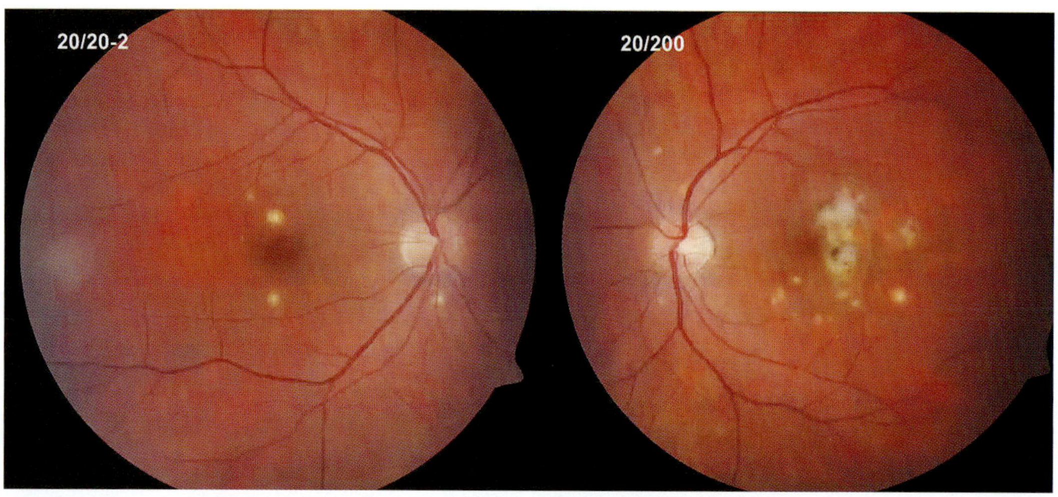

Fig. 54: Color fundus photos of both eyes show new punctate lesions around the maculae in both eyes.
Source: Uveitis Webinar - Grand Round 15. International Uveitis Study Group (IUSG). 2025. https://youtu.be/zWjjQGAAxh4?si=KrNaSnT3l5p4Mzkt.

Given active disease, she was started on prednisone 40 mg daily and given another injection of an anti-VEGF medication, bevacizumab 1.25 mg/0.05 mL in the right eye. After 1 week, she was less symptomatic and started a prednisone taper by 5 mg per week over several months. 2 years later, she developed increased blurriness in the right eye with development of new lesions in both eyes **(Fig. 54)**. While there is not an OCT scan through the lesion itself, a representative photograph is shown. There is an older, inactive lesion characterized by focal ellipsoid zone and retinal pigment epithelial disruption with increased choroidal transmittance **(Fig. 55)**.

While the lesion shown in **Figure 55** was inactive, there were other active lesions were identified on examination, necessitating restarting prednisone 50 mg daily and concurrent initiation of methotrexate 15 mg weekly given continued recurrences. 1 year later, she presented with even more lesions in both eyes despite treatment with methotrexate. She was switched to mycophenolate mofetil 1 g twice a day to increase immunosuppression dose. **Figures 56 and 57** show a color fundus photo progression of both eyes over 8 years of follow-up. The lesions did not disappear or regress over time.

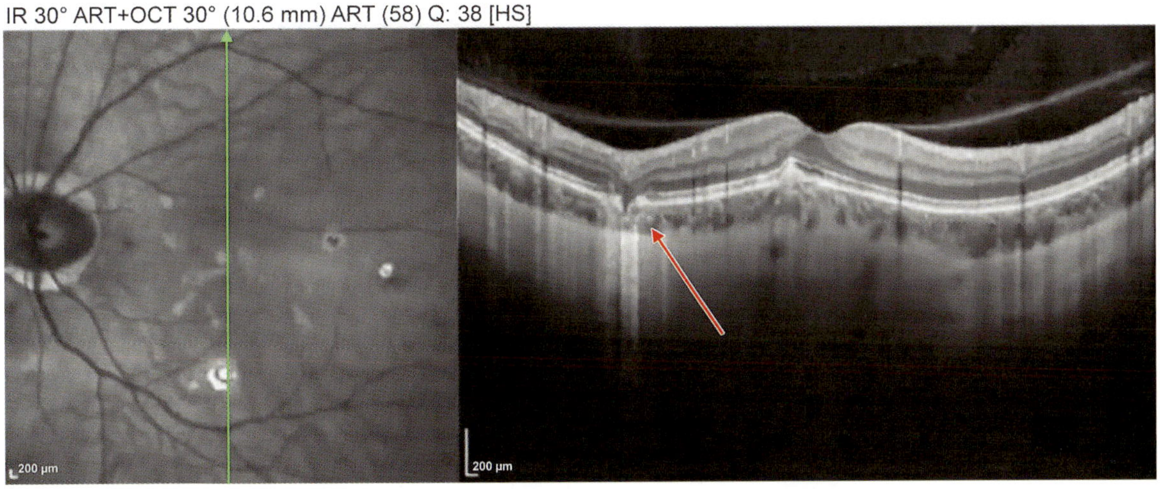

Fig. 55: An optical coherence tomography (OCT) scan showing an inactive lesion characterized by focal ellipsoid zone and retinal pigment epithelium disruption with increased choroidal transmittance (red arrow).
Source: Uveitis Webinar - Grand Round 15. International Uveitis Study Group (IUSG). 2025. https://youtu.be/zWjjQGAAxh4?si=KrNaSnT3l5p4Mzkt.

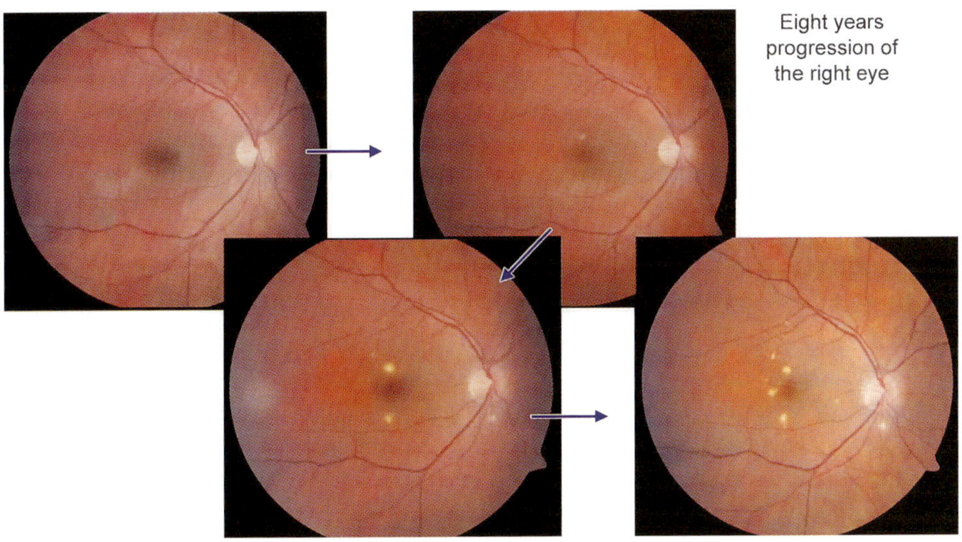

Fig. 56: Color fundus photos of the right eye over 8 years of follow-up showing continued development of punctate lesions around the macula.
Source: Uveitis Webinar - Grand Round 15. International Uveitis Study Group (IUSG). 2025. https://youtu.be/zWjjQGAAxh4?si=KrNaSnT3l5p4Mzkt.

She was subsequently lost to follow-up over the last 5 years to the present day. Hopefully this means she has been doing well and has not experienced a change in her vision. In short, PIC is a primary inflammatory choriocapillariopathy, which was formally categorized as a WDS. It is a multifocal chorioretinopathy and frequently affects young myopic women. It is characterized by inflammation of the retinal pigment epithelium and the inner choroid. Patients typically have scotomas, blurred vision, photopsias, floaters, photophobia, and metamorphopsia. It can present unilaterally, but usually it is a bilateral disease over the course of the disease.

Discussion

The SUN II criteria for PIC include multifocal, punctate inflammatory lesions <250 µm in size with posterior pole involvement (with or without peripheral lesions) and minimal anterior chamber and vitreous cells.[5] In addition, infections, most notably syphilis, and sarcoidosis need to be excluded as the etiology of the examination

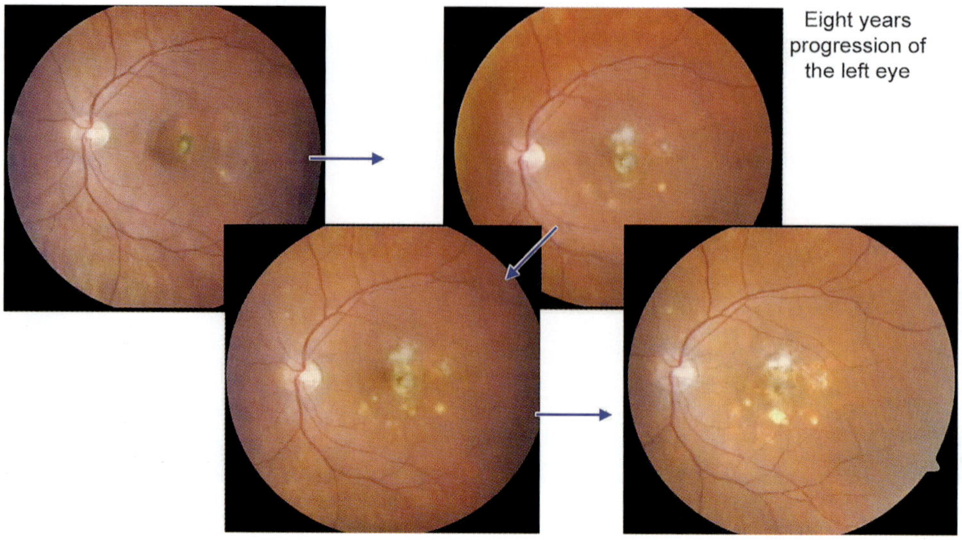

Fig. 57: Color fundus photos of the left eye over 8 years of follow-up showing continued development of punctate lesions around the macula and the presence of a choroidal neovascular membrane superior to the macula.
Source: Uveitis Webinar - Grand Round 15. International Uveitis Study Group (IUSG). 2025. https://youtu.be/zWjjQGAAxh4?si=KrNaSnT3l5p4Mzkt.

findings. If in an endemic area, tuberculosis must also be ruled out. The lesions may vary in size, but are typically circular, hypopigmented or yellow, and over time they evolve to appear atrophic with a clear margin. The lesions are deep and they can very frequently lead to macular neovascularization. An OCT or an OCTA is recommended in these patients to assess for a choroidal neovascular membrane (CNVM). When looking for a case, we searched for one that had a very long, chronic history. We did not have very good OCT images in the beginning of her clinical care, but we also wanted to show an FA, which is not ordered as frequently today. This case not only showed the progression but also illustrated many of the possible imaging modalities.

Is there a difference between PIC and MFC? Are they the same entity or different entities with differently sized lesions? Several manuscripts show that the same patient can have PIC in one eye and MFC in the other.[20] We are realizing that both are on the same disease spectrum but are phenotypically different. There are very classic features of PIC that may not be seen in MFC, but overall, they appear similarly on imaging and active lesions look the same on examination and imaging. Complication rates for CNVM are higher with PIC than in MFC. The patient population for both conditions is typically young, myopic females. In the United States, we also have presumed ocular histoplasmosis syndrome that can present with similar lesions, but there will be characteristic features that may not be present in PIC.

The MUV study working group recently published a paper on the multimodal features of PIC and MFC. There are two classic features on OCT: First when the retinal pigment epithelium is intact and the other occurs when the ellipsoid zone has a break. If the retinal pigment epithelium is intact, an inflammatory retinal pigment epithelial detachment (PED) can occur, and this lesion would be considered active. Another imaging finding on OCT that indicates activity is outer retinal disorganization or the presence of a SHRM. If there is a break in the ellipsoid zone, even if the lesion is small, the patient is symptomatic with a larger area of vision loss.

There are a couple of lessons that I would like to impart. Older OCT scans were limited to capturing a few RASER scans. With larger areas of the retina scanned, try to capture OCT slices through active lesions. OCT is the most sensitive imaging modality for detecting activity in PIC and MFC lesions. While these lesions resolve with treatment, unlike in a case of MEWDS, the ellipsoid zone may not reconstruct with a return of normal vision. These patients may have long-lasting visual impairment or scotomas. This is an important differentiation. It highlights the use of OCT to identify if a lesion is active and then subsequently monitor for change. Flares have two distinct forms. First, a new lesion can form, but with PIC and MFC, the same lesion in a previously affected area can reactivate. When obtaining OCT scans, there needs to be a focus even on the inactive lesions because a relapse may present in the exact same anatomic location.

The major cause of vision loss is from chronic lesions, which can be accompanied by choroidal neovascularization in the macula and subretinal fibrosis.[21,22] Subretinal fibrosis is not expansive, but even in focal scarring processes, it can lead to long-term visual impairment. OCT can also be used to determine if anti-VEGF treatment is required. While clinically there is an absence of exudation, OCTA can capture an increase in size of the neovascular net in the choriocapillaris. The value of OCTA lies in determining if SHRM lesions are inflammatory or due to CNVM formation. If the lesion has flow, anti-VEGF therapy should be administered. This raises the question of which clinical characteristics need to be considered when treating a patient with an intravitreal injection of an anti-VEGF agent. Is the patient symptomatic? Is the lesion or the complication of the inflammatory process visually impairing? Often, if neovascularization is present and accompanied by subretinal fluid on an OCT scan, the decision to administer in the injection is straightforward. If a lesion is enlarging, the start or escalation of immunosuppressive therapy is needed in addition to the anti-VEGF injection.

The duration of anti-VEGF injections also needs to be considered. As compared to wet macular degeneration where an anti-VEGF injection is given chronically every 2 or 3 months, in PIC the CNVM lesion does not necessarily need to be continuously treated. Typically, treatment includes one to three anti-VEGF injections. Underlying control of the inflammatory process is more important as the CNVM will regress once quiescence is achieved. Therefore, it is important to consider if chronic, immunosuppressive therapy is required. Some patients may respond to a short-acting intravitreal corticosteroid, such as the dexamethasone implant, or a high-dose, short course of oral prednisone to stabilize and achieve quiescence for many years. However, close follow-up, at least every 3 months, is needed to monitor the number of relapses and the impact on the visual acuity. If recurrent inflammatory lesions are present, then immunomodulatory therapy is warranted. There is no role for topical corticosteroids. While local corticosteroid intravitreal injections are an option, oral corticosteroids are more commonly used starting the taper at 1 mg/kg with a maximum dose of 60 mg/day.[23] Recurrent flares require immunosuppressive therapy. Most commonly, a first-line agent is an antimetabolite, including methotrexate or mycophenolate mofetil, depending on the patient's preference, age, medical comorbidities, and social factors.[24,25] Alcohol consumption should be discouraged with methotrexate use and patients in the reproductive age group should use contraception or consider an alternative agent if desiring to conceive. A second-line agent would be adalimumab. However, most patients with PIC have an acute, relapsing disease course.[26] These patients are at risk to be lost to follow-up if there is an intermittent disease course or if there is already the presence of a macular scar.

PEARLS FROM THE EXPERTS ON FREQUENTLY ASKED QUESTIONS

1. Can a patient be managed with anti-VEGF injections alone for inflammatory CNV formation or is dual therapy with immunosuppressive therapies needed to prevent progressive choroidal ischemia?

Answer: In relentless placoid choroidopathy, immunosuppression with mycophenolate mofetil was started at baseline, yet the patient developed a CNVM relatively early in his disease course. The progressive ischemia was aggressive in the first few months after presentation. After systemic side effects developed with the mycophenolate mofetil use, his rheumatologist stopped the medication. Evidence of change in the choriocapillary flow required the restart of immunomodulatory therapy. This made the diagnosis of relentless placoid chorioretinopathy clear. Conversely, patients with PIC have acute infiltrative lesions that show flow on OCTA imaging. After anti-VEGF treatment, the condition can be in remission for many years. The minority of PIC patients require immunomodulatory therapy. It is the sporadic nature of both PIC and MFC that makes the decision to start and to continue immunosuppressive therapy more difficult than in a chronic disorder, such as birdshot chorioretinitis. It is difficult when treating with immunosuppression to know whether the disease is quiescent or if the patient is between episodic flares. If there is an active CNV, combined therapy should be started, at least initially, to reduce inflammation.

2. Optical coherence tomography angiography (OCTA) imaging software may not be available in all clinics to detect the presence of a CNV in PIC. How would you suggest treating PIC when it is diagnosed with clinical findings and minimal imaging?

Answer: If imaging is not available, assessing for a change in vision and if a lesion is active by clinical appearance using handheld lenses at the slit lamp is the alternative option. However, OCT images allow for detection of active lesions, which can be treated with intravitreal corticosteroid injections. If a CNVM is present, an adjunctive anti-VEGF injection can be considered until the subretinal fluid resolves. An alternative to an intravitreal corticosteroid injection would be a taper of high dose oral prednisone for 2–4 weeks. Immunomodulatory therapy should be added if there are recurrent flares or a chronic course. Again, PIC is typically sporadic, so after the initiation of treatment, the patient should be monitored every 4 or 6 weeks to assess for change. With continued quiescence, visits can be spaced out over the duration of follow-up. Always obtain baseline fundus photos and autofluorescence images in cases of PIC to identify new lesions or detect enlarging lesions over time. It is important, if a CNVM is present to give the patient an Amsler grid for home monitoring and remind them to be seen urgently if there is a change.

3. What is the utility of initiating biologic immunosuppressive therapy in patients with a WDS?
Answer: Biologic immunosuppressive agents should be considered as second-line agents after treatment failure or side effect intolerability with an antimetabolite agent. Subcutaneous methotrexate has better bioavailability and can be an alternative to achieve disease control prior to switching to a biologic. Depending on the practice location, insurance prior authorization may be required before the start of a biologic therapy or it may be cost prohibitive, again relegating it to second-line status.

4. How important is ICG to diagnose and to monitor the response to therapy for WDS other than birdshot chorioretinitis?
Answer: Monitoring for activity in PIC does not require an ICG. For the placoid diseases, OCTA has been shown to correlate lesion activity with ICG images. OCTA can show choroidal ischemia, it is non-invasive, it does not require dye injection, and it can be repeated to assess the response to therapy. ICG is helpful if available on an ultra-widefield platform to show the peripheral extent of ischemia. For MEWDS, OCT images show hyporeflective spots with the overlying hyperreflective dots which are diagnostic. The reason ICG is important when assessing disease activity in birdshot chorioretinitis is that it is artificially placed in the WDS category due to the presence of spots. However, those lesions are deep in the choroid and below where the other forms of imaging are focused. OCTA, OCT, autofluorescence, and fluorescein angiography focus mainly at the level of the outer retina. OCTA is sufficient for monitoring choroidal lesions in birdshot chorioretinitis, which must resolve to achieve remission. OCT can identify degenerative changes in the inner and outer retina and hyporeflective lesions. These lesions do not correspond with the spots on color fundus photography or on ICG images. Choroidal thickness can also be monitored using extended depth OCT imaging to assess for clinical disease activity. However, OCT and OCTA alone are insufficient to monitor birdshot chorioretinitis, and again, ICG is the best imaging modality.

5. When monitoring a patient with birdshot chorioretinitis, does clinical quiescence require resolution of choroidal lesions on ICG testing? If the lesions remained, would you increase immunosuppressive therapy?
Answer: Yes, the lesions must disappear along with any retinal vasculitis seen on fluorescein angiography. This is a progressive, degenerative disease that progresses from past damage with accelerated chorioretinal aging. Most patients present in middle age with a hyporeflective, thinned choroid with outer retinal degeneration. Birdshot chorioretinitis is an extremely slow-progressing disease requiring long-term immunosuppression. Monitoring includes serial ICG imaging at each visit and a fluorescein angiogram at least yearly. Additionally, functional biomarkers, including visual field or ERG testing, can also be helpful to correlate structure with function. Bear in mind that ERG testing has a high inter-test variability. If clinical progression includes substantial pigment loss and choroidal thinning, it is difficult to reverse the process. The best prevention of visual decline is a preemptive reduction in choroidal inflammatory lesions.

6. How can you differentiate active lesions in birdshot chorioretinitis on ICG from scarring outside of the disappearance of active lesions?
Answer: An important observation is that the acute lesions regress with immunosuppressive therapy. Over time, lesions can become atrophic and permanent. Atrophic lesions appear wider or larger. Again, the most important aspect of disease management is to identify the lesions early and initiate treatment with corticosteroids as a bridge to non-corticosteroid immunosuppressive therapy. This aggressive treatment approach prevents cystoid macular edema formation, loss of the ellipsoid-zone, and ultimately, a decrease in the best corrected visual acuity and color perception. Those who present with changes at the level of the photoreceptors on OCT or hypoautofluorescent areas on imaging already have outer retinal damage. Hypocyanescent spots on ICG cannot be seen with any other type of imaging. On

histopathology, there are non-granulomatous clusters of T and B-cells with a mixed inflammatory reaction around the large choroidal veins. There is tropism for the location of the inflammation, which clinically represents a filling defect phenomenon on angiographic imaging. Hypocyanescence on ICG corresponds to focal areas of inflammation that resolve with immunosuppressive treatment. Given the chronic course of the disease and the necessity of immunosuppressive therapy, recurrent injections of the dexamethasone corticosteroid intravitreal implants should be avoided. Inflammation recurs between injections leading to progression of the disease.

7. How can you use MMI to differentiate between serpiginous choroiditis and serpiginous-like choroiditis due to tuberculosis?

Answer: Clinically, the presence of cells in the anterior chamber or vitreous should direct the clinician away from the diagnosis of serpiginous choroiditis. Lesions in serpiginous choroiditis are peripapillary with pseudopod-like extensions, as compared to tuberculosis where they are multifocal and extend across the posterior pole into the periphery. Active lesions will have a yellow, peripheral border adjacent to atrophic, pigmented lesions in serpiginous choroiditis. In tuberculosis, the lesions are round with peripheral yellow, active borders. Fluorescein angiography shows vascular leakage only in cases of tuberculosis. Positive tuberculosis testing through interferon gamma release assays, the Mantoux test, and chest radioimaging can help solidify the diagnosis.

8. In the case of APMPPE, was this simply an atypical disease course or did APMPPE lesions progress into relentless placoid choroiditis over time?

Answer: The clinical course on presentation was consistent with APMPPE, but then quickly took an atypical course due to the aggressive neovascularization that developed. Another point of differentiation is the older age at onset. The areas of ischemia several months into treatment reinforced that the diagnosis was more consistent with persistent placoid chorioretinopathy. APMPPE can progress to include multiple lesions in the fundus within the first week, but again, the significant ischemia and a very aggressive course of neovascularization in the subsequent months are not classically seen in cases of APMPPE.

FINAL WRAP-UP

The non-infectious posterior uveitides are a heterogenous group of conditions that should be considered individually when assessing a patient with inflammation in the posterior pole. Imaging modalities can determine the anatomic level of the inflammation and the presence of disease activity based on characteristic findings. Similarly, the disease course and treatment regimens differ between each disease. One commonality is the need for continued follow-up to assess for flares and secondary complications of the inflammation, which are not limited to cystoid macular edema, choroidal ischemia, and ellipsoid zone loss. Early institution of immunosuppressive therapy in chronic conditions, such as birdshot chorioretinitis, and in cases of recurrent flares improves long-term visual outcomes.

REFERENCES

1. Standardization of Uveitis Nomenclature (SUN) Working Group. Development of Classification Criteria for the Uveitides. Am J Ophthalmol. 2021:228:96-105.
2. Standardization of Uveitis Nomenclature (SUN) Working Group. Classification Criteria for Acute Posterior Multifocal Placoid Pigment Epitheliopathy. Am J Ophthalmol. 2021;228:174-81.
3. Standardization of Uveitis Nomenclature (SUN) Working Group. Classification Criteria for Birdshot Chorioretinitis. Am J Ophthalmol. 2021;228:65-71.
4. Standardization of Uveitis Nomenclature (SUN) Working Group. Classification Criteria for Multifocal Choroiditis with Panuveitis. Am J Ophthalmol. 2021;228:152-8.
5. Standardization of Uveitis Nomenclature (SUN) Working Group. Classification Criteria for Punctate Inner Choroiditis. Am J Ophthalmol. 2021;228:275-80.
6. Standardization of Uveitis Nomenclature (SUN) Working Group. Classification Criteria for Multiple Evanescent White Dot Syndrome. Am J Ophthalmol. 2021;228:198-204.
7. Standardization of Uveitis Nomenclature (SUN) Working Group. Classification Criteria for Serpiginous Choroiditis. Am J Ophthalmol. 2021;228:126-33.
8. Mudie LI, Reddy AK, Patnaik JL, Pecen P, Kim E, Cole K, et al. Evaluation of the SUN classification criteria for uveitides in an academic uveitis practice. Am J Ophthalmol. 2022;241:57-63.
9. Park HS, Kim M, Lee J, Choi EY, Lee J, Byeon SH, et al. Exploring the challenges of distinguishing punctate inner choroidopathy from multifocal choroiditis and panuveitis. Retina. 2024;44(7):1234-42.
10. Accorinti M, Berkenstock MK, Cicinelli MV, Davis JL, DE-LA-Torre A, Fabiani C, et al. Systematic Review of Clinical Utility of Multimodal Imaging in Noninfectious Posterior Uveitis: MUV Project Report 3. Am J Ophthalmol. 2025;279:56-77.
11. Invernizzi A, Agarwal A, Gangaputra S, Airaldi M, Carreno E, Munk MR, et al. Minimum Imaging Sets for Diagnosis,

Activity Assessment, and Complications in Noninfectious Posterior Uveitis - Multimodal Imaging in Uveitis (MUV) Task Force Report 9. Am J Ophthalmol. 2025;280:106-19.
12. Shelsta HN, Rao RR, Bhatt HK, Jampol LM. Atypical presentations of multiple evanescent white dot syndrome without white dots: a case series. Retina. 2011;31(5):973-6.
13. Cicinelli MV, Ramtohul P, Marchese A, Bandello F, Bailey Freund K, Miserocchi E, et al. Latest advances in white spot syndromes: New findings and interpretations. Prog Retin Eye Res. 2023;97:101207.
14. Klufas MA, Phasukkijwatana N, Iafe NA, Prasad PS, Agarwal A, Gupta V, et al. Optical coherence tomography angiography reveals choriocapillaris flow reduction in placoid chorioretinitis. Ophthalmol Retina. 2017;1(1):77-91.
15. Ramtohul P, Cabral D, Sadda S, Freund KB, Sarraf D. The OCT angular sign of Henle fiber layer (HFL) hyperreflectivity and the pathoanatomy of the HFL in macular disease. Prog Retin Eye Res. 2023;95:101135.
16. Feo A, Ramtohul P, Govetto A, Borrelli E, Sacconi R, Corradetti G, et al. En face OCT: Breakthroughs in understanding the pathoanatomy of retinal disease and clinical applications. Prog Retin Eye Res. 2025;106:101135.
17. Cheng JY, Santina A, Margines JB, Ochanski S, Ramtotohul P, Bousquet E, et al. Acute posterior multifocal placoid pigment epitheliopathy and placoid variant disease masquerading as age-related macular degeneration in the elderly. Retina. 2024. 44:1666-78.
18. Cheng JY, Freund KB, Sarraf D, et al. Acute posterior multifocal placoid pigment epitheliopathy and placoid variant diseases masquerading as age-related macular degeneration in the elderly: a case series. Retina. 2024;44(2):345-53.
19. Klufas MA, Phasukkijwatana N, Iafe NA, Prasad PS, Agarwal A, Gupta V, et al. Optical coherence tomography angiography reveals choriocapillaris flow reduction in placoid chorioretinitis. Ophthalmology Retina. 2017;1(1): 77-91.
20. Gilbert RM, Niederer RL, Kramer M, Sharief L, Sharon Y, Bar A, et al. Differentiating Multifocal Choroiditis and Punctate Inner Choroidopathy: A Cluster Analysis Approach. Am J Ophthalmol. 2020;213:244-51.
21. Gerstenblith AT, Thorne JE, Sobrin L, Do DV, Shah SM, Foster CS, et al. Punctate inner choroidopathy: a survey analysis of 77 persons. Ophthalmology. 2007;114(6):1201-4.
22. Brown J, Folk JC, Reddy CV, Kimura AE. Visual prognosis of multifocal choroiditis, punctate inner choroidopathy, and the diffuse subretinal fibrosis syndrome. Ophthalmology. 1996;103(7):1100-5.
23. Vienne-Jumeau A, Brézin Antoine P, Marie S, Florence R-S, Bousquet E. Corticosteroids Decrease the Incidence and Activity of Choroidal Neovascularization in Patients with Punctate Inner Choroidopathy or Multifocal Choroiditis. Ocular Immunol Inflam. 2024;32(5):602-8.
24. Daniel E, Thorne JE, Newcomb CW, Pujari SS, Kaçmaz RO, Levy-Clarke GA, et al. Mycophenolate Mofetil for Ocular Inflammation. Am J Ophthalmol. 2010;149(3):423-32.e1.
25. Kalogeropoulos D, Rahman N, Afshar F, Hall N, Lotery AJ. Punctate inner choroidopathy: A review of the current diagnostic and therapeutic approaches. Prog Retin Eye Res. 2024;99:101235.
26. Watzke RC, Packer AJ, Folk JC, Benson WE, Burgess D, Ober RR. Punctate inner choroidopathy. Am J Ophthalmol. 1984;98(5):572-84.

NOTE FROM EDITORS

This talk by Dr Janet Davis was given while MUV reports were being prepared. For the information of all our readers, the all the MUV reports are now published and can be assessed as follows:

1. Fabiani, C., Shantha, J., Gangaputra, S., Vitale, A., Thorne, J. E., Jabs, D. A., ... Gupta, V. (2025). Is it Time to Adopt a New Nomenclature and Classification for White Dot Syndromes Using Multimodal Imaging Techniques? Report 1 from Multimodal Imaging in Uveitis (MUV) Task Force. *Ocular Immunology and Inflammation*, *33*(4), 561–569. https://doi.org/10.1080/09273948.2024.2423870
2. Gupta V, Davis JL, Gangaputra S, Chee SP, Thorne JE, Agrawal R, Invernizzi A, Agarwal A, de Smet MD, Sarraf D, Jabs DA; Multimodal Imaging in Uveitis (MUV) Taskforce. Evidence and Consensus-Based Imaging Guidelines in Noninfectious Posterior Uveitis-Methodology of the Multimodal Imaging in Uveitis (MUV) Project Report 2. Am J Ophthalmol. 2025 Oct;278:257-265. doi: 10.1016/j.ajo.2025.06.033. Epub 2025 Jun 21. PMID: 40550447.
3. Accorinti M, Berkenstock MK, Cicinelli MV, Davis JL, DE-LA-Torre A, Fabiani C, Gangaputra S, Gupta V, Janetos TM, Leal I, Reynolds JM, Schlaen A. Systematic Review of Clinical Utility of Multimodal Imaging in Noninfectious Posterior Uveitis: MUV Project Report 3. Am J Ophthalmol. 2025 Nov;279:56-77. doi: 10.1016/j.ajo.2025.07.002. Epub 2025 Jul 12. PMID: 40659111.
4. Agarwal A, Agarwal A, Goldstein DA, Invernizzi A, Janetos TM, Cimino L, Nguyen QD, Jabs DA, Agrawal R, Fawzi A, Sarraf D, Gupta V; Multimodal Imaging in Uveitis (MUV) Taskforce. Evidence and Consensus-Based Imaging Guidelines in Serpiginous Choroiditis-Multimodal Imaging in Uveitis (MUV) Task Force Report 4. Am J Ophthalmol. 2025 Oct;278:81-92. doi: 10.1016/j.ajo.2025.05.052. Epub 2025 Jun 4. PMID: 40480346.
5. Gangaputra S, Agarwal A, Norel JO, Tsui E, Thorne JE, de-la-Torre A, Altaweel M, Biswas J, Sadda S, Invernizzi A, Agrawal R, Shantha JG, Accorinti M, Fawzi A, Jabs DA, Sarraf D, Gupta V; Multimodal Imaging in Uveitis (MUV) Task force. Evidence and Consensus-Based Imaging Guidelines in Multifocal Choroiditis With Panuveitis and Punctate

Inner Choroiditis-Multimodal Imaging in Uveitis (MUV) Taskforce Report 5. Am J Ophthalmol. 2025 Aug;276:272-285. doi: 10.1016/j.ajo.2025.04.018. Epub 2025 Apr 25. Erratum in: Am J Ophthalmol. 2025 Nov;279:588-590. doi: 10.1016/j.ajo.2025.08.027. PMID: 40288596.

6. Munk MR, Stillenmunkes R, Tillmann A, Jampol LM, Cicinelli MV, Lin P, Pepple KL, Freund KB, Tugal-Tutkun I, Habot-Wilner Z, Agarwal A, Gangaputra S, Agrawal R, Jabs DA, Sadda S, Sarraf D, Gupta V; Multimodal Imaging in Uveitis (MUV) Taskforce. Evidence and Consensus Based Imaging Guidelines in Multiple Evanescent White Dot Syndrome Multimodal imaging in Uveitis (MUV) Taskforce Report 6. Am J Ophthalmol. 2025 Oct;278:191-202. doi: 10.1016/j.ajo.2025.06.039. Epub 2025 Jun 24. PMID: 40571046.
7. Carreño E, Maghsoudlou P, Fonollosa A, Leal I, Schlaen A, Abraham AR, Dick AD, Agarwal A, Gangaputra S, Invernizzi A, Fawzi A, Miserocchi E, Agrawal R, Jabs DA, Sarraf D, Gupta V; Multimodal Imaging in Uveitis (MUV) Taskforce. Evidence and Consensus-Based Imaging Guidelines in Acute Posterior Multifocal Placoid Pigment Epitheliopathy (APMPPE) - Multimodal imaging in Uveitis (MUV) Taskforce Report 7. Am J Ophthalmol. 2025 Oct;278:38-51. doi: 10.1016/j.ajo.2025.06.007. Epub 2025 Jun 6. PMID: 40484301.
8. Pichi F, Miserocchi E, Grewal DS, Sharma S, Brézin AP, Bodaghi B, Agarwal A, Jabs DA, Fawzi A, Sarraf D, Gupta V; MULTIMODAL IMAGING IN UVEITIS (MUV) TASKFORCE. Evidence and Consensus-based Imaging Guidelines in Birdshot Chorioretinopathy: Multimodal Imaging in Uveitis (MUV) Taskforce Report 8. Am J Ophthalmol. 2025 Oct;278:271-281. doi: 10.1016/j.ajo.2025.06.029. Epub 2025 Jun 20. PMID: 40545009.
9. Invernizzi A, Agarwal A, Gangaputra S, Airaldi M, Carreno E, Munk MR, Pichi F, Shantha J, Agrawal R, Sadda S, Jampol LM, Smith JR, Jabs DA, Chee SP, Sarraf D, Gupta V; Multimodal Imaging in Uveitis (MUV) Task Force. Minimum Imaging Sets for Diagnosis, Activity Assessment, and Complications in Noninfectious Posterior Uveitis - Multimodal Imaging in Uveitis (MUV) Task Force Report 9. Am J Ophthalmol. 2025 Dec;280:106-119. doi: 10.1016/j.ajo.2025.07.029. Epub 2025 Aug 5. PMID: 40754260.
10. Agarwal A, Ramtohul P, Invernizzi A, Gangaputra S, Tsui E, Okada AA, Thorne JE, Smet MD, Bodaghi B, Pavesio C, Jabs DA, Sadda S, Sarraf D, Gupta V; MULTIMODAL IMAGING IN UVEITIS (MUV) TASKFORCE. Imaging Measures for the Assessment of Disease Activity in Noninfectious Posterior Uveitis - Multimodal Imaging in Uveitis (MUV) Taskforce: Report 10. Am J Ophthalmol. 2026 Mar 18;287:43-57. doi: 10.1016/j.ajo.2026.03.011. Epub ahead of print. PMID: 41861898.

CHAPTER 16

Systemic Therapy for Non-infectious Uveitis

Miguel Cordero-Coma, Israel Mendez, Jennifer Thorne, Emebet Getahun Tabor, John H Kempen, Jia-Horung Hung, Quan Dong Nguyen, Maggie Feng, Vishali Gupta, Marc de Smet, Reema Bansal, Alejandra de-la-Torre, Meghan Berkenstock

INTRODUCTION

Systemic therapy for non-infectious uveitis prevents ocular damage and vision loss, particularly in chronic or bilateral cases. Immunomodulatory agents, including corticosteroids, antimetabolites, calcineurin inhibitors, and biologics, have transformed the management of ocular inflammation by targeting underlying immune dysregulation. Early and individualized systemic treatment controls intraocular inflammation and reduces the cumulative burden of corticosteroid-related side effects. Understanding the immunopathogenesis of non-infectious uveitis allows clinicians to tailor therapy according to disease severity, anatomic location, and associated systemic conditions with improved long-term visual outcomes and quality of life.

THEMATIC LECTURE: PRACTICAL TIPS FOR SYSTEMIC THERAPY IN NON-INFECTIOUS UVEITIS

The management of non-infectious uveitis remains challenging for several reasons. First, it is a heterogeneous condition with many different clinical pictures under the same umbrella term.[1] Secondly, there is a lack of universally accepted therapeutic guidelines, as well as standardized criteria for treatment response and monitoring. Finally, therapeutic options remain limited, and many immunosuppressive agents are currently used off-label.

When comparing anterior with posterior pole-involving, non-infectious uveitis, patients with anterior uveitis have a limited disease course with a lower incidence of ocular complications.[2] The prognosis for inflammation restricted to the anterior chamber is better, and topical treatment is effective. This is why patients with anterior uveitis are treated initially with topical corticosteroids, and systemic therapy is reserved for select cases. On the other hand, non-anterior uveitis patients have a prolonged disease course with a higher incidence of ocular complications, a worse overall prognosis, and limited efficacy of topical treatments.[3-5] Systemic immunosuppressive therapy is the preferred initial treatment, leaving intraocular corticosteroid injections reserved for selected cases or to treat complications, such as macular edema **(Fig. 1)**.

The classic management of non-infectious uveitis is summarized in the stepladder algorithm shown in **Flowchart 1**. Corticosteroids are the initial common therapy for all patients. For those patients with severe, vision-threatening disease, immunosuppressive medications or even alkylating agents are used. Coadjuvant therapy with intravitreal or periocular corticosteroid injections or surgery is used by the clinician at their discretion.

As previously mentioned, corticosteroids were the mainstay of treatment, given the immediate anti-inflammatory effect.[6-9] However, the side effect profile is long, and as a class, corticosteroids display a tachyphylaxis phenomenon with increasing doses needed to maintain the same clinical effect with continued use.[6,7,10]

Analyzing causes of long-term vision loss from uveitis shows that macular damage remains the main risk factor.[2] The most important question to prevent complications is when should immunosuppression be started? The goal should be preservation of visual function starting in the early stages of the disease when inflammation is reversible.[11] Treatment delays result in irreversible structural damage, including atrophy of the external layers of the retina and fibrosis.

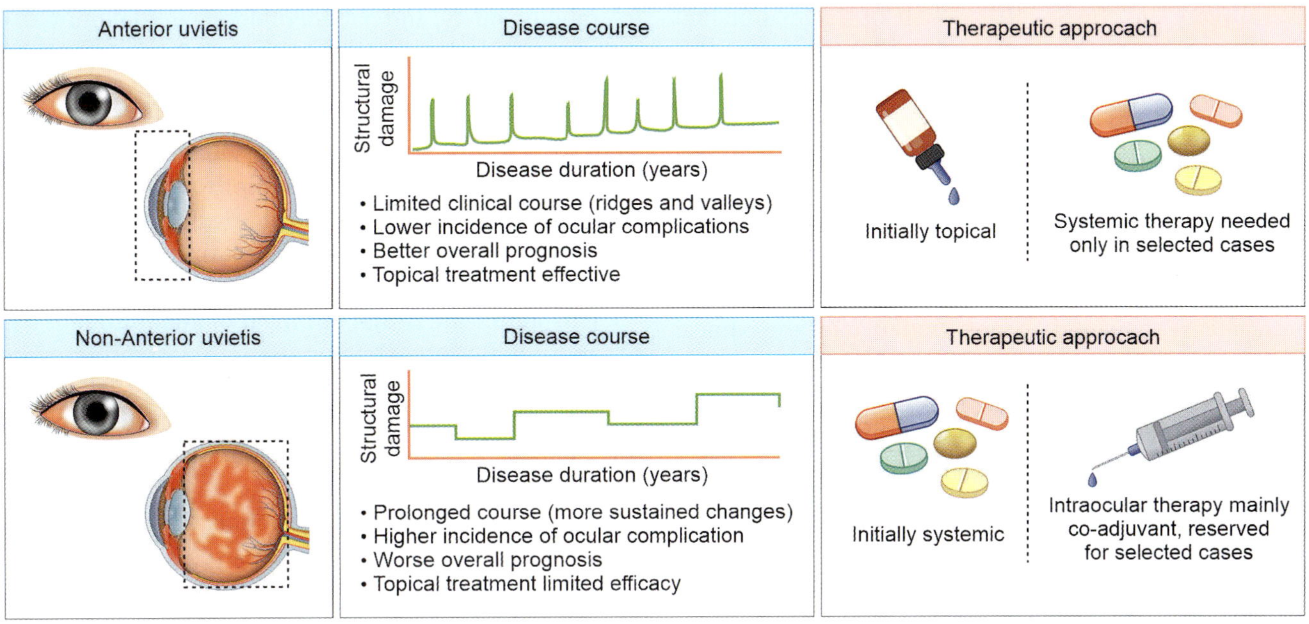

Fig. 1: A schematic diagram contrasting the locations of inflammation, disease course, and treatments for anterior versus non-anterior, non-infectious uveitis.

Source: Uveitis Course - Grand Rounds 16. International Uveitis Study Group (IUSG). June 14, 2025. Available at: https://youtu.be/2UVTU7oztTc?si=y7tNEsxDMokFr6uw.

Flowchart 1: A stepladder algorithm for management of non-infectious uveitis based on severity.

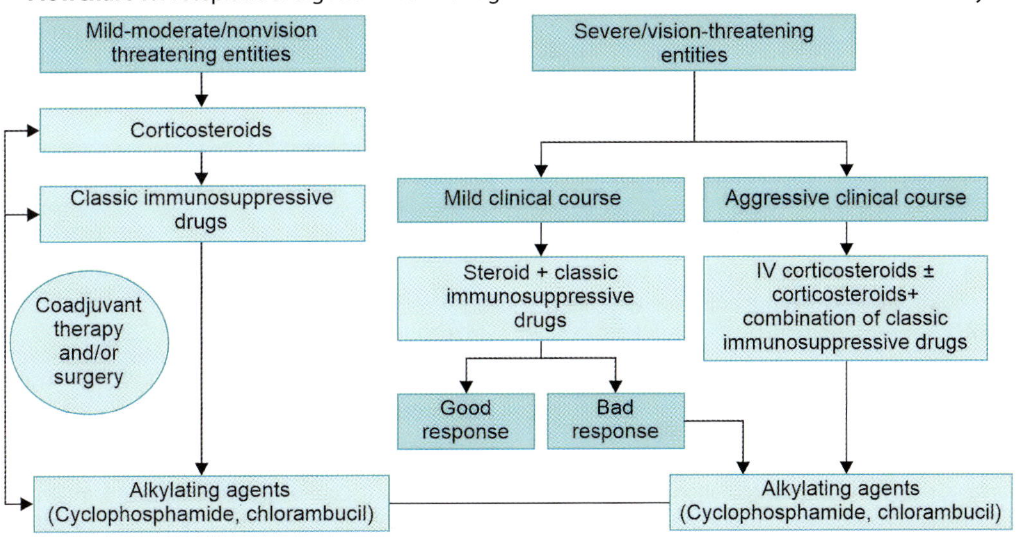

Source: Uveitis Course - Grand Rounds 16. International Uveitis Study Group (IUSG). June 14, 2025. Available at: https://youtu.be/2UVTU7oztTc?si=y7tNEsxDMokFr6uw.

The Fundamentals of Care for Uveitis (FOCUS) initiative published guideline indications for initiating systemic immunosuppressive therapy as summarized by four indications: ocular and anatomic, therapeutic, severity in adults, and severity in children.[12] The latter was specifically included regarding the treatment of juvenile idiopathic arthritis (JIA)-associated uveitis. These guidelines can help to decide when to start systemic immunosuppressive therapy, which can be challenging **(Box 1)**.

Many factors influence the choice of an immunosuppressive medication in patients with non-infectious uveitis.[13-15] Some of these factors are related to patient characteristics, such as the uveitis severity and location. Non-patient-related factors include failure or side effects from prior immunosuppressive drugs and cost.

Several years ago, the Spanish Society of Uveitis initiated a project to develop treatment recommendations for systemic immunosuppressive therapy for patients with both anterior and non-anterior uveitis. This was also supported by the Spanish Societies of Rheumatology, Immunology, and Internal Medicine. The project included a systematic review, meeting of expert panels, two Delphi rounds, and a final external evaluation.[16-18] The generated clinical statements provide evidence, a recommendation grade, a level of agreement, and guidance for the clinical care of patients with a complex disease history.

Regarding conventional immunomodulators and immunosuppressants, most are used off-label and have a more limited efficacy when compared to corticosteroids.[19-21] Furthermore, each has a specific side effect profile that can lead to discontinuation, as seen in **Table 1**. Efficacy is even lower when results are analyzed to include concurrent use of low doses of corticosteroids.[22-25]

Biologic agents filled the need for more effective, non-corticosteroid immunosuppression, first with anti-tumor necrosis factor (TNF) alpha inhibitors.[26-30] When comparing the discontinuation rates based on tolerability, safety, and patient preference, adalimumab or infliximab were stopped less frequently than conventional immunosuppressive medications **(Table 2)**.[31]

Beyond efficacy and tolerability, the third reason for worldwide use of biologic agents is quality of life. **Table 3** shows aspects of quality of life improved with the use of infliximab over traditional immunosuppressive agents, even in more severe cases of inflammation, such as Behçet's disease-associated uveitis.[32]

This led to the initial approval of adalimumab, then other biologic agents for patients with refractory or severe vision-threatening inflammation early in the disease course. Biologics replaced alkylating agents in these clinical scenarios, with the latter used only in select circumstances **(Flowchart 2)**.

Using the algorithm in **Flowchart 2**, deciding which patients should have treatment escalated to the use of biologic therapies and when to make the change becomes clearer. Factors to consider are the presence of inflammation refractory to conventional therapy, poor visual acuity, or bilateral disease in a working-age group. Additionally, other considerations requiring biologic agent use include systemic diseases associated with aggressive ocular inflammation, such as Behçet's disease, or in situations where conventional immunosuppressants or corticosteroids are contraindicated, such as in pregnancy and diabetes **(Table 4)**.

BOX 1: A summary of the four indications for starting systemic immunosuppressive therapy based on the FOCUS initiative.

Indications for initiating systemic therapy:
- *Ocular and anatomic* Acute sight-threatening, chronic persistent, macular involvement, binocular sight-threatening.
- *Therapeutic* Regional failure to respond to periocular/topical steroids, systemic failure to steroids, steroid intolerance, need for steroid-sparing effect.
- *Severity (adults)* VA worse than 20/100, Increase of vitreous haze >2, relapse of CME, disease that impacts quality of life
- *Severity (child's/JIA)* VA at presentation, posterior uveitis. glaucoma, advanced cataract, CME, synechiae, band keratopathy, hypotony, rubeosis iridis

(CME: cystoid macular edema; JIA: juvenile idiopathic arthritis; VA; visual acuity)

Source: Uveitis Course - Grand Rounds 16. International Uveitis Study Group (IUSG). June 14, 2025. Available at: https://youtu.be/2UVTU7oztTc?si=y7tNEsxDMokFr6uw.

TABLE 1: A summary of the efficacy over time of non-corticosteroid, systemic immunosuppressive therapies alone, and with concurrent use of low-dose prednisone.

Drug	*Success at 1 year*	*≤10 mg prednisone*	*Discontinued within 1 year*
Mycophenolate	73%	55%	12%
Cyclosporine	52%	36%	11%
Methotrexate	66%	58%	16%
Azathioprine	62%	47%	24%

Source: Uveitis Course - Grand Rounds 16. International Uveitis Study Group (IUSG). June 14, 2025. Available at: https://youtu.be/2UVTU7oztTc?si=y7tNEsxDMokFr6uw.

TABLE 2: A comparison of the reasons for medication discontinuation based on efficacy, tolerability, safety, and patient preference between methotrexate (MTX), mycophenolate mofetil (MMF), azathioprine (AZA), adalimumab (ADA), and infliximab (IFX).

IMT	*MTX*	*MMF*	*AZA*	*ADA*	*IFX*	*P-value*
Medication discontinued for any reason	159 (51.3%)	48 (53.3%)	29 (44.6%)	97 (43.1%)	24 (34.3%)	0.005
Discontinued for reasons other than efficacy (tolerability, safety, and patient preference)	131 (42.3%)	44 (48.9%)	24 (48.9%)	50 (22%)	13 (18.6%)	>0.0001

Source: Uveitis Course - Grand Rounds 16. International Uveitis Study Group (IUSG). June 14, 2025. Available at: https://youtu.be/2UVTU7oztTc?si=y7tNEsxDMokFr6uw.

TABLE 3: The National Eye Institute (NEI) 25 Visual Function Questionnaire showing areas of significant quality of life improvements in patients with Behçet's disease using infliximab biologic therapy.

NEI 25-item visual function questionnaire composite and subscale score in patients with Behçet's disease before and after receiving infliximab therapy	***p-value before versus after infliximab (IFX)***
General health	<0.0001
General vision	0.0001
Ocular pain	0.0002
Near activities	0.0001
Distance activities	0.0001
Social functioning	0.0001
Mental health	0.0001
Role difficulties	0.0001
Dependency	0.0001
Driving	0.0059
Color vision	0.0209
Peripheral vision	0.0004
Composite score	0.0001

Source: Uveitis Course - Grand Rounds 16. International Uveitis Study Group (IUSG). June 14, 2025. Available at: https://youtu.be/2UVTU7oztTc?si=y7tNEsxDMokFr6uw.

TABLE 4: A summary table of the factors for and against the use of biologics as the treatment choice for patients with non-infectious uveitis.

Treatment of Nina with biologic therapy	
Favors	***Against***
• Refractory to conventional therapy	• Good response
• Poor visual acuity (affected/ fellow eye)	• Good visual acuity (OU)
• Bilateral	• Unilateral
• Young working-age patients	• Old/retired/sedentary patients
• Theoretically aggressive associated diseases (i.e., Behçet's)	• Theoretically mild (less aggressive) associated disease
• Aggressive clinical courses	• Mild/moderate clinical courses
• Associated conditions that contra-indicate or complicate the use of corticosteroids or conventional immunomodulatory therapy (IMT) (e.g., diabetes and obesity)	• Absence of these conditions

Source: Uveitis Course - Grand Rounds 16. International Uveitis Study Group (IUSG). June 14, 2025. Available at: https://youtu.be/2UVTU7oztTc?si=y7tNEsxDMokFr6uw.

Flowchart 2: Current management of mild or severe, non-infectious uveitis in the era of biologic agent availability.

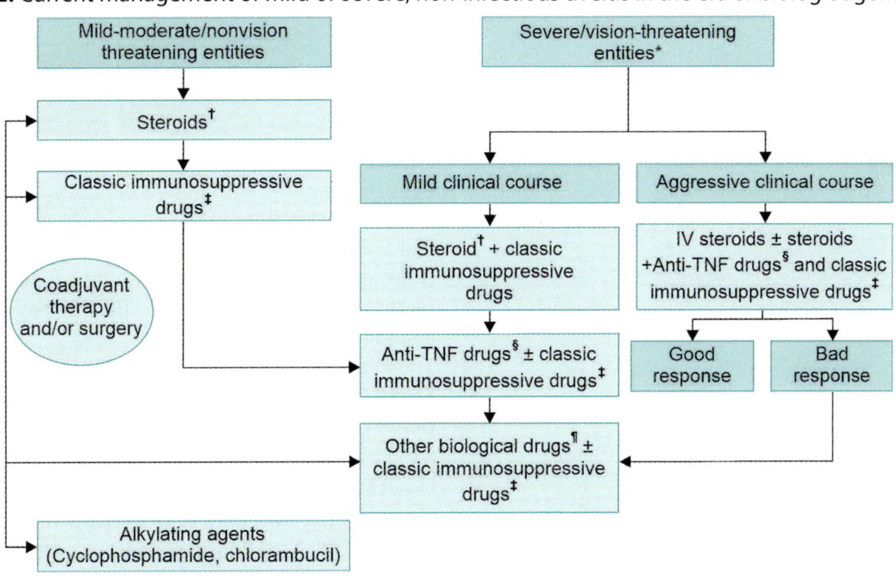

*Behceet disease, Juvenile Idiopathic Arthritis, Sympathetic Ophthalmia, Peripheral Ulcerative Keratitis, Scleritis, and Severe Choroidopathies (e.g. Serpiginous choroiditis)

†Topical, local, or regional and/or systemic

‡Methotrexate, azathioprine, mycophenolate mofetil, cyclosporine

§First-line anti-TNF drugs are infliximab and adalimumab

¶Other anti-TNF (golimumab, certolizumab), interferon, tocilizumab, rituximab

Source: Uveitis Course - Grand Rounds 16. International Uveitis Study Group (IUSG). June 14, 2025. Available at: https://youtu.be/2UVTU7oztTc?si=y7tNEsxDMokFr6uw.

TABLE 5: Summary tables showing the available biologic agents with evidence and recommendation level reported by the FOCUS initiative.

Originator biologic	***Evidence level***	***Recommendation level***
Antitumor necrosis factor (anti-TNF)		
Infliximab	2B AU, 3B IU, 3B-4 PU, and 5 PanU	B-C
Adalimumab	1B AU, 2B IU, 4 PU, and 5 PanU	A
Golimumab	4	C
Etanercept	2B	B
Certolizumab	-	D
Anti-interleukin 1		
Anakinra/canakinumab	4	C
Gevokizumab	2B	C
Anti-interleukin 2		
Daclizumab	2B-4	B
Anti-interleukin 6		
Tocilizumab	4	C
Sarilumab	-	D
Anti-interleukin 17		
Secukinumab	1B IU, 2B PU, and PanU	B
Anti-CD20		
Rituximab	2B	C
Anti-CD52		
Alemtuzumab	2B	C
Interferons		
Interferons alfa-2a and 2b	2B AU, 3B IU, 4 PU and PanU, 5 RV	B
Pegylated interferon alfa-2b	2B	C
Interferon beta	2B	C
Others		
IV immunoglobulins	2B	C

IU: intermediate uveitis, PU: posterior uveitis, PanU: panuveitis.
Source: Uveitis Course - Grand Rounds 16. International Uveitis Study Group (IUSG). June 14, 2025. Available at: https://youtu.be/2UVTU7oztTc?si=y7tNEsxDMokFr6uw.

The FOCUS initiative published tables listing the available biologic agents with their evidence and recommendation levels.[12] The only immunosuppressant with an A recommendation level was adalimumab due to the on-label approval and randomized controlled trial (RCT) data. However, there is an increased use of all of the biologics listed worldwide in **Table 5**.

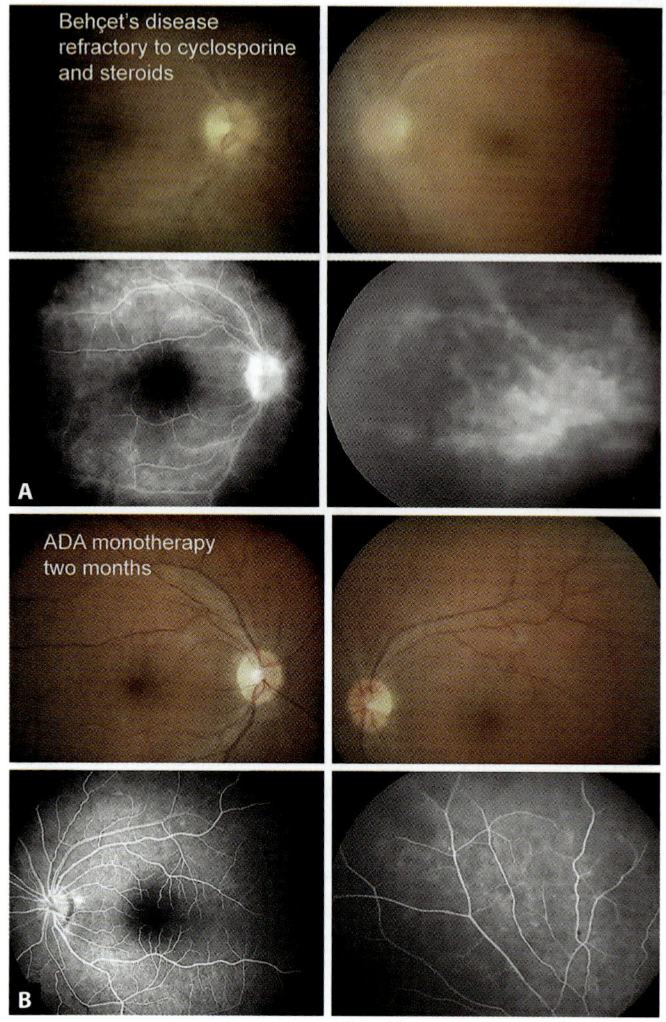

Figs. 2A and B: Color fundus photos (top, A) showing haze in both eyes in a patient with active Behçet's disease-associated uveitis. Fluorescein angiography of the right eye shows diffuse fern-like leakage (bottom, A). Two months after the start of adalimumab, there is less vitreous haze on color fundus photos (top, B) and minimal leakage on repeated fluorescein angiography in the left eye (bottom, B).
Source: Uveitis Course - Grand Rounds 16. International Uveitis Study Group (IUSG). June 14, 2025. Available at: https://youtu.be/2UVTU7oztTc?si=y7tNEsxDMokFr6uw.

Excluding issues unrelated to medical practice, such as higher costs, bureaucracy to obtain insurance approvals, and legal issues, here are some tips on how to proceed with immunosuppressive therapy in certain clinical scenarios. In a patient with panuveitis associated with Behçet's disease that is refractory to cyclosporine and corticosteroids, a TNF medication would be the next step in treatment if there were clinically active vitritis and retinal vasculitis. **Figures 2A and B** show the imaging results in a patient with this clinical picture after 2 months

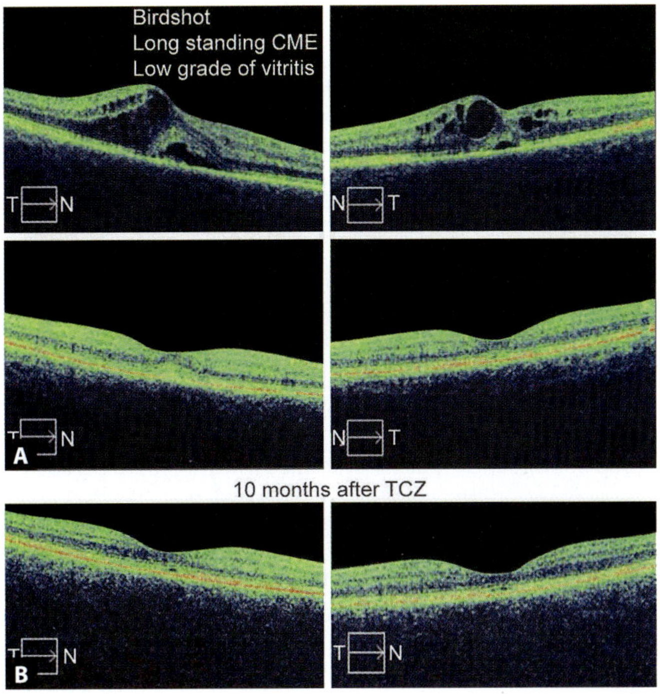

Figs. 3A and B: An OCT of the macula in a patient with Birdshot chorioretinitis showing the presence of cystoid macular edema (top) and gradual improvement and resolution of the edema after 10 months of tocilizumab monotherapy (bottom).
Source: Uveitis Course - Grand Rounds 16. International Uveitis Study Group (IUSG). June 14, 2025. Available at: https://youtu.be/2UVTU7oztTc?si=y7tNEsxDMokFr6uw.

of adalimumab therapy, showing a complete resolution of the clinical inflammation.

In the example of a patient with Birdshot chorioretinitis with long-standing cystoid macular edema and low-grade vitritis, the use of an interleukin 6 (IL-6) blocking biologic agent could be a better choice **(Figs. 3A and B)**. Long-standing edema evolves into atrophy, especially affecting the inner retina.

Another medically complex condition is Susac syndrome. In these cases, there needs to be an individualized therapeutic approach that is tailored to the patient. Treatment plans may require the use of all therapeutic modalities from traditional immunosuppressants to biologics to alkylating agents to control the underlying inflammation.

Once the decision to treat with an immunosuppressive agent has been made and the medication has been selected, the time needed to evaluate for efficacy is variable. The time until the full effect of the medication is obtained depends on the activity of an associated systemic disease, the location and severity of the uveitis, and the class of immunosuppressive medication. If 3–6 months have elapsed and inflammation is still present, questioning if the patient is administering the drug correctly at the appropriate dose and time is appropriate.[33,34] Time intervals will vary between agents, with a shorter time of action for biologics compared with classic immunosuppressive medications. There are paradoxical situations that occur with the use of immunosuppressive agents, such as having the quiet, better-seeing eye develop inflammation. In this case, a therapeutic response should be defined as quiescence in the better-seeing eye for preservation of visual function.

Assessing clinical efficacy requires assessment of the visual acuity in both eyes and a thorough clinical examination, scoring inflammation based on the Standardization in Uveitis Nomenclature (SUN) grading scales.[4] Additional imaging studies using a multimodal approach are needed. OCT scans can assess the central macular thickness, whereas a fluorescein angiogram can show details of the retinal vasculature.[35] Additional testing with autofluorescence, visual fields, and electroretinography should be performed at the discretion of the clinician. Posterior pole involving non-infectious uveitis requires a multimodal imaging approach to provide a comprehensive, in-depth evaluation for both monitoring and treatment decisions.

The concept of response to treatment remains ill-defined: complete, partial, or none. Current disease activity scales do take into account imaging test results, which are crucial for determining the response to treatment. Concepts including activity, worsening, and therapeutic failure would be beneficial as they give a more complete and comprehensive evaluation of the treatment of response and monitoring. In short, there is an unmet need regarding the development of a disease activity score in uveitis patients that incorporates data from many imaging and serologic tests to provide a complete assessment of clinical activity and the therapeutic response **(Fig. 4)**.[16,36-41]

Regarding monitoring safety, uveitis specialists can initiate the treatment independently or in a multidisciplinary approach. This includes checking for the presence of underlying infectious diseases before the initiation of immunosuppression, assessment of clinical inflammation prior to and after the start of treatment, and reminding the patient to follow dosing instructions and avoid live vaccines. This approach is important because it gives the opportunity to share the burden of management

Complete response	Partial response or improvement	No response
Grade 0 cells in both anterior and posterior segment in addition to absence of any other sign of intraocular inflammation on ophthalmologic, OCT, and FA examination	New onset from either baseline visit or when compared with previous clinical examination of any of the following: • A 2-step decrease in the SUN grading scheme (e.g., anterior chamber cells, vitreous haze) or decrease to grade 0 • Resolution of cystoid macular edema (1-mm central retinal thickness <300 mm and absence of intraretinal or subretinal fluid in OCT examination) • Absence of any retinal angiographic leakage in FA examination	Persistent intraocular inflammation without any finding consistent with the criteria of partial response or improvement

Fig. 4: A schematic showing proposed definitions for complete, partial, and no response to treatment in patients with non-infectious uveitis.
Source: Uveitis Course - Grand Rounds 16. International Uveitis Study Group (IUSG). June 14, 2025. Available at: https://youtu.be/2UVTU7oztTc?si=y7tNEsxDMokFr6uw.

with the patient and other medical specialists as prompt initiation of therapy leads to improved visual outcomes.

Therapeutic decision-making will be challenging. During the course of treatment, measurement of drug levels or antibody formation can be helpful in situations where there is a partial or no response.[36,42] Most of the research on this topic revolves around adalimumab, but this approach can be applied to many other biologic and non-biologic treatments. This clarifies the clinical situation by assessing for antibody formation, low drug levels, or if the patient is refractory to the mechanism of action of the drug when the response is less than expected. In the setting of low drug levels, making sure the drug is being taken correctly is also important. Monitoring of serum drug levels also gives the opportunity to establish a therapeutic range and aid in decision-making to optimize or discontinue an immunosuppressant. The goal is to plan ahead for unexpected events, such as altering dosing or switching agents to avoid a flare.[9,43]

How long to keep patients on immunosuppressive therapies is another difficult question. There has been work on drug retention rates on adalimumab, with >50% of patients at 60 months still taking the medication with concurrent immunomodulatory therapy.[44,45] Factors predictive of discontinuation included using adalimumab as a second or third-line agent due to efficacy and the development of adverse events.

In summary, there is solid evidence supporting the use of systemic immunosuppression in patients with non-infectious uveitis. Second, the goal is to preserve visual function through the early institution of immunosuppressive agents. The decision-making should be structured, standardized, and based on the available evidence. While this is not always possible, recommendations should be followed and treatment decisions should be supported with drug levels. Finally, treatment algorithms that incorporate drug levels and imaging results in the definition of response to therapy are needed.

CLASSIC, NON-INFECTIOUS ANTERIOR UVEITIS MANAGED WITH CORTICOSTEROIDS

Red Eye, Deeper Roots

Personal Data

A 14-year-old female presented from the emergency department with a 1-week history of right eye pain, redness, and light sensitivity.

History of Present Illness

The symptoms progressively worsened with the development of blurry vision in the right eye. She reported this was the first occurrence and she had no past medical, surgical, or trauma history. She was not taking any medications, and the review systems were completely unremarkable.

Physical Exam

On initial evaluation, the vision at near was J10 with pinhole improvement to J3 in the right eye and J1+ in the left eye. Her right eye was injected with the formation of a hypopyon **(Fig. 5)**.

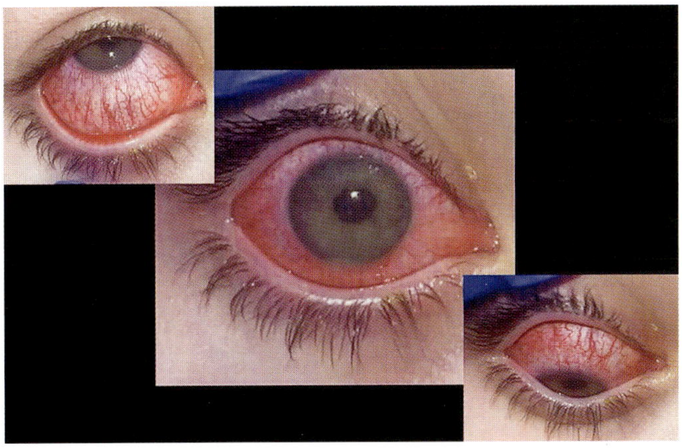

Fig. 5: An external color photograph of the right eye showing an inferior hypopyon and conjunctival injection.
Source: Uveitis Course - Grand Rounds 16. International Uveitis Study Group (IUSG). June 14, 2025. Available at: https://youtu.be/2UVTU7oztTc?si=y7tNEsxDMokFr6uw.

Slit Lamp Examination (Table 6)

Table 6 summarizes the initial examination findings.

Ancillary Testing

To assess for occult chorioretinal involvement or retinal vasculitis, a wide-field fluorescein angiogram was performed, which was normal in both eyes.

Uveitis Workup

The serologic workup had a negative syphilis IgG, RPR, QuantiFERON gold, and Lyme antibodies. A chest X-ray was also performed, which was normal. However, the patient was positive for the human leukocyte antigen B27 (HLA-B27) antigen.

Initial Treatment

At the top of the differential diagnosis for this patient was HLA-B27-associated anterior uveitis, Behçet's disease-associated anterior uveitis, or sarcoid-associated anterior uveitis. Endophthalmitis was less likely given the lack of precipitating risk factors and a normal posterior pole examination. The patient was started on one drop of prednisolone acetate 1% every hour while awake in the right eye with cyclopentolate 0.5% twice a day. Once the labs were negative for an underlying infectious process, the patient started oral prednisone 40 mg daily with a decrease every 3 days to suppress the inflammation faster: 30, 25, 20, 15, 12.5, 10, 7.5, 5, and 2.5 mg.

TABLE 6: Slit lamp examination of a patient having classic, noninfectious anterior uveitis managed with corticosteroids.

OD	*Parameter*	*OS*
J10 ph J3	BCVA	J1+
14 mm Hg	IOP	12 mm Hg
Reactive ptosis	Lids/Lashes	Normal
2+ injection	Conjunctiva	White and quiet
Inferior fine KPs	Cornea	Clear
3+ cell, <0.2 mm hypopyon versus fibrin collection inferiorly	Anterior chamber	Deep and quiet
Prominent vessels, no transillumination defects, fibrin across pupil, posterior synechiae clockwise from 1 to 4 o'clock	Iris	Normal
Hazy view	Lens	Clear
Hazy view with a red reflex	Vitreous	Normal
Grossly normal optic nerve, vessels, periphery, and macula	Fundus	Normal

(BCVA: best corrected visual acuity; IOP: intraocular pressure; KPs: keratic precipitates; ph: pinhole)

Follow-up

The patient was seen 4 weeks later, and the vision had improved to 20/25 in the right eye. She was taking prednisolone acetate 1% four times a day and continuing the oral prednisone taper. On examination, the synechiae was broken, and only pigment remained on the anterior capsule **(Fig. 6)**.

The treatment plan was to finish the oral prednisone and prednisolone acetate 1% tapers and to monitor for inflammation recurrence. Cyclopentolate drops were also discontinued. A rheumatology referral was placed to assess for occult spondyloarthropathy.

Discussion

A short burst of oral corticosteroids can be helpful in cases of fulminant HLA-B27 anterior uveitis to achieve quiescence faster. It is one of a handful of situations where a taper of oral corticosteroids for active inflammation should be done quickly. It is important to note that the most common cause of hypopyon formation in the United States is HLA-B27-associated anterior uveitis. However, in other parts of the world, Behçet's disease may be a

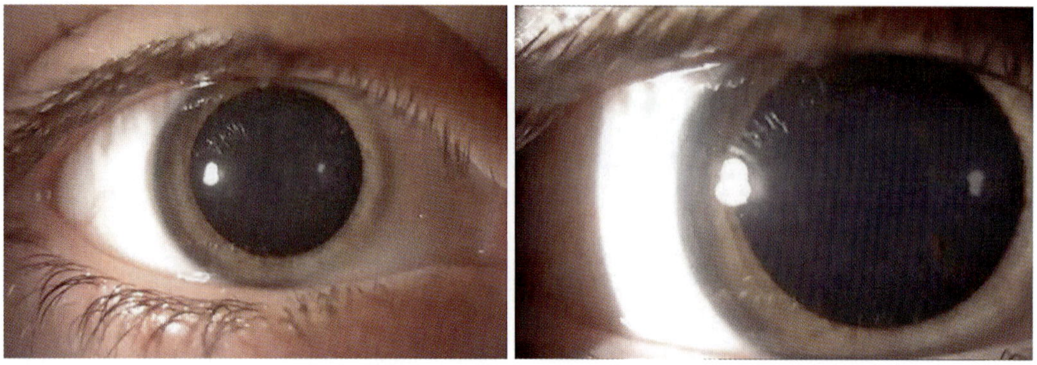

Fig. 6: An external color photograph of the right eye 4 weeks after presentation showing no posterior synechiae and resolution of the conjunctival injection.
Source: Uveitis Course - Grand Rounds 16. International Uveitis Study Group (IUSG). June 14, 2025. Available at: https://youtu.be/2UVTU7oztTc?si=y7tNEsxDMokFr6uw.

more likely diagnosis. In the case of Behçet's disease-associated uveitis with a hypopyon, treatment with high-dose prednisone is needed along with the concurrent start of an immunosuppressive agent, as corticosteroids alone will not lead to remission. The presence of a hypopyon and retinal vasculitis is an indication for starting with a biologic immunosuppressive agent over a conventional immunosuppressant. One severe episode of inflammation can lead to retinal infarction and irreparable structural damage. In this case, the fluorescein angiography showed no posterior involvement. Given the positive HLA-B27 antigen and no inflammation on fluorescein angiography, we would not start immunosuppression unless there were multiple, frequent, or severe flares.

A very important point for consideration regarding HLA-B27 positivity is the occult presence of an associated systemic disease. The Spondyloarthritis-Eye (SpEYE) and Dublin Uveitis Evaluation Tool (DUET) studies showed the underdiagnosis of rheumatologic manifestations of HLA-B27 positivity in patients with uveitis.[46,47] Therefore, it is important to investigate symptoms of arthritis, low back pain, and stiffness on a review of systems. Up to 50% of the patients either had spondyloarthritis or axial arthritis in the aforementioned studies. Early diagnosis prevents long-term sequelae of spinal curvature through immunosuppression, physical therapy, and exercise.

PANUVEITIS REQUIRING CORTICOSTEROID USE

Case Presentation

Personal Data

A 39-year-old male presented with blurred vision and floaters in both eyes for 2 months.

TABLE 7: Slit lamp examination of a patient having panuveitis requiring corticosteroid.

OD	***Parameter***	***OS***
6/36	BCVA	6/18
14 mm Hg	IOP	14 mm Hg
2+ injection	Conjunctiva	2+ injection
Endothelial dusting	Cornea	Endothelial dusting
2+ cell, 2+ flare	Anterior chamber	2+ cell, 2+ flare
Normal	Iris	Normal
Clear	Lens	Clear
2+ cell	Vitreous	2+ cell
Optic disc edema, small whitish chorioretinal lesions	Fundus	Optic disc edema, small whitish chorioretinal lesions

(BCVA: best corrected visual acuity, IOP: intraocular pressure; KPs: keratic precipitates)

History of Present Illness

The change in vision was accompanied by bilateral eye redness and photophobia. He had no past medical history or recent systemic illnesses.

Physical Examination

The best corrected vision was 6/26 in the right eye and 6/18 in the left eye. In both anterior chambers, 2+ cell and 2+ flare were noted. Posteriorly, optic nerve edema and white chorioretinal lesions were noted on fundoscopy.

Slit Lamp Examination

The slit lamp exam findings are summarized in **Table 7**.

Ancillary Testing

Optical coherence tomography scans of the retina showed macular and optic nerve edema with vitreous cells in the right eye. In the left eye, only vitreous cells were noted **(Fig. 7)**.

Uveitis Workup

Syphilis serologies and a tuberculin skin test were negative. A chest x-ray was also normal.

Initial Treatment

The patient started one drop of dexamethasone every hour in both eyes, atropine 1% twice per day in both eyes, prednisolone 20 mg daily, and calcium and vitamin D3 supplements to be taken daily.

Follow-up

Two weeks later, on re-evaluation, the vision in the right eye was 6/36 and 6/9 in the left eye. He had trace cells in both anterior chambers, and the chorioretinal lesions had resolved. He gradually tapered the dexamethasone eye drop weekly to a maintenance dose of once per day. The prednisolone was tapered to 5 mg/day as a maintenance dose.

Two weeks later, the best corrected vision in the right eye had improved from 6/36 to 6/9, and the left eye had improved from 6/18 to 6/6. There were no signs of inflammation, and the patient was advised to continue 5 mg of prednisolone per day and a drop of dexamethasone daily in both eyes as a maintenance dose until he could see an ophthalmologist while working abroad. Unfortunately, 3 months later, he returned with decreased vision in the right eye to 6/60 that corrected to 6/24. Similarly, in the left eye, there was a decrease to 6/18 with correction to 6/12. On slit lamp examination, there were fine keratic precipitates in both eyes and 2+ anterior chamber cells. Also noted were bilateral vitreous cells and snowballs. Further testing with OCT imaging showed cystoid macular edema in both eyes and choroidal elevation between the macula and the optic disc in the right eye only **(Fig. 8)**.

Given the clinical activity seen in both eyes, high-dose prednisolone was started orally at 60 mg/day for 1 week with the use of prednisolone acetate 1% every hour while awake in both eyes. Additionally, he was given calcium 600mg and vitamin D3 100 international units supplements to be taken orally once a day. One week later, the vision in the right eye improved to 6/60 and with correction to 6/12. The vision in the left eye also improved to 6/18 and to 6/9 with correction, with a concurrent improvement in the inflammation to 0.5+ cell in both anterior chambers. The oral prednisolone was tapered gradually over several weeks to a maintenance dose of 7.5 mg/day with one drop

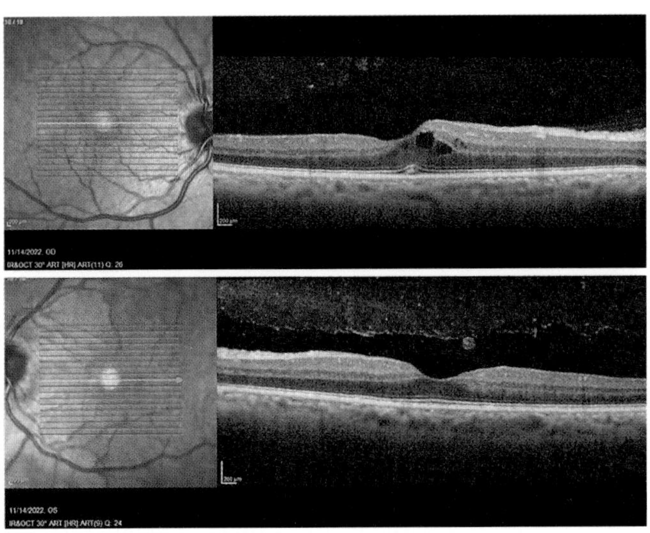

Fig. 7: An optical coherence tomography (OCT) scan of the retina in the right eye (top) shows macular edema and cells in the posterior vitreous, while the left eye scan (bottom) showed a preserved foveal contour with the presence of vitreous cells.
Source: Uveitis Course - Grand Rounds 16. International Uveitis Study Group (IUSG). June 14, 2025. Available at: https://youtu.be/2UVTU7oztTc?si=y7tNEsxDMokFr6uw.

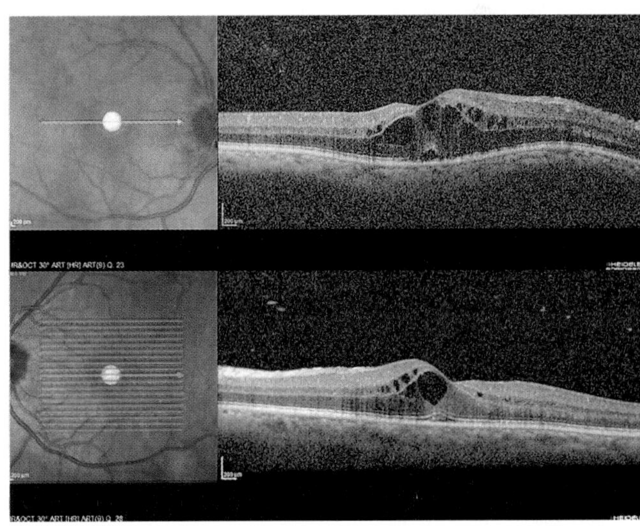

Fig. 8: An optical coherence tomography (OCT) scan of the macula in the right eye (top) showing macular edema with choroidal elevation between the macula and the optic disc. An OCT scan of the left eye also showed macular edema (bottom).
Source: Uveitis Course - Grand Rounds 16. International Uveitis Study Group (IUSG). June 14, 2025. Available at: https://youtu.be/2UVTU7oztTc?si=y7tNEsxDMokFr6uw.

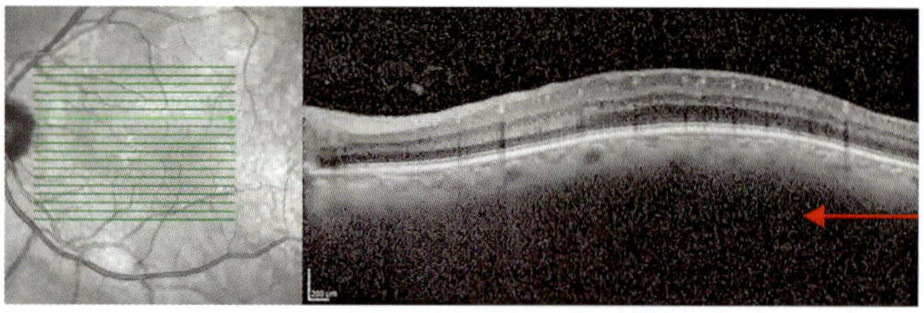

Fig. 9: An optical coherence tomography (OCT) scan through the macula of the left eye showing choroidal elevation and thickening (red arrow).
Source: Uveitis Course - Grand Rounds 16. International Uveitis Study Group (IUSG). June 14, 2025. Available at: https://youtu.be/2UVTU7oztTc?si=y7tNEsxDMokFr6uw.

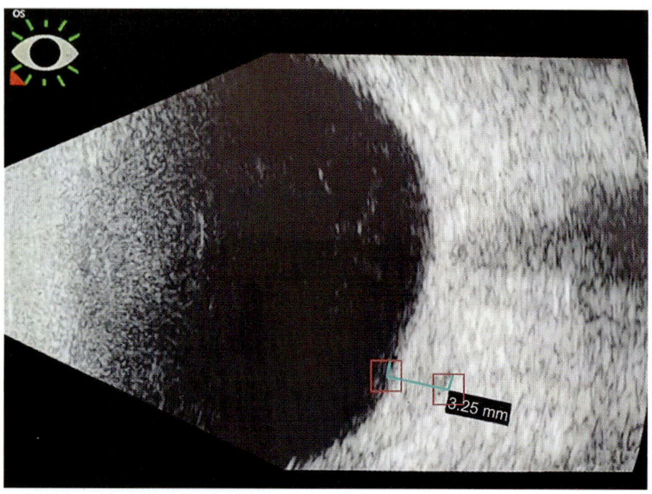

Fig. 10: A B-scan ultrasound of the left eye showing diffuse choroidal thickening that measured 3.25 mm. Vitreous debris is also noted.
Source: Uveitis Course - Grand Rounds 16. International Uveitis Study Group (IUSG). June 14, 2025. Available at: https://youtu.be/2UVTU7oztTc?si=y7tNEsxDMokFr6uw.

of dexamethasone in both eyes, resulting in control of the inflammation for 1 year.

He then presented with a headache and pain in the left eye. The vision in the right eye was 6/12 and 6/9 in the left eye. On examination, there was 1+ anterior chamber cell in the left eye, and both eyes had optic disc hyperemia. On OCT imaging, there was choroidal thickening noted in the macula **(Fig. 9)** of the left eye that measured 3.25 mm with a diffuse, hyperechoic signal on B-scan ultrasonography **(Fig. 10)**.

Repeat testing for tuberculosis with a purified protein derivative (PPD) test was negative, along with an interferon gamma release assay serologic test. He

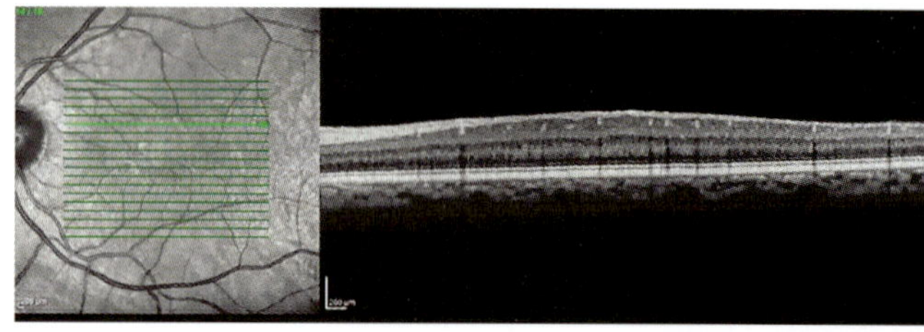

Fig. 11: An optical coherence tomography (OCT) scan of the left eye showing resolution of the choroidal thickening seen in **Figure 9**.
Source: Uveitis Course - Grand Rounds 16. International Uveitis Study Group (IUSG). June 14, 2025. Available at: https://youtu.be/2UVTU7oztTc?si=y7tNEsxDMokFr6uw.

was started on methotrexate 10 mg weekly for systemic immunosuppression, which was gradually increased weekly by 2.5 mg up to 20 mg weekly with folic acid supplementation. In addition, oral prednisolone 5 mg/day was continued. An OCT of the left eye clearly showed resolution of the choroidal thickening in addition to achieving clinical quiescence **(Fig. 11)**. The most recent follow-up occurred in May 2025 after 1 year of methotrexate use, and his vision with correction was 6/6 in both eyes with no sign of inflammation.

Discussion

This case illustrates how we often approach managing disease with just corticosteroids due to cost constraints in Ethiopia. While it works well to achieve quiescence in many patients, others require the start of non-corticosteroid immunosuppression. Herein, I will talk about conventional immunosuppression.

After excluding infectious etiologies start with the induction of high dose corticosteroids, either topically or with both topical and oral formulations, to quickly achieve control of the active inflammation. Once quiescence is achieved, gradually reduce the dose to see if the inflammation remains controlled, as in the first case. If not, the next step is to identify a minimal suppressive dose to continue, as in the second case. In chronic cases, the goal is to use the minimal suppressive corticosteroid dose with non-corticosteroid immunosuppressive agents. Vision is preserved through the use of maintenance dosing to prevent recurrent inflammation. Unfortunately, most of the immunosuppressive mediations used to treat ocular inflammation do not result in remission in all cases, except alkylating agents. Thus, control of inflammation is the goal using a combination of immunosuppressive agents.

Defining a safe, minimal, suppressive dose is not evidence-based. Previous literature on the development of cataracts from the Systemic Immunosuppressive Therapy for Eye Diseases Cohort Study (SITE) suggests that one drop of prednisolone acetate 1% every other day is a safe dose.[48] The risk of cataract formation with topical corticosteroid use increases in a dose-dependent manner.[49] In addition, a drop of prednisolone acetate 1% once a day has almost doubled the risk of elevated intraocular pressure.[48] Comparatively, oral prednisolone 7.5 mg/day, or preferably 5 mg/day, is well tolerated with no increased risk of intraocular pressure elevation per the Multicenter Uveitis Steroid Treatment (MUST) Trial. With the development of new non-corticosteroid immunosuppressive medications, tapering to 5 mg of oral prednisone per day is more achievable.[50] The paper entitled "Guidelines for the Use of Immunosuppressive Drugs in Patients with Ocular Inflammatory Disorders: Recommendations of an Expert Panel," by Jabs et al., contains a lot of information on how to manage oral corticosteroid tapering and non-corticosteroid immunosuppressant management.[6] I will talk about some of the principles and recommend it as a reference guide.

There are three major indications for the use of immunosuppressive therapies. First, if the suppressive dose of oral corticosteroids is higher than 7.5 mg/day (ideally 5 mg/day) or management with the equivalent of prednisolone acetate 1% requires two or more drops per day with the development of elevated intraocular pressures or cataract, then the start of a corticosteroid sparing agent is warranted.[6] Secondly, in rare cases where corticosteroid therapy fails to control the inflammation, non-corticosteroid therapy should be initiated. However, very carefully reconsider the possibility of an infectious etiology as corticosteroids are the strongest agent to induce control of inflammation. Finally, there are specific diseases that should be treated early or initially with immunosuppression. Examples include Behçet's disease-associated uveitis with posterior pole involvement, Birdshot retinochoroiditis, serpiginous choroiditis not associated with tuberculosis, necrotizing scleritis (which is associated with higher mortality in cases due to systemic vasculitis), and mucous membrane pemphigoid with cicatrizing conjunctivitis.[6] There are arguably others, such as multifocal choroiditis and panuveitis or sympathetic ophthalmia. The use of immunosuppressive drugs has increased with more experience and confidence in terms of the safety and preservation of vision over time.

The classes of non-corticosteroid immunosuppressive agents used include the antimetabolites, T-cell inhibitors, alkylating agents, and the calcineurin inhibitors: cyclosporine and tacrolimus. The antimetabolites are relatively contraindicated in patients with liver disease, and the calcineurin inhibitors are relatively contraindicated in patients with renal disease and hypertension. At an age of ≥55 years, the risk of immunosuppressive agent discontinuation tripled in the SITE study.[50]

Table 8 is a summary slide that Dr. Douglas Jabs created for the MUST trial based on the aforementioned paper discussing the expert opinion on the use of immunosuppressants.[6,51] Escalating to the highest tolerated dose, with the exception of the alkylators, and

TABLE 8: Non-biologic, non-corticosteroid immunosuppressive drug dose recommendations for use in the treatment of ocular inflammatory disorders.

Drug	***Initial dose***	***Typical range***
Azathioprine	2 mg/kg/day	100–200 mg/day
Methotrexate	15 mg/week	15–25 mg/week
Mycophenolate	1 gm BID	1–1.5 g BID
Cyclosporine (Neoral)	2 mg/kg BID	1.5–2.5 mg/kg BID
Cyclosporine (Sandimmune)	2.5 mg/kg BID	1.5–2.5 mg/kg BID
Tacrolimus	1 mg BID	0.03–0.08 mg/kg/day
Cyclophosphamide	2 mg/kg/day	100–200 mg/day
Chlorambucil	0.1 mg/day	6–12 mg/day

Courtesy: MUST Research Group.

Source: Jabs DA, Rosenbaum JT, Foster CS, Holland GN, Jaffe GJ, Louie JS, et al. Guidelines for the use of immunosuppressive drugs in patients with ocular inflammatory disorders: recommendations of an expert panel. Am J Ophthalmol. 2000;130(4):492-513.

Source: Uveitis Course - Grand Rounds 16. International Uveitis Study Group (IUSG). June 14, 2025. Available at: https://youtu.be/2UVTU7oztTc?si=y7tNEsxDMokFr6uw.

then lowering to the dose that still achieves quiescence has been the trend. For example, I use methotrexate dosing of 20 mg/week, whereas the First-line Antimetabolites as Steroid-sparing Treatment Trial (FAST) used 25 mg weekly.[52]

The next question is *which agent should I use?* The FAST trial was led by Dr. Nisha Acharya, who initially polled the American Uveitis Society and found that methotrexate and mycophenolate mofetil were the two most popular agents.[52] She and her colleagues from around the world compared methotrexate and mycophenolate in a randomized clinical trial, and methotrexate was proven to be non-inferior. It is also cheaper than mycophenolate. Another antimetabolite, azathioprine, has not been compared with anything other than in the SITE study.[53] It is popular in less developed countries and is reasonably inexpensive. In summary, methotrexate and azathioprine are the inexpensive options, and in the SITE study, the efficacy of all of the antimetabolites was similar. Methotrexate was slightly better, but this difference was not statistically significant. T-cell inhibitors and calcineurin inhibitors have also been successfully used to treat ocular inflammation. The efficacy of cyclosporine, per the SITE data, is less than that of the antimetabolites.[53] However, this may be due to increased use at the National Eye Institute location in the study, and since every visit was part of a protocol, they may have been more aggressive about documenting +0.5 anterior chamber cells. If you counted 0.5+ cells as a success, cyclosporine performed better. Many would argue that you should combine a calcineurin inhibitor with an antimetabolite if you are going to use combination therapy. However, this is becoming less popular with the availability of biologic agents.

The primary result of the FAST trial was treatment success in 66.7% in the methotrexate group versus 57.1% in the mycophenolate group [95% confidence interval (CI), −5.3–21.8%]; odds ratio (OR) 1.5 (95% CI: 0.81 to 2.81); $p = 0.20$.[52] Note that the OR for success by 6 months was considerable. There were 50% higher odds of success with methotrexate. However, the confidence interval crossed 1.0, and the result was not statistically significant. However, it did formally prove that methotrexate was non-inferior.

Moving on to alkylating agents, which arguably are the only class of immunosuppressive agents that induce remission. Slightly less than two-thirds of patients tolerate therapy per the SITE data.[50] Most of the data were from patients treated for mucous membrane pemphigoid. There is a short-term, high-dose approach with chlorambucil where the dose is escalated quickly and is stopped once the patient begins to become aplastic on complete blood count (CBC) studies. Remission occurs shortly thereafter. The use of alkylators is limited due to a high incidence of sterility, in as many as half of patients. It requires weekly monitoring with a CBC and urinalysis. There is also an increased risk of cancer, which was not found in the SITE studies.[50] Due to these potential side effects, the class is a less popular treatment option.

In our case, it was not clear early on that immunosuppression was needed. It seemed that with low-dose topical and oral corticosteroids, the patient could be managed with continued quiescence. Anatomically, panuveitis cannot be managed with topical therapy alone. However, as severity increased with time, it became clear that additional therapy would be needed. We view methotrexate as the first-line antimetabolite, based on the FAST study, the cost, and its availability in Ethiopia. After initiation of methotrexate, we assess for tolerance through symptom query and monitoring for toxicity from laboratory tests. If the initial drug fails, we can either try another agent in the same class, change to a calcineurin inhibitor or a T-cell inhibitor, or advance to a biologic. Anecdotally, we are not seeing an increase in infections in Ethiopia with the use of methotrexate and azathioprine. In contrast, more infections may occur if we had access to TNF inhibitors, as one out of three patients has developed disseminated tuberculosis.

Another consideration with immunosuppression use is the time to efficacy. As seen in both the SITE Study and the FAST trial, conventional agents take longer to work. In the FAST Trial, it took 4 months or longer before there was a 50% success rate in achieving quiescence. The primary outcome was achieving quiescence at 6 months. Therefore, 4–6 months is the time period needed to see if an antimetabolite is effective in controlling inflammation.[52] This may require the use of high-dose corticosteroids in the interim to maintain control of the inflammation. This trend drives an increase in TNF inhibitor use since, as a class, they are faster in achieving treatment success.[54]

What baseline testing is needed prior to starting conventional immunosuppressive agents? First, obtain laboratory testing to assess for potential contraindications. For antimetabolites, check for hepatitis B and C. Clinically assess for hypertension or serologically for renal disease when considering cyclosporine and tacrolimus use. Address if pregnancy could be present or is contemplated in the next few months. For azathioprine, check thiopurine methyltransferase levels to assess for a homozygous deficiency, which could lead to decreased drug metabolization and aplastic anemia or leukopenia. Unfortunately, this test is not widely available across the globe. In addition to the above, baseline testing should also include liver enzymes and a CBC.

Regarding pregnancy, there is a review by the European League Against Rheumatism on the use of immunosuppressive therapy.[55] Many of our patients are reproductive-age women. Looking at the rates of intermediate, posterior, and panuveitis alone, 60–65% are female. If starting immunosuppressive therapy, avoidance of pregnancy through contraception or complete abstinence should be discussed. Both the United States Food and Drug Administration (FDA) and the European Medicines Agency require labels that warn against using immunosuppressive therapy in pregnancy. Some agents, such as methotrexate, mycophenolate, and alkylators, are frankly contraindicated. Methotrexate has been used off-label to induce abortions, leading to fetal loss or malformations. Even males have been advised to wait 3 months after stopping antimetabolites before impregnating their partner. Cyclosporine and tacrolimus have not been associated with excess malformations. Tacrolimus does have a Food and Drug Administration (FDA) warning label, but there was a transplant study registry that showed no excess malformations. Azathioprine also has not been found to be associated with malformations or adverse pregnancy outcomes. Although, the label still warns against use in pregnancy. Therefore, these would be options if a patient were pregnant and needed more treatment than corticosteroids alone. Corticosteroids have traditionally been thought to be a safe approach during pregnancy. However, there are suggestions that there is a higher risk of preterm birth at doses even in the 5–10 mg range. There is also an increased risk of maternal infection. There is a placental enzyme that partially protects the fetus against the effects of corticosteroids. All Janus kinase (JAK) inhibitors should be avoided in pregnancy, as there is insufficient data to evaluate them. There was some concern about reproductive issues in men taking JAK inhibitors, which did not reach statistical significance in more recent studies. Other agents considered relatively safe during pregnancy, although less commonly used for the treatment of uveitis, include sulfasalazine, hydroxychloroquine, colchicine, and intravenous immunoglobulins. Anti-TNF inhibitors also appear to have a generally favorable safety profile in this setting. Although crude analyses initially suggested a higher rate of congenital malformations, this association was not observed after adjustment for disease severity and other methodological factors. Sulfasalazine has also been reported to affect male fertility by reducing sperm count and motility; however, this effect is reversible and may decrease the likelihood of conception during treatment.

For the longitudinal follow-up of these patients, at each visit, it is important to query about treatment side effects and to encourage patients to mention even minor things. Additionally, it is ideal to follow the weight if a patient is taking oral corticosteroids. This is especially important in children on oral corticosteroids, which is a treatment that should be limited due to many side effects, including short stature from early epiphyseal closure. Sometimes in Ethiopia, due to resource restrictions, we monitor height as well. Repeating laboratory studies to assess for changes in liver enzymes and a CBC should be conducted at least every 3 months, or more frequently if there are abnormalities or an immunosuppressive agent was recently started. Consider magnesium testing for patients taking calcineurin inhibitors. The paper by Jabs et al. provides a detailed framework for clinical and laboratory monitoring tailored to each immunosuppressive agent. In clinical practice, laboratory testing is commonly performed at baseline, at 1 month, at 2 months, and subsequently every three months. In patients with stable and consistently normal laboratory results for more than one year, some clinicians may extend the monitoring interval to every six months.

Once a successful, suppressive regimen is established at the lowest dose possible, treatment should continue for at least 2 years of quiescence or for longer. We have little data on the rates of remission of all of the uveitides, with most of the literature focusing on intermediate uveitis and chronic anterior uveitis. Even in these conditions, the remission rate is not high and is similarly low for anterior scleritis. Dose adjustments may be required due to side effects or switching agents if a drug is not well tolerated. During maintenance therapy, occasional flares may occur related to immune stimulation, such as trauma, immunization, and illness. The minimal suppressive dose may need to be changed under these circumstances, whether that is a temporary discontinuation for an infection to heal or increased dosing for recurrent flares. A major flare should be treated with a full reinduction of oral corticosteroids at 1 mg/kg of ideal body weight, and a smaller flare with a partial reinduction. A rule of thumb is to double the corticosteroid dose at which the patient was last quiet if a flare occurs during a taper.

The MUST trial established systemic therapy as the first-line maintenance therapy for posterior pole involving uveitis.[51] Not only was it non-inferior to long-acting intraocular implants, but came with a lower cost. The 7-year results show the visual acuity in the cohort receiving systemic immunosuppression was superior to those receiving a long-acting corticosteroid implant. The FAST trial has well-established methotrexate as the first-line agent unless there are systemic or lifestyle contraindications.[52] The data from the SITE study mirror those of the MUST trial 7-year results, where there was an initial improvement in vision with induction and then stability of improvement in most uveitides over time.

A commonly posed question is: What is the safety of systemic immunosuppression? The SITE Study looked at the long-term incidence of death and cancer.[50] Given 10 years of median follow-up time, methotrexate, azathioprine, mycophenolate, cyclosporine, and TNF inhibitors are safe with respect to both mortality and cancer. Furthermore, data from the MUST papers argue well for short-term safety, even in the follow-up phase of the study.[51] More infections requiring treatment occurred in the systemic arm, but this trend may have been the result of treatment bias.

In short, we want to choose the treatment that achieves clinical quiescence and avoids complications as much as possible. Complications can be managed if there is no better treatment option given patient-specific limitations. However, use of systemic immunosuppression has been associated with the development of fewer intraocular complications, such as cataract and elevated intraocular pressures.[56] While some complications are reversible with surgery, treatment of macular edema with additional local corticosteroid therapies as adjunctive treatments can improve vision based on clinical observation studies. However, the clinician must be patient and give conventional immunosuppressive drugs the appropriate time to reach full effect.

In summary, systemic immunosuppression should be considered the first-line treatment. Methotrexate is a reasonable first choice worldwide, and while not as effective, it is safer than using high-dose oral corticosteroids. With monitoring and dose adjustments, conventional immunosuppressants can effectively treat ocular inflammation.[50,51,56,57] Usage requires a level of skill and attention by the physician for monitoring and cooperation by the patient. Carefully consider pregnancy and monitoring for side effects on an individual basis. Despite a several-month lag to attain full efficacy, the best corrected visual acuity can be maintained, and ocular complications can be prevented with use. With more treatment options available after approval of biologic medications, there are additional treatment strategies at our disposal, as described in the next case.

NONINFECTIOUS UVEITIS MANAGED WITH BIOLOGIC THERAPY

Case Presentation

Personal Data

A 16-year-old female developed decreased vision in the left eye more than the right eye for 2 weeks.

History of Present Illness

The change in vision was accompanied by flashes in both eyes. Her prior ophthalmic history was limited to astigmatism in both eyes and hyperopia in the right eye and myopia in the left eye. Her past medical history was remarkable for acute T-cell lymphoblastic leukemia, for which she was on chemotherapy for the past 6 months. She also had a history of bilateral hip osteonecrosis related to systemic corticosteroid use.

Physical Examination

The visual acuity was 20/30 in both eyes, and 1+ cells were seen in the anterior vitreous of the left eye. The fundus exam showed temporal macular hemorrhages in the right eye and multiple retinal infiltrates peripherally with adjacent hemorrhages in both eyes **(Figs. 12A and B)**.

Slit Lamp Examination

The slit lamp examination is summarized in **Table 9**.

Ancillary Testing

Fundus autofluorescence images showed hyper-autofluorescence in the areas of exudates and hypoautofluorescence in areas of hemorrhage **(Figs. 13A and B)**. Fluorescein angiography showed early and late blocking in areas of retinal hemorrhage and late leakage in areas with exudation in the periphery with adjacent non-perfusion **(Figs. 14 and 15)**. OCT scans of the retina showed outer retinal damage with thinning and loss of the retinal contour with a preretinal membrane and subretinal fluid in the right eye. The OCT scans of the macula in the left eye showed temporal retinal thinning, disorganization,

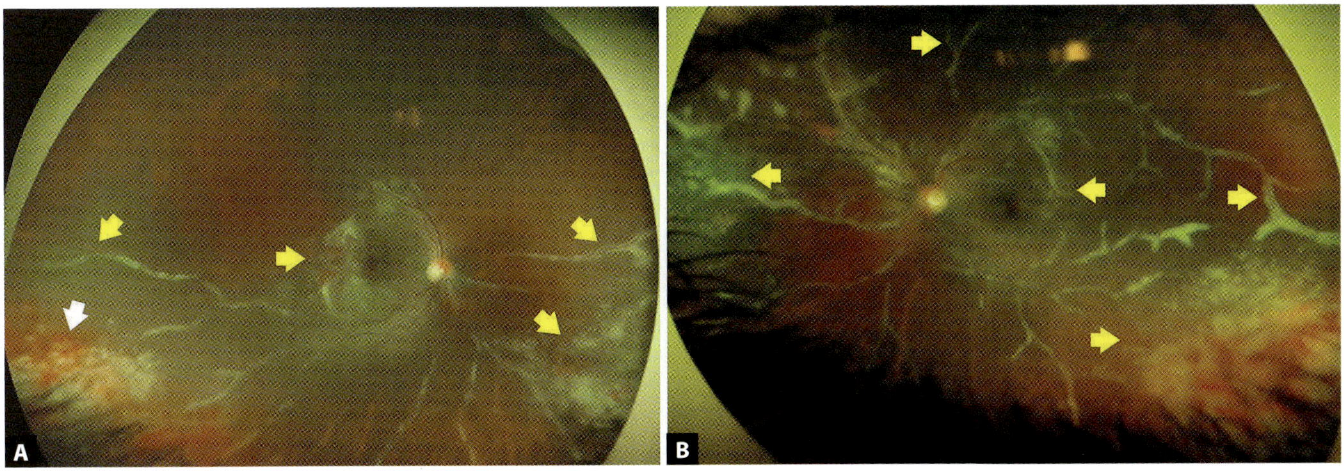

Figs. 12A and B: Color fundus photos of both eyes showing exudates surrounding the vessels with surrounding hemorrhages (yellow arrows).
Source: Uveitis Course - Grand Rounds 16. International Uveitis Study Group (IUSG). June 14, 2025. Available at: https://youtu.be/2UVTU7oztTc?si=y7tNEsxDMokFr6uw.

TABLE 9: Slit lamp examination of a patient having noninfectious uveitis managed with biologic therapy.

OD	***Parameter***	***OS***
20/30	BCVA	20/30-2
16 mm Hg	IOP	20 mm Hg
White and quiet	Conjunctiva	White and quiet
Clear	Cornea	Clear
Deep and quiet	Anterior chamber	Deep and quiet
Round and reactive	Iris	Round and reactive
Clear	Lens	Clear
Normal	Vitreous	1+ cell
Hemorrhages temporal to the macula. Multiple retinal infiltrates surrounding the vessels into the periphery with adjacent hemorrhages	Fundus	Infiltrates along blood vessels with surrounding hemorrhages in the periphery

(BCVA: best corrected visual acuity; IOP: intraocular pressure)

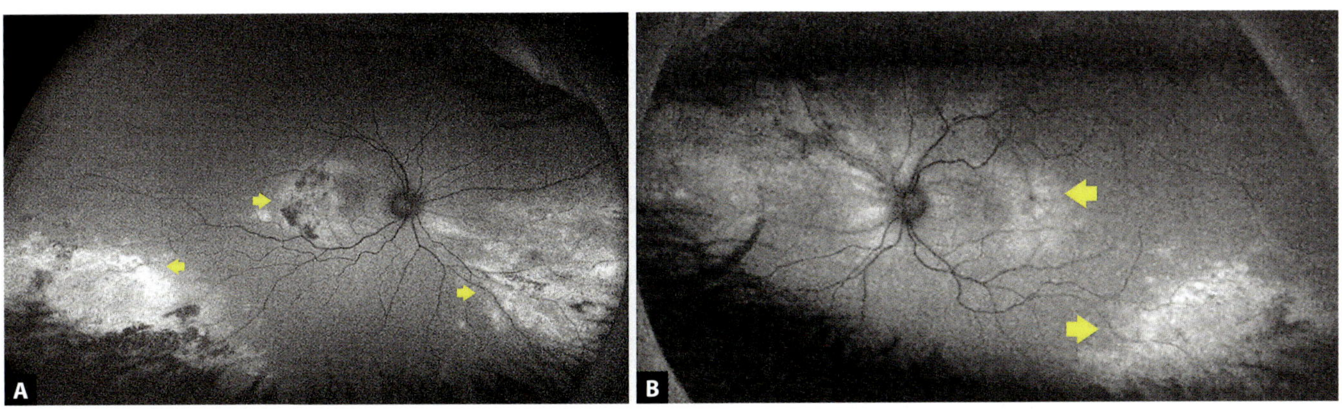

Figs. 13A and B: Fundus autofluorescence images of both eyes showing hyperautofluorescence in the areas of exudates (yellow arrows) and hypoautofluorescence in areas of hemorrhage.
Source: Uveitis Course - Grand Rounds 16. International Uveitis Study Group (IUSG). June 14, 2025. Available at: https://youtu.be/2UVTU7oztTc?si=y7tNEsxDMokFr6uw.

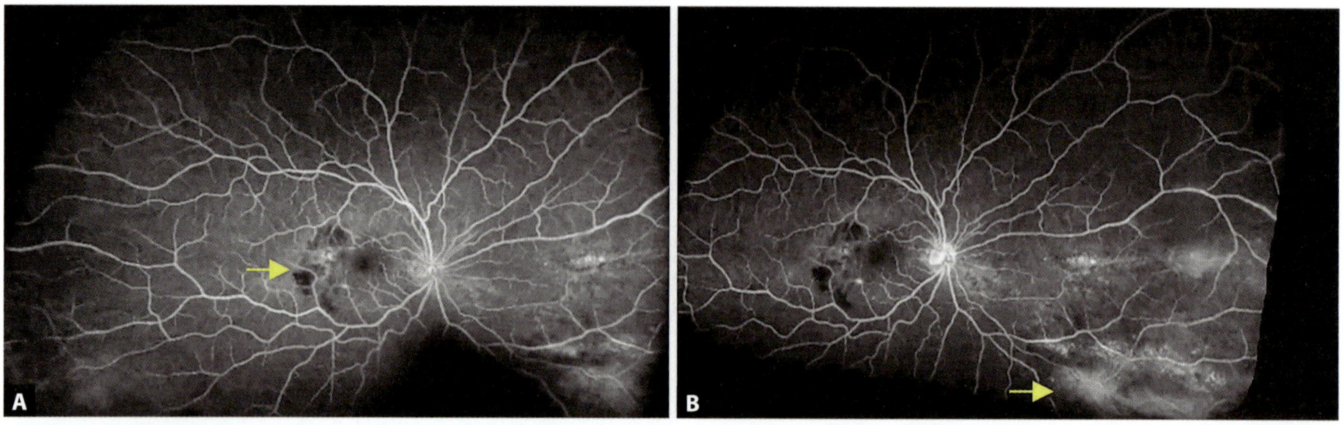

Figs. 14A and B: Fluorescein angiography of the right eye showing early and late blocking in areas of retinal hemorrhage (yellow arrow, left) and in the left eye, late leakage in areas with exudation in the periphery (yellow arrow, right).
Source: Uveitis Course - Grand Rounds 16. International Uveitis Study Group (IUSG). June 14, 2025. Available at: https://youtu.be/2UVTU7oztTc?si=y7tNEsxDMokFr6uw.

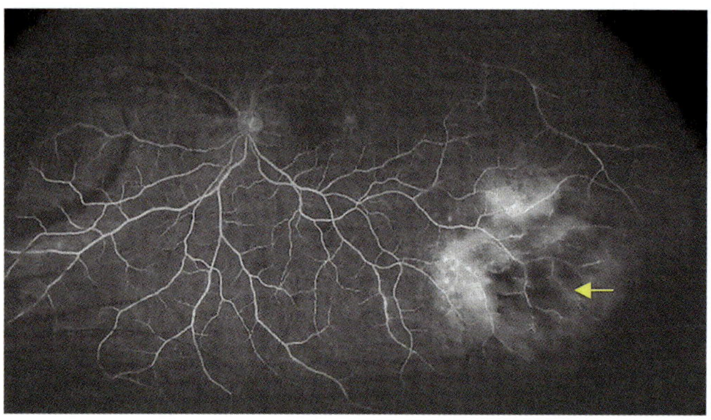

Fig. 15: Fluorescein angiography of the left eye showing peripheral capillary nonperfusion in areas adjacent to vessels with exudation and late leakage (yellow arrow).
Source: Uveitis Course - Grand Rounds 16. International Uveitis Study Group (IUSG). June 14, 2025. Available at: https://youtu.be/2UVTU7oztTc?si=y7tNEsxDMokFr6uw.

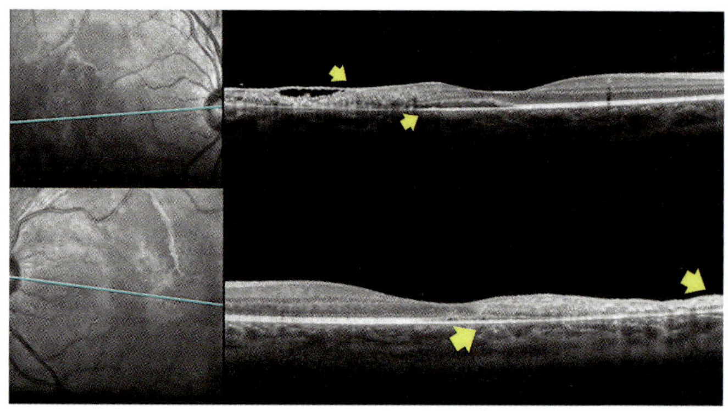

Fig. 16: An optical coherence tomography (OCT) scan of the retina of the right eye (above) showing outer retinal damage with loss of retinal structure and epiretinal membrane formation (top yellow arrow). Subretinal fluid was also present (bottom yellow arrow). In the left eye, temporal retinal thinning with fluid separation in the central fovea is denoted by yellow arrows (bottom image).
Source: Uveitis Course - Grand Rounds 16. International Uveitis Study Group (IUSG). June 14, 2025. Available at: https://youtu.be/2UVTU7oztTc?si=y7tNEsxDMokFr6uw.

and a mild, shallow fluid separation in the central fovea **(Fig. 16)**.

Uveitis Workup

At the top of the differential diagnosis were infectious etiologies, namely *Cytomegalovirus* (CMV) retinitis, versus inflammatory etiologies, such as Behçet's disease-associated uveitis. Other diagnoses that were considered were acute retinal necrosis, progressive outer retinal necrosis, syphilitic retinitis, or leukemic retinopathy. Laboratory testing showed leukopenia with a very low CD4 count. Additional testing was negative and included HLA-B27, B51, and A29. There were also negative results for the QuantiFERON, syphilis serologies, HIV, toxoplasma antibodies, and PCR for varicella zoster and herpes simplex. She was serologically positive for CMV immunoglobulin G (IgG) and immunoglobulin M (IgM) antibodies, with CMV deoxyribonucleic acid (DNA) also detected. An anterior chamber paracentesis and injection of intravitreal foscarnet in both eyes was performed. A positive PCR result for CMV in the aqueous sample confirmed the diagnosis of CMV retinitis.

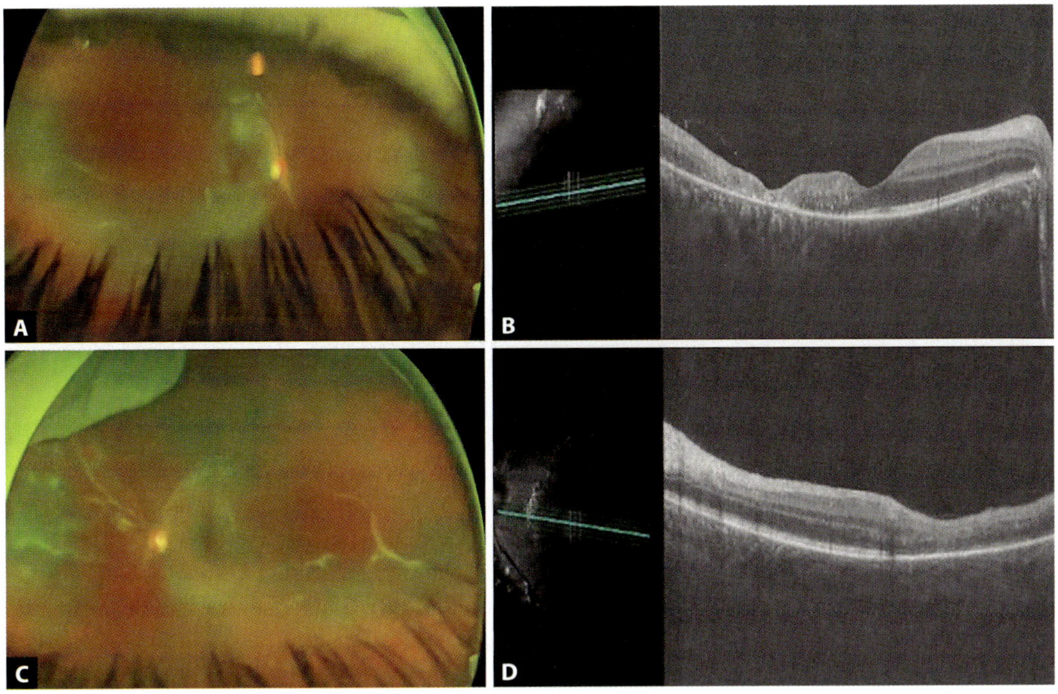

Figs. 17A to D: Color fundus photos of the right (top left) and left eye (bottom left) showing decreased retinal infiltrates along the vasculature. Optical coherence tomography (OCT) scans of the right eye (top right) show loss of retinal contour with atrophy nasal to the macula, with resolution of the subretinal fluid. An OCT scan of the left eye (bottom right) shows atrophy temporal to the macula without subretinal fluid after 2 weeks of treatment.
Source: Uveitis Course - Grand Rounds 16. International Uveitis Study Group (IUSG). June 14, 2025. Available at: https://youtu.be/2UVTU7oztTc?si=y7tNEsxDMokFr6uw.

Initial Treatment

Intravitreal foscarnet injections were administered in both eyes every 3 days. Only two injections were required in total, as intravenous ganciclovir 5 mg/kg every 12 hours was initiated at the same time. The treatment was then changed to oral valganciclovir 900 mg twice a day prior to discharge from the hospital.

Follow-up

Two weeks later, there was a decrease in the retinal infiltrates along the vasculature with an absence of subretinal fluid in both eyes **(Figs. 17A to D)**.

After 6 weeks, the patient's vision returned to 20/20 in both eyes, and valganciclovir 900 mg twice a day was continued. On posterior pole examination, the retinal infiltrates were nearly resolved and replaced with scarring. By 10 weeks after presentation, there was scarring in the periphery with resolution of all retinal infiltrates **(Fig. 18)**.

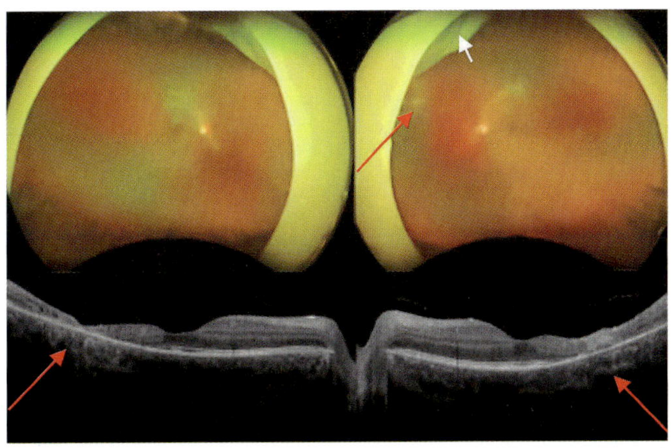

Fig. 18: Color fundus photos of both eyes after 10 weeks of treatment (top) showing no retinal exudates and peripheral scarring (red arrow). Optical coherence tomography (OCT) scans of the right (left bottom) and left eyes (right bottom) show continued resolution of subretinal fluid and retinal atrophy (red arrows).
Source: Uveitis Course - Grand Rounds 16. International Uveitis Study Group (IUSG). June 14, 2025. Available at: https://youtu.be/2UVTU7oztTc?si=y7tNEsxDMokFr6uw.

However, 3 months later, the patient experienced blurry vision in the left eye for 1 week, leading to a repeated evaluation in the clinic. She had discontinued valganciclovir after completing her course of chemotherapy. The visual acuity in the right eye was 20/20 and 20/30 in the left eye. Slit lamp examination showed 0.5+ cells in the anterior vitreous in both eyes. A dilated fundus exam showed no retinal infiltrates, only scarring in the right eye. There was also a lack of infiltrates in the left eye with inactive scars. However, there were new pink elevated areas temporal to the macula from subretinal fluid **(Fig. 19)**.

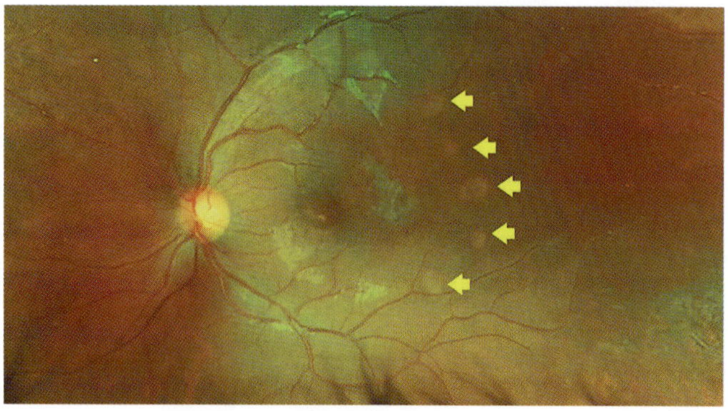

Fig. 19: A color fundus photograph of the left macula showing areas of subretinal fluid temporally (yellow arrows).
Source: Uveitis Course - Grand Rounds 16. International Uveitis Study Group (IUSG). June 14, 2025. Available at: https://youtu.be/2UVTU7oztTc?si=y7tNEsxDMokFr6uw.

Fluorescein angiography was repeated in both eyes and showed late leakage of the optic discs and small vessel capillary leakage in the peripheral retinas. Additionally, hyperfluorescence of the subretinal fluid pockets and capillary non-perfusion in the periphery were noted **(Figs. 20A and B)**. OCT scans of the retina showed intraretinal fluid in both eyes with subretinal fluid only in the left eye **(Figs. 21A and B)**.

Laboratory testing was repeated and showed both the white blood cell count and the CD4+ count had increased to the normal range, and no CMV DNA was detected in the serum. The differential diagnosis had changed, given the new clinical picture to include reactivation of CMV retinitis, immune recovery uveitis (IRU), and leukemic retinopathy. With normal white blood cell and CD4+

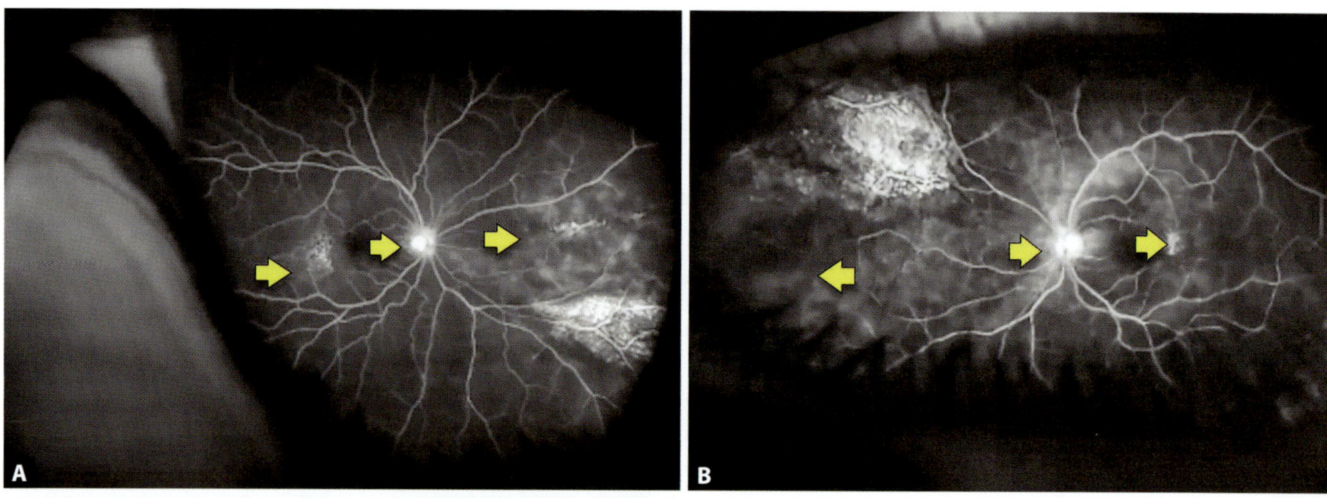

Figs. 20A and B: Fluorescein angiography images of the right (left) and left eye (right) that show bilateral, late optic disc leakage (center arrows). In the right eye, there is capillary leakage (yellow arrows). In the left eye, there is capillary non-perfusion (left arrow) and hyperfluorescence of the subretinal fluid pockets temporal to the macula (right arrow).
Source: Uveitis Course - Grand Rounds 16. International Uveitis Study Group (IUSG). June 14, 2025. Available at: https://youtu.be/2UVTU7oztTc?si=y7tNEsxDMokFr6uw.

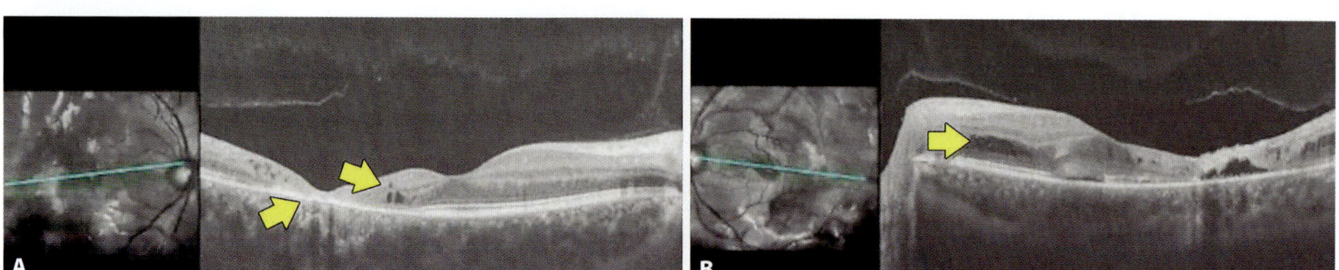

Figs. 21A and B: Optical coherence tomography (OCT) scans of the right eye (left) and the left eye (right) show areas of new intraretinal edema bilaterally (yellow arrows).
Source: Uveitis Course - Grand Rounds 16. International Uveitis Study Group (IUSG). June 14, 2025. Available at: https://youtu.be/2UVTU7oztTc?si=y7tNEsxDMokFr6uw.

counts, leukemic retinopathy and active retinitis from CMV were much less likely. The patient was diagnosed with IRU, and valganciclovir 900 mg twice a day was restarted. While systemic corticosteroids are the gold standard treatment for IRU, given the history of osteonecrosis, this class of medication was contraindicated. A better choice was a biologic agent: Either a TNF inhibitor or an IL-6 inhibitor. The patient was admitted and given 1 g of intravenous methylprednisolone for 2 days with transition to a rapid oral corticosteroid taper while concurrently starting tocilizumab 8 mg/kg intravenously per month.

After three cycles of tocilizumab, there was a marked decrease in leakage in the periphery on fluorescein angiography in both eyes, with an absence of subretinal fluid in the right eye. After seven infusions, the leakage had almost completely resolved and the vision in the right eye remained at 20/25, but improved to 20/20 in the left eye.

While IRU has been reported in patients with acquired immunodeficiency syndrome (AIDS) after the start of combination antiretroviral therapy, there are nowadays more cases of IRU seen in patients on chemotherapy and with non-AIDS immunodeficiencies. IRU is a late sequelae of CMV retinitis, with the greatest risk factor being increasing CD4+ cell counts to a level of ≥100 cells/µL or a decreasing number of human immunodeficiency virus copies.[58-60]

The first-line treatment for cystoid or intraretinal edema associated with IRU is corticosteroid therapy: topically or systemically.[61,62] In the literature, intravitreal injection of aflibercept has also been attempted with a third-line option of systemic IL-6 inhibition. The rationale supporting IL-6 inhibition in uveitic macular edema secondary to non-infectious uveitis is rooted in the STOP-Uveitis Study conducted by Dr. Yasir Sepah.[63] The findings of the study showed there was a significant reduction of cystoid macular edema at 6 months after the initiation of tocilizumab infusions.

In summary, CMV retinitis can occur in patients with an immune deficiency, and IRU arises with recovery of the immune system as CD4+ cell counts normalize. IL-6 receptor antagonists, such as tocilizumab, offer a therapeutic approach for IRU.

Discussion

This case illustrates several different points. The diagnosis of CMV retinitis and IRU was straightforward. The challenge lay in how to treat the patient based on available options, given the absolute contraindication to oral corticosteroids with the history of osteonecrosis. In our initial work with IRU, we published that using a local corticosteroid injection is possible.[64] However, that was not appropriate for this patient because of her very young age and the higher risk of developing ocular hypertension and cataracts. The patient's parents also did not want to proceed with a periocular or intravitreal corticosteroid injection. As we know from the literature, the use of immunomodulatory therapies such as mycophenolate, methotrexate, and cyclosporine does not have a strong record of treating uveitic macular edema. Since the macular edema was significant and acute, we focused on starting a biologic agent. Adalimumab is the only currently approved biologic medication for the treatment of non-infectious intermediate, posterior, and panuveitis based on the efficacy shown in the VISUAL Studies.[65,66] However, resolution of uveitic macular edema with the use of adalimumab can take months.

What about another anti-TNF inhibitor, infliximab? While infliximab can decrease small vessel leakage, there is not as much in the literature on the effect on macular edema. Given the patient's comorbidities and the above findings on macular edema resolution with TNF inhibitors, we chose to treat with tocilizumab. The STOP-Uveitis study and several studies from both Spain and France support role of IL-6 inhibition in treating uveitis.[63,67,68] Even intravitreal IL-6 inhibitors have been investigated for the treatment of uveitis and macular edema.[69] Systemic IL-6 inhibitor therapy has also shown significant benefits in treating uveitic macular edema with an acceptable safety profile.[68]

What about other biologic agents? Again, the only biologic that has been approved in the United States for the treatment of non-infectious uveitis is adalimumab. However, uveitis specialists often employ other agents off-label, including IL-17, IL-1, and IL-23 inhibitors. We also have prescribed JAK inhibitors, such as tofacitinib, but studies have shown variable efficacy of this drug class in controlling intraocular inflammation. We learned from the HUMBOLDT study that the JAK inhibitor, filgotinib, showed significant ability to control both macular edema and uveitis.[70] Unfortunately, the trial was terminated for business reasons. Fortunately, other trials are assessing the efficacy of another JAK inhibitor, brepocitinib, which is a JAK1-tyrosine kinase 2 inhibitor with promising phase 2 results in the NEPTUNE study. Currently, the phase 3 CLARITY trial is ongoing in the United States, Europe, South America, and Asia.

This case showed the appropriateness of the use of biologic agents, even if off-label. Biologics are still considered second-line therapies, except in cases of Behçet's disease-associated uveitis involving the posterior segment. The main reason for second line status is cost. The ADVISE trial compares adalimumab to conventional immunosuppressants. If biologic therapy shows greater efficacy when the results are released, treatment options will move more toward using TNF inhibitors earlier in the disease process. If there is macular edema or subretinal fluid, the IL-6 inhibitors have robust data to support their efficacy. Interferon-alpha has been reported to successfully treat uveitic macular edema, but side effects can limit tolerability.

PEARLS FROM THE EXPERTS ON FREQUENTLY ASKED QUESTIONS

1. When an insufficient response is observed to a TNF inhibitor, should one switch to another agent within the same class or to a drug with a different mechanism of action?

Answer: If there is an insufficient response to adalimumab, after you have increased to weekly dosing and given it at least 3 months to work, then it is okay to change to infliximab. Infliximab allows for changes in both the dose and the infusion interval. If you have tried two anti-TNF inhibitors, then you should switch classes.

2. How commonly does HLA-B27-associated uveitis present as intermediate or posterior uveitis?

Answer: Posterior uveitis alone is not associated with HLA-B27 positivity, and less than 10% of cases can present as intermediate uveitis.

3. In the second presented case, was sarcoidosis ruled out? What is the recommendation of usage of calcium along with oral corticosteroids in patients with sarcoid uveitis, given the association with hypercalcemia in that disease state?

Answer: A chest X-ray was performed to assess for sarcoidosis, and it was negative. We do recommend the addition of calcium 1,000 mg and vitamin D 800 international units per day to any patient taking oral corticosteroid therapy, with rare exceptions.

4. Once an immunosuppressive medication is started, how long is it continued?

Answer: First, understand the stepwise approach. Initiate therapy with an antimetabolite, and if the ocular inflammation remains uncontrolled, then escalate to the prescription of a TNF inhibitor. Before deciding if an immunosuppressive agent is not effective, wait for at least 3 months at the maximum tolerated dose. Secondly, once quiescence is achieved, a patient is asked to continue on the immunosuppressive agent for at least 2 years. If they remain quiet for that duration, which includes lack of macular edema, then a taper off of the medication over the next 3–6 months is warranted. Some of the uveitides require continued treatment indefinitely to preserve vision, especially where macular-threatening lesions are present. These can include sympathetic ophthalmia, Birdshot chorioretinitis, and serpiginous choroiditis.

5. Do rheumatologists treat uveitis patients on the recommendation of the ophthalmologist? What does off-label use of a medication mean?

Answer: Uveitis specialists vary in whether they prescribe immunosuppressive agents themselves or in conjunction with a rheumatologist or other internal medicine specialist. The only FDA-approved immunosuppressive agent to treat non-infectious intermediate, posterior, and panuveitis in the United States is adalimumab. Nonetheless, antimetabolites, such as methotrexate, are prescribed off-label to treat ocular inflammation and are less expensive than biologic medications. Once a medication is FDA approved, it can be prescribed, even if the indication is outside of the disease states for which the approval was issued. Insurers can refuse to pay for a drug that is prescribed for an off-label use, which would require the patient to pay for the medication out-of-pocket. As a reminder, we concurrently prescribe 1mg of folic acid to be taken daily with methotrexate use. The caveat is to take the folic acid daily except on the day of the week when the methotrexate is taken, since it is a competitive inhibitor and can lead to decreased methotrexate efficacy when taken together.

6. In the second case that was presented, could the serous retinal detachment be due to central serous chorioretinopathy? Are certain immunosuppressant medications more effective in treating serous retinal detachments?

Answer: Yes, central serous chorioretinitis (CSCR) should always be included as a possible cause of a serous retinal detachment in the setting of systemic corticosteroid use. However, the patient presented with anterior and vitreous cells, which were suggestive of active inflammation as the cause of the subretinal fluid. Inflammatory cells should not be present in a case of CSCR. Both anti-TNF inhibitors and tocilizumab can effectively treat cases of non-infectious uveitis. They are second-line agents, except in Behçet's disease-associated uveitis involving the posterior segment, due to cost. Depending on the results of the ADVISE Trial, if adalimumab is more effective than traditional immunosuppressants, there may be a shift toward using TNF inhibitors earlier in treatment. If there is macular edema or subretinal fluid on examination, the IL-6 inhibitors and interferons are effective treatments. However, interferons cause many side effects and are not readily available.

7. What is the safest biologic to use in tuberculosis-endemic countries where it may be risky to use adalimumab or other TNF inhibitors?

Answer: The first step in treatment is to take all precautions with thorough testing for latent tubercular infection and to screen for risk factors for infection. A discussion with an infectious disease specialist on the risk versus benefit ratio of treatment with a TNF inhibitor should occur. It is important to know if the patient can safely be treated through antitubercular treatment prior to the initiation of biologic therapy or during use based on serologic testing and risk factors. In enemic areas, TNF inhibitors may not be the best therapeutic option. IL-6 inhibitors have shown efficacy, but again, testing for latent tuberculosis and determining the risk for the development of the infection are required prior to any biologic agent initiation. In short, there is no safe immunosuppressive agent if chemoprophylaxis is not administered in patients with latent tuberculosis, including corticosteroids.

The patient in the second case acquired tuberculosis after starting a TNF inhibitor, which was disappointing due to the high out-of-pocket cost. These agents may naturally be used less due to resource limitations. Another consideration is pregnancy with the use of immunosuppressants. The data support using azathioprine or cyclosporine rather than systemic corticosteroids. Prior to the start of any of these medications, always get a formal, high-risk obstetrics consult to ensure that the latest medical literature and maternal-fetal risks are presented to the patient. Ask them for recommendations because, even though azathioprine may be reasonably safe in the literature, there may be contraindications or other systemic considerations that need to be weighed. Another third-line agent that was not discussed is the melanotropin peptide. The mechanism of action is unknown, and there is currently no way to assess medication levels. Sometimes there are medical questions outside of what ophthalmologists are expected to know, so consultation with another service may be needed.

8. How long after latent or even active tuberculosis treatment with four drugs can a TNF inhibitor be started?

Answer: The infectious disease group at Stanford University advises that once antitubercular therapy is started to wait for 6 weeks for initiation of a TNF inhibitor. In a patient with active tuberculosis, within a week of the start of ATT, corticosteroids can be prescribed. Reactivation of tuberculosis is a greater concern with TNF inhibitors due to potency and the effect on granuloma formation, which explains the need for a delay of treatment until ATT has time to become effective. Even despite treatment, some uveitis specialists will not use a TNF inhibitor in a patient with a history of active tuberculosis. Coordination with a rheumatologist is needed for starting, supervising, and monitoring the medication. Given the high-risk situation for tuberculosis reactivation, it is a clinical dilemma, and rheumatology may also counsel against use. Local therapy, including the dexamethasone implant, is a reasonable option in patients with systemic contraindications to the use of immunosuppressive agents.

FINAL WRAP-UP

Systemic immunosuppressive therapies can be employed to effectively manage intraocular inflammation. With appropriate baseline screening for infectious diseases and periodic laboratory monitoring, these medications can be used safely over time. Consultations are required from other medical specialists in complex situations that are not limited to pregnancy, a history of tuberculosis, and in the setting of active systemic malignancies. Long term studies have shown that the use of systemic immunosuppressive agents for the treatment of non-infectious uveitis has better visual outcomes compared to the use of local corticosteroid treatments alone.

REFERENCES

1. Salazar-Méndez R, Yilmaz T, Cordero-Coma M. Moving forward in uveitis therapy: preclinical to phase II clinical trial drug development. Expert Opin Investig Drugs. 2016;25(2):195-214.
2. Tomkins-Netzer O, Talat L, Bar A, Lula A, Taylor SR, Joshi L, et al. Long-term clinical outcome and causes of vision loss in patients with uveitis. Ophthalmology. 2014;121(12):2387-92.

3. Guly GM, Forrester JV. Uveitis: a review. BMJ. 2010;341: c4976:821-6.
4. Jabs DA, Nussenblatt RB, Rosenbaum JT; Standardization of Uveitis Nomenclature (SUN) Working Group. Standardization of uveitis nomenclature for reporting clinical data. Results of the First International Workshop. Am J Ophthalmol. 2005;140(3):509-16.
5. Servat JJ, Mears KA, Black EH, Huang JJ. Biological agents for the treatment of uveitis. Expert Opin Biol Ther. 2012;12(3):311-28.
6. Jabs DA, Rosenbaum JT, Foster CS, Holland GN, Jaffe GJ, Louie S, et al. Guidelines for the use of immunosuppressive drugs in patients with ocular inflammatory disorders: recommendations of an expert panel. Am J Ophthalmol. 2000;130(4):492-513.
7. Huscher D, Thiele K, Gromnica-Ihle E, Hein G, Demary W, Dreher R, et al. Dose-related patterns of glucocorticoid-induced side effects. Ann Rheum Dis. 2009;68(7):1119-24.
8. Agrawal H, Doan H, Pham B, Khosla A, Babu M, McCluskey P, et al. Systemic immunosuppressive therapies for uveitis in developing countries. Indian J Ophthalmol. 2020;68(9):1852-62.
9. Cordero-Coma M, Calleja S, Llorente M, Rodríguez E, Franco M, Ruiz de Morales JG. Serum cytokine profile in adalimumab-treated refractory uveitis patients: decreased IL-22 correlates with clinical responses. Ocul Immunol Inflamm. 2013;21(3):212-9.
10. Lee FF, Foster CS. Pharmacotherapy of uveitis. Expert Opin Pharmacother. 2010;11(7):1135-46.
11. Maksymowych WP. Disease modification in ankylosing spondylitis. Nat Rev Rheumatol. 2010;6(2):75-81.
12. Dick AD, Tundia N, Sorg R, Zhao C, Chao J, Joshi A, et al. Guidance on noncorticosteroid systemic immunomodulatory therapy in noninfectious uveitis: Fundamentals Of Care for UveitiS (FOCUS) Initiative. Ophthalmology. 2018;125(5):757-73.
13. Foster CS, Kothari S, Anesi SD, Vitale AT, Chu D, Metzinger JL, et al. The Ocular Immunology and Uveitis Foundation preferred practice patterns of uveitis management. Surv Ophthalmol. 2016;61(1):1-17.
14. Agarwal R, Lee C, Phatak S, Pavesio C. Immunopharmacotherapy of non-infectious uveitis: where do we stand?. Expert Opin Biol Ther. 2014;14(12):1719-22.
15. Pasadhika S, Rosenbaum JT. Update on the use of systemic biologic agents in the treatment of noninfectious uveitis. Biologics. 2014;8:67-81.
16. Espinosa G, Muñoz-Fernández S, García Ruiz de Morales JM, Herreras JM, Cordero-Coma M. Document of treatment recommendations for non-infectious anterior uveitis. Med Clin (Barc). 2017;149(12):552.e1-12.
17. Gómez-Gómez A, Loza E, Rosario MP, Espinosa G, García-Ruiz de Morales JM, et al. Efficacy and safety of immunomodulatory drugs in patients with non-infectious intermediate and posterior uveitis, panuveitis and macular edema: A systematic literature review. Seminars in Arthritis and Rheumatism. 2020;50(6):1299-306.
18. Cordero-Coma M, Calleja S, et al. Efficacy and safety of immunomodulatory drugs in patients with anterior uveitis: a systematic literature review. Medicine (Baltimore). 2016;95(17):e3558.
19. Duru N, van der Goes MC, Jacobs JW, Andrews TJ, Boers M, Buttgereit F, et al. EULAR evidence-based and consensus-based recommendations on the management of medium to high-dose glucocorticoid therapy in rheumatic diseases. Ann Rheum Dis. 2013;72(12):1905-13.
20. Vegas-Revenga N, Martín-Varillas JL, Calvo-Río V, González-Mazón I, Sánchez-Bilbao L, Beltran E, et al. Intravenous methylprednisolone induces rapid improvement in non-infectious uveitis: a multicentre study of 112 patients. Clin Exp Rheumatol. 2022;40(1):142-9.
21. Rathinam SR, Gonzales JA, Thundikandy R, Kanakath A, Murugan S, Vedhanayaki R, et al. Effect of corticosteroid-sparing treatment with mycophenolate mofetil vs methotrexate on inflammation in patients with uveitis: a randomized clinical trial. JAMA. 2019;322(10):936-45.
22. Daniel E, Thorne JE, Newcomb CW, Pujari SS, Kaçmaz RO, Levy-Clarke GA, et al. Risk of hypotony in patients with uveitis: results from the Multicenter Uveitis Steroid Treatment (MUST) Trial and Follow-up Study. Am J Ophthalmol. 2010;149(3):423-32.e1-2.
23. Kacmaz RO, Kaçmaz RO, Kempen JH, Newcomb CW. Risk factors for cataract in uveitis. Ophthalmology. 2010;117(3):576-84.
24. Gangaputra S, Newcomb CW, Liesegang TL, Kaçmaz RO, Jabs DA, Levy-Clarke GA, et al. Risk of glaucoma in patients with uveitis: results from the MUST Trial and Follow-up Study. Ophthalmology. 2009;116(11):2188-98.e1.
25. Pasadhika S, Kempen JH, Newcomb CW, Liesegang TL, Pujari SS, Rosenbaum JT, et al. Ocular complications in patients with uveitis: results from the Systemic Immunosuppressive Therapy for Eye Diseases (SITE) Cohort Study. Am J Ophthalmol. 2009;148(4):500-9.e2.
26. Takeuchi M, Kezuka T, Sugita S, Keino H, Namba K, Kaburaki T, et al. Evaluation of the long-term efficacy and safety of infliximab treatment for uveitis in Behçet's disease: a multicenter study. Ophthalmology. 2014;121(10):1877-84.
27. Okada AA, Goto H, Ohno S, Mochizuki, Ocular Behçet's Disease Research Group of Japan. Multicenter study of infliximab for refractory uveoretinitis in Behçet's disease. Arch Ophthalmol. 2012;130(5):592-8.
28. Kruh JN, Yang P, Suelves AM, Foster CS. Infliximab for the treatment of refractory noninfectious uveítis: a study of 88 patients with long-term follow-up. Ophthalmology. 2014;121(1):358-64.
29. Artornsombudh P, Gevorgyan O, Payal A, Siddique SS, Foster CS. Infliximab treatment of patients with birdshot retinochoroidopathy.Ophthalmology. 2013;120(3):588-92.
30. Díaz-Llopis M, Salom D, Garcia-de-Vicuña C, Cordero-Coma M, Ortega G, Ortego N, et al. Treatment of refractory

uveitis with adalimumab: a prospective multicenter study of 131 patients. Ophthalmology. 2012;119(8):1575-81.
31. Shunyakova J, Patnaik JL, Xia J, Hassman LM, Pecen PE, Palestine AG, et al. Immunomodulatory Therapy Discontinuation for Reasons Other Than Efficacy in the Treatment of Ocular Inflammation. Ocul Immunol Inflamm. 2025:1-4.
32. Sakai T, Watanabe H, Kuroyanagi K, Akiyama G, Okano K, Kohno H, et al. Health- and vision-related quality of life in patients receiving infliximab therapy for Behçet's uveitis. Br J Ophthalmol. 2013;97(3):338-42.
33. Levy-Clarke G, et al. Expert panel recommendations for the use of immunosuppressive drugs in patients with ocular inflammatory disorders. Ophthalmology. 2014;121(4):785-96.
34. Diaz-Llopis M, Salom D, García-de-Vicuña C, Cordero-Coma M. Treatment of refractory uveitis with biologic agents. Survey of Ophthalmology. 2015;60(5):575-89.
35. Ossewaarde-van Norel J, Rothova A, Los LI, Berendschot TTJM. Long-term outcome of treatment with methotrexate for noninfectious uveitis. American Journal of Ophthalmology. 2012;154(2):233-9.
36. Cordero-Coma M, Calleja-Antolín S, Garzo-García I, Nuñez-Garnés AM, Álvarez-Castro C, et al. Adalimumab for treatment of noninfectious uveitis: immunogenicity and clinical relevance of measuring serum drug levels and antidrug antibodies. Ophthalmology. 2016;123(12):2618-25.
37. Espinosa G, Herreras JM, Muñoz-Fernández S, García Ruiz de Morales JM, Cordero-Coma M. Recommendations statement on the immunosuppressive treatment of non-infectious, non-neoplastic, non-anterior uveitis. Med Clin (Barc). 2020;155(5):220.e1-12.
38. Llorenç V, Serrano A, Mesquida M, Lin P, Esquinas C, Sainz-de-la-Maza M, Metea C, et al. Swept-source optical coherence tomography objective composite activity score for uveitis. Acta Ophthalmol. 2021;99(7):756-64.
39. Pato E, Martín-Martínez MA, Castelló A, Méndez-Fernández R, Muñoz-Fernández S, Cordero-Coma M, et al. Development of an activity disease score in patients with uveitis (UVEDAI). Rheumatol Int. 2017;37(4):647-56.
40. Tallouzi MO, Mathers JM, Moore DA, Bucknall N, Calvert MJ, Murray PI, et al. Development of a core outcome set for clinical trials in non-infectious uveitis of the posterior segment. Ophthalmology. 2021;128(8):1209-21.
41. Bradley LD, Ward A, Hsueh MCY, Liu J, Copland DA, Dick AD, et al. Quantitative assessment of experimental ocular inflammatory disease. Front Immunol. 2021:12:630022.
42. Sejournet L, Keverez S, Mathis T, Kodjikian L, Jamilloux Y, Seve P. Therapeutic drug monitoring guides the management of patients with chronic non-infectious uveitis treated with adalimumab: a retrospective study. Br J Ophthalmol. 2022;106(10):1380-6.
43. Calleja S, Cordero-Coma M, Rodriguez E, Llorente M, Franco M, Ruiz de Morales JG. Adalimumab specifically induces CD3+ CD4+ CD25^high^ Foxp3+ CD127− T-regulatory cells and decreases vascular endothelial growth factor plasma levels in refractory immuno-mediated uveitis: a non-randomized pilot intervention study. Eye (Lond). 2012;26(3):468-77.
44. Llorenç V, Mesquida M, Sainz de la Maza M, Adán A, Blanco-Fernández J, Calvo-Río V, et al. Drug retention rate and causes of discontinuation of adalimumab in uveitis: real-world data from the Biotherapies in Uveitis (BioÚvea) Study Group. Ophthalmology. 2020;127(6):814-25.
45. Sharma SM, Damato E, Hinchcliffe AE, Andrews CD, Mynit K, Lee R, Dick AD. Long-term efficacy and tolerability of TNFα inhibitors in the treatment of non-infectious ocular inflammation: an 8-year prospective surveillance study. Br J Ophthalmol. 2021;105(9):1256-62.
46. Haroon M, O'Rourke M, Ramasamy P, Murphy CC, FitzGerald O. A novel evidence-based detection of undiagnosed spondyloarthritis in patients presenting with acute anterior uveitis: the DUET (Dublin Uveitis Evaluation Tool). Ann Rheum Dis. 2015;74(11):1990-5.
47. van Bentum RE, Verbraak FD, Wolf S, Ongkosuwito J, Boers M, Tan HS, et al. High Prevalence of Previously Undiagnosed Axial Spondyloarthritis in Patients Referred With Anterior Uveitis and Chronic Back Pain: The SpEYE Study. J Rheumatol. 2022;49(7):680-7.
48. Daniel E, Pistilli M, Kothari S, Khachatryan N, Kacmaz RO, Gangaputra SS, et al. Risk of ocular hypertension in adults with noninfectious uveítis. Ophthalmology. 2017;124(8):1196-208.
49. Papaliodis GN, Rosner BA, Dreger KA, Fitzgerald TD, Artornsonbudh P, Kothari S, et al. Incidence of and risk factors for cataract in anterior uveítis. Am J Ophthalmol. 2023;254:221-32.
50. Kempen JH, Newcomb CW, Washington CL, Foster CS, Sobrin L, Thorne JE, et al. Use of immunosuppression and the risk of subsequent overall or cancer mortality. Ophthalmology. 2023;130(12):1258-68.
51. Writing committee for the multicenter uveítis steroid treatment (MUST) Trial and Follow-up study research group; Kempen JH, Altaweel MM, Holbrook JT, Sugar EA, Thorne JE, et al. Between long-lasting intravitreous fluocinolone acetonide implant versus systemic anti-inflammatory therapy and visual acuity at 7 years among patients with intermediate, posterior, or panuveitis. J Am Med Assoc. 2017;317(19):1993-2005.
52. Bui AD, Kong CL, Rathinam SR, Gonzales JA, Thundikandy R, Kanakath A, et al. Time to Uveitis Control with Methotrexate and Mycophenolate Mofetil. Ophthalmology. 2022;129(6):721-23.
53. Kempen JH, Daniel E, Gangaputra S, Dreger K, Jabs DA, Kaçmaz RO, et al. Methods for identifying long-term adverse effects of treatment in patients with eye diseases: the Systemic Immunosuppressive Therapy for Eye Diseases (SITE) cohort study. Ophthalmic Epidemiol. 2008;15(1):47-55.

54. Liu R, Cifuentes-Gonzales C, Gangputra S, Purera I, Rojas-Carabali W, La Distia Nora R, et al. A survey of diagnostic and anagement practices in retinal vasculitis: intermation uveítis study group (IUSG) retinal vasculitis study (ReViSe)-Report5. Ocul Immunol Inflamm. 2025;1-9.
55. Ruegg L, Pluma A, Hamroun S, Cecchi I. EULAR recommendations for use of antirheumatic drugs in reproduction, pregnanacy, and lactation: 2024 update. Ann Rheum Dis. 2025;84(6):910-26.
56. Pistilli M, Joffe MM, Gangaputra SS, Pujari SS, Jabs DA, Levy-Clarke GA, et al. Visual Acuity Outcome over Time in Non-Infectious Uveitis.Ocul Immunol Inflamm. 2021;29(6):1064-71.
57. Buchanich JM, Newcomb CW, Washington TL, Foster CS, Sobrin L, Thorne JE, et al. Use of immunosuppression and subsequent cáncer incidence: cohort study. BMJ Oncol. 2023;2(1):e000037.
58. Nguyen QD, Foster CS. Risk of vision loss in patients with uveitis. American Journal of Ophthalmology. 2000;129(5): 634-9.
59. Urban B, akunowicz-Łazarczyk A, Michalczuk M. Immune recovery uveitis: pathogenesis, clinical symptoms, and treatment. Mediators Inflamm. 2014;2014:971417.
60. Kempen JH, Daniel E, Dunn JP, Foster CS, Gangaputra S, Hanish A, et al. Overall and cancer mortality among patients with ocular inflammation treated with immunosuppressive drugs: the Systemic Immunosuppressive Therapy for Eye Diseases (SITE) cohort study. Ophthalmology. 2006; 113(4):684-94.
61. Hu J, Coassin M, Stewart JM. Fluocinolone acetonide implant (Retiset) for chronic cystoid macula edema in two patients with AIDS and a history of cytomegalovirus retinitis. Ocul Immunol Inflamm. 2011;19(3):206-9.
62. Rothova A, Ten Berge JCEM, Vingerling JR. Intravitreal aflibercept for treatment of macular oedema associated with immune recovery uveítis. Acta Ophthalmol. 2020;98(7):e922-3.
63. Sepah Y, Sadiq MA, Chu DS, Dacey M, Gallemore R, Dayani P, et al. Primary (Month-6) Outcomes of the STOP-Uveitis Study: Evaluating the Safety, Tolerability, and Efficacy of Tocilizumab in Patients With Noninfectious Uveitis. Am J Ophthalmol. 2017;183:71-80.
64. Akhavanrezayat A, Uludag Kirimli G, Matsumiya W, Khojasteh H, Or C, Karaca I, et al. The Role of Corticosteroids and Immunomodulatory Therapy in the Management of Infectious Uveitis. Ocul Immunol Inflamm. 2024;32(8):1832-43.
65. Jaffe GJ, Dick AD, Brézin AP, Nguyen QD, Thorne JE, Kestelyn P, et al. Adalimumab in Patients with Active Noninfectious Uveitis. N Engl J Med. 2016;375(10):932-43.
66. Sheppard J, Joshi A, Betts KA, Hudgens S, Tari S, Chen N, et al. Effect of Adalimumab on Visual Functioning in Patients With Noninfectious Intermediate Uveitis, Posterior Uveitis, and Panuveitis in the VISUAL-1 and VISUAL-2 Trials. JAMA Ophthalmol. 2017;135(6):511-8.
67. Leclercq M, Jacquot R, Charbonnier C, Desbois AC, Maalouf G, Touhami S, et al. Comparative Effectiveness of Intravenous versus Subcutaneous Tocilizumab for Refractory Uveitis: A Retrospective Analysis. Ophthalmology. 2025;132(10):1134-41.
68. Vegas-Revenga N, Calvo-Río V, Mesquida M, Adán A, Hernández MV, Beltrán E, et al. Anti-IL6-Receptor Tocilizumab in Refractory and Noninfectious Uveitic Cystoid Macular Edema: Multicenter Study of 25 Patients. Am J Ophthalmol. 2019;200:85-94.
69. Heissigerová J, Callanan D, de Smet MD, Srivastava SK, Karkanová M, Garcia-Garcia O, et al. Efficacy and Safety of Sarilumab for the Treatment of Posterior Segment Noninfectious Uveitis (SARIL-NIU): The Phase 2 SATURN Study. Ophthalmology. 2019;126(3):428-37.
70. Srivastava SK, Watkins TR, Nguyen QD, Sharma S, Scales DK, Dacey MS, et al. Filgotinib in Active Noninfectious Uveitis: The HUMBOLDT Randomized Clinical Trial. JAMA Ophthalmol. 2024;142(9):789-97.

NOTE FROM EDITORS

As an update, the editors recommend readers to go through the *Multimodal Imaging in Uveitis (MUV) Report No. 10*, which discusses the imaging measures for assessment of disease activity in non-infectious posterior uveitis. The full text is available to all, as the article is open access.

1. Agarwal A, Ramtohul P, Invernizzi A, Gangaputra S, Tsui E, Okada AA, Thorne JE, Smet MD, Bodaghi B, Pavesio C, Jabs DA, Sadda S, Sarraf D, Gupta V; MULTIMODAL IMAGING IN UVEITIS (MUV) TASKFORCE. Imaging Measures for the Assessment of Disease Activity in Noninfectious Posterior Uveitis - Multimodal Imaging in Uveitis (MUV) Taskforce: Report 10. Am J Ophthalmol. 2026 Mar 18;287:43-57. doi: 10.1016/j.ajo.2026.03.011. Epub ahead of print. PMID: 41861898.

CHAPTER 17

Local Therapy for Non-infectious Uveitis

Quan Dong Nguyen, Eugenia Ramos-Davila, Maria Carmela Saturno, Marc de Smet, Ngoc Trong Tuong Than, Jia-Horung Hung, Maggie Feng, Vishali Gupta, Reema Bansal, Alejandra de-la-Torre, John H Kempen, Meghan Berkenstock

INTRODUCTION

Local therapy for non-infectious uveitis is usually given as an adjunct with systemic treatment to prevent visual loss and structural damage from active intraocular inflammation. Rarely, when systemic drugs are contraindicated or poorly tolerated, local therapy becomes the mainstay of treatment. Various options for local therapy include corticosteroids (topical, periocular, intravitreal, and suprachoroidal), intravitreal anti-vascular endothelial growth factor (anti-VEGF) agents, methotrexate, and biologic agents. While the use of these medications prevents the development of systemic side effects and addresses compliance issues with a longer duration of action, they have the limitations of causing significant ocular complications.

THEMATIC LECTURE: PEARLS AND CLUES IN MANAGING A PATIENT WITH NON-INFECTIOUS UVEITIS WITH LOCAL THERAPY

When discussing therapeutic principles in the local management of uveitis, it is important to start with the route of administration, which includes topical, periocular, intravitreal, or suprachoroidal formulations. All of these agents can be used as primary therapy or adjunctive treatments with concurrent use of systemic corticosteroids or immunosuppressive medications. The goal of treatment is to reduce inflammation to a grade zero level (with no vitreous or anterior chamber cells) in order to preserve visual function and limit ocular comorbidities.[1] The traditional approach to achieve rapid control of immune-mediated inflammation using systemic medications includes starting an intravenous or oral corticosteroid with a taper to ≥7.5 mg/day to avoid the development of side effects.[2,3] Depending on the inflammatory disease process or if long-term control is needed, a non-corticosteroid immunosuppressive agent is started concurrently to facilitate the tapering of the corticosteroid. If there are contraindications to systemic immunosuppression or ocular comorbidities that have not resolved with systemic treatment, local therapy can be considered as an adjunctive option.

If we look specifically at local corticosteroids, there are several agents to choose from, as well as routes of administration. Beyond the sub-Tenon injection of 1 mL of triamcinolone (40 mg/mL), several intravitreal implants containing triamcinolone, dexamethasone, and fluocinolone at varying concentrations are available for use **(Fig. 1)**.[4] The newest addition to the local therapy armamentarium is the suprachoroidal triamcinolone formulation, which is delivered on a 30-gauge microneedle. Several trials have assessed the efficacy of each formulation, as noted in **Figure 1**. The Periocular versus Intravitreal Corticosteroids for Uveitic Macular Edema (POINT) trial showed the superiority of an intravitreal triamcinolone acetonide injection and the dexamethasone implant over the periocular injection of triamcinolone.[5] The efficacy of the surgical intravitreal fluocinolone implant was compared to systemic immunosuppressive agents for the treatment of vision-threatening, non-infectious intermediate uveitis, posterior uveitis, or panuveitis in the Multicenter Uveitis Steroid Treatment (MUST) trial.[3] Eyes that were randomized into the fluocinolone surgical implant group had higher rates of cataract formation, glaucoma, and ocular hypertension. At 7 years, the systemic treatment arm showed vision improvement of 7.1 letters. However, the (Retisert®) implant will no longer be manufactured after April 2026.

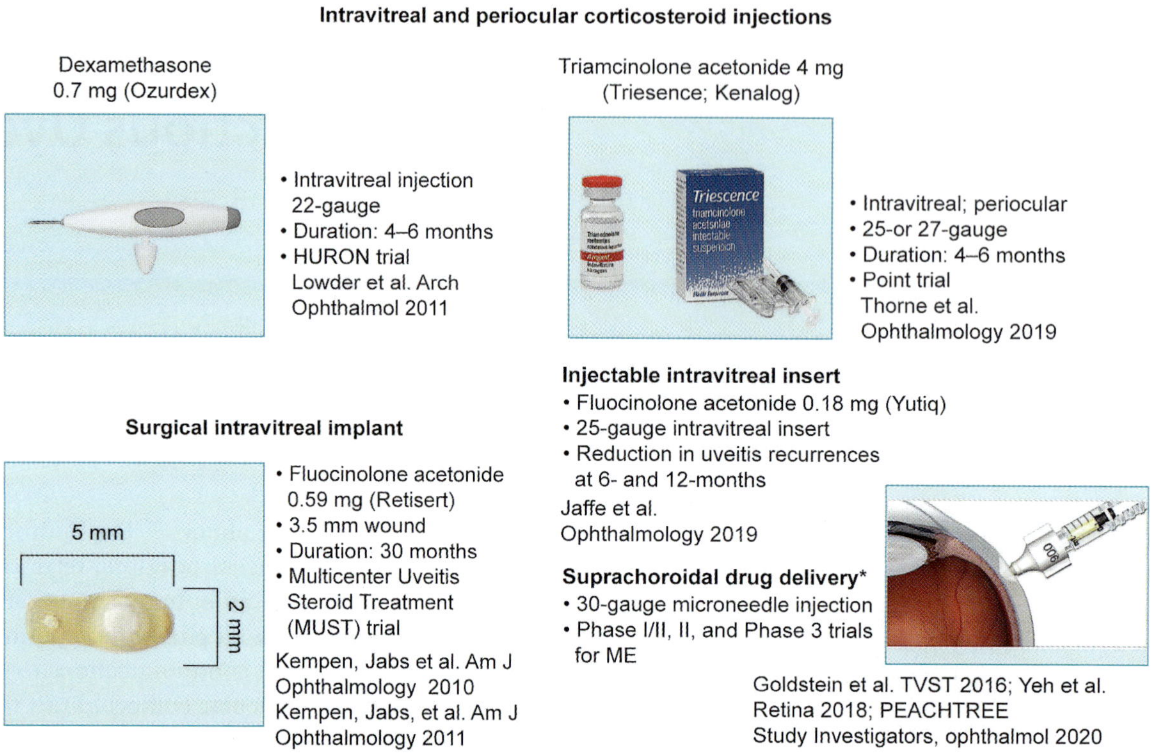

Fig. 1: A schematic showing local corticosteroid routes of administration and formulations available for use to treat non-infectious intermediate, posterior, and panuveitis or macular edema (ME).
Source: Uveitis Course - Grand Rounds 17. International Uveitis Study Group (IUSG). September 13, 2025. Available from: https://youtu.be/y3z7sP5bOUs?si=OWmVOWonkdVQ7nZC.

In addition to corticosteroids, there are several alternative anti-inflammatory drugs available for intravitreal injection to treat non-infectious uveitides. Varying doses of methotrexate, adalimumab, infliximab, complement inhibitors, and rituximab have been used in clinical trials. Intravitreal methotrexate has been used to treat intraocular lymphoma and may be a promising alternative to intravitreal corticosteroid injections, given the lack of an increased intraocular pressure response or cataract formation. Currently, studies have found that intravitreal methotrexate administered as a monotherapy may not be adequate to achieve remission, but rather can be used as an adjunctive treatment.[4] Based on the studies by Taylor and colleagues, Khalil and colleagues, and the Intravitreal Therapy for Uveitic Macular Edema- Ranibizumab versus Methotrexate versus the Dexamethasone Implant (MERIT) Trial (the first two studies showed favorable results but the MERIT Trial did not), intravitreal methotrexate has been used to treat cystoid macular edema and intermediate uveitis.[6-8] Another use has been in the treatment of paradoxical worsening of tubercular uveitis after the start of anti-tuberculosis therapies (ATT). However, corneal epitheliopathy may occur after intravitreal methotrexate injections and warrants close follow-up to assess for ocular surface changes.

We have learned from the VISUAL I and II studies that systemic adalimumab is effective in treating non-infectious intermediate, posterior, and panuveitis by decreasing the recurrence of inflammation.[9,10] It is currently used throughout the world as the only approved biologic for the treatment of non-infectious uveitis by several regulatory bodies. Systemic administration has been associated with the development of side effects and an increased risk of infection. What about intravitreal adalimumab? The first paper on the topic was published by Androudi and colleagues in 2010.[11] The case series showed that intravitreal adalimumab (0.5 mg/0.05 mL) was ineffective in reducing central retinal thickness or improving best-corrected visual acuity in patients with refractory uveitic macular edema. On the other hand, the paper by Hamam and colleagues showed efficacy of intravitreal adalimumab using a higher concentration.[12] Without a randomized control trial, the evidence is unclear on the appropriate dosing, effectiveness, and duration of effect.

What about intravitreal infliximab for the treatment of non-infectious uveitis? A paper from Markomichelakis and colleagues reported a prospective, non-comparative, interventional pilot study examining control of intraocular inflammation during an Adamantiades-Behçet disease-associated uveitis flare using a 1 mg/0.05 mL dose.[13] The best corrected visual acuity improved, and the anterior chamber and vitreous cell levels decreased. However, cystoid macular edema persisted in 9 of 11 affected eyes. While no adverse events were reported in the study, the development of retinal toxicity or autoantibody formation, which was reported previously by Giganti and colleagues, were not assessed.[14] More studies are needed to understand the pathophysiology of the retinal toxicity, even at 0.05 mg doses. For this reason, intravitreal administration of infliximab is not currently used.

In addition to controlling of intraocular inflammation, local therapies can be used to treat macular edema, which causes vision loss in up to 41% of patients with uveitis.[15,16] Whether in combination with systemic immunosuppressives or as a single agent, local therapy can treat uveitic macular edema that may persist despite the control of inflammation in 50% of eyes. In the MUST trial, 62% of eyes treated systemically required regional corticosteroid injections for macular edema.[17] Furthermore, uveitic macular edema can occur with each anatomic subtype. The pathophysiology includes several factors, including the production of inflammatory cytokines, the chronic breakdown of the inner and outer blood-retinal barriers, and tractional vitreomacular adhesions. In a large series of 842 eyes (529 patients with uveitis) by Lardenoye and colleagues, 33% developed macular edema, with a higher risk associated with older age, chronic inflammation, and certain uveitides: Birdshot chorioretinitis, Adamantiades-Behçet disease-associated uveitis, and sarcoidosis.[18] The study also reported macular edema as the leading cause of visual impairment or blindness in cases of intermediate uveitis or posterior uveitis. Additional risk factors identified from the current medical literature include male sex, retinal vascular inflammation, and drug-associated macular edema with the use of tamoxifen and fingolimod, the latter of which is hypothesized to be inflammatory in origin.

How does the use of local corticosteroid therapy compare to the use of systemic immunosuppressive agents? Taking a closer look at the 7-year MUST trial data, the primary outcome measure, best corrected visual acuity, was better in the systemic treatment arm.[3] However, the treatment exposure was not balanced over the 7-year follow-up with the fluocinolone group receiving <2 implants on average. The finding raised the question if sufficient treatment was administered in the fluocinolone group, although a large minority of eyes never relapsed after implant therapy, and many participants declined re-implantation. The MUST trial showed that while both arms were effective, the fluocinolone implant was more effective at controlling early inflammation and macular edema , but its effectiveness diminished over time as the availability of fluocinolone lessened. Specific to the fluocinolone implant group, there was an increased rate of cataract, glaucoma, and ocular hypertension.

The next study that needs to be discussed is the POINT trial.[5] As alluded to previously, it was a multicenter trial with 1:1:1 randomization to periocular triamcinolone acetonide, intravitreal triamcinolone acetonide, and the intravitreal dexamethasone implant. The key takeaway was that the intravitreal delivery of triamcinolone or dexamethasone were superior in decreasing the central retinal thickness at 8 weeks compared to periocular administration. This effect was observed through the 24-week follow-up period, and in the safety analysis, intraocular pressures were similar across all groups, over six months' follow-up.

Another briefly mentioned study was the MERIT trial, which was a randomized, head-to-head comparison of intravitreal methotrexate, intravitreal ranibizumab, and the intravitreal dexamethasone implant for the treatment of uveitic macular edema.[6] Intravitreal methotrexate was not effective compared to ranibizumab, which showed a mild decrease in central retinal thickness but without improvement in the best visual acuity. The dexamethasone group showed a statistically greater reduction in central retinal thickness and a statistically significant improvement in visual acuity. This advocates for a large study with adequate power, rather than individual case series.

Flowchart 1 shows an algorithm for treating uveitic macular edema prepared by James P. Dunn of the Wills Eye Hospital, that outlines the complexity of treatment.[19] By assessing the location of the inflammation, the presence of a choroidal neovascular membrane, and disease activity can provide therapeutic direction.

When considering the use of local versus systemic therapy, consider if the etiology is infectious or if there

Flowchart 1: An algorithm outlining macular edema treatment strategies based on the anatomic location of inflammation, disease activity, and the presence of choroidal neovascularization.

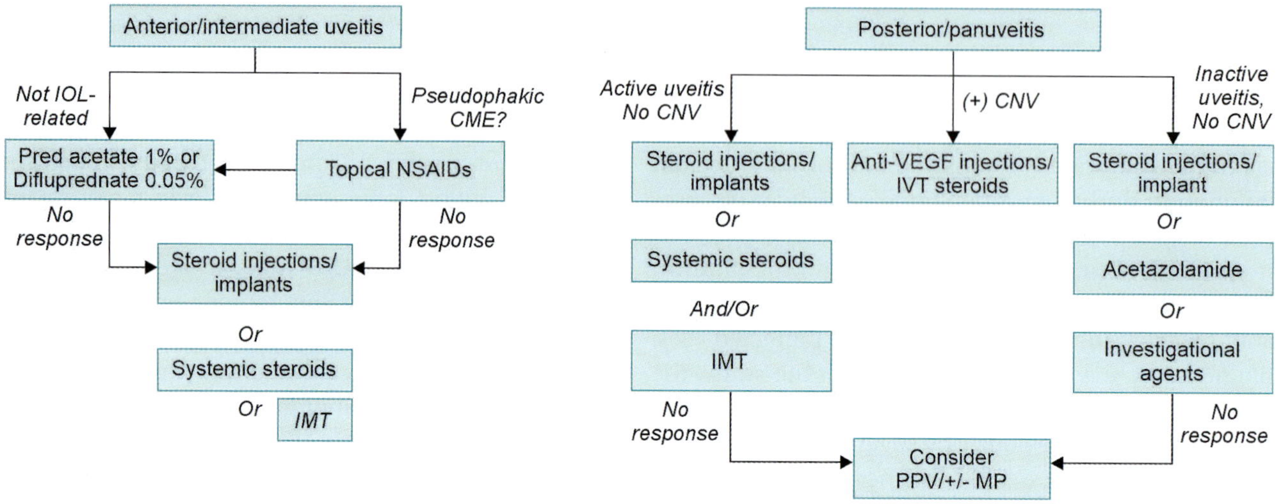

(CME: cystoid macular edema, IOL: intraocular lens, Pred: prednisolone, NSAIDs: non-steroidal anti-inflammatory drugs, IMT: immunosuppressive therapy, PPV: pars plana vitrectomy, MP: membrane peel, Anti-VEGF: anti-vascular endothelial growth factor, CNV: choroidal neovascular membrane, IVT: intravitreal)

Source: Uveitis Course - Grand Rounds 17. International Uveitis Study Group (IUSG). September 13, 2025. Available from: https://youtu.be/y3z7sP5bOUs?si=OWmVOWonkdVQ7nZC.

is the presence of an underlying systemic disease. Avoid injection of a corticosteroid or other anti-inflammatory agent intravitreally or via a periocular route in the setting of an active ocular infection. The exception is for control of inflammation during paradoxical worsening after the initiation of ATT (only if oral corticosteroid treatment is not feasible). The presence of an underlying inflammatory disease requiring treatment, or bilateral ocular involvement, should favor the use of systemic therapy to address inflammation across all affected organs.

Several trials are ongoing that assess the effectiveness of new agents for the local treatment of non-infectious uveitis. In addition to uveitic macular edema, the treatment of post-surgical macular edema requires discussion. There is an unmet need for such treatment, as macular edema is still the leading cause of post-operative vision loss in patients with uveitis. The challenge is that there are no established treatment guidelines for post-surgical macular edema, and some cases are refractory to all current therapies. In a paper by Shulman and colleagues, topical dexamethasone cyclodextrin eye drops (OCS-01) were shown to be effective in treating macular edema.[20] OCS-01 is a formulation of dexamethasone coated by a cyclodextrin nanoparticle, which is hydrophilic and increases the penetration of the lipophilic molecule into the anterior chamber. The same investigational product was studied in the DIAMOND study, a Phase 3, double-masked, randomized, control trial, showed a significant decrease in central retinal thickness and an increase in best corrected visual acuity in patients with diabetic macular edema.[21] This was the first time that a topical-based formulation demonstrated efficacy in treating diabetic macular edema. Based on these results, the Uveitis Division at the Byers Eye Institute at Stanford University is the lead location conducting the multicenter LEOPARD study to assess the change in both uveitic and post-surgical macular edema using OCS-01. The primary endpoints are central subfield thickness reduction on optical coherence tomography (OCT) at week 12 compared with baseline and the mean change in ETDRS best-corrected visual acuity letter score at week 12.

Another agent currently in clinical trials is the interleukin-6 (IL-6) inhibitor, vamikibart. The STOP-Uveitis trial was the first randomized trial to assess the effectiveness of this class of pharmacologic agents, specifically the systemic administration of tocilizumab, in treating non-infectious uveitis and uveitic macular edema.[22] Subsequently, Vamikibart was developed a localized version. It is a recombinant, fully humanized IgG2 monoclonal antibody engineered for intravitreal delivery to block both cis and trans-signaling pathways. Adverse events are limited, given the lower systemic exposure and rapid systemic clearance with a half-life of 7 days. Intravitreal vamikibart is currently under investigation in another clinical trial for the treatment of diabetic macular edema. The topline results of both of these Phase 3, randomized, double-masked, sham-controlled studies, MEERKAT and SANDCAT, will be presented next month at the 2025 American Academy of Ophthalmology meeting in Orlando, Florida. Two other IL-6 inhibitors to mention are KSI-501 and KSI-101. These are bispecific, antibody-biopolymer conjugates that target both IL-6 and VEGF receptors. The cumulative result is inhibition of angiogenesis and normalization of the inner and outer blood-retinal barriers with greater effect than with administration of either agent alone. Currently intravitreal KSI-501 is in clinical trial for both diabetic macular edema and macular edema secondary to inflammation.

The final agent that will be discussed is laquinimod. It is the first synthetic small molecule immunomodulator to target the aryl hydrocarbon receptor on antigen-presenting cells.[23] Administration skews the immune response toward an anti-inflammatory phenotype, and the LION study is an open-label, prospective, single-center Phase 1 trial of the safety, tolerability, and distribution of the drug in an eyedrop formulation over 2 weeks. Phase 2 and 3 studies of the oral formulation of laquinimod for the treatment of multiple sclerosis revealed a favorable safety and tolerability profile with significant decreases in relapses as an endpoint. These studies raised the question if laquinimod could provide anti-inflammatory treatment for uveitis. Could it penetrate the anterior chamber or even into the vitreous? Based on the current preliminary results from the LION study, there is a dose-dependent reduction in the anterior chamber cell. Enrolled subjects had normal eye pressures and underwent a pars plana vitrectomy for an unrelated condition. Subjects were divided into three different daily dose levels (0.6, 1.2, and 1.8 mg) with instillation for 14 days prior to surgery. In short, we questioned if a topical solution of laquinimod led to a sufficient concentration in the vitreous humor. With increasing dose strength, concentration increased linearly in both the anterior chamber and the vitreous. Even with topical delivery, low levels were identified in the plasma. The safety profile was also favorable across the three doses. The LION study supports further investigation of the therapeutic potential of laquinimod for the treatment of uveitis and other ocular inflammatory diseases.

There remains a substantial need for well-controlled, randomized, prospective studies to evaluate emerging local therapeutic options for non-infectious uveitis and uveitic macular edema. Future studies will examine the effectiveness of new IL-6 inhibitors, TNF-alpha inhibitors, and JAK-1 inhibitors. Local therapies, including intravitreal or topical formulations of adalimumab, laquinimod, and perhaps OCS-01, may have a role in treating uveitis and macular edema in the future. These agents will provide a therapeutic approach that combines local and systemic treatments to reduce inflammation and achieve complete quiescence.

USE OF TOPICAL STEROIDS

Case Presentation

Personal Data

A 41-year-old male presented with an acute onset of redness, pain, and photophobia in the right eye.

History of Present Illness

The symptoms started 2 days prior. He had no past medical history; however, there was a maternal history of rheumatoid arthritis. The review of systems was positive for chronic low back pain, which he associated with a mechanical injury.

Physical Examination

The best corrected visual acuity was 20/40 in the right eye and 20/20 in the left eye. The anterior chamber of the right eye contained 4+ cells, a hypopyon, and posterior synechiae at 3 o'clock **(Fig. 2)**. Examination of the left eye was unremarkable.

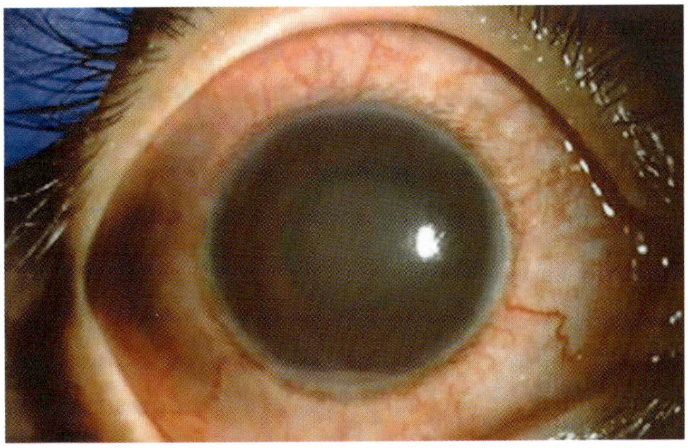

Fig. 2: An external photograph of the right eye showing conjunctival injection and the presence of a hypopyon in the anterior chamber.
Source: Uveitis Course - Grand Rounds 17. International Uveitis Study Group (IUSG). September 13, 2025. Available from: https://youtu.be/y3z7sP5bOUs?si=OWmVOWonkdVQ7nZC.

TABLE 1: Slit lamp examination of a patient having acute onset redness, pain, and photophobia in the right eye.

OD	Parameter	OS
20/40	BCVA	20/20
14 mm Hg	IOP	12 mm Hg
Normal	Lids/Lashes	Normal
2+ injection	Conjunctiva	White and quiet
Inferior fine KPs	Cornea	Clear
4+ cells, 2+ flare with a 1-mm hypopyon	Anterior chamber	Deep and quiet
Synechiae at 3 o'clock	Iris	Normal
Clear	Lens	Clear
0.4	Optic nerve	0.4
Normal	Vitreous	Normal
Normal	Fundus	Normal

(BCVA: best corrected visual acuity; IOP: intraocular pressure; KPs: keratic precipitates)

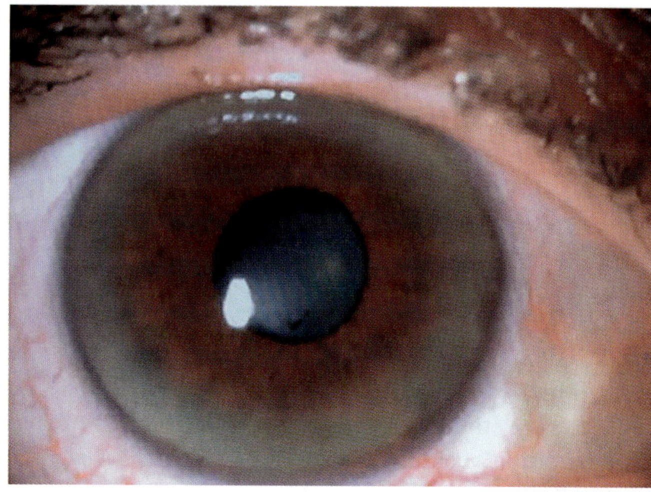

Fig. 3: An external photograph of the right eye 1 month after treatment showing resolution of the hypopyon and posterior synechiae. Residual pigment can be seen on the anterior lens capsule.

Source: Uveitis Course - Grand Rounds 17. International Uveitis Study Group (IUSG). September 13, 2025. Available from: https://youtu.be/y3z7sP5bOUs?si=OWmVOWonkdVQ7nZC.

Slit lamp examination: Slit lamp examination is discussed in **Table 1**.

Ancillary testing: A retinal OCT scan of the macula showed no signs of cystoid macular edema and a very mild epiretinal membrane in the right eye.

Uveitis workup: A laboratory work-up was sent that included testing for the human leukocyte antigen (HLA)-B27 antigen, reverse sequence testing for syphilis via Treponema pallidum antibodies followed by non-specific testing, and a chest X-ray to assess for sarcoidosis.

Initial treatment: A weekly taper of prednisolone acetate 1% was prescribed starting with one drop every hour while awake for 1 week followed by decrements of one eye drop per week. Atropine 1% twice a day for 2 weeks was added due to the presence of a significant amount of flare and synechiae formation.

Follow-up: One month later, there was moderate improvement in the patient's symptoms, but discomfort persisted in the right eye. The laboratory work-up was positive for the HLA-B27 antigen. Despite the use of prednisolone acetate 1% three times a day, there were still inferior, fine keratic precipitates on the corneal endothelium and 2+ anterior chamber cells. The synechiae were broken leaving pigment on the anterior capsule **(Fig. 3)**.

Given persistent inflammation after a prednisolone acetate 1% taper, the patient was switched to difluprednate 0.05% starting four times a day for a week in the right eye with weekly decrements. A referral to rheumatology was placed to assess for systemic manifestations associated with HLA-B27 positivity. A month later, he had decreased the difluprednate 0.05% to once a day in his right eye and was asymptomatic. A rheumatologic evaluation revealed no spondyloarthritis, and the vision in the right eye had improved to 20/20. Throughout the clinical course, the intraocular pressure remained normal and at the last visit, the anterior chamber remained quiet. The patient stopped the difluprednate drops without a recurrence of the anterior uveitis. However, the average recurrence rate in patients with acute anterior uveitis associated with HLA-B27 positivity is approximately one episode per year.[24,25] He continues to return every 6–12 months for re-evaluation and has been reminded to return sooner if new symptoms develop.

Discussion

The route of administration of local corticosteroids is based on the anatomic location of the inflammation. Topical therapy, in the form of eye drops, is effective for inflammation limited to the anterior chamber and the anterior vitreous. Periocular corticosteroid injections, including periocular and sub-Tenon, can be used to deliver a depot in patients that cannot administer drops reliably or in patients who have developed cystoid macular edema. The mainstay of corticosteroid eye drop treatment is prednisolone acetate 1%. Always remind patients that it is a suspension, which requires shaking prior to use. An alternative is difluprednate 0.05%, which has a fluorinated chemical structure to enhancing penetration into the vitreous humor. In a study by Sheppard and colleagues, difluprednate was found to be twice as potent as prednisolone acetate 1%.[26] Thus, difluprednate can be useful to reduce the number of times a corticosteroid drop needs to be taken during a taper. It can also treat either cystoid macular edema or intermediate uveitis, in which the inflammation is mostly in the anterior vitreous.

In addition to the site of inflammation, you also need to choose the correct formulation. In the United States, insurance companies have drug formularies with preferred agents that are covered to steer prescriptions toward a particular topical agent. Prednisolone sodium phosphate 1% is covered by several payors, but the phosphate base will limit penetration through the corneal interface when compared to prednisolone acetate 1%. Similarly, fluorometholone avoids causing a corticosteroid-induced increase in the intraocular pressure.[27] These pharmacokinetic properties limit the use of both agents in the treatment of anterior chamber inflammation. If a patient has a history of corticosteroid response, consider loteprednol 0.5%, which effectively treats anterior chamber inflammation with less of an impact on the intraocular pressure based on the presence of an ester at C-20 on the hydrocarbon backbone.[28]

While corticosteroids are potent and inexpensive, their side effects are considerable and include cataracts, glaucoma, secondary infections, and delayed wound healing in the post-operative period. Most adverse events can be managed with additional prophylaxis for secondary infections, close monitoring of intraocular pressures with a low threshold for adding anti-glaucoma medications, and assessment of lens status at each follow-up.[29]

No clinician wants to create a more serious problem than the initial condition for which the patient presented. In an amblyogenic-age-range child, monitor the lens status and refractive error.[30] If you notice a change or if other local side effects develop, transition to corticosteroids-sparing immunosuppressive therapy is warranted.[31,32] In short, topical administration of corticosteroids plays a large role in controlling inflammation centered anteriorly in the eye and avoids the plethora of systemic side effects of oral corticosteroids, which include premature closure of the epiphyses, thinning of the skin, hyperglycemia, and hyperlipidemia. However, it has increased local therapy risks, especially for cataract and elevated intraocular pressure.

Inadequately treated intraocular inflammation can lead to the development of ocular complications. Severe cases of inflammation require immediate use of high dose corticosteroids at the treatment onset. Do not to be reluctant to prescribe an adequate corticosteroid dose for fear of side effects. Allowing inflammation to smolder to lower intraocular pressure, or avoiding more frequent dosing to prevent a rise in intraocular pressure, can lead to a protracted taper at doses higher than acceptable.[33] Alternatively, continued inflammation can lead to a failure to achieve quiescence and the development of chronic sequelae including peripheral anterior synechiae and glaucoma. As noted in children with chronic anterior uveitis, even a long-term, moderate dose of a corticosteroid can result in cataract when administering >2 drops of prednisolone acetate 1% per day.[30] While tapering as fast as possible should be part of the treatment strategy, using the correct corticosteroid formulation and completely quieting the inflammation should be the first goal.

So how do we taper topical corticosteroids? Wait until complete quiescence is achieved, as starting a taper while it is only beginning to improve or stabilize can prolong the inflammation.[30] Have a zero tolerance for cells or macular edema. Specifically ask the patient, what happens if you miss a dose? Most patients will forget at least one drop administration and if that missed dose is enough to allow symptoms to return, then it is too soon to taper. In this case, slow the taper and reassess for residual inflammation in the anterior chamber or macular edema on OCT testing.

Another point is to taper to the lowest potency corticosteroid formulation. A traditional corticosteroid taper is by one-drop decrement per week. If the taper starts with difluprednate drops, a switch to prednisolone acetate 1% can be made if ophthalmic side effects occur. Similarly, a switch allows return to the specific drop previously used for maintenance therapy. Again, adjust the taper speed based on the cell grade and flare, with close follow-up every few weeks. Also, remember that children have a robust inflammatory response. If there is chronic inflammation, the patient likely has had long standing disease, and it may take longer for a medication to have an effect. Slow tapers reduce the total number of drops the patient takes and avoid prescribing repeated tapers that can lead to rebound inflammation after each discontinuation. Taking fewer drops also decreases the overall cost and exposure to preservatives that can lead to ophthalmic sequelae, including dry eyes and other ocular surface conditions. Finally, do not be afraid of maintenance dosing.[30] This is a common issue that we see at a tertiary referral center, where the long-term goal prior to referral was to taper off corticosteroids. However, not every patient can taper off corticosteroid drops and may require staying at a low dose of two or fewer drops of prednisolone acetate 1% per day to prevent flares.

What if side effects start to occur at the current dose or you cannot taper to two drops or less per day? Then you need to think about starting corticosteroid-sparing systemic immunosuppressive agents. Based on data from the Systemic Immunosuppressive Therapy for Eye Diseases (SITE) Cohort Study, the mean annual incidence rates for ocular hypertension with a pressure over 21 mm Hg or over 30 mm Hg were 14% and a 5% per eye per year, respectively.[34] Statistically significant risk factors for a pressure over 30 mm Hg included the presence of anterior chamber cells, a history of ocular hypertension or use of intraocular pressure-lowering drops, surgery in the other eye for uncontrolled pressures, and topical corticosteroid use greater than eight times a day. Collectively, the data provide ample reasons to control anterior chamber inflammation, lower the intraocular pressure if it increases, and taper the corticosteroid drops as quickly as possible.

Data supporting the use of two or fewer drops of prednisolone acetate 1% per day as a maintenance dose to lower ocular complications was published by Thorne and colleagues.[30] The risk of cataract was independently associated with topical corticosteroid use in children with non-infectious, juvenile idiopathic arthritis-associated uveitis. Those taking two or fewer drops per day had a 0 per eye-year incidence of cataract formation. Hence if three drops of prednisolone acetate 1% are required for maintenance dosing, then start considering the initiation of a systemic agent. The SITE study showed a similar result, but in subjects using prednisolone acetate 1% at two or more drops per day, there was a higher incidence of cataract.[31,32] Interestingly, the use of oral prednisone at a dose of ≥7.5 mg/day or topical corticosteroid drops administered less than two times per day were not associated with an increased risk of cataract development.

Beyond cataracts in children, you need to be mindful of elevated intraocular pressure. The SITE study showed that those taking two to three drops of prednisolone acetate 1% per day had a two to three-fold increase in the incidence of elevated intraocular pressures.[35] When the dose increased to four or more drops per day, the risk of elevated intraocular pressures was nine-fold higher. In contrast, the use of systemic immunosuppressive therapies or ≥7.5 mg of prednisone daily was not associated with a higher risk of presenting with an elevated intraocular pressure. Subjects taking ≥7.5 mg of prednisone per day had a similar risk to subjects not taking oral corticosteroids. Overall, the incidence of any observed intraocular pressure elevation to ≤21 mm Hg or ≤30 mm Hg were 33.4% and 14.8%, respectively.

Corticosteroid use in pregnancy is another topic that we encounter with young female patients. Corticosteroid eye drops are listed as a category C due to a lack of well-controlled studies. Intraocular pressure often falls during pregnancy, which may provide a protective effect against the intraocular pressure-raising effects of topical corticosteroids.[36] Oral corticosteroid use has been associated with an increased risk of birth defects in lab animals, but there are no human studies that have demonstrated this from topical administration.[37]

Finally, another commonly encountered issue associated with insurance coverage is the use of brand versus generic corticosteroid drop formulations. While generic medications are cheaper, they may be less effective. While generic drugs contain the same active ingredient as their brand-name equivalents, they are not required to produce identical therapeutic outcomes. There can be differences in solubility, penetration, pH, and bottle-tip design that affect the effectiveness of a generic topical corticosteroid.[38-41] If a flare occurs in a patient with previously well-controlled disease, ask if they recently changed from a trade to a generic formulation.

In summary, the risk of ocular hypertension and uveitic glaucoma with topical corticosteroid use increases in a dose-dependent relationship. On average, there is no increased risk of elevated intraocular pressure with the use of oral prednisone at doses of 7.5 mg or less per day. There is no increased risk of elevated intraocular pressure with daily prednisolone acetate 1%, but the risk progressively increases with increased frequency of use. Patients with uveitis should be assessed not only for ocular hypertension, but for cataract development at each visit. If there is uncontrolled inflammation or the development of ocular complications, initiate systemic corticosteroid and immunosuppressive therapies.

INTRAVITREAL THERAPY FOR NONINFECTIOUS UVEITIS

Case Presentation

Case 1

Personal data: A 25-year-old woman developed a slight, bilateral decrease in visual acuity.

History of present illness: Symptoms began started 3 months prior. She had no prior medical history.

Physical examination: The best corrected visual acuity was 20/25 in the right eye and 20/60 in the left eye. The anterior chambers contained no cells or flare. However, the posterior poles contained multiple, well-defined, hypopigmented lesions, and a choroidal neovascular membrane in the left eye **(Fig. 4)**.

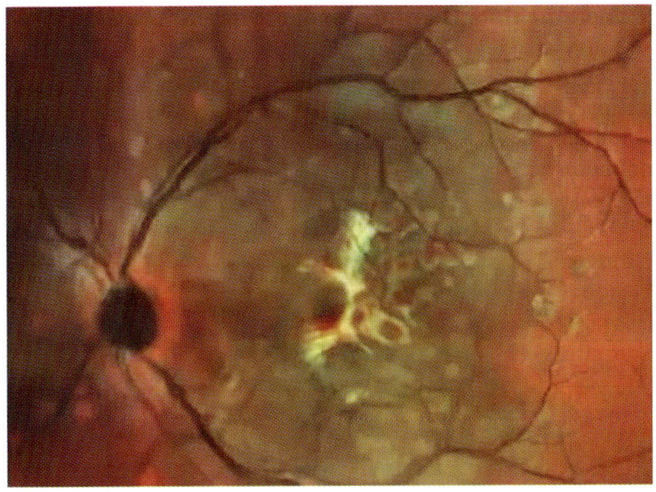

Fig. 4: A Heiderlberg tricolor fundus photo of the left eye showing a macular scar with the development of a choroidal neovascular membrane.
Source: Uveitis Course - Grand Rounds 17. International Uveitis Study Group (IUSG). September 13, 2025. Available from: https://youtu.be/y3z7sP5bOUs?si=OWmVOWonkdVQ7nZC.

Slit lamp examination ***(Table 2):*** Slit lamp examination is discussed in **Table 2**.

TABLE 2: Slit lamp examination of a patient having noninfectious uveitis.

OD	*Parameter*	*OS*
20/25	BCVA	20/60
13 mm Hg	IOP	12 mm Hg
Normal	Lids/Lashes	Normal
White and quiet	Conjunctiva	White and quiet
Clear	Cornea	Clear
Deep and quiet	Anterior chamber	Deep and quiet
Normal	Iris	Normal
Clear	Lens	Clear
Normal	Vitreous	Normal
Multiple well-defined hypopigmented chorioretinal lesions	Fundus	Multiple well-defined hypopigmented chorioretinal lesions, a macular scar with active choroidal neovascular (CNV) membrane

(BCVA: best corrected visual acuity; IOP: intraocular pressure)

Ancillary testing: Multimodal imaging was performed, beginning with fluorescein angiography, which showed multiple, hypofluorescent lesions with surrounding hyperfluorescent staining in both eyes. Late leakage within the macula from the choroidal neovascular membrane (CNV) was noted in the left eye **(Fig. 5)**. Indocyanine green angiography showed hypocyanescent lesions in the choroid with pinpoint surrounding areas of hypercyanescence **(Fig. 6)**. OCT scans of the left eye revealed hyper-reflective subretinal material **(Fig. 7)**, which confirmed the presence of an active CNV.

Uveitis workup: Serologic testing for systemic infectious and inflammatory disorders were negative, including syphilis, tuberculosis, and sarcoidosis.

Initial treatment: Based on the clinical examination and the imaging results, a working diagnosis of punctate inner choroidopathy (PIC) was made and the patient refused systemic therapy. For treatment of the CNV, 3 monthly intravitreal injections of ranibizumab were administered.

Follow-up: 2 months after the last injection, she presented with reactivation of the CNV in the left eye. However, she remained steadfast in her decision to not start systemic therapy. The decision was made to perform an intravitreal injection of 400 mg of methotrexate (0.1 mL). Over the subsequent 20 months, the visual acuity returned to 20/25 in the left eye without the recurrence of a flare.

This case illustrates why intravitreal therapy can be an alternative treatment strategy in patients with uveitis. Due to the ocular anatomy, intravitreal administration can lead to higher local drug concentrations, minimize systemic side effects, and it is useful when the disease is unilateral or asymmetric.[42] Finally, it is an option for a patient that declines systemic therapy. Besides uncontrolled

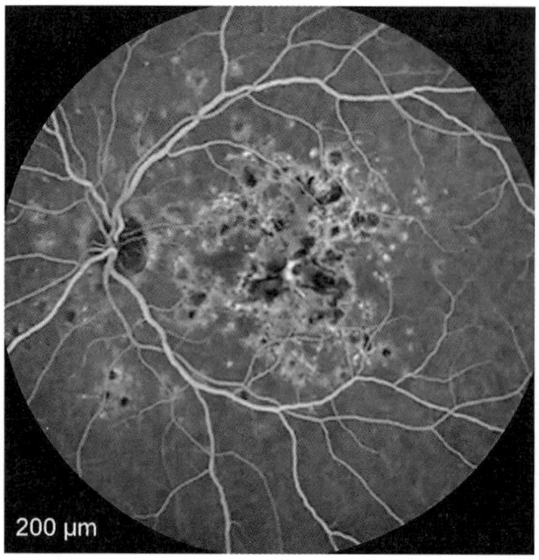

Fig. 5: A late phase fluorescein angiogram of the left eye showing multiple hypofluorescent lesions with hyperfluorescent borders and leakage in the macula from the choroidal neovascular membrane.
Source: Uveitis Course - Grand Rounds 17. International Uveitis Study Group (IUSG). September 13, 2025. Available from: https://youtu.be/y3z7sP5bOUs?si=OWmVOWonkdVQ7nZC.

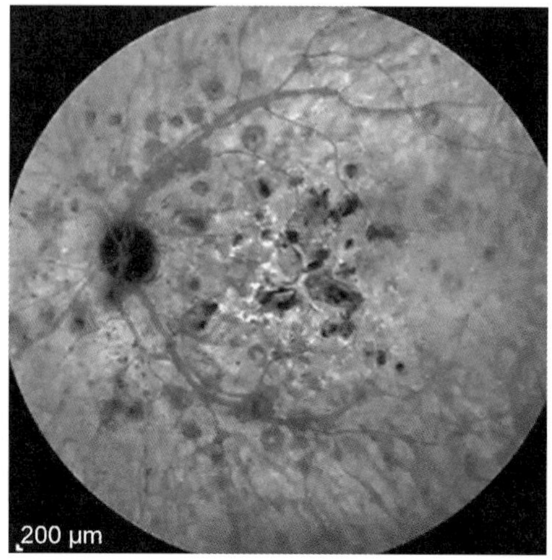

Fig. 6: An indocyanine green angiogram showing hypocyanescent lesions in the choroid with pinpoint surrounding areas of hypercyanescence.
Source: Uveitis Course - Grand Rounds 17. International Uveitis Study Group (IUSG). September 13, 2025. Available from: https://youtu.be/y3z7sP5bOUs?si=OWmVOWonkdVQ7nZC.

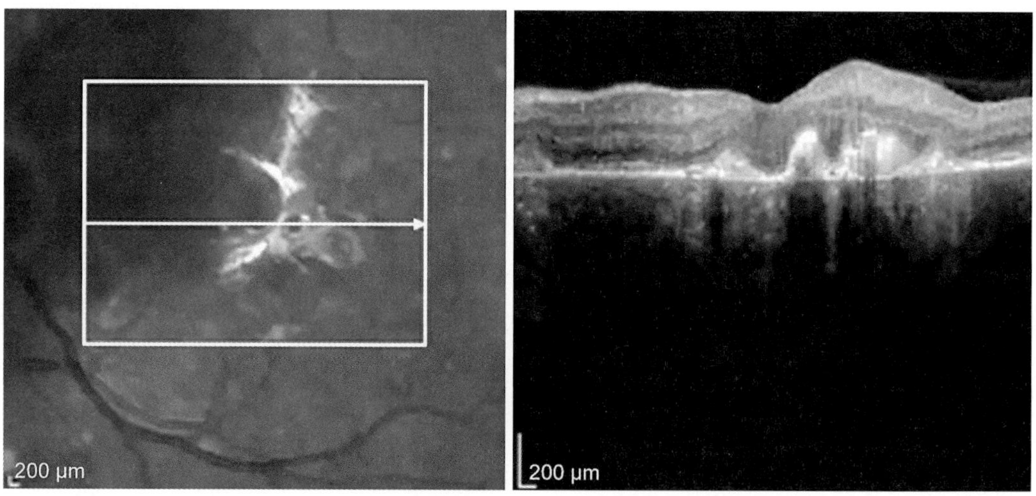

Fig. 7: An optical coherence tomography (OCT) scan through the macula of the left eye showing hyperreflective subretinal material suggestive of a choroidal neovascular membrane.
Source: Uveitis Course - Grand Rounds 17. International Uveitis Study Group (IUSG). September 13, 2025. Available from: https://youtu.be/y3z7sP5bOUs?si=OWmVOWonkdVQ7nZC.

intraocular inflammation, intravitreal drug delivery (typical corticosteroid depots or implants) can treat the most common complications of uveitis, which are CNV and cystoid macular edema. Specifically, the pathogenesis of a CNV is related to several factors—genetic, damage to the outer retina, choriocapillaris ischemia, or uncontrolled intraocular inflammation.[43]

As seen in **Figures 8A and 8B**, the main diagnoses associated with the development of an inflammatory CNV are PIC and multifocal choroiditis. While reported prevalences vary by the disease state, the location and morphology of the inflammatory CNV are important to note. Not only can a subfoveal CNV form, but extrafoveal and peripapillary areas can be affected **(Table 3).**[44]

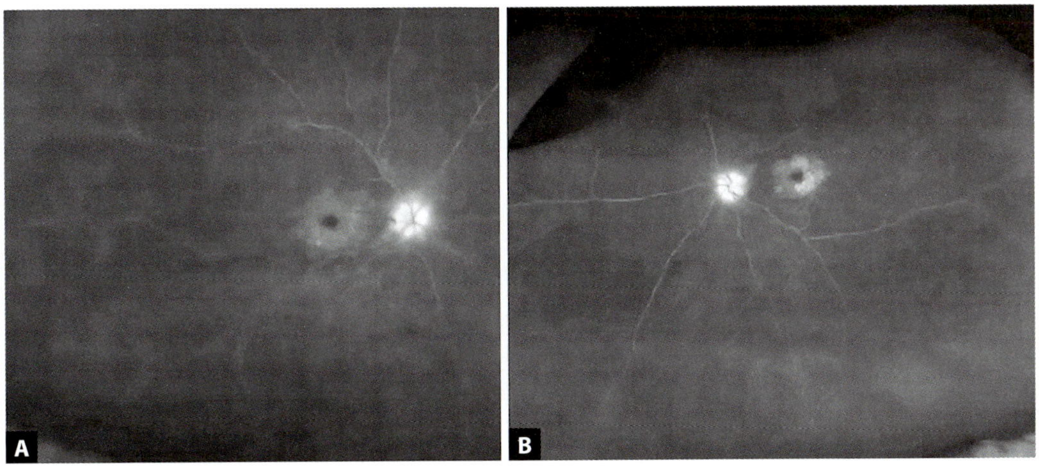

Figs. 8A and B: A fluorescein angiogram of the right (A) and left (B) eyes showing late optic disc, macular, and small vessel leakage.
Source: Uveitis Course - Grand Rounds 17. International Uveitis Study Group (IUSG). September 13, 2025. Available from: https://youtu.be/y3z7sP5bOUs?si=OWmVOWonkdVQ7nZC.

TABLE 3: Prevalence, location, and morphology of choroidal neovascular membranes by several conditions affecting the posterior pole.

	Multifocal choroiditis	***Punctate inner choroidopathy***	***Serpiginous choroiditis***	***Vogt-Koyanagi-Harada disease***
Prevalence	14% cases	71% cases	1.4% cases	2.4%
Location of choroidal neovascular membrane (CNV)	Associated with inflammatory lesions in the subfoveal or extrafoveal region	Highly focal; associated with inflammatory lesions in the macula	CNV is located near chorioretinal lesions in peripapillary, subfoveal, or extrafoveal areas	Usually extrafoveal; can be subfoveal and associated with a chorioretinal scar
Morphology	CNV appear as subretinal elevations and subretinal fluid with or without associated hemorrhage, closely resembling inflammatory lesions	CNV appear as subretinal elevations and subretinal fluid with or without hemorrhage, closely resembling inflammatory lesions	CNV lesions are deep with associated chorioretinal fibrosis and pigment clumping	CNV lesions are deep, associated with subretinal or intraretinal fluid, with hemorrhage and exudation

Source: Uveitis Course - Grand Rounds 17. International Uveitis Study Group (IUSG). September 13, 2025. Available from: https://youtu.be/y3z7sP5bOUs?si=OWmVOWonkdVQ7nZC.

Treatment strategies include using an anti-VEGF medication alone or in combination with systemic immunosuppressive therapies.[44,45] Alternatively, intravitreal corticosteroid and intravitreal immunosuppressive agents can be administered. As noted in **Table 4**, Servillo et al. summarized the results of several studies that assessed the efficacy of anti-VEGF therapy in treating inflammatory CNVs.[43] While some studies found an improvement of visual acuity and a reduction of central macular thickness, others only reported visual acuity stabilization.

Managing inflammation should be the mainstay of treating inflammatory CNVs, as we know that several proinflammatory cytokines, such as IL-1 and IL-6, lead to greater secretion of VEGF by the retinal pigment epithelial cells.[46] Several papers have shown data that the addition of systemic corticosteroid therapy can improve visual outcomes, reduce the incidence and the recurrence of inflammatory CNVs, and decrease the number of required anti-VEGF injections. In the same way, systemic immunosuppressants started early in the disease course reduce the occurrence and the recurrence of inflammatory CNVs.

What about intravitreal corticosteroids? They are an older drug class that not only decreases inflammation but also reduces VEGF production. However, usage is limited by the development of intraocular side effects. Some

TABLE 4: Intravitreal antivascular endothelial growth factor treatments used to treat inflammatory choroidal neovascular membranes by study with the associated follow-up times and the total number of injections.

Study (design)	*Type of uveitis (number of eyes)*	*Group compared/anti-VEGF agent (number of eyes injected)*	*Outcomes*	*Follow-up*	*Injections (range)*
Tran et al. 2008 (retrospective)	PIC/iMFC (6) SC (2) SO (1) VKH (1)	Bevacizumab (10)	VA ↑ 0.62–0.45 logMAR CMT ↓ 326–267 µm	7.5 months	2.5 (1–4)
Cornish et al. 2011	PIC/iMFC (9)	Bevacizumab (6) Ranibizumab (3)	VA ↑ 0.26 LogMar	14.9 months	2.34 (1–6)
Iannetti et al. 2013 (retrospective)	Posterior uveitis (6) Panuveitis (2)	Bevacizumab (8)	VA ↑ 0.57 ± 0.17–0.30 ± 0.28 LogMar CMT ↓ from 402.8 ± 114.1 – 300.5 ± 91 µm	19.2 months	3.75 (3–6)
Barth et al. 2018 (retrospective)	PIC/iMFC (15)	Bevacizumab (13) Ranibizumab (2)	VA improvement in 8/16 eyes VA stabilization in 4/16 eyes	15 months	3.5 (1–9)
Menezo et al. 2010 (retrospective)	PIC/iMFC (10)	Ranibizumab (9) Switch from ranibizumab to bevacizumab (1)	VA stabilization in 9/10 eyes	12.5 months	1.9 (1–5)

(VEGF: vascular endothelial growth factor; PIC: punctate inner choroidopathy; iMFC: idiopathic multifocal choroiditis; SC: serpiginous choroiditis; SO: sympathetic ophthalmia; VKH: Vogt-Koyanagi-Harada disease; VA: visual acuity; CMT: central macular thickness; logMAR: log10(minimum angle of resolution)

Source: Uveitis Course - Grand Rounds 17. International Uveitis Study Group (IUSG). September 13, 2025. Available from: https://youtu.be/y3z7sP5bOUs?si=OWmVOWonkdVQ7nZC.

previous studies have combined immunosuppressants or intravitreal corticosteroid and intravitreal anti-VEGF injections with clinical resolution of the CNV.[47-52] As Dr Nguyen alluded to earlier, an area for further research is the use of intravitreal injection of non-corticosteroid immunosuppressants. Only one paper reported a good response with the use of intravitreal methotrexate to treat an inactive inflammatory CNV. However, there are promising results in animal models where the incidence of endophthalmitis and ocular hypertension are less with injection of intravitreal methotrexate into rabbit eyes compared to intravitreal corticosteroid administration.[42] In human studies, the anti-inflammatory effect of intravitreal methotrexate has been studied in subjects with Behçet disease complicated by refractory retinal vasculitis.[53] Results showed high tolerability, even in those with a history of corticosteroid response. Overall, 86% of subjects showed an improvement in visual acuity, while 57% had a decrease in retinal vascular leakage on fluorescein angiography. Concurrently, there was a reduction of IL-6 and IL-8 levels in the aqueous humor compared to pretreatment levels.

Sirolimus, a macrolide antibiotic, has also been studied for intravitreal injection given its anti-inflammatory properties through preventing Th1 and Th17 T-cell differentiation.[54] In vitro studies have shown sirolimus decreases endothelial cell proliferation and VEGF secretion in retinal pigment epithelial cells. Alternatively, Sirolimus as a Therapeutic Approach for Uveitis (SAVE), was an open label, randomized, prospective study that assessed the in vivo efficacy of 352 µg of sirolimus administered intravitreally or 1,320 µg subconjunctivally in patients with intermediate, posterior, or panuveitis. Injections were performed at 0, 60, and 120 days with a primary endpoint of a two-step reduction in vitreous haze with 70% of these patients achieving this reduction by 12 months without serious adverse events reported.[54]

Case 2

Personal data: A 72-year-old male developed a bilateral decrease in visual acuity.

History of present illness: The change in vision occurred shortly after the cataract surgery. He had a past medical

TABLE 5: Slit lamp examination of a patient having bilateral decrease in visual acuity.

OD	***Parameter***	***OS***
20/60	BCVA	20/60
12 mm Hg	IOP	13 mm Hg
Normal	Lids/Lashes	Normal
White and quiet	Conjunctiva	White and quiet
Clear	Cornea	Clear
Deep and quiet	Anterior chamber	Deep and quiet
Normal	Iris	Normal
Posterior chamber intraocular lens	Lens	Posterior chamber intraocular lens
Normal	Vitreous	Normal
Macular edema	Fundus	Macular edema

(BCVA: best corrected visual acuity; IOP: intraocular pressure)

history of low vitamin D levels and diverticulitis requiring a colostomy 2 years prior. He was treated with a dexamethasone implant with only a transient response.

Physical examination: The best corrected visual acuity was 20/60 in both eyes. The anterior chambers contained no cells or flare. However, the posterior poles showed macular edema on biomicroscopy.

Slit lamp examination: Slit lamp examination is discussed in **Table 5**.

Ancillary testing: Multimodal imaging was performed starting with fluorescein angiography, which showed late optic disc, small-vessel, and macular leakage **(Fig. 8)**. OCT scans of both maculas showed the presence of subretinal fluid and cystoid macular edema **(Fig. 9)**.

Uveitis workup: Serologic testing for syphilis was negative.

Initial treatment: The patient was started on a combination of systemic and intravitreal therapies: mycophenolate 1 g twice a day and intermittent dexamethasone 0.7 mg intravitreal injections during flares.

In summary, an intravitreal anti-VEGF injection is the first-line therapy to treat an inflammatory CNV. However, managing the underlying inflammation is essential to control an inflammatory CNV. Intravitreal therapy provides effective control of inflammation while minimizing systemic side effects. While there are promising results with the use of non-corticosteroid immunosuppressant medications administered intravitreally, the clinical evidence is still limited.

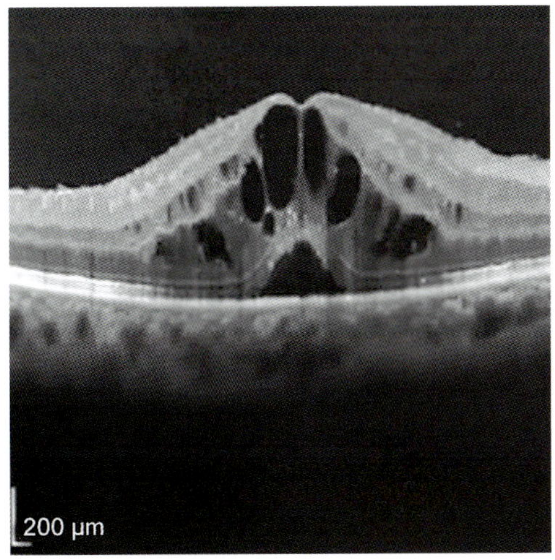

Fig. 9: An optical coherence tomography (OCT) scan of the right eye through the macula showing the presence of subretinal fluid and cystoid macular edema.
Source: Uveitis Course - Grand Rounds 17. International Uveitis Study Group (IUSG). September 13, 2025. Available from: https://youtu.be/y3z7sP5bOUs?si=OWmVOWonkdVQ7nZC.

Discussion

Many new treatments that are currently in clinical trials will provide additional therapies for future use. Maximizing the patient's systemic health can also be beneficial for treating the underlying inflammation. In this case, the patient had very low vitamin D levels as a side effect of his intestinal surgeries. Several studies have shown low vitamin D levels lead to a pro-inflammatory state, and most recently, have been associated with an increased risk of developing proliferative vitreoretinopathy in patients with retinal detachments.[55,56] We added daily vitamin D supplementation in addition to starting mycophenolate mofetil for immunosuppression. Once vitamin D supplementation is started, the treatment goal is not only to return levels to the normal range but also to achieve the highest levels within the therapeutic range. In contrast, the first case was more difficult to treat after the patient refused systemic immunosuppression. Since her disease was not severe with multiple ocular complications, intravitreal methotrexate was effective in controlling the inflammation. This highlights that the development of an inflammatory CNV can be treated through intravitreal therapy alone provided that the treatment is not an anti-VEGF agent alone. While an anti-VEGF agent will treat early neovascularization, a CNV is a secondary phenomenon of inflammation. As discussed, treatment of the inflammation with systemic corticosteroids and immunosuppressive medications can at least decrease the risk of CNV recurrence by 50% and achieve faster resolution.[50,51] An increase in immunosuppression dosing is also needed if a new CNV develops, as it is a marker of continued inflammation.

SUPRACHOROIDAL CORTICOSTEROID INJECTION CASES

Case Presentation

Case 1

Personal information: A 62-year-old male with chronic macular edema in the left eye presented for a repeat evaluation.

History of present illness: He failed multiple prior therapies, including oral prednisone with the return of macular edema when the dose was tapered. Both corticosteroids and non-steroidal anti-inflammatory (NSAID) drops had minimal effects. Similarly, only a partial response was achieved using oral acetazolamide.

Physical examination: While the anterior chamber was quiet, there was macular edema in the left eye only.

Slit lamp examination: Slit lamp examination is discussed in **Table 6**.

Ancillary testing: An OCT of the macula showed cystoid macular edema and subretinal fluid in the left eye **(Fig. 10)**.

Uveitis workup: Prior serologic testing for syphilis was negative.

Initial treatment: Since the patient wanted to taper off prednisone and the macular edema was unilateral, the decision was made to use a local treatment. A triamcinolone acetonide suprachoroidal injection was performed. This is an office-based procedure, and the medication is provided in a kit that includes a syringe, medication vial, and two microneedles. Normally, the injection is attempted with the 900 microneedle but often changing to the 1,100 microneedle is required. Topical anesthetics can be used, but subconjunctival lidocaine provides better analgesia. Both appropriate anesthesia and slow injection are key to delivering the medication into the small, potential suprachoroidal space.

Follow-up: Only 1 day after the injection, nearly all of the macular edema resolved **(Figs. 11 and 12)**. The remaining edema was secondary to epiretinal membrane formation.

TABLE 6: Slit lamp examination of a patient having chronic macular edema in the left eye.

OD	Parameter	OS
20/20	BCVA	20/30
13 mm Hg	IOP	20 mm Hg
Normal	Lids/lashes	Normal
White and quiet	Conjunctiva	White and quiet
Clear	Cornea	Clear
Deep and quiet	Anterior chamber	Deep and quiet
Normal	Iris	Normal
2+ Nuclear sclerosis	Lens	2+ nuclear sclerosis
Normal	Vitreous	Normal
Normal	Fundus	Cystoid macular edema

(BCVA: best corrected visual acuity; IOP: intraocular pressure)

There was no recurrence over the following year, and the best corrected visual acuity improved to 20/20 without an elevation in the intraocular pressure.

Case 2

Personal data: A 60-year-old female presented for evaluation of continued macular edema in the right eye.

History of present illness: She had already undergone a vitrectomy for a retinal detachment, and the macular edema was refractory to several local therapies including a sub-Tenon triamcinolone injection, an intravitreal bevacizumab injection, an intravitreal fluocinolone implant, and multiple intravitreal dexamethasone implants, which showed a transient improvement for only 2 months prior to a recurrence.

Physical examination: The best corrected visual acuity was 20/200 in the right eye and 20/20 in the left eye. On biomicroscopy, the vitreous was surgically absent in the right eye and there was continued macular edema noted.

Slit lamp examination: Slit lamp examination is discussed in **Table 7**.

Ancillary testing: An OCT of the macula showed cystoid macular edema and subretinal fluid in the right eye **(Fig. 11)**.

Uveitis workup: Prior serologic testing for syphilis was negative.

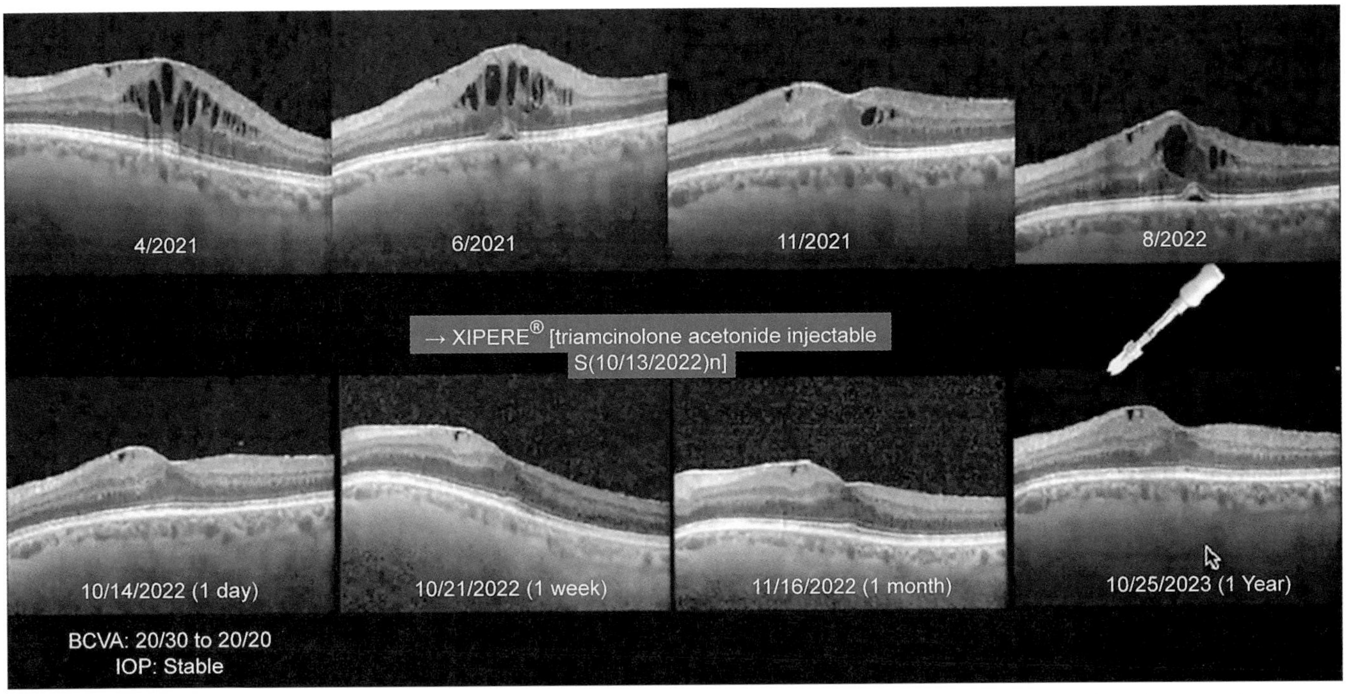

Fig. 10: A montage image of optical coherence tomography (OCT) scans showing continued cystoid macular edema in the left eye through the macula prior to the administration of suprachoroidal triamcinolone (superior) and after the injection (inferior).
Source: Uveitis Course - Grand Rounds 17. International Uveitis Study Group (IUSG). September 13, 2025. Available from: https://youtu.be/y3z7sP5bOUs?si=OWmVOWonkdVQ7nZC.

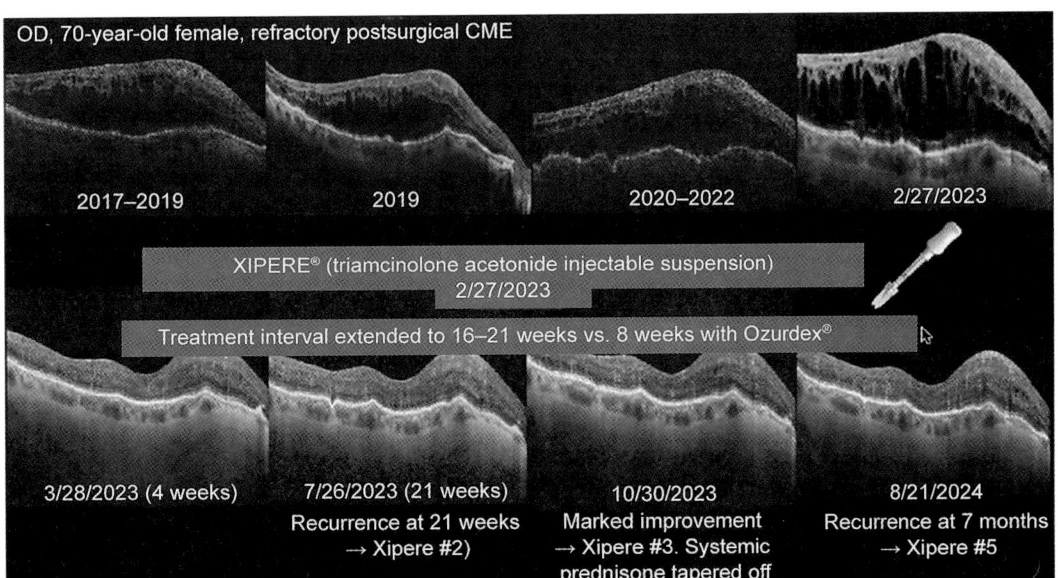

Fig. 11: A montage image of continued cystoid macular edema in the right eye on optical coherence tomography (OCT) scans through the macula prior to the administration of suprachoroidal triamcinolone (superior) and after the injection (inferior).
Source: Uveitis Course - Grand Rounds 17. International Uveitis Study Group (IUSG). September 13, 2025. Available from: https://youtu.be/y3z7sP5bOUs?si=OWmVOWonkdVQ7nZC.

Initial treatment: Given that the intravitreal fluocinolone implant (0.19 mg) was insufficient to treat the chronic macular edema, a suprachoroidal triamcinolone injection was planned.

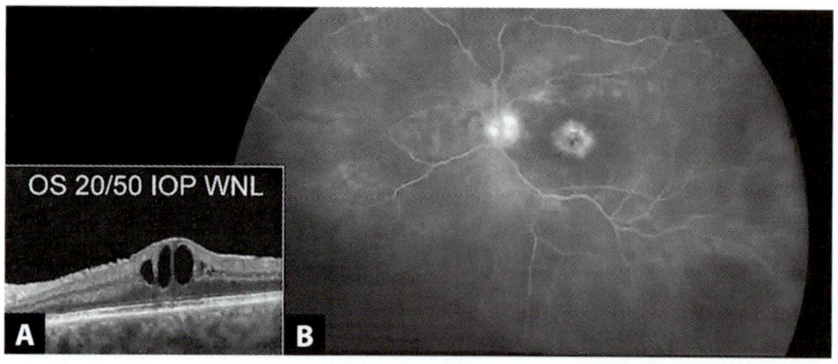

Figs. 12A and B: A late phase fluorescein angiography image of the left eye showing optic disc and macular leakage with small vasculitis (B). An optical coherence tomography (OCT) scan of the macula of the left eye (A) showed the presence of cystoid macular edema.
Source: Uveitis Course - Grand Rounds 17. International Uveitis Study Group (IUSG). September 13, 2025. Available from: https://youtu.be/y3z7sP5bOUs?si=OWmVOWonkdVQ7nZC.

TABLE 7: Slit lamp examination of a patient having macular edema in the right eye.

OD	*Parameter*	*OS*
20/200	BCVA	20/20
21 mm Hg	IOP	11 mm Hg
Normal	Lids/Lashes	Normal
White and quiet	Conjunctiva	White and quiet
Clear	Cornea	Clear
0.5+ cell, no flare	Anterior chamber	Deep and quiet
Normal	Iris	Normal
Posterior chamber intraocular lens	Lens	1+ nuclear sclerosis
Absent, dexamethasone implant inferiorly	Vitreous	Normal
Cystoid macular edema	Fundus	Normal

(BCVA: best corrected visual acuity; IOP: intraocular pressure)

Follow-up: The macular edema resolved but ultimately recurred and required reinjection every 16–21 weeks, which is longer than the prior 8-week interval required with the dexamethasone implant **(Fig. 11)**. She had an improvement in the best corrected visual acuity and there was no intraocular pressure elevation.

Case 3

Personal data: A 79-year-old female presented for re-evaluation for sclerokeratitis complicated by peripheral ulcerative keratitis in the left eye.

TABLE 8: Slit lamp examination of a patient having sclerokeratitis complicated by peripheral ulcerative keratitis in the left eye.

OD	*Parameter*	*OS*
20/25	BCVA	20/50
9 mm Hg	IOP	8 mm Hg
Normal	Lids/lashes	Normal
White and quiet	Conjunctiva	White and quiet
Clear	Cornea	Peripheral opacity with pannus (inactive temporal peripheral ulcerative keratitis)
Deep and quiet	Anterior chamber	Deep and quiet
Normal	Iris	Normal
Posterior chamber intraocular lens	Lens	Posterior chamber intraocular lens
Normal	Vitreous	Normal
Flat	Fundus	Cystoid macular edema

(BCVA: best corrected visual acuity; IOP: intraocular pressure)

History of present illness: She had a past medical history of rheumatoid arthritis refractory to multiple systemic immunosuppressive therapies, including methotrexate and etanercept. She finally achieved control of the arthritis and the sclerokeratitis with the start of rituximab. A diagnosis of osteoporosis limited use of high-dose corticosteroids. She had also developed chronic macular edema that was refractory to treatment with topical NSAIDs, topical dorzolamide, oral prednisone, and oral acetazolamide.

Physical examination: The best corrected visual acuity was 20/25 in the right eye and 20/50 in the left eye. On biomicroscopy, the peripheral ulcerative keratitis was inactive, and both eyes were white and quiet. Continued macular edema was noted in the left eye.

Slit lamp examination: Slit lamp examination is discussed in **Table 8**.

Ancillary testing: On fluorescein angiography, there was late optic disc and macular leakage with small vessel vasculitis in the left eye **(Fig. 12)**. On OCT scans of the macula of the left eye, there was the presence of cystoid macular edema **(Fig. 12)**.

Uveitis workup: Prior serologic testing for syphilis was negative.

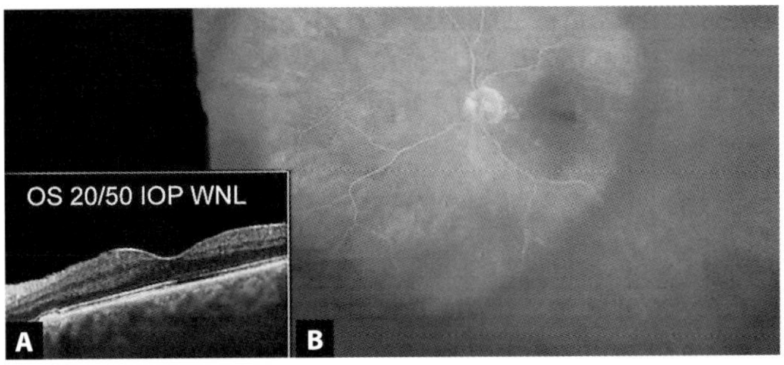

Figs. 13A and B: A late phase fluorescein angiography image of the left eye showing resolution of the optic disc and macular leakage (B). There is also no retinal vascular leakage. An optical coherence tomography (OCT) scan of the macula of the left eye (A) showed resolution of the cystoid macular edema.
Source: Uveitis Course - Grand Rounds 17. International Uveitis Study Group (IUSG). September 13, 2025. Available from: https://youtu.be/y3z7sP5bOUs?si=OWmVOWonkdVQ7nZC.

Initial treatment: Again, the suprachoroidal triamcinolone injection was a suitable option since her systemic disease was controlled and the inflammation was restricted to the posterior pole in one eye.

Follow-up: After one suprachoroidal triamcinolone injection, the macular edema, optic disc leakage, and retinal vasculitis resolved with no recurrence for over 1 year **(Figs. 13A and B)**.

Discussion

Uveitic macular edema can be treated with periocular triamcinolone acetonide injections (typically 40 mg in 1 mL); intravitreous triamcinolone acetonide injections (preservative free is best; typically 4 mg in 0.1 mL); intraocular implants such as the dexamethasone pellet (Ozurdex) or fluocinolone acetonide 0.18 or 0.19 mg implants. Biologics with IL-6 inhibiting activity and interferons also have good effect. Regarding intraocular treatments, the The PeriOcular vs. INTravitreal corticosteroids for uveitic macular edema (POINT) Trial[5] demonstrated that both intravitreous triamcinolone acetonide and the dexamethasone pellet were superior to periocular injections of triamcinolone acetonide 40 mg without detectably higher side effects within the limitations of only six months' follow-up. The subsequent Macular Edema Ranibizumab versus Intravitreal Anti-inflammatory Therapy Trial (MERIT) Trial demonstrated that the dexamethasone pellet was superior to both methotrexate and ranibizumab, and that methotrexate had no appreciable effect on vision, whereas ranibizumab's was very small.

The newest route of corticosteroid administration is into the suprachoroidal space.[57] This technique prevents the systemic side effects associated with oral corticosteroids and provides penetration to the posterior pole, unlike most topical agents. Periocular and sub-Tenon injections have variable drug diffusion across the sclera, and the corticosteroid depot may actually accumulate under the conjunctiva and not within Tenon's capsule. Intravitreal corticosteroid injections are an excellent way to control uveitis; however, drug delivery into the vitreous may lead to anterior segment side effects, which include cataract and elevated intraocular pressures. Finally, subretinal injection is possible, but highly invasive.

How can we deliver a drug into the suprachoroidal space? There are two methods. One is catheter-based infusion, which is not yet commercially available at the time of publication.[58,59] The other is via a microneedle injection, as seen in **Figure 14**. Suprachoroidal triamcinolone injection was approved by the United States Food and Drug Administration (FDA) in 2021 under the trade name, Xipere®. The proprietary micro-injector system creates a path into the suprachoroidal space, which is a potential space that when opened, allows for equal diffusion of the drug throughout the posterior pole.

When choosing approaches to treat macular edema, the clinician should first make sure that all infectious etiologies have been ruled out. Then he/she should review previous therapies and assess patient risk factors, including underlying systemic diseases requiring treatment or ocular conditions such as end-stage glaucoma. The clinician should control the inflammation and consider the start of immunosuppression early in the disease course. The first treatment is starting topical drops, which are either NSAIDs or difluprednate, as mentioned previously. If cases are unilateral and have mild to moderate inflammation, then he/she should consider treatment with intravitreal corticosteroids. In cases where cystoid macular edema or inflammation are refractory to this route of administration, the clinician can consider using a suprachoroidal triamcinolone injection.

The pivotal trial for FDA approval of the suprachoroidal triamcinolone injection was the Phase 3 PEACHTREE study with the subsequent follow-up or extension studies: AZALEA and MAGNOLIA, respectively.[60-62] Additional studies of suprachoroidal triamcinolone include the Tanzanite study, which evaluated the need for repeat aflibercept injections when used in combination versus aflibercept alone for the treatment of macular edema secondary to a retinal vein occlusion.[63]

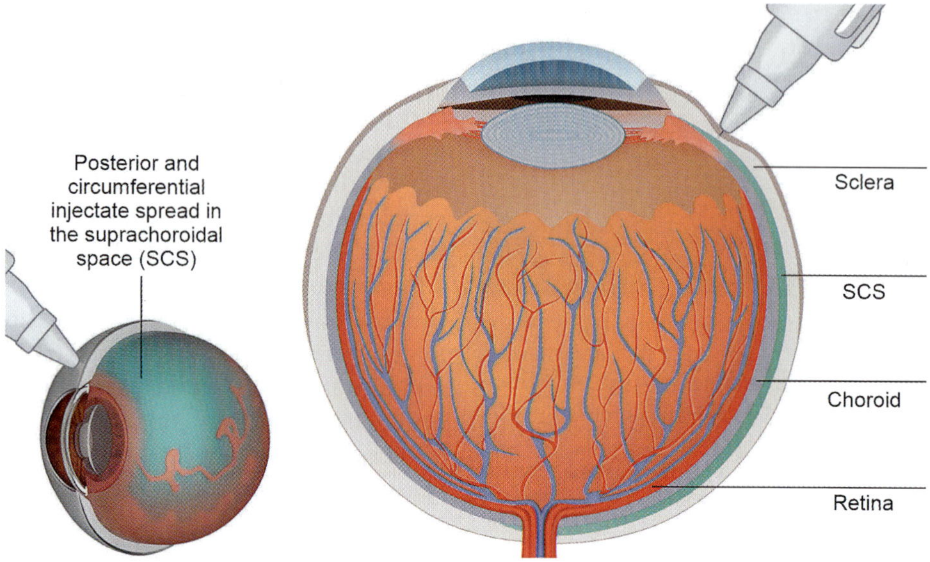

Fig. 14: A schematic drawing showing the temporal placement of the microneedle to inject triamcinolone into the suprachoroidal space. *Source:* Uveitis Course - Grand Rounds 17. International Uveitis Study Group (IUSG). September 13, 2025. Available from: https://youtu.be/y3z7sP5bOUs?si=OWmVOWonkdVQ7nZC.

In the PEACHTREE study, suprachoroidal triamcinolone was compared to sham injections in a masked, randomized fashion.[60] Suprachoroidal triamcinolone was injected on day zero and week 12 with follow-up through week 24. The primary endpoint was gaining >15 letters from baseline at week 24. Overall, 47% of eyes receiving suprachoroidal triamcinolone achieved this goal versus 16% in the sham arm. The rates of elevated intraocular pressure and cataract were similar between the treatment and sham groups, and compared to other corticosteroid administrations, the percentage of patients with increased intraocular pressure was lower. There were no systemic side effects observed. The sham arm also required rescue therapy of a suprachoroidal triamcinolone injection faster.

In a post hoc analysis of the PEACHTREE trial, a suprachoroidal triamcinolone injection showed decreased central subfield thickness and improvement in the best corrected visual acuity, regardless of the anatomical sites of the uveitis.[64] In summary, the PEACHTREE study shows that the >15 letter gain can be achieved in 47% of patients receiving suprachoroidal triamcinolone injections. There was also an average of 150 μm reduction in central subfield thickness, and rescue therapy was needed in only 13–17% of patients. While the PEACHTREE protocol dictated that subjects receive two injections: one at a baseline and the other one at 12 weeks, the real-world data about the effect of repeated injections were published in the AZALEA Trial. Pooled data show that there are 16% of patients (6 of 38 eyes) that experience an intraocular pressure rise of >10 mm Hg, but only 5% experience an intraocular pressure elevation of up to 30 mm Hg. Furthermore, there is a rapid visual acuity gain of two to three lines, and on average, a 100–150 central subfield thickness reduction. These data points can help you estimate and counsel your patient on the benefits of the suprachoroidal triamcinolone injection.

The durability of these effects was demonstrated in the MAGNOLIA extension study.[65] The median time to rescue was 257 days in the suprachoroidal injection arm and about 50% of eyes require no rescue injection for 9 months on average. This specific drug-delivery design confines the medication to the suprachoroidal space leading to clinical durability. More recent data suggest suprachoroidal injections can also be effective with or without systemic therapy, including corticosteroids or immunosuppressive therapies.

There are no randomized controlled data comparing the efficacy of suprachoroidal versus intravitreal or subtenon triamcinolone administrations.[66] The closest comparison came from a post hoc analysis by Singer and colleagues that showed suprachoroidal triamcinolone injection outperformed rescue therapies, which included intravitreal or periocular triamcinolone.[64] A recent meta-analysis by Liu and colleagues assessed the net intraocular pressure change of different routes of triamcinolone acetonide from clinical trials.[67] At week 24, compared to the placebo, the suprachoroidal injection triamcinolone had the highest risk of intraocular pressure elevation. This finding is a reminder that intraocular pressure elevation should always be monitored even if the Phase 3 trial reported a small percentage of subjects with this complication.

A recent study by Gundlach and colleagues visualized the change in the suprachoroidal space using anterior segment OCT immediately after the XIPERE® injection.[68] The space is confined anteriorly in the eye and does not extend posteriorly as early as 5 minutes after the injection. While anterior segment OCT scans showed an early anterior placement of the suprachoroidal space, a study by Hedgeland and colleagues used cadaver or a non-human primate eyes to illustrate drug placement using different approaches of suprachoroidal injection.[69] Higher concentrations of the injected dye were found in the posterior pole up to 20 minutes after injection. The take-home point is that suprachoroidal triamcinolone administration can effectively treat uveitic macular edema, adding another treatment to the periocular, intravitreous, and systemic therapy options discussed earlier. The advantage of the suprachoroidal approach is is the greater exposure of the retinal pigment epithelium, choroid, and sclera, leading to a clinical effect. Conversely, there is lower lens, iris, and vitreous exposure, as demonstrated in cadaveric and animal experimental models. Nonetheless, intraocular pressure should still be monitored throughout the treatment course. Final practical tips include use of subconjunctival lidocaine for anesthesia, even though the patient will still feel pressure. Avoid using the 900 microneedle and first select the 1,100 microneedle to enter into the suprachoroidal space on the first try.

PEARLS FROM THE EXPERTS ON FREQUENTLY ASKED QUESTIONS

1. Do you advise on the use of intravitreal methotrexate in cases of ocular tuberculosis or pseudo-serpiginous choroiditis? Can you highlight the retinal pigment epithelial complication associated with intravitreal methotrexate use and comment on the role of topical folinic acid in cases of keratitis after long-standing use of intravitreal methotrexate injections in cases of lymphoma?

Answer: To treat ocular tuberculosis, we need to treat the underlying disease with ATT. We also need to understand the concept of using anti-inflammatory agents is related to the case of paradoxical worsening of inflammation after the start of ATT due to a secondary inflammatory response. Several local treatment options have been reported in the literature to treat this inflammation, including dexamethasone implants or intravitreal methotrexate injections. A methotrexate dose of 400 μg is administered in the case of paradoxical worsening of ocular tuberculosis and to treat primary vitreoretinal lymphoma. To limit the development of side effects, methotrexate should not be administered more frequently than every 72 hours. There are reports in the literature of intravitreal methotrexate toxicity as illustrated by electroretinogram changes in animal models.[70] An important point prior to injection is understanding what phenotype of ocular tuberculosis is being treated. Intravitreal methotrexate can be used off-label in serpiginous-like choroiditis with paradoxical worsening. Multiple injections are required and the dexamethasone implant is more practical, as it lasts for at least 8 weeks. The additional question was on the application of topical folic acid in cases of corneal toxicity from intravitreal methotrexate use. Compounded topical folic acid reduced keratopathy, but oral formulations were ineffective.

An additional point is that no other chemotherapeutic agent is given in a fixed dose, rather it depends on body surface area and the patient's weight. Our eyes vary from 3 to ≥15 mL. The initial paper that reported intravitreal use of methotrexate aimed for 100 μg per milliliter, which requires measurement of axial length. To calculate the vitreous volume, you use the equation for a sphere: the length of the lens plus the vitreous length divided by 2 gives the radius, which is then entered into the equation $4/3\pi(r)$.[3] This approach allows for dosage adjustment to avoid intraocular toxicity. It should be administered weekly (e.g., for primary vitreoretinal lymphoma), and if measured, levels of IL-10 disappear within a month. If there is a good response to treatment, you can extend to monthly treatment. If there is a very myopic eye, 100 μg in 10 milliliters would not be therapeutic, whereas in a hyperopic eye, 3 milliliters would be overtreatment.

2. When administering longer-acting local corticosteroid therapies, when do you stop treatment and wait until the uveitis or macular edema relapses prior to retreatment?

Answer: In one of the cases presented today, the patient received 10–14 dexamethasone implant injections. This suggests that there is a recurrent disease underlying the flare that needs to be treated with a combination of both systemic immunosuppression and local corticosteroid therapies. This is key to avoiding a situation in which the disease is left without treatment after the local therapy wears off. When treating a patient with uveitis, stay ahead of the inflammation and give local therapies to augment the anti-inflammatory response or treat ocular complications, such as macular edema, until you feel confident the disease is controlled, and likely to remain controlled after the local treatment wears off.

3. Should local therapy be managed differently than systemic therapy, as most uveitis specialists attempt a taper of the immunosuppressant medication after several years of quiescence?

Answer: In the past, it was felt that after quiescence was achieved with immunosuppressive treatment for 2–3 years, the medication could be tapered or discontinued. Recently, the ADJUST trial showed that this timeframe is insufficient for the class of patients recruited for that study and that recurrence is still possible.[71] We now have patients that remain on immunosuppressive therapies for three or more years, as it seems a subset of patients will have a recurrence of inflammation. The key is to continue to closely follow the patient and tailor the duration of therapy to the individual patient's disease course. In the MUST trial, subjects receiving systemic and local therapies were treated the same. If the patient went several years without treatment and there were many side effects, the fluocinolone implant was not replaced unless there was a reactivation. This was done since the same approach would have been taken in those on systemic therapy. Indeed, 45% of subjects never relapsed, going into 7 years of follow-up. If there is a recurrence, restart the immunosuppressant and continue it for another 1–2 years after regaining quiescence. For local therapy for uveitic macular edema, follow the patient and readminister if macular edema recurs. The time from injection to recurrence of the macular edema gives the interval for retreatment.

When managing noninfectious uveitis, two clinical entities typically require long-term therapy. The first includes choroidal inflammatory conditions associated with vascular leakage, such as Vogt–Koyanagi–Harada disease and sympathetic ophthalmia. In these cases, indocyanine green angiography and fluorescein angiography should be repeated to evaluate for subclinical activity. If subclinical inflammation is detected, continuation of immunosuppressive therapy is recommended. The principle of assessing for subclinical disease activity before tapering off treatment is essential. In the absence of angiographic leakage, a gradual tapering of treatment may be considered after at least two years of disease quiescence. The second entity is retinal vasculitis, which presents a greater diagnostic challenge. Fluorescein angiography—particularly with wide-field imaging—often reveals some degree of small-vessel leakage. However, much of this leakage may reflect structural or mechanical vascular alterations rather than ongoing inflammation, supporting the concept of a vasculopathy. This finding does not warrant indefinite immunosuppressive therapy, as it is not typically associated with macular edema nor indicative of active inflammatory disease. Accordingly, peripheral small-vessel leakage alone should not be considered a criterion for continuation of immunosuppressive treatment.

4. Is there experience using the suprachoroidal triamcinolone injection off-label as a treatment to control intraocular inflammation? Is the effect equal across the posterior pole with even distribution of the drug to prevent asymmetric inflammation on the side of the eye opposite of the injection site?

Answer: Yes, in cases where the initial indication for use was to treat macular edema, there was centrally located perivascular leakage. Some improvement in the leakage or even resolution early on in the treatment interval occurred, which then recurred as the triamcinolone concentration decreased. Suprachoroidal triamcinolone injections require close monitoring and repeated treatments to control the intraocular inflammation, similar to the other intraocular depot corticosteroid treatments. Another situation is that in which chorioretinal lesions, such as those in multifocal choroiditis, show a reduction in size after treatment. There is a lack of long-term data if the regressed lesions remain stable and regarding the probabilities of the regressed lesions remaining stable and of avoiding the occurrence of new lesions.

Previously, 4 mg of triamcinolone could be placed at the level of the arcades via a catheter and macular edema resolved for over 6 months. Having a corticosteroid depot posteriorly theoretically increases the concentration around the macula with an extended effect. A potential avenue for therapeutic invention is developing a technique to perform this depot placement. This may require a larger needle since triamcinolone is a suspension.

FINAL WRAP-UP

Local therapy can be quite effective for managing unilateral cases of uveitis and treating secondary inflammatory complications, particularly macular edema. Close monitoring for the recurrence of active disease is essential to prevent breakthrough inflammation that may lead to structural damage. Similarly, the use of corticosteroid agents requires regular monitoring of the intraocular pressure and lens status. While the armamentarium of drug classes and routes of administration have expanded in recent years, numerous additional therapeutic agents remain under active development.

REFERENCES

1. Letko E, Yeh S, Foster CS, Pleye U, Brigell M, Grosskreutz Cl, et al. Efficacy and safety of intravenous secukinumab in noninfectious uveitis requiring steroid-sparing immunosuppressive therapy. Ophthalmology. 2015;122(5): 939-48.
2. Writing committee for the multicenter uveitis steroid treatment (MUST) Trial and Follow-up study research group, Kempen JH, Altaweel MM, Holbrook JT, Sugar EA, Thorne JE, et al. Between long-lasting intravitreous fluocinolone acetonide implant versus systemic anti-inflammatory therapy and visual acuity at 7 years among patients with intermediate, posterior, or panuveitis. J Am Med Assoc. 2017;317(19):1993-2005.
3. Chu DS, Johnson SJ, Mallya UG, Davis MR, Sorg RA, Duh MS. Healthcare costs and utilization for privately insured patients treated for non-infectious uveitis in the USA. J Ophthalmic Inflamm Infect. 2013;3(1):64.
4. Tan HY, Agarwal A, Lee CS, Chhablani J, Gupta V, Khatri M, et al. Management of noninfectious posterior uveitis with intravitreal drug therapy. Clin Ophthalmol. 2016;10:1983-2020.
5. Multicenter Uveitis Steroid Treatment Trial (MUST) Research Group; Gonzales J, Acharya NR, Sugar EA, Burke AE, Vitale AT, Gupta V, et al. Macular Edema Ranibizumab versus Intravitreal Anti-inflammatory Therapy Trial: 24-Week Outcomes of Uveitic Macular Edema Re-treatment. Ophthalmology. 2025;132(5): 527-37. doi: 10.1016/j.ophtha.2024.11.021. Epub 2024 Nov 28. PMID: 39612949; PMCID: PMC12018142.
6. Thorne JE, Sugar EA, Holbrook JT, Burke AE, Altaweel MM, Vitale AT, et al. Periocular Triamcinolone vs. Intravitreal Triamcinolone vs. Intravitreal Dexamethasone Implant for the Treatment of Uveitic Macular Edema: The PeriOcular vs. INTravitreal corticosteroids for uveitic macular edema (POINT) Trial. Ophthalmology. 2019;126(2):283-95.
7. Multicenter Uveitis Steroid Treatment Trial (MUST) Research Group, Writing Committee, Acharya NR, Vitale AT, Sugar EA, Holbrook JT, Burke AE, et al. Intravitreal Therapy for Uveitic Macular Edema-Ranibizumab versus Methotrexate versus the Dexamethasone Implant: The MERIT Trial Results. Ophthalmology. 2023;130(9):914-23.
8. Khlalil HE, El Gendy HA, Youssef HA, Haroun HE, Gheita TA, Bakir HM. The effectiveness of intraocular methotrexate in the treatment of posterior uveitis in Behcet's disease patients compared to retrobulbar steroids injection. J Ophthalmol. 2016:2016:1678495.
9. Taylor SR, Banker A, Schlaen A, Couto C, Matthe E, Joshi L, et al. Intraocular methotrexate can induce extended remission in some patients in noninfectious uveitis. Retina. 2013;33(10):2149-54.
10. Jaffe GJ, Dick AD, Brézin AP, Nguyen QD, Thorne JE, Kestelyn P, et al. Adalimumab in Patients with Active Noninfectious Uveitis. N Engl J Med. 2016;375(10):932-43.
11. Nguyen QD, Merrill PT, Jaffe GJ, Dick AD, Kurup SK, Sheppard J, et al. Adalimumab for prevention of uveitic flare in patients with inactive non-infectious uveitis controlled by corticosteroids (VISUAL II): a multicentre, double-masked, randomised, placebo-controlled phase 3 trial. Lancet. 2016;388(10050):1183-92.
12. Androudi A, Tsironi E, Kalogeropoulos C, Theodoridou A, Brazitikos P. Intravitreal adalimumab for refractory uveitis-related macular edema. Ophthalmology. 2010;117(8):1612-6.
13. Hamam RN, Barikian AW, Antonios RS, Abdulaal MR, Alameddine RM, El Mollayess G, et al. Intravitreal adalimumab in active noninfectious uveitis: A pilot study. Ocul Immunol Inflamm. 2016;24(3):319-26.
14. Markomichelakis N, Delicha E, Masselos S, Sfikakis PP. Intravitreal infliximab for sight-threatening relapsing uveitis in Behcet disease: a pilot study in 15 patients. Am J Ophthalmol. 2012;154(3):534-41.e1.
15. Giganti MM, Beer PM, Lemanski N, Hartman C, Schartman J, Falk N. Adverse events after intravitreal infliximab (Remicade). Retina. 2010;30(1):71-80.
16. Dodds EM, Lowder CY, Meisler DM. Posterior segment inflammation in HLA-B27+ acute anterior uveitis: clinical characteristics. Ocul Immunol Inflamm. 1999;7(2):85-92.
17. Rodriguez A, Akova YA, Pedroza-Seres M, Foster CS. Posterior segment ocular manifestations in patients with HLA-B27-associated uveitis. Ophthalmology. 1994;101(7):1267-74.
18. Multicenter Uveitis Steroid Treatment Trial Research Group, Kempen JH, Altaweel MM, Holbrook JT, Jans DA, Louis TA, et al. Randomized comparison of systemic anti-inflammatory therapy versus fluocinolone acetonide implant for intermediate, posterior, and panuveitis : the multicenter uveitis steroids treatment trial. Ophthalmology. 2011;118(10):1916-26.
19. Lardenoye CW, van Kooij B, Rothova A. Impact of macular edema on visual acuity in uveitis. Ophthalmology. 2006;113(8):1446-9.

20. Bagheri N, Wajda B, Durrani A, Calvo C (Eds). The Wills Eye Manual. 7th edition. Lippincott Williams and Wilkins, 2016.
21. Shulman S, Jóhannesson G, Stefánsson E, Loewenstein A, Rosenblatt A, Habot-Wilner Z. Topical dexamethasone-cyclodextrin nanoparticle eye drops for non-infectious Uveitic macular oedema and vitritis - a pilot study. Acta Ophthalmol. 2015;93(5):411-5.
22. Stefansson E, Loftsson T, Larsen M, Papp A, Kaarniranta K, Munk MR, et al. Topical treatment of diabetic macular edema using dexamethasone ophthalmic suspension: A randomized, double-masked, vehicle-controlled study. Acta Ophthalmol. 2023;101(1):22-33.
23. Sepah YJ, Sadiq MA, Chu DS, Dacey M, Gallemore R, Dayani P, et al. Primary (Month-6) Outcomes of the STOP-Uveitis Study: Evaluating the Safety, Tolerability, and Efficacy of Tocilizumab in Patients With Noninfectious Uveitis. Am J Ophthalmol. 2017;183:71-80.
24. Xu M, Zhu B, Cao X, Li S, Li D, Zhou H, et al. OSBP-Related protein 5L maintains intracellular IP3/Ca2+ signaling and proliferation in T-cells by facilitating PIP2 hydrolysis. J Immunol. 2020;204(5):1134-45.
25. Brodie JT, Thotathil AZ, Jordan CA, Sims J, Niederer RL. Risk of Recurrence in Acute Anterior Uveitis. Ophthalmology. 2024;131(11):1281-9.
26. Monnet D, Breban M, Hudry C, Dougados M, Brézin AP. Ophthalmic findings and frequency of extraocular manifestations in patients with HLA-B27 uveitis: a study of 175 cases. Ophthalmology. 2004;111(4):802-9.
27. Sheppard JD, Toyos MM, Kempen JH, Kaur P, Foster CS. Difluprednate 0.05% versus prednisolone acetate 1% for endogenous anterior uveitis: a Phase 3, multicenter, randomized study. Invest Ophthalmol Vis Sci. 2014;55(5):2993-3002.
28. Awan MA, Agarwal PK, Watson DG, McGhee CN, Dutton GN. Penetration of topical and subconjunctival corticosteroids into human aqueous humour and its therapeutic significance. Br J Ophthalmol. 2009;93(6):708-13.
29. Cohen CR, Davis J, DeBarge R, Foley J, Foster CS, Fox K, et al. Controlled evaluation of loteprednol etabonate and prednisolone acetate in the treatment of acute anterior uveitis. Am J Ophthalmol. 1999;127(5):537-44.
30. Duvall B, Kershner RM. Ophthalmic Medications and Pharmacology, 2nd edition. CRC Press. 2006.
31. Thorne JE, Woreta FA, Dunn JP, Jabs DA. Risk of Cataract Development among Children with Juvenile Idiopathic Arthritis-Related Uveitis Treated with Topical Corticosteroids. Ophthalmology. 2020;127(4S):S21-S26.
32. Papaliodis GN, Rosner BA, Dreger KA, Fitzgerald TD, Artornsonbudh P, Kothari S, et al. Incidence of and risk factors for cataract in anterior uveitis. Am J Ophthalmol. 2023:254:221-32.
33. Minkus CL, Pistilli M, Dreger KA, Fitzgerald TD, Payal AR, Begum H, et al. Risk of cataract in intermediate uveitis. Am J Ophthalmol. 2021:229:200-9.
34. Friedman NJ, Kaiser PK. Ocular pharmacology. In: Essentials of Ophthalmology. Philadelphia: Elsevier; 2007:25-32.
35. Daniel E, Pistilli M, Kothari S, Khachatryan N, Kacmaz RO, Gangaputra SS, et al. Risk of ocular hypertension in adults with noninfectious uveitis. Ophthalmology. 2017;124(8):1196-1208.
36. Kothari S, Foster CS, Pistili M, Liesgang TL, Daniel E, Sen HN, et al. The risk of intraocular pressure elevation in pediatric noninfectious uveitis. Ophthalmology. 2015;122(10):1987-2001.
37. Qureshi IA. Intraocular pressure: association with menstrual cycle, pregnancy and menopause in apparently healthy women. Chin J Physiol. 1995;38(4):229-34.
38. Bhatia J, Sadiq M, Chaudhary TA, Bhatia A. Eye changes and risk of ocular medications during pregnancy and their management. Pak J Ophthalmol. 2007;23(1):1-6.
39. Fiscella RG, Jensen M, Van Dyck G. Generic prednisolone suspension substitution. Arch Ophthalmol. 1998;116(5):703.
40. Food and Drug Administration. (2014). Content and Format of Labeling for Human Prescription Drug and Biological Products; Requirements for Pregnancy and Lactation Labeling (final rule) 79 FR 72063. Federal Register 2014, FR Doc. 2014-28241 Filed 12-3-14. [online] Available from https://www.federalregister.gov/articles/2014/12/04/2014-28241/content-and-format-of-labeling-for-human-prescription-drug-and-biological-products-requirements-for [Last accessed February 2025].
41. Chambers WA. Ophthalmic generics—are they really the same? Ophthalmology. 2012;119:1095-6.
42. Mammo ZN, Flanagan JG, James DF, Trope GE. Generic versus brand-name North American topical glaucoma drops. Can J Ophthalmol. 2012;47:55-61.
43. Modorati G, Miserocchi E. Intravitreal injection therapy in the treatment of noninfectious uveitis. Dev Ophthalmol. 2012;51:110-21.
44. Servillo A, Scandale P, Oldoni G, Begar PG, Bandello F, Miserocchi E, et al. Inflammatory choroidal neovascularization: An evidence-based update. Surv Ophthalmol. 2025;70(3):451-66.
45. Agarwal A, Invernizzi A, Singh RB, Foulsham W, Aggarwal K, Handa S, et al. An update on inflammatory choroidal neovascularization: epidemiology, multimodal imaging, and management. J Ophthalmic Inflamm Infect. 2018;8(1):13.
46. Mateo-Montoya A, Baglivo E, de Smet MD. Intravitreal methotrexate for the treatment of choroidal neovascularization in multifocal choroiditis, Eye (Lond). 2013;27(2):277-8.
47. Alves CH, Fernandes R, Santiago AR, Ambrosio AF. Microglia contribution to the regulation of the retinal and choroidal vasculature in age-related macular degeneration. Cells. 2020;9(5):1217.
48. Vienne-Jumeau A, Brézin AP, Seminel M, Ribeaudeau-Saindelle F, Bousquet E. Corticosteroids Decrease the

Incidence and Activity of Choroidal Neovascularization in Patients with Punctuate Inner Choroidopathy or Multifocal Choroiditis. Ocul Immunol Inflamm. 2024;32(5):602-608.
49. Wu W, Li S, Xu H, Liu Y, Wang Y, Lai TYY, et al. Treatment of punctate inner choroidopathy with choroidal neovascularization using corticosteroids and intravitreal ranibizumab. Biomed Res Int. 2018:2018:1585803.
50. Niederer RL, Gilber R, Lightman SL, Tomkins-Netzer O. Risk factors for developing choroidal neovascular membrane and visual loss in punctate inner choroidopathy. Ophthalmology. 2018;125(2):288-94.
51. Airaldi M, Monteduro D, Tondini G, Pichi F, De Simone L, Cornish E, et al. Immunomodulatory Treatment Versus Systemic Steroids in Inflammatory Choroidal Neovascularization Secondary to Idiopathic Multifocal Choroiditis. Am J Ophthalmol. 2024;262:62-72.
52. Neri P, Pichi F, Pirani V, Arapi I. Systemic Immunosuppression Is Highly Effective in the Long-term Control of Inflammatory non-infectious Uveitic Choroidal Neovascularization: A Comparative Study. Ocul Immunol Inflamm. 2021;29(6):1132-6.
53. Pai SA, Hebri SP, Lootah AM. Management of recurrent inflammatory choroidal neovascular membrane secondary to Vogt-Koyanagi-Harada syndrome, using combined intravitreal injection of bevacizumab and triamcinolone acetate. Indian J Ophthalmol. 2012;60(6):551-2.
54. Bae JH, Lee SC. Effect of intravitreal methotrexate and aqueous humor cytokine levels in refractory retinal vasculitis in Behcet disease. Retina. 2012;32(7):1395-402.
55. Ibrahim MA, Sepah YJ, Watters A, Bittencourt M, Vigil EM, Do DV, et al. One-Year Outcomes of the SAVE Study: Sirolimus as a Therapeutic Approach for UVEitis. Transl Vis Sci Technol. 2015;4(2):4.
56. Grotting LA, Davoudi S, Palenzuela D, Papaliodis GN, Sobrin L. Association of Low Vitamin D Levels with Noninfectious Anterior Uveitis. JAMA Ophthalmol. 2017;135(2):150-3.
57. Ness S, Mitsiades R, Poulaki V. Association of Low Serum Vitamin D Levels with Proliferative Vitreoretinopathy after Rhegmatogenous Retinal Detachment Repair. Ophthalmol Retina. 2025:S2468-6530(25)00350-1.
58. Wan CR, Muya L, Kansara V, Ciulla TA. Suprachoroidal Delivery of Small Molecules, Nanoparticles, Gene and Cell Therapies for Ocular Diseases. Pharmaceutics. 2021;13(2):288.
59. Kicinska AK, Rekas M. Alternative application of an iTrack microcatheter and canaloplasty: case report and literature review. Expert Opin Drug Deliv. 2023;20(9):1201-8.
60. Rotenstreich Y, Sher I, Lawrence M, Mangelus M, Ingerman A, Barak Y. A Novel Device for Suprachoroidal Drug Delivery to Retina: Evaluation in Nonhuman Primates. Transl Vis Sci Technol. 2023;12(6):3.
61. Yeh S, Khurana RN, Shah M, Henry CR, Wang RC, Kissner JM, et al. Efficacy and Safety of Suprachoroidal CLS-TA for Macular Edema Secondary to Noninfectious Uveitis: Phase 3 Randomized Trial. Ophthalmology. 2020;127(7):948-55.
62. Shah M, Albini T, Nguyen Q, Wykoff C, Barakat M, Khurana RN, et al. Safety and Efficacy of CLS-TA by Anatomic Location of Inflammation: Results from the Phase 3 PEACHTREE Clinical Trial. Ocul Immunol Inflamm. 2024;32(8):1556-63.
63. Henry CR, Shah M, Barakat MR, Dayani P, Wang RC, Khurana RN, et al. Suprachoroidal CLS-TA for non-infectious uveitis: an open-label, safety trial (AZALEA). Br J Ophthalmol. 2022;106(6):802-6.
64. Campochiaro PA, Wykoff CC, Brown DM, Boyer DS, Barakat M, Taraborelli D, et al. Suprachoroidal Triamcinolone Acetonide for Retinal Vein Occlusion: Results of the Tanzanite Study. Ophthalmol Retina. 2018;2(4):320-8.
65. Singer MA, Merrill P, Yeh S, Hall C, Kapik B, Ciulla TA. Suprachoroidal triamcinolone acetonide versus rescue therapies for the treatment of uveitic macular oedema: A post hoc analysis of PEACHTREE. Clin Exp Ophthalmol. 2022;50(1):23-30.
66. Merrill PT, Henry CR, Nguyen QD, Reddy A, Kapik B, Ciulla TA. Suprachoroidal CLS-TA with and without Systemic Corticosteroid and/or Steroid-Sparing Therapy: A Post-Hoc Analysis of the Phase 3 PEACHTREE Clinical Trial. Ocul Immunol Inflamm. 2023;31(8):1579-86.
67. Smith JR, Thorne JE, Flaxel CJ, Jain N, Kim SJ, Maguire MG, et al. Treatment of noninfectious uveitis macular edema with periocular and intraocular corticosteroid therapies: a report by the American Academy of Ophthalmology. Ophthalmology. 2024;131(9):1107-20.
68. Liu K, Yi J, Xu J, Zhang L, Su N. Risk of intraocular pressure elevation associated with triamcinolone acetonide administration via different routes in macular edema: a systematic review and network meta-analysis of randomized controlled trials. BMC Ophthalmol. 2025;25(1):150.
69. Gundlach BS, Tsui I, Tsui E. Visualization of the Suprachoroidal Space with Swept-Source Anterior Segment OCT before and after Suprachoroidal Triamcinolone Acetonide Injection. Ophthalmol Retina. 2025;9(11):e105.
70. Hedgeland M, Camacho Gonzalez S, Stampoulis D, Lee V, Powell K, Qiu Y, et al. Evaluation of Suprachoroidal Injection in Cadaveric and Preclinical Models. Transl Vis Sci Technol. 2025;14(3):20.
71. Aly E, Ebrahim A. Apoptosis and electroretinogram after intravitreal injection of methotrexate in an experimental rabbit model. Gen Physiol Biophys. 2016;35(2):231-6.
72. Acharya NR, Ramanan AV, Coyne AB, Dudum KL, Rubio EM, Woods SM, et al. Stopping of adalimumab in juvenile idiopathic arthritis-associated uveitis (ADJUST): a multicenter, double-masked, randomised controlled trial. Lancet. 2025;405(10475):303-13.

CHAPTER

18 Drug-induced Uveitis

James P Dunn, Eugenia Ramos-Davila, James T Rosenbaum, Jennifer Hu, Lucia Sobrin, Wenbo Ding, Maggie Feng, Nimesh Patel, Vishali Gupta, Marc de Smet, Reema Bansal, Alejandra de-la-Torre, John H Kempen, Meghan Berkenstock

INTRODUCTION

Drug-induced uveitis is a rare cause of ocular inflammation. Proposed mechanisms include direct toxicity through a breakdown of the blood-retinal barrier, indirectly through deposition of immune complexes, or via microvascular disruption. While the cause of nearly 0.5% of all uveitis cases, clinicians still need to be aware of the drug classes that are associated with the development of this condition. Understanding the ocular manifestations and therapeutic options to treat drug-induced uveitis can promote early diagnosis and prevent ocular complications.

THEMATIC LECTURE: KEEPING AN EYE ON OCULAR ADVERSE EVENTS OF IMMUNOTHERAPIES AND TARGETED CANCER THERAPIES

The era of immunotherapy started with the United States Food and Drug Administration (FDA) approval of the chimeric monoclonal antibody rituximab for the treatment of B-cell non-Hodgkin lymphomas in 1997.[1] This was followed by the release of the first small-molecule kinase inhibitor, imatinib, in 2001. The first checkpoint inhibitor, ipilimumab, was released in 2011 followed by MEK-kinase (MEK) and B-RAF (BRAF) kinase inhibitors in 2014.[2] The ocular adverse events, including uveitis, associated with the use of each of these antineoplastic drug classes will be discussed.

Checkpoint inhibitors are fully humanized, monoclonal antibodies that exert antitumor activity by activating T-cells in lymph nodes or at the tumor site.[3] First, they promote activation of naive T-cells in the draining lymph nodes nearest to the tumor.[4] Once proteins from the cancer cell surface are released into the peripheral circulation, dendritic cells (DC) and other antigen-presenting cells uptake the antigen, process it, and display it on a major histocompatibility complex (MHC) II molecule. The DC then migrates to the nearest draining lymph node, where the tumor antigen is presented to the naive T-cells. Two signals are required for full, CD8+ cytotoxic T-cell activation. The first is the interaction of the T-cell receptor with the MHC molecule on the DC. The second is a costimulatory signal of the CD28 receptor on the T-cell surface binding CD80/CD86, also known as the B7 receptor, on the DC **(Fig. 1)**. A competitive inhibitor of this interaction is the binding of cytotoxic T cell-associated protein-4 (CTLA-4) on the T-cell surface with B7 on the DC, if this occurs, an anergistic T-cell response occurs leading to immune tolerance, formation of T-regulatory cells, and continued tumor growth. Blocking of the CTLA-4 antigen by an anti-CTLA-4 checkpoint inhibitor leads to continued T-cell activation and tumor lysis. Even if an antigen-educated, cytotoxic T-cell exits the lymph node, it can still be deactivated in the tumor bed. The effector T-cell response begins with the release of the activated CD8+ lymphocytes into the peripheral circulation, where they hone to and infiltrate the tumor, leading to malignant cell apoptosis.

The second mechanism of action of checkpoint inhibitors occurs within the tumor. This time, the T-cell receptor binds the MHC I molecule on the cancer cell surface.[4] However, to evade immune recognition, the tumor cells also upregulate a surface protein, programmed death ligand 1 (PD-L1). If the programmed death-1 (PD-1) receptor on the T-cell surface binds the PD-L1 molecule on the malignant cell, the T-cell deactivates leading to

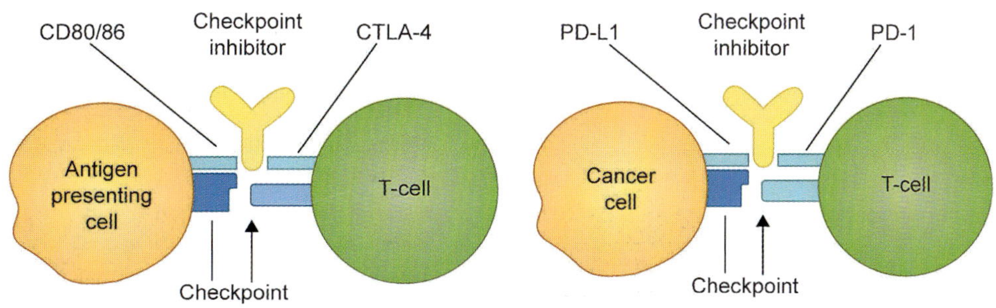

Fig. 1: A schematic showing the mechanism of action of CTLA-4 inhibitors in lymph nodes and PD-1/PD-L1 inhibitors at the tumor cell surface. (CTLA-4: cytotoxic T cell-associated protein-4; PD-1: programmed death-1; PD-L1: programmed death ligand 1)
Source: Uveitis Course - Grand Rounds 18. International Uveitis Study Group (IUSG). October 11, 2025. Available from: https://youtu.be/pNJBcK5iP2s?si=kxQm2qSQy-qd5OQg.

immunosuppression. Blockage of either the PD-1 or the PD-L1 receptors by a checkpoint inhibitor monoclonal antibody allows for a continued cytotoxic T-cell response and tumor cell lysis.

A third checkpoint inhibitor mechanism of action involves inhibition of lymphocyte activation gene-3 (LAG-3), promoting CD8+ T-cell differentiation and inhibiting T-regulatory cell immunotolerance to tumor antigens.[4]

During many of the initial clinical trials of checkpoint inhibitors, patients with preexisting autoimmune disorders were not enrolled given the concern for an increased risk of developing immune-related adverse events (IRAEs). However, the development of IRAEs are common and occur in 70–90% of patients affecting multiple organ systems.[3,5] The most common systemic IRAEs include fatigue, skin rash, lymphopenia, and transaminemia. These IRAEs stem from overactive immune responses that start days to weeks after the initiation of checkpoint inhibitor therapy and can continue after drug cessation. Most are low-grade (grade 1 or 2) and can be treated with local or systemic corticosteroids, while allowing continuation of the checkpoint inhibitor.[3,6] However, robust inflammation may rarely require the start of noncorticosteroid immunosuppressive agents, especially with the development of inflammatory arthritis or colitis. If a higher grade (grade 3 or 4) event occurs, the checkpoint inhibitor may need to be temporarily or permanently discontinued. The grading scale for adverse events is provided in **Table 1** later in this chapter.

Ocular IRAEs are rare and occur in 1–3% of patients. The unique environment within the eye provides immune privilege through several mechanisms.[3,6,7] The intraocular structures lack efferent lymphatic drainage as well as the presence of the blood-retinal barrier. In addition, the upregulation of Fas-ligand and the expression of PD-L1 in retinal pigment epithelial cells leads to apoptosis of aberrant T-cell responses and promotion of T-regulatory cells within the uveal tract. Inflammation of any ocular structure can develop with checkpoint inhibitor use, which requires a detailed discussion of IRAEs.

Starting with the ocular surface, inflammatory keratitis, episcleritis, blepharitis, and/or conjunctivitis have been reported.[8-13] Corneal inflammation can lead to ulceration, perforation, and in the case of prior transplantation, graft rejection. One of the most common side effects is keratoconjunctivitis sicca, occurring in up to 40% of patients. Corneal ulceration due to severe surface dryness was reported in one clinical trial. When treating ocular surface IRAEs, bear in mind that these patients are immunocompromised and can still develop opportunistic infections, such as herpes zoster keratitis. Keratoconjunctivitis sicca should be treated with preservative-free artificial tears at least four times a day with additional management strategies including punctal plugs, serum tears, or bandage contact lenses added as needed. Blepharitis should be managed with baby shampoo lid scrubs followed by application of warm compresses twice daily. Episcleritis responds well to topical non-steroidal anti-inflammatory or corticosteroid eye drops. Inflammatory keratitis and conjunctivitis can be treated with topical corticosteroids; however, more advanced therapies may be needed in the setting of ulceration.

The most common orbital IRAE is myasthenia gravis.[6,14] Patients with new-onset ptosis and ocular motility abnormalities require a prompt work-up including serologic testing for acetylcholine antibodies

TABLE 1: An adaption of the Common Terminology Criteria for Adverse Events Grading Scale (Version 5) for corneal ulcer, dry eye, keratitis, and uveitis.

Ocular AE	*Grade 1*	*Grade 2*	*Grade 3*	*Grade 4*
Corneal ulcer	-	-	Corneal ulcer without perforation in the affected eye	Perforation in the affected eye
Dry eye	Asymptomatic; clinical or diagnostic observations only; symptoms relieved by lubricants	Symptomatic; moderate decrease in visual acuity (best-corrected visual acuity 20/40 and better or three lines or less decreased vision from known baseline)	Symptomatic with marked decrease in visual acuity (best-corrected visual acuity worse than 20/40 or more than three lines of decreased vision from known baseline, up to 20/200); limiting self-care ADL	-
Keratitis (corneal inflammation)	Asymptomatic; clinical or diagnostic observations only; intervention not indicated	Symptomatic; moderate decrease in visual acuity (best-corrected visual acuity 20/40 and better or three lines or less decreased vision from known baseline)	Symptomatic with marked decrease in visual acuity (best-corrected visual acuity worse than 20/40 or more than three lines of decreased vision from known baseline, up to 20/200); corneal ulcer; limiting self-care ADL	Perforation; best-corrected visual acuity of 20/200 or worse in the affected eye
Uveitis	Anterior uveitis with trace cells	Anterior uveitis with 1+ or 2+ cells	Anterior uveitis with 3+ or greater cells; intermediate posterior or panuveitis	Best-corrected visual acuity of 20/200 or worse in the affected eye

(ADL: activities of daily living; AE: adverse event)
Source: Uveitis Course - Grand Rounds 18. International Uveitis Study Group (IUSG). October 11, 2025. Available from: https://youtu.be/pNJBcK5iP2s?si=kxQm2qSQy-qd5OQg.

and referral to neurology to initiate of intravenous corticosteroids. Additional treatments can include pyridostigmine, plasmapheresis, and intravenous immunoglobulin infusions. Death from respiratory failure secondary to myasthenia gravis has been reported, requiring ophthalmologists to be aware of this potentially fatal condition when assessing a patient on checkpoint inhibitors. Orbital inflammatory syndrome, thyroid-like ophthalmopathy, and dacryoadenitis can also occur. In the setting of a new-onset cranial nerve palsy, a drug-induced IRAE should always be a diagnosis of exclusion. Neuroimaging is required to rule out metastatic disease.

Another potentially blinding complication associated with checkpoint inhibitor use is polymyalgia rheumatica and giant cell arteritis.[15] The average time to onset is within the first five cycles of treatment. If a patient presents with transient visual obscurations and temple pain, an erythrocyte sedimentation rate (ESR) and C-reactive protein (CRP) should be obtained. The prompt start of oral or intravenous corticosteroids, in addition to referral for a temporal artery biopsy, is warranted to prevent both visual and systemic morbidity.

The most commonly reported IRAE is uveitis, which can affect any chamber of the eye. It is always bilateral with variable amounts of anterior chamber cells with optic nerve and/or macular edema.[16-22] As in non-checkpoint inhibitor-associated cases of uveitis, patients typically present with redness, pain, blurred vision, and photophobia. The median time to onset is 6–12 weeks after the first infusion. A diagnostic workup is always required, as drug-induced uveitis is a diagnosis of exclusion. A minimal workup should include both treponemal and non-treponemal syphilis serologies, human leukocyte antigen B27 (HLA-B27) antigen testing, and a chest X-ray to assess for sarcoidosis; serum angiotensin-converting enzyme and lysozyme levels can be assayed, but the results are variable in IRAEs. Posterior pole manifestations include placoid retinal lesions, retinal vasculitis, multifocal choroiditis, and a birdshot-like choroiditis. Cases of Vogt-Koyanagi-Harada-like panuveitis with the development of a sunset-glow fundus appearance and extraocular manifestations including hearing loss, meningismus, vitiligo, and poliosis have been reported **(Figs. 2 and 3)**.[16]

Management of uveitis includes topical corticosteroids for primarily anterior inflammation and intravitreal,

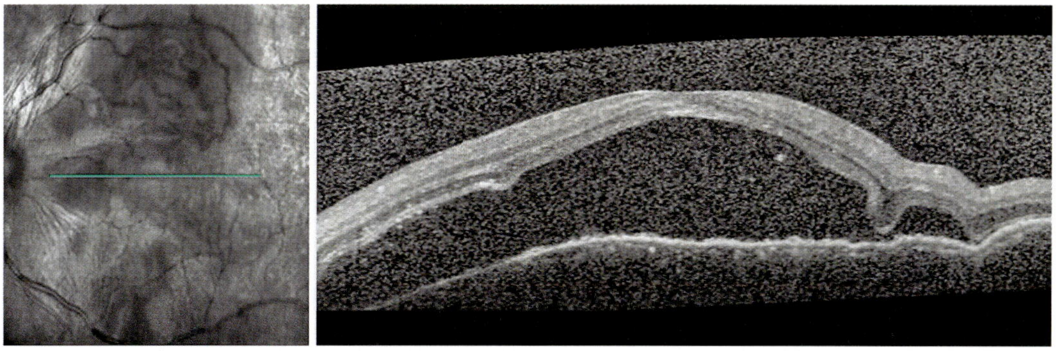

Fig. 2: An optical coherence tomography (OCT) scan through the macula of a left eye showing a thickened choroid and the presence of subretinal fluid in a patient with Vogt-Koyangi-Harada-like panuveitis.
Source: Uveitis Course - Grand Rounds 18. International Uveitis Study Group (IUSG). October 11, 2025. Available from: https://youtu.be/pNJBcK5iP2s?si=kxQm2qSQy-qd5OQg.

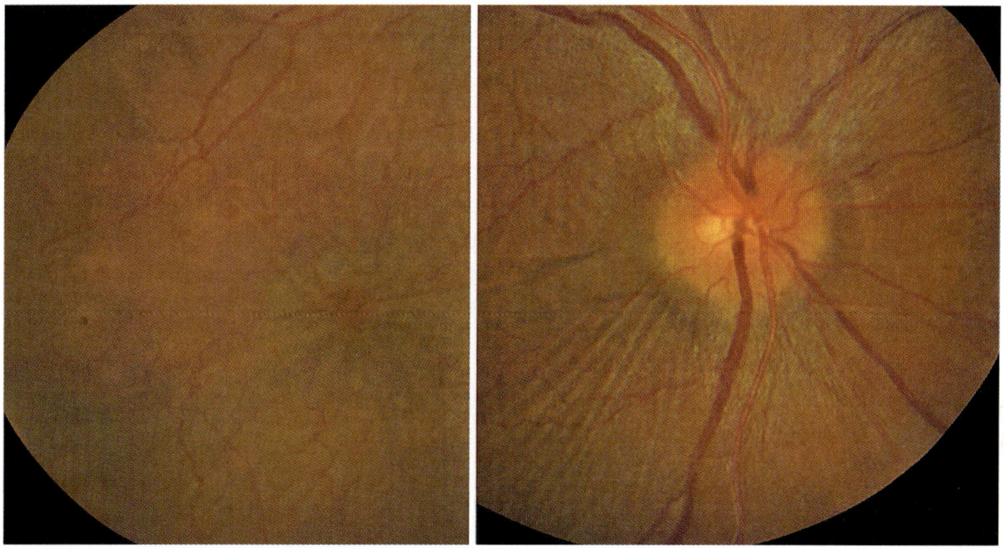

Fig. 3: A color fundus photo of a right eye showing striae radially surrounding the optic nerve and the macula in a case of Vogt-Koyanagi-Harada disease-like panuveitis.
Source: Uveitis Course - Grand Rounds 18. International Uveitis Study Group (IUSG). October 11, 2025. Available from: https://youtu.be/pNJBcK5iP2s?si=kxQm2qSQy-qd5OQg.

oral, or periocular corticosteroids in cases of posterior pole involvement.[19] Intravenous corticosteroids should be administered in cases with robust, vision-threatening inflammation, and tapered after transition to oral prednisone.[20] Treatment should primarily be focused through local routes of corticosteroid administration to avoid the need to stop or delay checkpoint inhibitor infusions. When oral prednisone is prescribed at doses higher than 10 mg daily, the checkpoint inhibitor may be temporarily held by the oncologist. Corticosteroids inhibit T-cell activation and decrease immunotherapy efficacy. In rare cases, uveitis can persist despite the discontinuation of the checkpoint inhibitor, and non-corticosteroid immunosuppressive medications may be required to achieve quiescence. Every attempt to control the uveitis should be made prior to discontinuing the checkpoint inhibitor.

The pathophysiology underlying the development of uveitis with checkpoint inhibitor use remains speculative. The leading hypothesis is that activation of T-cells primed against antigens with epitopic similarity to uveal antigens results in continued intraocular inflammation.[19] Specific to cases of melanoma, both cutaneous and choroidal, the release of melanin and melanin-associated proteins with tumor lysis may facilitate the generation of inflammation in the uveal tract. Melanin-associated proteins have been shown to induce experimental autoimmune uveitis in animal models.

A final IRAE to mention is the development of optic neuritis. As opposed to optic nerve inflammation associated with demyelinating diseases, checkpoint inhibitor-associated optic neuritis is most commonly bilateral and painless.[23] Any change in color vision or visual fields should prompt neuroimaging and referral to neurology. Treatment revolves around the start of intravenous corticosteroids and at least temporary cessation of the checkpoint inhibitor.

MEK and BRAF inhibitors are signal transduction protein kinases that become constitutively active upon mutation, resulting in sustained downstream activation of gene transcription, cell motility, and tumor proliferation with metastasis.[24] While these agents have initial high response rates, the responses are short-lived with a median time to progression of 5.1–8.8 months. The addition of a MEK inhibitor to a BRAF inhibitor extends median response duration from 5.6 to 9.5 months for melanomas. About 20% of patients develop an IRAE with BRAF inhibitor use. The most common IRAE is uveitis, which can be anterior, intermediate, or panuveitis.[17,25-29] As with checkpoint inhibitor-induced uveitis, treatment predominantly includes topical, intravitreal, periocular, and systemic corticosteroids without cessation of the BRAF inhibitor. The onset of uveitis with this class of medications is bilateral and occurs later in treatment (mean 5.6 months) than with checkpoint inhibitors. As with the checkpoint inhibitor class, this is a true drug-induced uveitis by the Naranjo scale-which helps assess causality of drug adverse events where there is a reasonable time period for absorption of the drug, development of an adverse event, and then recurrence of an adverse event on re-exposure to the drug.[30] Rechallenge with the same or another BRAF inhibitor within the class can facilitate recurrence of uveitis.

MEK inhibitors are associated with the development of another IRAE, a multifocal, central serous choroidopathy-like collection of subretinal fluid called MEK-associated retinopathy or MEKAR.[29,31-33] It occurs within a few days of the treatment start and is always bilateral. The thickness of the detachment on optical coherence tomography (OCT) scans of the retina is dose-dependent. MEKAR self-resolves over time, with dose reductions, or treatment discontinuation. However, the development of a retinal vein occlusion, which was reported in early clinical trials (and led to the exclusion of patients with advanced glaucoma from later FDA approval studies), is an ocular reason for dose holds, reductions, or discontinuation. The pathophysiology of the subretinal fluid accumulation in MEKAR is not well understood. Inhibition of the MEK pathway can lead to a variety of intracellular changes that include alterations in cytoskeletal dynamics, intra- and extracellular water transport, oxidative damage, and dysfunction of the outer blood-retinal barrier with loosening of the tight junctions. The same interruption of the tight junctions in the non-pigmented epithelium of the ciliary body is the proposed mechanism for the development of anterior uveitis.

The final class of medications to discuss are the antibody drug conjugates (ADCs). These medications have been a revolutionary addition in oncology and have provided treatment options for cancer patients resistant to other therapies. With over 150 new agents in clinical development and trials worldwide, all ophthalmologists need to know the adverse events associated with ADC use and how to treat them. ADCs deliver antineoplastic molecules directly to cancer cells, providing cytotoxic effects with cellular specificity. ADCs are fully humanized monoclonal antibodies composed of a Fab portion that binds to an overexpressed protein on the cancer cell surface and a linker that is cleavable or non-cleavable that attaches the cytotoxic payload or warhead to the antibody **(Fig. 4)**.[34,35] There can be variable amounts of cytotoxic payloads attached to the antibody ranging from one to eight, which is called the drug-antibody ratio (DAR). Depending on the mechanism of action of the cytotoxic

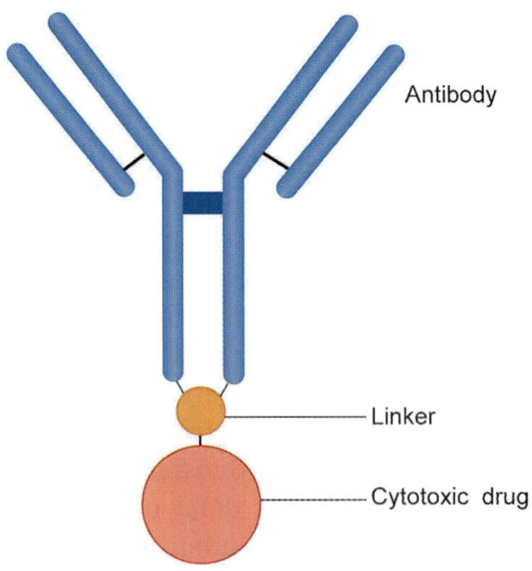

Fig. 4: A schematic diagram of the structure of an antibody drug conjugate A monoclonal antibody is attached to a variable amount of cytotoxic payload molecules through a linker protein. *Source:* Uveitis Course - Grand Rounds 18. International Uveitis Study Group (IUSG). October 11, 2025. Available from: https://youtu.be/pNJBcK5iP2s?si=kxQm2qSQy-qd5OQg.

payload, cellular division is prevented through microtubule disruption, DNA damage, or RNA modification.

Once the ADC binds to the target receptor, it is internalized into the cell via endocytosis. It is degraded in the lysosome, releasing the cytotoxic payload into the cytoplasm. The cytotoxic payload can then migrate to the nucleus or interfere with other intracellular pathways depending on the mechanism of action, thereby decreasing cell proliferation. Despite the "lock and key" or specific antigen targeting, aberrant delivery to other tissues can occur if the receptor is expressed on otherwise normal tissues.[35] There are several methods of delivery to nonmalignant cells leading to the development of adverse events. Binding of the ADC to receptors expressed on nonmalignant cells is called on-target delivery. Conversely, off-target delivery occurs when the cytotoxic payload is released after malignant cell apoptosis and and is taken up by adjacent normal cells through plasma membrane diffusion. Alternatively, cells routinely sample the surrounding interstitial fluid in a process called macropinocytosis. In tissues with rich blood flow, such as at the corneoscleral limbus, the ADC is delivered through the capillary bed into the interstitial space. There the process of macropinocytosis allows for uptake of the ADC into the corneal stem cells, which undergo apoptosis as they differentiate into surface epithelial cells and migrate anteriorly and centrally. This leads to the formation of pseudomicrocysts, which are visible on slit lamp examination **(Fig. 5)**. Pseudomicrocysts represent ADC-related phagocytosis or intracellular drug accumulation in corneal basal epithelial cells.[36] In vivo confocal microscopy shows hyperreflective intracellular inclusions that represent apoptotic corneal epithelial cells on histology. The number of pseudomicrocysts correlates with the cumulative dosage and the duration of therapy and are reversible 2 weeks to 8 months after cessation of the ADC.

Mitigation strategies were developed to decrease the incidence of adverse events and to avoid cessation of the ADC to continue treatment of the underlying malignancy.[37] Despite the use of these protocols, reductions or delays in ADC dosing should be based on the type of adverse event and the severity grade based on the Common Terminology Criteria for Adverse Events (CTCAE) scale **(Table 1)**, which was developed by the National Cancer Insitute.[38] The use of a standardized grading scale allows for the relaying of the best-corrected visual acuity and slit-lamp findings to the oncologist and enables collective treatment decisions. Grade 1 events are the least severe, and the immunotherapy agent should be held if a grade 2 adverse event occurs until it improves to a grade 1. Through early detection and continued follow-up, grade 2 events can be identified early in the clinical course and treated before they escalate to a grade 3 or grade 4 event, which requires cessation of the immunotherapy agent.

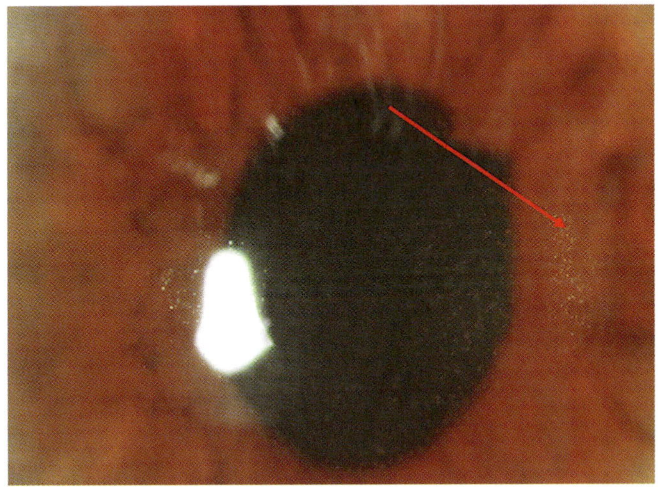

Fig. 5: A slit lamp photograph showing the development of pseudomicrocysts in the visual axis in a patient on an antibody drug conjugate (red arrow).
Source: Uveitis Course - Grand Rounds 18. International Uveitis Study Group (IUSG). October 11, 2025. Available from: https://youtu.be/pNJBcK5iP2s?si=kxQm2qSQy-qd5OQg.

The percentage of patients who develop adverse events ranges from 0 and 90% depending on the ADC. The most common ocular adverse events include keratopathy, dry eye syndrome, limbal stem cell dysfunction, and conjunctivitis. These events can occur in isolation, overlap, or develop cumulatively. ADCs encountered in clinical practice that are associated with a high percentage of adverse events include tisotumab, mirvetuximab, and belantamab. Belantamab, a fourth-line drug recently approved by the FDA for use in combination with conventional chemotherapeutic agents, will be briefly discussed in the context of multiple myeloma treatment. Belantamab targets B-cell maturation antigen and has the highest percentage of adverse events, which is predominately the formation of pseudomicrocysts. Specific mitigation protocols and required examination schedules for each ADC are available on the manufacturer's website.

Tisotumab is a second- or third-line drug for the treatment of cervical cancer that targets tissue factor.

Microtubule-disrupting agent monomethyl auristatin E (MMAE) is the cytotoxic payload is attached via a cleavable linker. Tissue factor is expressed on the ocular surface resulting in adverse events involving conjunctival inflammation from on-target delivery. Thus, patients require a slit-lamp examination every cycle for the first 9 cycles. In the Phase 3 InnovaTV 204 trial, 53% of patients developed ocular adverse events, which were mostly grade 1 or 2 and predominately confined to the conjunctiva and/or the cornea.[37] Only 2% were Grade 3 events and all were ulcerative keratitis. The median time to onset of adverse events was 1.4 months (interquartile range: 0.7–2.0) and 86% resolved within 30 days after the last dose. The median time to resolution was 0.7 months (interquartile range: 0.3–1.6). Reassuringly, the longer treatment duration did not lead to higher-grade events. **Figure 6** shows keratinization of the conjunctival surface, which is treatable with a taper of topical corticosteroids. A grade 3 event is the development of subconjunctival fibrosis and symblepharon **(Figs. 7A and B)**, which requires discontinuation of the ADC.

To limit the delivery of the ADC to the ocular surface, vasoconstrictive eye drops are applied prior to the infusion along with placement of cold packs over the eyes.[35] Prophylactic corticosteroid drops are then administered for 72 hours post-infusion. The avoidance of refractive contact lenses and the use of frequent preservative-free artificial tears throughout the treatment cycle decreased the risk for developing a corneal ulcer or dry eye syndrome. If a corneal ulcer develops, ADC discontinuation is required (grade 3 event), and higher-order management strategies are needed including performing a culture and starting topical antibiotics. Higher-order management with amniotic membrane placement or patch grafting in cases of thinning or perforation should be considered in cases of sterile keratitis.

Mirvetuximab is a second- or third-line agent in the treatment of ovarian cancer that has failed platinum-based therapies that targets folate-receptor alpha (FRα). The cytotoxic payload is maytansinoid DM4 (derivative

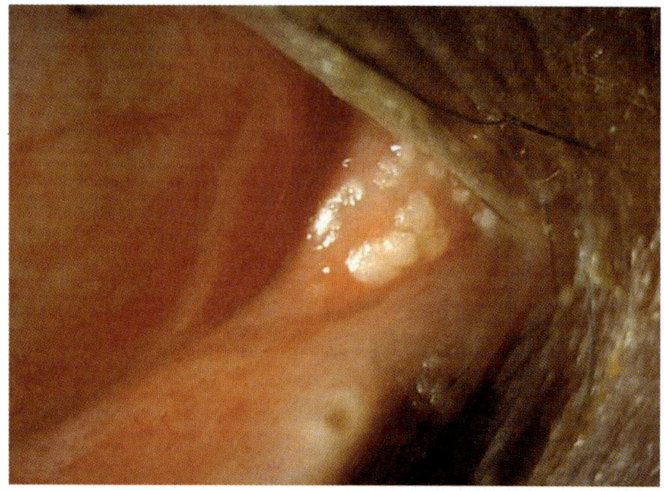

Fig. 6: A slit lamp photograph showing the development of squamous epithelial plaques in the right caruncle of a patient on tisotumab.
Source: Uveitis Course - Grand Rounds 18. International Uveitis Study Group (IUSG). October 11, 2025. Available from: https://youtu.be/pNJBcK5iP2s?si=kxQm2qSQy-qd5OQg.

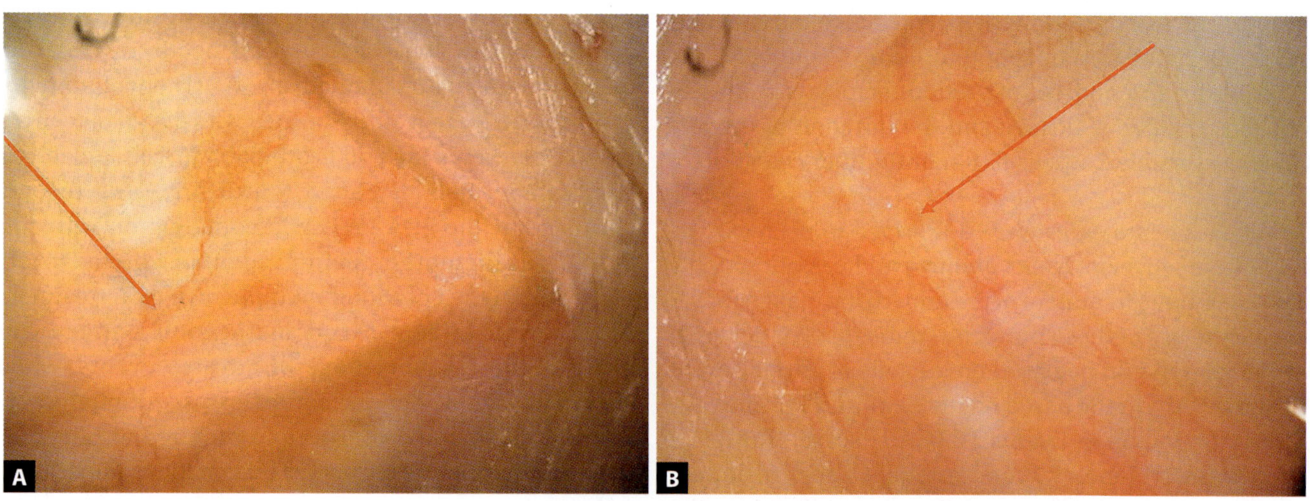

Figs. 7A and B: A slit lamp photograph showing a normal forniceal contour in the right eye (red arrow, left) compared to the early formation of a symblepharon with the development of subepithelial fibrosis in the left eye (red arrow, right).
Source: Uveitis Course - Grand Rounds 18. International Uveitis Study Group (IUSG). October 11, 2025. Available from: https://youtu.be/pNJBcK5iP2s?si=kxQm2qSQy-qd5OQg.

of maytansine-4) or auristatin metabolite [monomethyl auristatin F (MMAF)] and attached via a cleavable linker. Ocular examinations are needed at baseline and prior to every other cycle. Ocular toxicities occur in the cornea despite the absence or minimal expression of FRα on the ocular surface.[39,40] Grade 1 or 2 keratopathy is reversible, and the most common events are blurred vision (40%), keratopathy (30%), and dry eye (25%). There were no grade 3 or 4 events in clinical trials.[41] No retinal toxicity was reported despite the expression of FRα in the retinal pigment epithelium. However, cases of anterior uveitis were reported in clinical trials. If a grade 2 event occurs, hold the ADC and reassess weekly until the adverse event improves to grade 1. Topical corticosteroids are administered through day 10 of the infusion cycle as a mitigation strategy. Based on a large data study by Kim et al., the real-world cumulative incidence of developing uveitis with any ADC at 3 years is 0.33 and 0.14% for formation of a corneal ulcer.[35] The development of an adverse event was associated with a statistically significant increase in survival.[42] Thus, ocular adverse events should be treated without permanently stopping the ADC unless they are high-grade.

In summary, always refer to the current prescribing information for the most up-to-date dose modification and management guidance with new clinical data. The oncology care team should monitor patients through asking an ocular review of symptoms. Close communication between oncologists and ophthalmologists is needed to determine if an IRAE occurs, the grade of the adverse event, and if a dose delay, reduction, or drug discontinuation is needed.[43] In order to control the underlying metastatic disease, try to avoid discontinuation of an immunotherapy agent whenever possible. Also, remind patients to have intraocular pressures and lens status monitored to detect glaucoma and cataract formation with corticosteroid use.

Ocular toxicities are often associated with other systemic IRAES that dictate the course of treatment. Nonetheless, ophthalmologists should be vigilant for life-threatening complications, which may require cessation of immunotherapy, such as myasthenia gravis, giant cell arteritis, or metastases masquerading as uveitis. With more experience, the list of IRAEs is likely to increase, and they should always be included in the differential diagnosis when seeing a cancer patient with new ocular symptoms. With the increased use, continued development of new agents, and more clinical indications, it is important for all ophthalmologists to understand and identify IRAEs. While the percent of patients with ocular adverse events varies by drug class, IRAEs can be blinding and require prompt diagnosis and treatment. Over time, the CTCAE grading of ocular complications will change to decouple visual acuities and clinical findings.[44] Algorithms for the diagnosis and management of these ocular adverse events can be found in several recent papers by Chang et al. and the National Comprehensive Cancer Network guidelines, which can be found in the works cited in this chapter.[45,46]

TUMOR NECROSIS FACTOR ALPHA INHIBITOR-INDUCED UVEITIS

Case Presentation

Personal Information

A 50-year-old female has had blurred vision and floaters in both eyes for 7 months.

History of Present Illness

She had previously been treated with difluprednate 0.05% twice a day in both eyes without any improvement in her symptoms. On review of systems, she reported fatigue and lower-extremity paresthesia.

Physical Examination

The best-corrected visual acuity in both eyes was 20/40. While the anterior chambers were quiet, there were 2+ vitreous cell, vitreous condensations, and snowballs present bilaterally. Only peripheral, atrophic chorioretinal scars were noted **(Fig. 8)**.

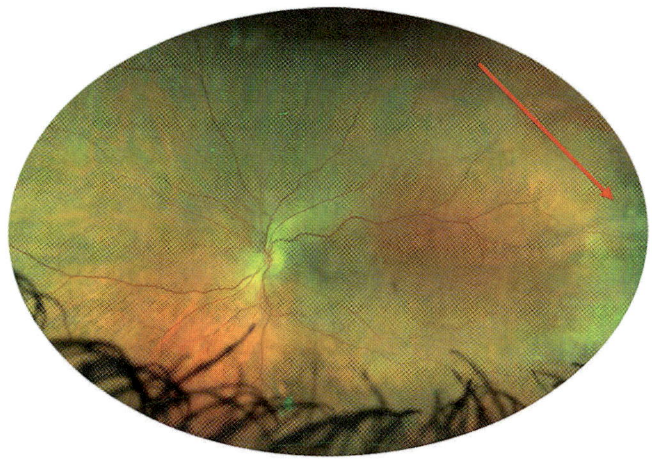

Fig. 8: A color fundus photo of the left eye showing peripheral chorioretinal scars (red arrow).
Source: Uveitis Course - Grand Rounds 18. International Uveitis Study Group (IUSG). October 11, 2025. Available from: https://youtu.be/pNJBcK5iP2s?si=kxQm2qSQy-qd5OQg.

TABLE 2: Slit lamp examination of a patient having tumor necrosis factor alpha inhibitor-induced uveitis.

OD	***Parameter***	***OS***
20/40	BCVA	20/40
19 mm Hg	IOP	20 mm Hg
Normal	Lids/Lashes	Normal
White and quiet	Conjunctiva	White and quiet
Clear	Cornea	Clear
Deep and quiet	Anterior chamber	Deep and quiet
Normal	Iris	Normal
Clear	Lens	Clear
2+ cell, vitreous condensations, and snowballs	Vitreous	2+ cell, vitreous condensations, and snowballs
Peripheral chorioretinal scars	Fundus	Peripheral chorioretinal scars

(BCVA: best-corrected visual acuity; IOP: intraocular pressure; KPs: keratic precipitates; OD: right eye; OS: left eye)

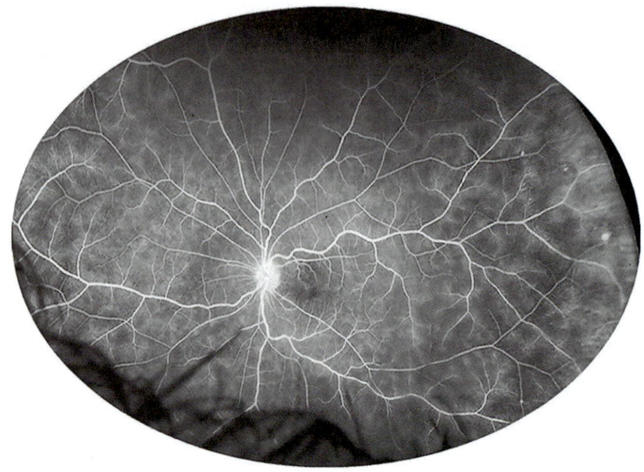

Fig. 9: A fluorescein angiogram of the left eye showing late, diffuse, small vessel leakage and staining of the peripheral temporal scarring. Optic disc leakage is also present.
Source: Uveitis Course - Grand Rounds 18. International Uveitis Study Group (IUSG). October 11, 2025. Available from: https://youtu.be/pNJBcK5iP2s?si=kxQm2qSQy-qd5OQg.

Slit Lamp Examination

Slit lamp examination findings in a patient with tumor necrosis factor alpha inhibitor-induced uveitis are summarized in **Table 2**.

Ancillary Testing

Fluorescein angiography was performed in both eyes and showed late, diffuse, small vessel leakage, optic disc leakage, and staining of the peripheral scarring **(Fig. 9)**. An indocyanine green angiography study did not reveal choroidal lesions and normal perfusion bilaterally **(Fig. 10)**. OCT scans through the macula of both eyes showed no macular edema and the presence of mild epiretinal membranes **(Fig. 11)**.

Uveitis Workup

Serologic testing for the HLA-B27 antigen and Lyme titers, and reverse sequence testing for syphilis via Treponema pallidum antibodies were negative. A chest X-ray was also normal. Given the peripheral paresthesias on the review of systems, an MRI of the brain and orbits was ordered with and without contrast to assess for lesions suggestive of multiple sclerosis, which was negative. Since the patient was 50 years old, primary intraocular lymphoma remained on the differential diagnosis along with undifferentiated intermediate uveitis.

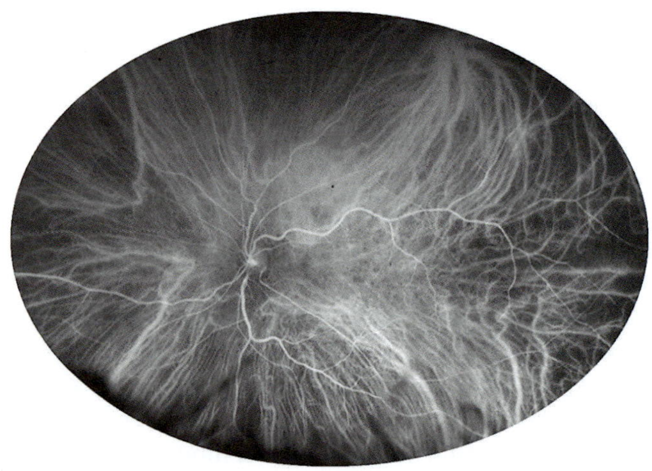

Fig. 10: An indocyanine green angiogram of the left eye showing no choroidal lesions and normal perfusion.
Source: Uveitis Course - Grand Rounds 18. International Uveitis Study Group (IUSG). October 11, 2025. Available from: https://youtu.be/pNJBcK5iP2s?si=kxQm2qSQy-qd5OQg.

Initial Treatment

While there was no macular edema, fluorescein angiography showed diffuse vascular leakage; with vitreous cells and condensations blurring her vision. She was tapered off difluprednate by one drop a day per week. Concurrently, oral prednisone was started at 60 mg daily for 2 weeks and tapered by 5 mg decrements weekly.

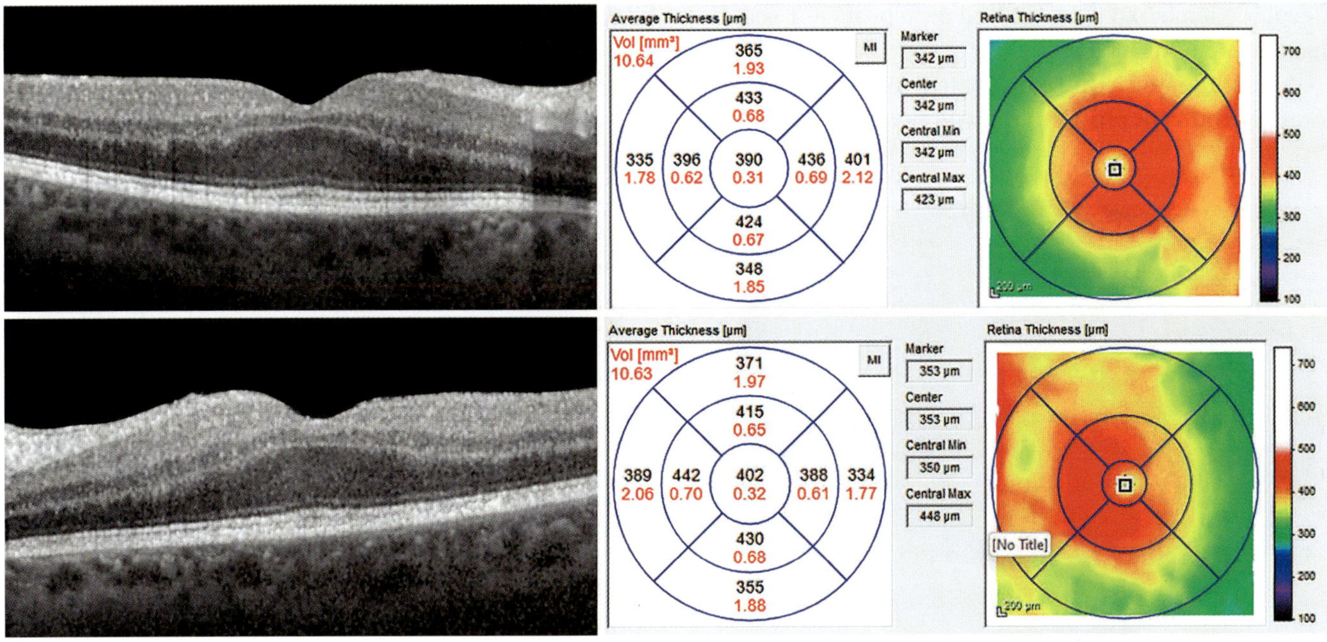

Fig. 11: Macular optical coherence tomography (OCT) scans of the right eye (superior) and the left eye (inferior) showing the absence of cystoid macular edema and the presence of mild epiretinal membranes.
Source: Uveitis Course - Grand Rounds 18. International Uveitis Study Group (IUSG). October 11, 2025. Available from: https://youtu.be/pNJBcK5iP2s?si=kxQm2qSQy-qd5OQg.

When re-examined 1 month later, her vision had improved to 20/25 in the right eye and 20/30 in the left eye. While there was less leakage on repeat fluorescein angiography, it remained present in both eyes. She was started on adalimumab 40 mg subcutaneously every other week and tapered off the prednisone by 5 mg/week.

Follow-up

Three months later, she returned with a drop in her vision to 20/20 in both eyes with new keratic precipitates on the cornea of both anterior chambers with 2+ cell in the right eye and 1+ cell in the left eye. There was also an increase in vitreous cells in the right eye to 3+ and continued 2+ cells in the left eye. The vitreous condensations and the number of snowballs also increased **(Fig. 12)**. On fluorescein angiography, there was more, diffuse, small vessel leakage and the presence of cystoid macular edema was noted on OCT scans in the left eye **(Figs. 13 and 14)**. With the paradoxical development of anterior chamber cells and more vitreous condensations, adalimumab was discontinued. The patient was referred for a pars plana vitrectomy of the right eye to rule out primary intraocular lymphoma as the cause of the intermediate uveitis. The vitreous biopsy was negative for a monoclonal B cell population, and nonspecific inflammation was noted. She was started on mycophenolate mofetil 1,000 mg twice a day; 4 months later, the vision had improved to 20/30 in the right eye and 20/25 in the left eye with 1+ vitreous cells noted on examination and resolution of the anterior chamber reaction in both eyes **(Fig. 15)**. The cystoid

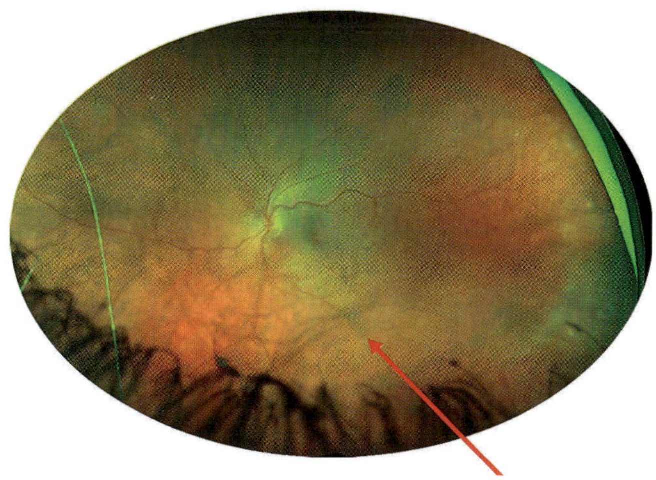

Fig. 12: A color fundus photo of the left eye showing more vitreous condensations at the 3-month follow-up after the start of adalimumab (red arrow).
Source: Uveitis Course - Grand Rounds 18. International Uveitis Study Group (IUSG). October 11, 2025. Available from: https://youtu.be/pNJBcK5iP2s?si=kxQm2qSQy-qd5OQg.

macular edema had also resolved on repeat OCT scans of the macula in the left eye.

In conclusion, the paradoxical worsening of the intermediate uveitis bilaterally was attributed to adalimumab-induced uveitis. An alternative explanation was a treatment failure with adalimumab. However, the patient did have improvement while on the prednisone taper and only developed an anterior chamber reaction when treated with the adalimumab, which was not present prior in her disease course. More importantly, there was a 2-step reduction in vitreous cells and resolution of vitreous condensations in both eyes with the start of mycophenolate without concomitant prednisone use. While the development or worsening of intraocular inflammation is an uncommon adverse effect associated with TNF-inhibitors, it has been posited that a cytokine disequilibrium with an increase in other inflammatory cytokines, such as interferons, leads to inflammation.[47] The highest risk of drug-induced uveitis has been associated with the use of etanercept, a soluble TNF-α receptor that traps the circulating cytokine.[47] Etanercept is associated with a threefold higher risk of drug-induced uveitis compared to adalimumab and almost a two-fold increase compared with infliximab.[48] Anterior uveitis is the most common clinical presentation; however, there have been reports of intermediate or posterior uveitis and scleritis. The time to onset of inflammation varies widely, ranging from 2 and 24 months after treatment initiation.[49]

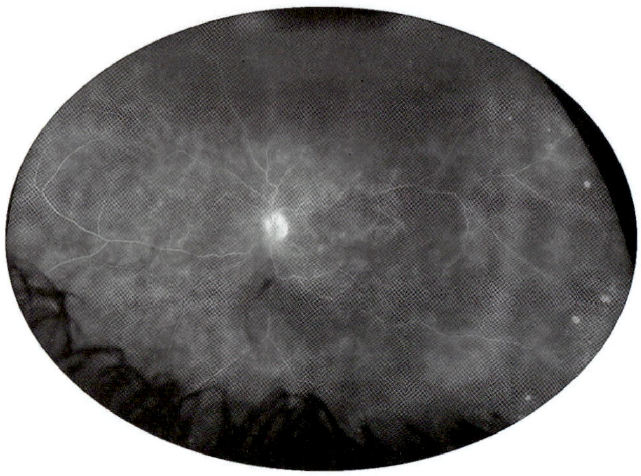

Fig. 13: A fluorescein angiogram of the left eye showing more late, diffuse, small vessel leakage with blockage by the increase in vitreous condensations.

Source: Uveitis Course - Grand Rounds 18. International Uveitis Study Group (IUSG). October 11, 2025. Available from: https://youtu.be/pNJBcK5iP2s?si=kxQm2qSQy-qd5OQg.

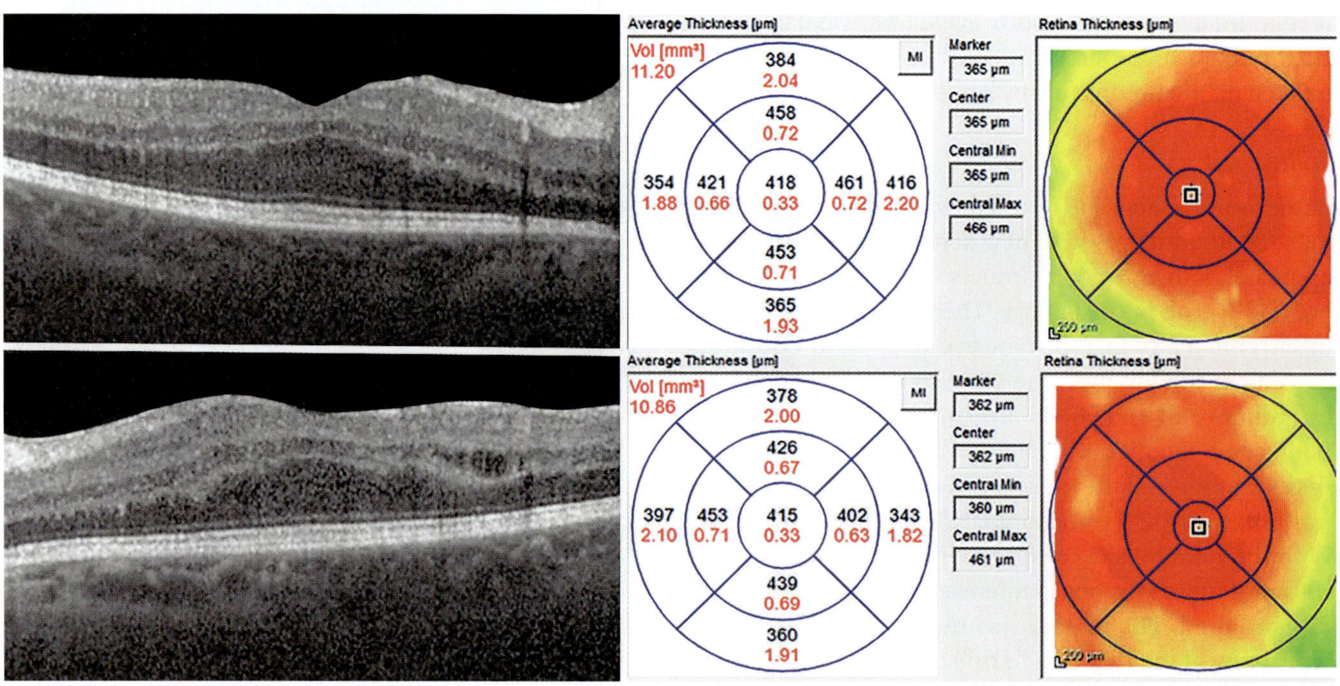

Fig. 14: Macular optical coherence tomography (OCT) scans of the right eye (superior) and the left eye (inferior) showing the presence of cystoid macular edema in the left eye.

Source: Uveitis Course - Grand Rounds 18. International Uveitis Study Group (IUSG). October 11, 2025. Available from: https://youtu.be/pNJBcK5iP2s?si=kxQm2qSQy-qd5OQg.

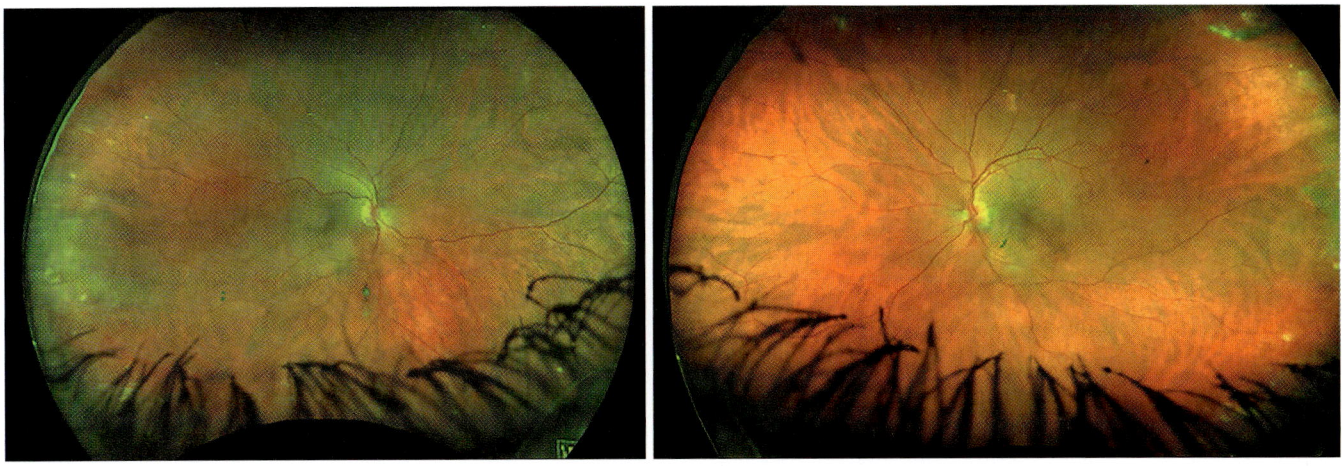

Fig. 15: Color fundus photos of both eyes 4 months after the start of mycophenolate mofetil showing clearer media without vitreous condensations and stable temporal peripheral chorioretinal scarring.
Source: Uveitis Course - Grand Rounds 18. International Uveitis Study Group (IUSG). October 11, 2025. Available from: https://youtu.be/pNJBcK5iP2s?si=kxQm2qSQy-qd5OQg.

Discussion

How do you assess whether epidemiologic factors are causally related to disease? 60 years ago, Sir Bradford Hill, a British epidemiologist and statistician, proposed a set of factors he used to determine causality in an epidemiologic evaluation. We know that just because there is a correlation, this does not necessarily indicate causation. This is the basis of the Bradford Hill criteria, which are still used today. I will not dwell on each criterion, but the strength of the association, the consistency, the specificity, the temporal relationship, a dose response curve, the plausibility, coherence, experimental evidence, and analogy were important to assess.[50] It is not critical to satisfy all criteria to argue for causation after an epidemiologic exposure.

Not counting biosimilars, there are five main TNF-α inhibitors. One is the soluble receptor, etanercept, which has the Fc portion of an immunoglobulin molecule attached to receptors. It acts like a sponge and irreversibly binds to soluble TNF-α molecules. The other drugs in the class bind to cell surface receptors, activate complement, and induce cell lysis. Of the four monoclonal antibodies, the first was infliximab, a chimeric human-murine antibody. Adalimumab and golimumab are fully humanized monoclonal antibodies. Certolizumab differs because of the polyethylene glycol moiety attached to the Fab fragment, making it less likely to cross the placenta when prescribed to pregnant women.

These chemical differences also equate to functional differences. Etanercept has the least risk of reactivating tubercular infections, but also has less efficacy in inflammatory bowel disease, sarcoidosis, and arguably, uveitis. Comparatively, the monoclonal antibodies are efficacious for each of those indications. Previously, the nomenclature for tumor necrosis factor beta (TNF-β) was lymphotoxin, which has since been abandoned. It is not necessary to refer to TNF as TNF-α, but note that the soluble receptor, etanercept, will also bind TNF-β. As mentioned, infliximab has the greatest likelihood of inducing neutralizing antibodies due to its chimeric composition. One advantage of infliximab is its intravenous administration, the use of a loading dose, and a very rapid onset of action.

My (JR) group was arguably the first to do a large registry-based study on whether TNF inhibitors induce uveitis. We used a registry maintained at Oregon Health & Science University. When the data were reviewed in 2007, there were 43 cases of uveitis attributable to etanercept, 14 with infliximab, and two with adalimumab.[51] When adjusting for the frequency of prescription, we concluded that etanercept was more likely to induce uveitis than the other two monoclonal antibodies. Often, these agents were prescribed for diseases like ankylosing spondylitis or psoriatic arthritis that were associated with concurrent intraocular inflammation. If the analysis was restricted to diseases like rheumatoid arthritis, which is not associated with the development of uveitis, we still found that etanercept was more likely to induce uveitis.

A better approach would be a national registry that captures an entire population's use of TNF-inhibitors compared to our registry that lacked universal reporting of toxicities. A Swedish registry reported in 2007 the rates of new-onset uveitis with the use of adalimumab, etanercept, and infliximab. Jacobsson et al. found that adalimumab use led to roughly a 50% reduction in the odds of developing uveitis, whereas etanercept doubled the chance of inducing uveitis.[48]

Finally, a recent meta-analysis included 18 studies on TNF-inhibitor-induced uveitis in over 11,000 patients.[52] Adalimumab, when compared to etanercept, had a 70% less likelihood of being associated with the development of uveitis. Etanercept also had a higher risk for inducing uveitis than either golimumab or infliximab. There is a precedent for TNF inhibitors causing paradoxical reactions, as in sarcoidosis, psoriasis, and inflammatory bowel disease. This includes either new onset of disease or worsening of preexisting inflammation. While a definitive explanation remains unclear, the immune system can be thought of as having checks and balances to carefully coordinate between homeostasis and inflammation. Introduction of a TNF-inhibitor could tip that balance, and the evidence does strongly support the concept that etanercept can cause intraocular inflammation and is less efficacious in treating of uveitis.

TABLE 3: Slit lamp examination of a patient having Ibrutinib-Related Uveitis

OD	*Parameter*	*OS*
20/70	BCVA	20/40
12 mm Hg	IOP	11 mm Hg
Normal	Lids/Lashes	Normal
White and quiet	Conjunctiva	White and quiet
Fine KP (endothelial dusting)	Cornea	Fine KP (endothelial dusting)
2+ cell, no flare	Anterior chamber	1–2+ cell, no flare
Normal	Iris	Normal
Posterior chamber intraocular lens	Lens	Posterior chamber intraocular lens
0.4	Optic nerve	0.4
Normal	Vitreous	Normal
Macular edema, epiretinal membrane	Fundus	Macular edema, epiretinal membrane

(BCVA: best-corrected visual acuity; IOP: intraocular pressure; KP: keratic precipitates; OD: right eye; OS: left eye)

IBRUTINIB-RELATED UVEITIS

Case Presentation

Personal Data

A 75-year-old male with chronic lymphocytic leukemia (CLL) presented with blurred vision in both eyes.

History of Present Illness

He was treated with ibrutinib 420 mg/day for 9 years along with monthly intravenous immunoglobulin infusions. Four years prior, he developed post-traumatic anterior uveitis that resolved with a corticosteroid taper only to recur as an anterior and intermediate uveitis 1 month later. The inflammation resolved with topical corticosteroid treatment, but posterior synechiae remained on examination. He underwent uncomplicated cataract extraction in both eyes 2 years prior, and no macular edema or anterior uveitis was seen at multiple follow-up visits over the following 2 years. The patient was seen by an outside provider one week before presentation, and the ibrutinib was discontinued at that time.

Physical Examination

The best-corrected visual acuity was 20/70 in the right eye and 20/40 in the left eye. The anterior chamber of the right eye contained 2+ cells and 1–2+ cells in the left eye. Examination of the fundus showed bilateral epiretinal membranes and macular edema that was greater in the right eye.

Slit lamp examination: Slit lamp examination findings in a patient with ibrutinib-related uveitis are summarized in **Table 3**.

Ancillary Testing

Optical coherence tomography imaging of both eyes showed epiretinal membranes and the presence of cystoid macular edema **(Fig. 16)**.

Uveitis Workup

Medical records were obtained from the patient's prior ophthalmologist, which showed negative serologic testing for the HLA-B27 antigen, negative reverse sequence testing for syphilis via Treponema pallidum antibodies, and a negative chest X-ray.

Initial Treatment

A taper of prednisolone acetate 1% was prescribed starting at one drop four times a day followed by weekly decrements of one drop. In addition, he was started on one drop of bromfenac daily. Ibrutinib was restarted at 420 mg daily.

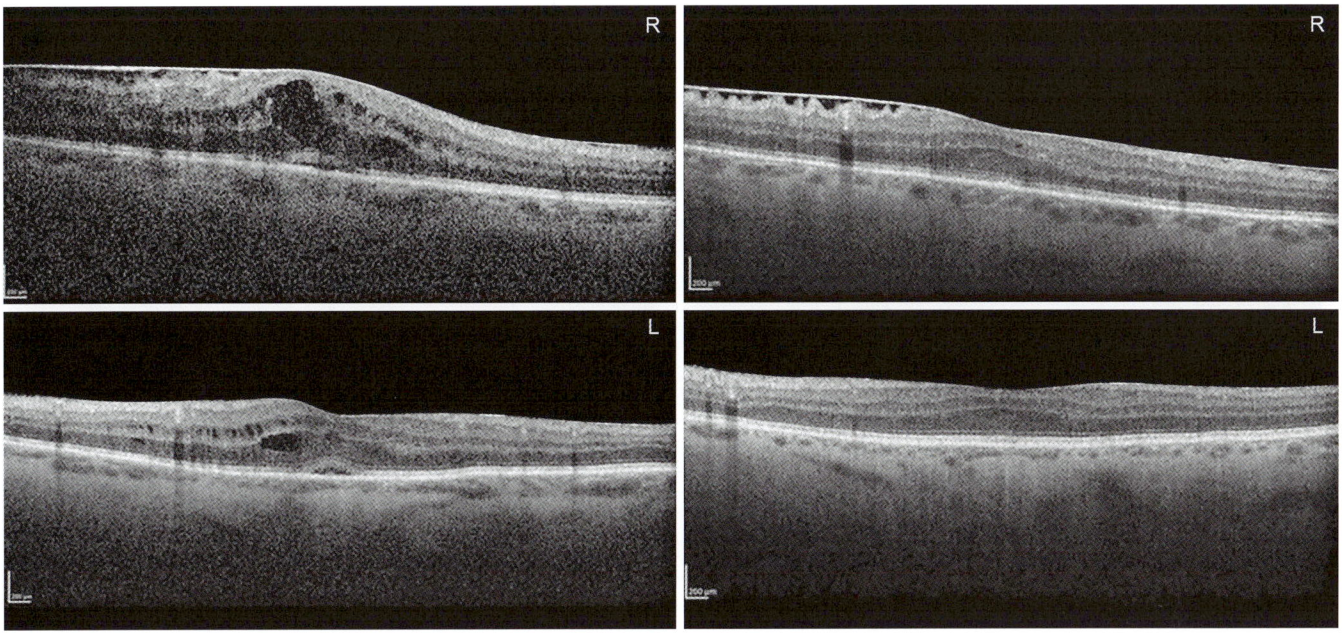

Fig. 16: A macular OCT scan of the right eye (top left) and the left eye (bottom left) at presentation showing the presence of cystoid macular edema and epiretinal membrane formation greater in the right eye. A small amount of subretinal fluid can also be seen in the baseline scan of right eye. Repeat OCT scans 3 months after treatment show a persistent epiretinal membrane in the right eye (top right) and resolution of the cystoid macular edema in both eyes.
Source: Uveitis Course - Grand Rounds 18. International Uveitis Study Group (IUSG). October 11, 2025. Available from: https://youtu.be/pNJBcK5iP2s?si=kxQm2qSQy-qd5OQg.

Follow-up

Three months later, the best-corrected visual acuity in the right eye improved to 20/25-1 and 20/20-2 in the left eye. The epiretinal membranes appeared stable on dilated fundus examination. OCT testing showed a markedly decreased central subfield thickness of the macula in both eyes **(Fig. 16)**.

Discussion

Ibrutinib is an oral Bruton tyrosine kinase (BTK) inhibitor used primarily to treat CLL.[53,54] Binding of the drug to the BTK protein stops downstream phosphorylation and results in decreased proliferation and increased apoptosis of malignant B cells. Systemic side effects include the development of a peripheral neuropathy, diarrhea, bleeding, fatigue, and autoimmune skin, rheumatologic, and blood disorders. The onset of ibrutinib-associated IRAEs usually occurs 1–3 years after the initiation of treatment. Ibrutinib also inhibits other small molecule kinases through targeting epidermal growth factor receptors, MEK, and IL-2-inducible kinase in T-cells. The most common ocular IRAEs are anterior and intermediate uveitis with variable amounts of optic disc edema and cystoid macular edema.[55] Patients with a preexisting history of uveitis are at an increased risk for developing ibrutinib-associated inflammation.[56] Additional ocular IRAEs include dry eyes, subconjunctival hemorrhages, and branch artery occlusions. While the mechanism of these complications is unknown, it has been posited that concurrent inhibition of non-BTK pathways may contribute.[57] The most important consideration in treating a patient with ibrutinib-associated uveitis is whether this is a grade 1 or 2 adverse event and if it is responsive to corticosteroids without the need to stop the drug.

WHEN THE CURE CLOUDS THE VISION: UNRAVELING ANTIBIOTIC-ASSOCIATED UVEITIS

Case Presentation

Personal Data

A 67-year-old woman with no past ocular history presented with 3 weeks of acute onset, painless vision loss in both eyes.

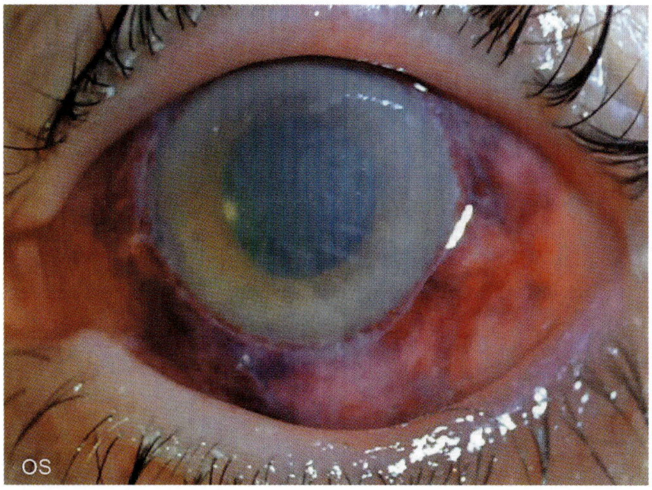

Fig. 17: A slit lamp photograph of the left eye showing corneal edema and folds in Descemet membrane. Subconjunctival hemorrhage seen is a result of intravitreous injections given prior to the photograph.
Source: Uveitis Course - Grand Rounds 18. International Uveitis Study Group (IUSG). October 11, 2025. Available from: https://youtu.be/pNJBcK5iP2s?si=kxQm2qSQy-qd5OQg.

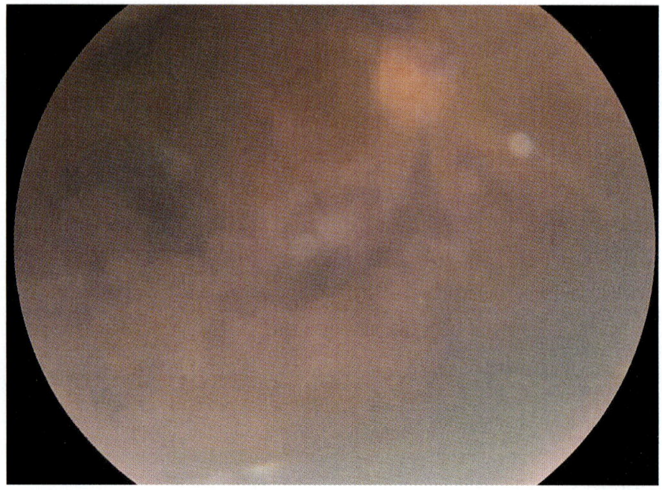

Fig. 18: A color fundus photo of the right eye showing hemorrhages along the vascular arcades.
Source: Uveitis Course - Grand Rounds 18. International Uveitis Study Group (IUSG). October 11, 2025. Available from: https://youtu.be/pNJBcK5iP2s?si=kxQm2qSQy-qd5OQg.

History of Present Illness

She had undergone uncomplicated cataract surgery in the right eye 28 days prior. One day after cataract surgery in the left eye, she developed rapidly progressive, painless bilateral vision loss. She was taking prednisolone acetate 1%, ketorolac 0.5%, and ofloxacin 0.3% drops in the left eye four times a day. She was also prescribed atropine 1% daily in both eyes.

Physical Examination

Visual acuity was no light perception (NLP) in the right eye and light perception in the left eye. Subconjunctival hemorrhages, corneal edema, and Descemet folds were present bilaterally **(Fig. 17)**. A pupillary membrane extended from the iris posteriorly to the ciliary body in both eyes. The posterior chamber examination was hazy due to the presence of the pupillary membranes, but showed numerous hemorrhages along the arcades in both eyes **(Fig. 18)**.

Slit Lamp Examination

Slit lamp examination findings in a patient with antibiotic-associated uveitis are summarized in **Table 4**.

TABLE 4: Slit lamp examination of a patient having unraveling antibiotic-associated uveitis.

OD	***Parameter***	***OS***
NLP	BCVA	LP
38 mm Hg	IOP	16 mm Hg
Normal	Lids/Lashes	Normal
Subconjunctival hemorrhages	Conjunctiva	Subconjunctival hemorrhages
Descemet folds and edema	Cornea	Descemet folds and edema
Trace cell, no flare	Anterior chamber	Trace cell, no flare
Pupillary membrane, pharmacologically dilated	Iris	Pupillary membrane, pharmacologically dilated
Posterior chamber intraocular lens	Lens	Posterior chamber intraocular lens
No cells	Vitreous	No cells
Numerous hemorrhages along the arcades with a hazy view	Fundus	Numerous hemorrhages along the arcades with a hazy view

(BCVA: best-corrected visual acuity, IOP: intraocular pressure; KPs: keratic precipitates; NLP: no light perception; LP: light perception; OD: right eye; OS: left eye)

Ancillary Testing

Due to the poor view, a B-scan ultrasound of each eye was performed, which showed thickening of the ocular coats and vitreous membranes **(Fig. 19)**. An anterior chamber ultrasound biomicroscopic examination showed low reflective membranes across the pupil and extending from the iris to the ciliary body **(Fig. 20)**.

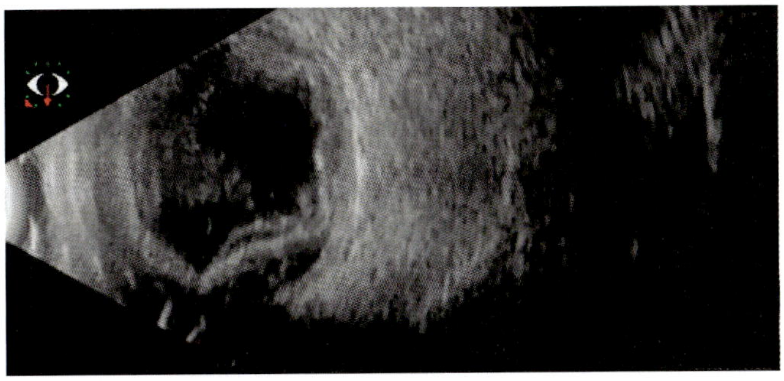

Fig. 19: A B-scan ultrasound image of the left eye showing the presence of choroidal thickening, subretinal fluid, and vitreous membranes.
Source: Uveitis Course - Grand Rounds 18. International Uveitis Study Group (IUSG). October 11, 2025. Available from: https://youtu.be/pNJBcK5iP2s?si=kxQm2qSQy-qd5OQg.

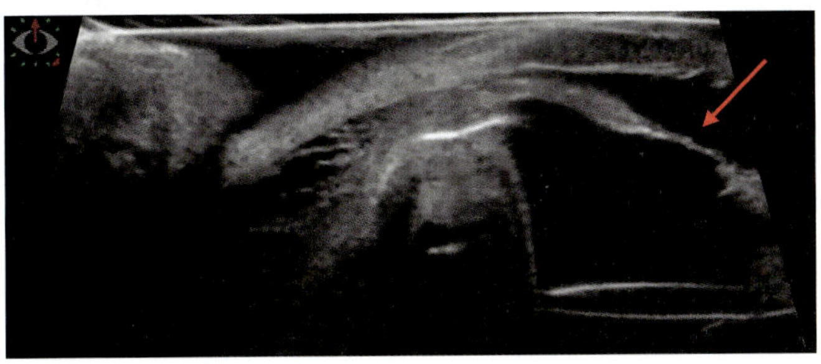

Fig. 20: An ultrasound biomicroscopy image of the anterior segment showing pupillary membrane formation with extension from the iris to the ciliary body (red arrow).
Source: Uveitis Course - Grand Rounds 18. International Uveitis Study Group (IUSG). October 11, 2025. Available from: https://youtu.be/pNJBcK5iP2s?si=kxQm2qSQy-qd5OQg.

Uveitis Workup

An anterior chamber paracentesis was performed, and the aqueous fluid was sent for polymerase chain reaction (PCR) testing for cytomegalovirus (CMV), varicela zoster virus, and herpes simplex (HSV) given the concern for the development of acute retinal necrosis. The sample was negative, and serologic testing for viral etiologies was only positive for HSV. Further laboratory studies were ordered to assess for underlying autoimmune disorders including antineutrophil cytoplasmic antibodies (ANCA), antinuclear antibodies (ANA), ESR, and CRP. All were negative along with serologic testing for syphilis including rapid plasma reagin (RPR) and fluorescent treponemal antibody (FTA)-absorption and blood cultures. Similarly, a complete blood count and complete metabolic panel were normal.

Initial Treatment

Given the rapid progression and unclear etiology, intravitreal injections of vancomycin (1 mg/0.1 mL), ceftazidime (2.25 mg/0.1 mL), and ganciclovir (2 mg/0.1 mL) were performed bilaterally on the day of presentation. This accounts for the subconjunctival hemorrhages noted on the slit lamp photograph in **Figure 17**. With negative viral PCR results obtained from the aqueous sample and negative serologic testing, a pars plana vitrectomy was performed. The aspirate was sent for bacterial and fungal cultures, which were also negative. Operative records were obtained and both cataract surgeries were reported as uncomplicated with intercameral vancomycin (1.0 mg/0.1 mL) administered at the end of each case. No other adverse postoperative events were noted at the surgery center. In the setting of marked postoperative inflammation, retinal hemorrhages, and a negative infectious work-up, the diagnosis of hemorrhagic occlusive retinal vasculitis (HORV) secondary to the administration of intraocular vancomycin was made.

Follow-up

The patient was started on one drop per hour of prednisolone acetate 1% and prednisone 40 mg daily by mouth. Despite these treatments, the vision decreased to NLP in both eyes with the development of hypotony.

Discussion

Antibiotic-associated uveitis represents a diverse group of inflammatory syndromes triggered by systemic or intraocular administration. Among these, HORV is one of the better-characterized conditions, typically linked to intracameral vancomycin or mixed into the irrigation bottle for prophylaxis against endophthalmitis during otherwise uneventful cataract surgery. There is also a case of a patient that developed inflammation without retinal vasculitis after cataract surgery and then was given an intravitreal injection of vancomycin for possible bacterial endophthalmitis. The patient subsequently developed HORV. Patients typically have a normal postoperative day-one examination before developing delayed, painless, rapidly progressive vision loss at a median of 8 days after surgery due to the extensive vasculitis and resulting ischemia. HORV can occur whether the patient is exposed to vancomycin in one eye only, administered in both eyes, or into the second eye sequentially. There are some interesting features of HORV. In some cases of bilateral vancomycin exposure, HORV develops only in the second eye. That observation has led to speculation that sensitization in the first eye led to the development of HORV on exposure in the second eye from immune system priming to the vancomycin. In some bilateral HORV cases, the reaction in the second eye was more severe, and the onset was quicker. On retrospection, there was probably HORV developing in the first eye that received vancomycin, but it was mild and presented as a few intraretinal hemorrhages in the periphery that were missed during the postoperative examinations. Then the second eye developed much more dramatic findings, which led to the diagnosis of HORV in both eyes.

These observations led to the proposed pathophysiology of HORV being exposure sensitization after the first surgery and triggering of the immune response after the second surgery. However, as previously mentioned, HORV can occur under circumstances of unilateral exposure. In consultation with immunologists, Witkin et al. proposed that HORV is a type III hypersensitivity reaction, similar to leukocytoclastic vasculitis, in which antigen-antibody complexes deposit in small vessels.[58] Skin testing was performed on patients included in the original case series, and no hypersensitivity to vancomycin was observed. However, skin testing is designed to identify type I and some type IV hypersensitivities, not a type III reaction. While not definitive, there is very strong evidence that vancomycin is the causative agent, as all these patients had only this exposure in common. Additionally, there is evidence of a dose-response, as those exposed to vancomycin in the irrigation solution bottle had a milder clinical presentation given the lower drug concentration. This contrasts with intracameral vancomycin injection at the end of our case. Some patients, unfortunately, received additional vancomycin in the postoperative period for the suspicion of bacterial endophthalmitis. This additional exposure, including the patient we presented, had the worst outcomes with NLP vision. While not definitive, there is very strong evidence that vancomycin is the causative agent of HORV.

While there are patients that develop NLP vision, the final visual acuity ranges considerably. Mild cases can present with 20/20 vision, but the majority have 20/200 or worse. The initial clinical presentation is mild-to-moderate anterior chamber inflammation without a hypopyon. The patient we presented had the development of membranes and robust anterior chamber inflammation, but had also been through vitrectomy and multiple procedures prior to her first visit at our clinic, which might have influenced her severe presentation. The vitreous inflammation is typically mild, and the most important finding is hemorrhagic, occlusive retinal vasculitis on dilated fundus examination. Fluorescein angiography shows significant peripheral nonperfusion and blocking intraretinal hemorrhages throughout the periphery. A work-up for underlying autoimmune and infectious diseases is required, and was negative in all reported cases. With the extensive ischemia, patients can rapidly develop neovascular glaucoma and therefore need to be very carefully monitored with gonioscopy.

The treatment for this condition is first to control the inflammation with both topical prednisolone acetate 1% and oral prednisone. In a 36 patient case series published by Witkin et al., several patients were administered intravitreal corticosteroids, and anecdotally, had better final visual acuities.[58] This method of treatment is a consideration when attempting to control the inflammation quickly. The other treatment consideration is the ischemia and prevention of neovascular glaucoma. Intravitreal injection of anti-vascular endothelial growth factor (VEGF) agents followed by panretinal photocoagulation should be implemented. Avoiding additional vancomycin exposure is very important, and it is important to distinguish HORV from bacterial endophthalmitis (for which intravitreal vancomycin would be appropriate).

Since it was first described in 2017, there has been a shift in cataract surgeons' use of vancomycin. An American Society of Cataract and Refractive Surgery member survey in 2014 showed 36% of surgeons used intracameral antibiotics at the end of the case and 22% specifically used vancomycin.[59] After the publication of the Witkin et al. paper in 2017, the FDA issued an alert on the development of HORV with vancomycin use for cataract surgery prophylaxis. When the survey was repeated in 2021, there was a significantly increased number of surgeons administering other intracameral antibiotics, such as moxifloxacin, but the use of vancomycin had decreased despite the 2017 paper acknowledging that HORV was an extremely rare event. Is there a risk of HORV with other antibiotics? The only other antibiotic with which HORV has been reported is with intracameral moxifloxacin based on a case series of two patients.[60] One patient had a very good outcome with a final visual acuity of 20/20. The second case had a final visual acuity of 20/300 with a fundus appearance to that of vancomycin-associated-associated HORV patients. While this case series was an isolated report, it is possible that HORV can develop with the use of other intracameral antibiotics.

Although antibiotic-associated uveitis occurs only rarely with intracameral moxifloxacin, oral moxifloxacin can cause uveitis. Of all of the fluoroquinolones, moxifloxacin causes a very distinct clinical phenotype. Patients who develop moxifloxacin-associated uveitis often take the medication for pneumonia or a urinary tract infection and develop a dramatic, bilateral, acute iris transillumination (BAIT).[61] A less severe form known as bilateral acute depigmentation of the iris (BADI) has also been reported.[62] There is some debate in the literature whether some of the BAIT cases are all due to moxifloxacin or whether they are a reaction to the underlying viral or bacterial entity that is causing the infection for which they were treated. In the larger case series, most but not all patients who developed BAIT have received oral moxifloxacin. We will concentrate on oral moxifloxacin as the likely cause in most cases where a patient presents with an acute anterior uveitis with diffuse transillumination defects. The pupils often do not respond to light, and onset is typically 7–10 days after the start of the oral fluoroquinolone. A proposed mechanism of action is a direct toxic effect of the fluoroquinolone on the pigmented iris tissue. While the acute inflammation is managed with topical steroids, the transillumination defects persist resulting in chronic and often debilitating photophobia.

What is the evidence in the literature that moxifloxacin is the causative agent? After all, it is a very commonly prescribed class of antibiotics. There was a case–control study by Eadie et al. that included 26,000 patients and looked over a 15-year period at the risk of developing uveitis with different fluoroquinolones.[63] Moxifloxacin was associated with the highest rate of new-onset uveitis cases. Ciprofloxacin was associated with a lower relative risk. Finally, levofloxacin was not significantly associated with the development of uveitis. This large-scale study provides additional evidence that moxifloxacin is the predominant agent in this class associated with developing intraocular inflammation. Again, BAIT is a rare complication and does not necessarily preclude the use of oral fluoroquinolones.

The third antibiotic-induced uveitis to mention is rifabutin-associated uveitis, which has another distinctive appearance. It commonly causes the formation of a hypopyon, which mimics HLA-B27-associated uveitis. Rarely, intermediate and posterior uveitis develops without anterior chamber cells or the development of a hypopyon.[64] Compared to the other medications discussed, the onset is delayed and occurs weeks to months after the initiation of therapy. The risk is compounded by concurrent use of other medications metabolized through the hepatic cytochrome P-450 pathway, such as clarithromycin or fluconazole, which inhibit rifabutin metabolism and elevate drug concentrations. While topical corticosteroids are the mainstay of treatment, rifabutin may need to be discontinued to fully control intraocular inflammation.

The last antibiotic class that may induce uveitis is the sulfonamides, primarily sulfamethoxazole-trimethoprim. The uveitis is typically bilateral, anterior, and nongranulomatous. The largest series was published by Tildon et al. in 1991.[65] The onset typically occurs within a few weeks of initiating therapy, and the condition responds well to topical corticosteroids. In patients who develop uveitis after use of a sulfonamide, other agents in the class should be avoided, as the cases of uveitis in this series often occurred in the setting of Stevens–Johnson syndrome with elevated liver function tests or erythema multiforme.

In conclusion, it is important to take a thorough history in patients with uveitis, particularly medication use. Some forms of antibiotic-associated uveitis can be visually devastating or debilitating, requiring early intervention and further exposure to the antibiotic. Intervention often involves stopping the offending agent and preventing future exposure. Even with treatment, the effects can be irreversible, making it very important for the clinician to identify and distinguish medication-induced uveitis from other causes of ocular inflammation.

PEARLS FROM THE EXPERTS ON FREQUENTLY ASKED QUESTIONS

1. Was the case of ibrutinib-induced uveitis new in onset or an exacerbation of preexisting uveitis?

Answer: Given the negative serologic work-up and the absence of other risk factors, this appeared to be true ibrutinib-related uveitis. The patient's previous episode of uveitis was associated with trauma.

2. How long can uveitis last after infusion of alendronic acid or other bisphosphonates?

Answer: Most cases are typically self-limited with only anterior chamber inflammation and respond quickly to topical corticosteroid therapy. The onset is more rapid when the bisphosphonate is given intravenously, and the patient may require maintenance, low-dose corticosteroid drop therapy for several months or even a year until the drug is fully excreted and loses effectiveness. The occurrence of drug-induced uveitis is rare. If a patient is concerned that the development of intraocular inflammation is a potential side effect of a bisphosphonate, it is important to note that the morbidity and mortality associated with hip fractures in older patients is substantial. Physicians should emphasize that potential, rare side effects can occur with any prescribed drug. Thus, the relative risks of a mild uveitis that responds well to topical corticosteroids must be compared to the morbidity and mortality caused by a hip fracture from untreated osteoporosis. Bisphosphates have also been associated with the development of a drug-induced scleritis.

3. Has HORV been reported to occur following intravitreal injection of vancomycin to treat bacterial endophthalmitis and should the use of it be avoided in this context?

Answer: In a case series of 36 patients, there was one patient who had cataract surgery and did not have intraretinal hemorrhages suggestive of HORV. The patient then developed inflammation postoperatively and received intravitreal vancomycin after which HORV was diagnosed. However, vancomycin is one of the best antibiotics to use in the setting of suspected bacterial endophthalmitis because of its broad antibacterial coverage. We have used intravitreal vancomycin for years to treat endophthalmitis, and HORV may have occurred but was obscured due to the severity of bacterial endophthalmitis or misattributed to the infection itself. Nonetheless, HORV is quite rare, and intravitreal vancomycin injection to treat possible endophthalmitis should not be discouraged.

4. In a patient who develops chronic uveitis in the setting of an underlying malignancy, would you treat with immunosuppressive therapy?

Answer: This is a difficult decision, and you have to weigh the risks and benefits of treatment. If the patient is responding well to the immunotherapy and there are no other treatment options for the cancer, then it becomes a collective discussion with the oncologist regarding whether to start immunosuppressive therapy to preserve vision but at the cost of possibly reducing the lifespan. Can immunotherapy be started without jeopardizing the benefit of the ibrutinib for CLL patients with ibrutinib-associated uveitis? Can you control the IRAEs locally with periocular or intravitreal corticosteroid injections or corticosteroid drops without starting immunosuppressive therapy? While the latter approach is preferred, deciding on a treatment plan requires careful interaction between the oncology team and the ophthalmologist about what is the best overall approach for the patient.

5. Can topical medications, such as hypotensive agents derived from sulfonamides, also induce uveitis?

Answer: There are case reports of uveitis attributed to carbonic anhydrase inhibitors since they have a sulfonamide group in their chemical structure. However, the topical antihypertensive that is been most associated with uveitis is brimonidine, which can cause a granulomatous anterior uveitis. There have also been cases of choroidal detachment following the use of oral acetazolamide and sudden hypotony with topiramate use, but not uveitis with either drug. Metoprolol has also been associated with uveitis, leading to a shift to the use of other drugs in the beta-blocker class.

6. Can BAIT occur with use of topical fluoroquinolone drops?

Answer: A posited reason for the development of BAIT with oral formulations is that a higher concentration of the drug accumulates in the anterior chamber. However, there have been rare reports of BAIT occurring with topical moxifloxacin use as well. Another possible explanation for the occurrence with systemic administration is anterior chamber-acquired immune deviation.

7. Are there other agents that can cause uveitis that were not already discussed?

Answer: Vaccines can cause a drug-induced uveitis, most commonly due to the influenza vaccine. Cases of uveitis have developed after administration of the tetanus-diphtheria-pertussis, human papillomavirus, measles mumps and rubella, yellow fever, varicella zoster, hepatitis A and B, COVID-19, and the Bacille Calmette-Guérin vaccines. Anterior uveitis and posterior segment inflammation have been reported, including the development of acute posterior multifocal placoid pigment epitheliopathy, multifocal evanescent white dot syndrome, and Vogt-Koyanagi-Harada disease.

FINAL WRAP-UP

Though uncommon, drug-associated uveitis should remain in your differential diagnosis when evaluating a patient with ocular inflammation. The clinical presentation can mimic infectious, autoimmune, and postoperative uveitis, making the diagnosis challenging. A detailed medication history and careful evaluation of the timing of the inflammation onset is essential for the diagnosis. Clinicians should be familiar with the drug classes and vaccines that are associated with the development of uveitis and in the case of antineoplastic agents, IRAEs.

REFERENCES

1. Bhatti MT, Salama ARS. Neuro-ophthalmic side effects of molecularly targeted cancer drugs. Eye (Lond). 2018;32(2):287-301.
2. Niro A, Strippoli S, Alessio G, Sborgia L, Reechimurzo N, Guida M. Ocular Toxicity in Metastatic Melanoma Patients Treated With Mitogen-Activated Protein Kinase Inhibitors: A Case Series. Am J Ophthalmol. 2015;160(5):959-67.
3. Baraibar I, Melero I, Ponz-Sarvise M, Castanon E. Safety and Tolerability of Immune Checkpoint Inhibitors (PD-1 and PD-L1) in Cancer. Drug Saf. 2019;42(2):281-94.
4. Mellman I, Coukos G, Dranoff G. Cancer immunotherapy comes of age. Nature. 2011;480(7378):480-9.
5. Danlos FX, Voisin AL, Dyevre V, Michot JM, Routier E, Taillade L, et al. Safety and efficacy of anti-programmed death 1 antibodies in patients with cancer and pre-existing autoimmune or inflammatory disease. Eur J Cancer. 2018;91:21-9.
6. Dalvin LA, Shields CL, Orloff M, Sato T, Shields JA. Checkpoint Inhibitor Immune Therapy: Systemic Indications and Ophthalmic Side Effects. Retina. 2018;38 (6):1063-78.
7. Zhou R, Caspi RR. "Ocular immune privilege." F1000 Biol Rep. 2010;2:39.
8. AstraZeneca Pharmaceuticals LP. Imfinzi (Durvalumab) Injection, for Intravenous Use [Prescribing Information]. Wilmington, DE: AstraZeneca Pharmaceuticals LP; 2017.
9. Baughman DM, Lee CS, Snydsman BE, Jung HC. Bilateral uveitis and keratitis following nivolumab treatment for metastatic melanoma. Med Case Rep (Wilmington). 2017;3(2):8.
10. Bristol-Myers Squibb Company. Yervoy Injection [Prescribing Insert]. Princeton, NJ. Bristol-Myers Squibb Company; 2017.
11. EMD Serono Inc. Bavencio (Avelumab) Injection, for Intravenous Use [Prescribing Information]. Rockland, MD: EMD Serono, Inc. and Pfizer, Inc.; 2017.
12. Merck & Company Inc. Keytruda (Pembrolizumab) for Injection [Prescribing Information]. Whitehouse Station, NJ: Merck & Co, Inc.; 2017.
13. Nguyen AT, Elia M, Materin MA, Sznol M, Chow J. Cyclosporine for dry eye associated with nivolumab: a case progressing to corneal perforation. Cornea. 2016;35: 399-401.
14. Antoun J, Titah C, Cochereau I. Ocular and orbital side-effects of checkpoint inhibitors: a review article. Curr Opin Oncol. 2016;28(4):288-94.
15. Goldstein BL, Gedmintas L, Todd DJ. Drug-associated polymyalgia rheumatica/giant cell arteritis occurring in two patients after treatment with ipilimumab, an antagonist of CTLA-4. Arthritis Rheumatol. 2014;66:768-9.
16. Arai T, Harada K, Usui Y, Irisawa R, Tsuboi R. Case of acute anterior uveitis and Vogt-Koyanagi-Harada syndrome-like eruptions induced by nivolumab in a melanoma patient. J Dermatol. 2017;44(8):975-6.
17. Conrady CD, Larochelle M, Pecen P, Palestine A, Shakoor A, Singh A. "Checkpoint inhibitor-induced uveitis: a case series." Graefes Arch Clin Exp Ophthalmol. 2018; 256(1):187-91.
18. Kanno H, Ishida K, Yamada W, Nishida T, Takahashi N, Mochizuki K, et al. Uveitis induced by programmed cell death protein 1 inhibitor therapy with nivolumab in metastatic melanoma patient. J Infect Chemother. 2017;23(11):774-7.
19. Moorthy RS, Moorthy MS, Cunningham ET. "Drug Induced Uveitis." Curr Opin Opht. 2028;29(6):588-603.
20. Samra KA, Valdes-Navarro M, Lee S, Swan R, Foster CS, Anesi SD. A case of bilateral uveitis and papillitis in a patient treated with pembrolizumab. Eur J Ophthalmol. 2016;26(3):e46-8.
21. Thomas M, Armenti ST, Ayres MB, Demirci H. Uveal effusion after immune checkpoint inhibitor therapy. JAMA Ophthalmol. 2018;136(5):553-6.
22. Parikh RA, Chaon BC, Berkenstock MK. Ocular Complications of Checkpoint Inhibitors and Immunotherapeutic Agents: A Case Series. Ocul Immunol Inflamm. 2021;29(7-8):1585-90.
23. Francis JH, Jaben K, Santomasso BD, Canestraro J, Abramson DH, Chapman PB, et al. Immune Checkpoint Inhibitor-Associated Optic Neuritis. Ophthalmology. 2020;127(11):1585-9.
24. Ryu S, et al. "Therapeutic Inhibitors against Mutated BRAF and MEK for the Treatment of Metastatic Melanoma." Chonannam Med J. 2017;53(3):173-77.
25. Draganova D, Kerger J, Caspers L, Willermain F. Severe bilateral panuveitis during melanoma treatment by dabrafenib and trametinib. J Ophthalmic Inflamm Infect. 2015;5:17-9.
26. Guedj M, Queant A, Funck-Brentano E, Kramkimel N, Lellouch J, Monnet D, et al. Uveitis in patients with late-stage cutaneous melanoma treated with vemurafenib. JAMA Ophthalmol. 2014;132:1421-5.
27. Liu CY, Francis JH, Brodie SE, Marr B, Pulido JS, Marmor MF, et al. Retinal toxicities of cancer therapy drugs: biologics, small molecule inhibitors, and chemotherapies. Retina. 2014;34(7):1261-80.
28. Welsh SJ, Corrie PG. Management of BRAF and MEK inhibitor toxicities in patients with metastatic melanoma. Ther Adv Med Oncol. 2015;7:122-36.
29. Joshi L, Karydis A, Gemenetzi M, Shao EH, Taylor SJR. Uveitis as a result of MAP kinase pathway inhibition. Case Rep Ophthalmol. 2013;4:279-82.

30. Naranjo CA, Busto U, Sellers EM, Sandor P, Ruiz I, Roberts EA, et al. A method for estimating the probability of adverse drug reactions. Clin Pharmacol Ther. 1981;30(2):239-45.
31. McCannel TA, Chmielowski B, Finn RS, Goldman J, Ribas A, Wainberg ZA, et al. Bilateral subfoveal neurosensory retinal detachment associated with MEK inhibitor use for metastatic cancer. JAMA Ophthalmol. 2014;132(8):1005-9.
32. Schoenberger SD, Kim SJ. Bilateral multifocal central serous-like chorioretinopathy due to MEK inhibition for metastatic cutaneous melanoma. Case Rep Ophthalmol Med. 2013;(2013):673796.
33. Urner-Bloch U, Urner M, Stieger P, Galliker N, Winterton N, Zubel A, et al. Transient MEK inhibitor-associated retinopathy in metastatic melanoma. Ann Oncol. 2014; 25(7):1437-41.
34. de Bono JS, Concin N, Hong DS, Thistlethwaite FC, Machiels JP, Arkenau HT, et al. Tisotumab vedotin in patients with advanced or metastatic solid tumours (InnovaTV 201): a first-in-human, multicentre, phase 1-2 trial. Lancet Oncol. 2019;20(3):383-93.
35. Kim SK, Ursell P, Coleman RL, Monk BJ, Vergote I. Mitigation and management strategies for ocular events associated with tisotumab vedotin. Gynecol Oncol. 2022;165(2):385-92.
36. Dalvin LA, Berkenstock MK, Pasricha ND. Corneal Changes From Antibody-Drug Conjugates. JAMA Ophthalmol. 2025;143(6):515-6.
37. Coleman RL, Lorusso D, Gennigens C, González-Martín A, Randall L, Cibula D, et al.; innovaTV 204/GOG-3023/ENGOT-cx6 Collaborators. Efficacy and safety of tisotumab vedotin in previously treated recurrent or metastatic cervical cancer (innovaTV 204/GOG-3023/ENGOT-cx6): a multicentre, open-label, single-arm, phase 2 study. Lancet Oncol. 2021;22(5):609-19.
38. National Cancer Institute. Common Terminology Criteria for Adverse Events (CTCAE- Version 5.0). United States Department of Health and Human Services; 2017.
39. Matulonis UA, Birrer MJ, O'Malley DM, Moore KN, Konner J, Gilbert L, et al. Evaluation of Prophylactic Corticosteroid Eye Drop Use in the Management of Corneal Abnormalities Induced by the Antibody-Drug Conjugate Mirvetuximab Soravtansine. Clin Can Res. 2019;25(6):1727-36.
40. Corbelli E, Miserocchi E, Marchese A, Guiffre C, Berchicci L, Sacconi R, et al. Ocular Toxicity of Mirvetuximab. Cornea. 2019;38(2):229-32.
41. Moore KN, Vergote I, Oaknin A, Colombo N, Banerjee S, Oza A, et al.; FORWARD I: a phase III study of mirvetuximab soravtansine versus chemotherapy in platinum-resistant ovarian cancer. Future Oncol. 2018;14:1669-78.
42. Kim SH, Marshall RF, Wai KM, Rahimy E, Vingopoulos F, Mishra K, et al. Ocular Adverse Events of Antibody Drug Conjugates and Association With Survival From a Real-World Database. Cornea. 2025. [Online ahead of print]
43. Ali A, Shah AA, Jeang LJ, Fallgater K, George TJ, DeRemer D. Emergence of ocular toxicities associated with novel anticancer therapeutics: What the oncologist needs to know. Can Treat Rev. 2022;105:102376.
44. Berkenstock MK, Saji S, Farooq AV, Pasricha N. (2025). Antibody-Drug Conjugates and Ocular Toxicities: A Call for Standardized Guidelines. [online] Available from https://www.aao.org/education/clinical-statement/antibody-drug-conjugates-ocular-toxicities-call-st [Last accessed February, 2026].
45. Thompson JA, Schneider BJ, Brahmer J, Achufusi A, Armand P, Berkenstock MK, et al. NCCN Clinical Practice Guidelines in Oncology (NCCN Guidelines®): Management of Immunotherapy-Related Toxicities. Version 1.2025. National Comprehensive Cancer Network; 2025. Available at: https://www.nccn.org.
46. Chang E, Liu R, Keyhanian K, Huynh K, Berkenstock MK, Bhatti MT, et al. Consensus disease definitions for ophthalmic immune related adverse events of immune checkpoint inhibitors. J Immunother Cancer. 2025;13(4):e011049.
47. Wendling D, Paccou J, Berthelot JM, Flipo RM, Guillaume-Czitrom S, Prati C, et al. New onset of uveitis during anti-tumor necrosis factor treatment for rheumatic diseases. Semi Arth Rheum. 2011;41(3):503-10.
48. Lie E, Lindström U, Zverkova-Sandström T, Olsen LC, Forsblad-d'Elia H, Askling J, et al. Tumour necrosis factor inhibitor treatment and occurrence of anterior uveitis in ankylosing spondylitis: results from the Swedish biologics register. Annal Rheum Dis. 2017;76(9):1515-21.
49. Nicolela Susanna F, Pavesio C. A review of ocular adverse events of biological anti-TNF drugs. J Ophthalmic Inflamm Infect. 2020;10(1):11.
50. Hill AB. The environment and disease: association and causation. Proc R Soc Med 1965;58:295-300.
51. Lim LL, Fraunfelder FW, Rosenbaum JT. Do tumor necrosis factor inhibitors cause uveitis? A registry-based study. Arthritis Rheum. 2007;56(10):3248-52.
52. Zhao X, Xie Q, He X, Lu Y, Li M, Shuai S. Risk of new-onset and recurrent uveitis with different biologics for ankylosing spondylitis: a network meta-analysis. Front Immunol. 2025;16:1556313.
53. Pottier C, Fresnais M, Gilon M, Jérusalem G, Longuespée R, Sounni NE. Tyrosine kinase inhibitors in cancer: breakthrough and challenges of targeted therapy. Cancers. 2020;12(3):731.
54. Dubovsky JA, Beckwith KA, Natarajan G, Woyach JA, Jaglowski S, Zhong Y, et al. Ibrutinib is an irreversible molecular inhibitor of ITK driving a Th-1 selective pressure in T lymphocytes. Blood. 2013;122:2539-49.
55. Chiu ZK, Goh JKS, Ling C, Ling M-L, Hall AJ. Ibrutinib-related uveitis. A case series. AJO Case Rep 2022;25:101300.

56. Shaikh H, Dkattab A, Faisal MS, Chilkulwar A, Albrethsen M, Sadashiv S, et al. Case series of unique adverse events related to the use of ibrutinib in patients with B-cell malignancies-a single institution experience and review of the literature. J Oncol Pharm Pract. 2018;25:1265-70.
57. Wanner D, Bohn J-P, Rudzki J, Stockhammer G, Steurer. Autoimmune myelitis in a CLL patient undergoing treatment with ibrutinib. Ann Hematol. 2019;98:205-7.
58. Witkin AJ, Chang DF, Jumper JM, Charles S, Eliott D, Hoffman RS, et al. Vancomycin-Associated Hemorrhagic Occlusive Retinal Vasculitis: Clinical Characteristics of 36 Eyes. Ophthalmology. 2017;124(5):583-95.
59. Chang DF, Rhee DJ. Antibiotic prophylaxis of postoperative endophthalmitis after cataract surgery: results of the 2021 ASCRS member survey. J Cataract Ref Surg. 2022;48(1)3-7.
60. Pan WW, Miller AR, Young BK, Johnson MW, Sassalos TM. Hemorrhagic Occlusive Retinal Vasculitis Associated With Triamcinolone-Moxifloxacin Use During Uncomplicated Cataract Surgery. JAMA Ophthalmol. 2023;141(1):99-101.
61. Hui BTK, Capewell N, Ansari Y, Liu X. Bilateral acute anterior uveitis and iris atrophy caused by moxifloxacin. BMJ Case Reports CP. 2020;13(6):e233528.
62. da Costa DS, Gameiro Filho AR, Barbosa AL, Brasil MVM. Bilateral Acute Iris Transillumination Syndrome after Topical Moxifloxacin/Dexamethasone Initially Misdiagnosed as Uveitis: Case Report. Case Rep Ophthalmol. 2023;14(1):39-46.
63. Eadie B, Etminan M, Mikelberg FS. Risk for Uveitis With Oral Moxifloxacin: A Comparative Safety Study. JAMA Ophthalmol. 2015;133(1):81-4.
64. Sood S, Du J, Chen A, Medina A, Do BK. Segmental retinal arteritis in a case of presumed bilateral rifabutin-associated hypopyon uveitis. Am J Ophthalmol Case Rep. 2024;36:102170.
65. Tilden ME, Rosenbaum JT, Fraunfelder FT. Systemic sulfonamides as a cause of bilateral, anterior uveitis. Arch Ophthalmol. 1991;109(1):67-9.

Index

Page numbers followed by *f* refer to figure, *fc* refer to flowchart, and *t* refer to table.

J

K

L

M

N

O

P

Q

R

S

T

U

V